Developmental Neuropsychology

Developmental Neuropsychology

Otfried Spreen
University of Victoria
Victoria, B.C.

Anthony H. Risser
Consulting Neuropsychology Services
Peoria, IL

Dorothy Edgell
Queen Alexandra Centre for Children's Health
Victoria, B.C.

New York   Oxford
OXFORD UNIVERSITY PRESS
1995

Oxford University Press

Oxford   New York   Toronto
Delhi   Bombay   Calcutta   Madras   Karachi
Kuala Lumpur   Singapore   Hong Kong   Tokyo
Nairobi   Dar es Salaam   Cape Town
Melbourne   Auckland   Madrid

and associated companies in
Berlin   Ibadan

Library of Congress Cataloging-in-Publication Data
Spreen, Otfried.
Development neuropsychology / Otfried Spreen
Anthony H. Risser, Dorothy Edgell.
p. cm.
ISBN 0-19-506736-3. — ISBN 0-19-506737-1
1. Pediatric neuropsychology. 2. Developmental disabilities.
3. Developmental neurology. I. Risser, Anthony H.
II. Edgell, Dorothy. III. Title.
RJ486.5.S68   1995
618.92'8—dc20   94-5698

9 8 7 6 5 4 3 2

Printed in the United States of America
on acid-free paper

Preface

This book is addressed to neuropsychologists and neurologists working with children as well as to students of psychology, education, and other child-care professions. We have attempted to write the book so that it poses no difficulties in understanding for the clinical psychologist without background in neurology or the pediatrician without background in psychology.

Adult human neuropsychology has developed in tandem with adult neurology during the past 150 years. An impressive amount of well-documented clinical observation, experimental study and systematic clinical research has been embodied in several major textbooks. Developmental neuropsychology does not have the same tradition, nor is an easy translation of the work with adults into a developmental framework possible. Rather, developmental work has its origins in various related fields such as pediatrics, embryology, and animal research. Application of the knowledge from these areas to psychology and particularly to neuropsychology has been slow and fairly recent. As Segalowitz (1992) pointed out, it is ironic that Freud, Piaget, and Gesell, the major theorists of child development, were biologically oriented, but did not include a scheme of brain maturation in their descriptions of the childhood period. They realized that they did not have enough information to map brain growth onto psychological growth, or vice versa.

This situation has changed dramatically. A wealth of information has become available during recent years, emanating from many disciplines concerned with the development of the nervous system. These include clinical and experimental neuropsychology, pediatrics, neurology, psychiatry, biology, and ethology as well as more specialized disciplines, such as behavioral embryology, developmental neurobiology, and teratology. Much of the research basic to developmental neuropsychology can be found in the highly technical literature of neurobiology, in disease-oriented medical publications, and in the many journals devoted to psychological development and education. In this book we have attempted to integrate this information, rephrasing technical terms or explaining studies as necessary, without trying to provide exhaustive coverage of background issues. Our main goal is an increased understanding of normal and abnormal development in early and middle childhood and adolescence and relate it to the development of nervous system and behavioral disorders during the prenatal, perinatal, and postnatal periods.

Part I of the book provides the background material essential to an understanding of the growth of the nervous system, information gathered in minute detail over many decades by neurobiologists, mostly from animal studies. It includes a chapter on normal cognitive development basic to the understanding of neuropsychological issues.

Part II reviews some conceptual and clinical issues related to human development such as newborn and infant assessment, critical periods, neural plasticity, and the disconnection syndromes. It also provides an introduction to the epidemiology and classification of developmental disorders and a discussion of the advantages and disadvantages of various research designs.

Part III enters the clinical arena more fully. It reviews information gathered by clinicians caring for the human fetus, embryo, or newborn, and presents overviews of the potentially damaging events and conditions like anoxia, trauma, or intoxication that may affect the normal growth of the child. Of necessity, the tools of the clinician differ sharply from those available to the neurobiologist. Instead of dissection and experimentation, the results of clinical observation and measurement, or at best of radiological studies and other clinical procedures, have to be relied upon.

Part IV describes the functional disabilities frequently associated with damage to the developing nervous system. Once again, the focus of interest and the tools of assessment differ. When functional disorders are discovered, the educator, psychiatrist, or clinical psychologist must focus on the problem and on the immediate environment of the child, on how he or she is treated by peers or teachers, how achievement tests rank the child in the classroom, and so forth. Compared with these questions, the problem of a difficult birth or a maternal infection during the first trimester of pregnancy may seem rather remote. Although such remote events have been invoked as an explanation of many functional disabilities in middle childhood, the relationship remains elusive and tenuous. Yet the exploration of such relationships remains the ultimate aim of this book.

Two major obstacles to the development of a coherent framework for developmental neuropsychology are:

(a) The constantly changing picture of the developing child with age. While some generalizations to the adult with a specific type of brain lesion can be made, the effects of lesions in children vary greatly with age. Our book stresses that child development does not include just infancy and childhood, but the full prenatal period as well.

(b) The constant interaction of the developing individual with the environment. Consider the difficulty of comparing, for example, studies of severely malnourished children living in abject poverty in rural parts of Mexico with studies of learning disabled children from affluent families attending a specialized private school in Toronto. This range and the attendant diversity of available services and remediation efforts make generalizations even to children within a specific age range extremely difficult.

In addition to age and environmental factors, the more traditional concerns of clinical neuropsychology have to be considered:

(a) What type of brain damage has occurred and what specific area of the CNS has been affected? While these questions can be answered for postnatal injuries as well as they can in adult neuropsychology, prenatal and perinatal damage tends to be less localized and affects larger parts of the CNS. In contrast to the adult, brain damage sustained by the infant raises additional questions of compensation and plasticity that make the outcome much less predictable.

(b) What psychological functions are affected by damage to the CNS? This question is also likely to lead to more qualified and complex answers than in the adult. Many psychological functions examined in the adult like reading and writing have not even developed in the young child to a point where they can be tested. Language may not be available except in rudimentary forms. Hence, the prediction of long-term outcome becomes a matter of probability that cannot be answered unless a long-term follow-up is conducted. Retrospective studies of individuals with specific disorders of function tend to be fraught with problems since causes other than the organic impairment must be ruled out; furthermore, such studies provide no answer to the question of how many children with a similar lesion developed normally or near-normally and hence were omitted from the sample for retrospective study.

Clinical neuropsychologists are well aware of these many interacting factors, but in daily practice they must make use of the tools available and interpret them as well as possible. In assessing a handicapped infant, developmental neuropsychologists may use only a few formal tests, such as the Denver or the Bailey developmental scales, supplemented with observations of their own and those of the parents and caregivers working with the child.

We are encouraged by the many ongoing and recently published studies and the increasing sophistication in study design, statistical analysis, subject description, psychological measurement and neurological examination. A few exemplary studies, particularly those from the NIH Collaborative Perinatal Study, have even attempted the multivariate analysis of a large number of dependent and independent variables, the statistician's nightmare. If the results of such studies are less impressive for those of us who want clearcut answers, if we learn for example that head circumference at age one, contributed −.26 (i.e., only approximately 7 per cent of the total variance) to the discrimination between seven-year-old learning disabled and control children (Nichols and Chan, 1981), we should keep in mind that in a study of 30,000 children and in the context of numerous other variables, this is indeed a meaningful finding that must be interpreted in the context of other interacting variables to achieve predictive significance.

The predictive significance of research findings almost always remains a matter of probability. It is predictive only for the group, not for each individual with his or her own unique background. Many times in this book we took refuge in the term "interactive" in describing the effects of a particular prenatal, perinatal or postnatal event. The term is not meant to be evasive; rather it refers to the fact that the genetic history, the socioeconomic status of the mother and father, the medical history of pregnancy, and the numerous stress factors during pregnancy and birth all contribute to the state of the newborn and hence to the measurements taken at birth or during the first few months. After birth, family size, early infant experience and a host of other environmental factors continue to shape the individual. Childhood illnesses, bumps and falls, nutrition, early childhood education, physical care, and treatment among others contribute to the making of the individual in middle childhood, the time when most childhood problems reach the clinical psychologist. The relationship between brain and behavior, especially in children, is mitigated by these and other moderator variables, including social and cultural factors, remediation, and intrinsic compensation mechanisms (Fletcher and Taylor 1984, Spreen 1989). It is not surprising then that only the major damaging events or conditions clearly show a profound influence on the development of the child while most other negative events apparently contribute only mildly to the eventual outcome.

While gathering material for this book, we were struck both by the richness of detailed research in many areas and by the lack of integration. Research in basic developmental neurobiology proceeds largely in a field by itself; few serious attempts to relate the information to clinical research or the long-term outcome of pathological conditions have been made. Studies of the clinical disorders of the perinatal period are usually designed to answer questions raised by the practicing obstetrician or pediatrician but pay little attention to long-term psychological sequelae except in their most severe form (e.g., mental retardation). Follow-up studies usually are short-term; for example, the outcome of certain infections during pregnancy is assessed in the newborn or in infancy and early childhood. On the other hand, the disorders of psychological function discussed in Part IV are usually studied as a current problem in terms of how it affects a child's life at that time; the origin of such conditions during the prenatal and perinatal periods is often either assumed or studied retrospectively. For example, learning disorders or hyperactivity may be attributed to "minimal brain damage" of unspecified origin with or without a search of hospital records or a report from the parents. Assessment instruments developed for adults with brain injury cannot simply be expected to yield similar data and insights in children, especially if these instruments have been modified to fit the child's cognitive abilities. Fletcher and Taylor (1984) have pointed to this problem of drawing conclusions from tests by describing the "similar skill fallacy," the "special sign fallacy" and the "differential sensitivity fallacy," all based on our knowledge of adult neuropsychology. Chapter 8 is devoted to a discussion of assessment problems in infancy and early childhood, and Chapter 10 reviews briefly the various research designs pertinent to long-term studies in developmental neuropsychology.

Since the appearance of the first edition of this book, developmental neuropsychology has attracted increasing interest in the literature. There are two new journals directly devoted to the topic (*Developmental Neuropsychology*, Vol. 1, 1984 and *Child Neuropsychology*, Vol. 1, 1994). A number of authors have written or edited books on the subject (Boller and Grafman, Vol. 6, 1992, Hynd and Willis 1988, Lavigne and Burns 1981, Njiokiktjien 1988, Novick and Arnold 1988, Obrzut and Hynd 1986, Rapin and Segalowitz 1992, Reynolds and Fletcher-Janzen 1989, Rourke et al. 1983), and a series of "Advances" (Tramontana and Hooper 1992) is on its way. Most of these books combine basic information on developmental neuropsychology with assessment and other clinical issues and case presentations. In contrast, this text aims to integrate developmental research from a wide variety of sources without adding detailed clinical case descriptions or discussions of assessment (which are well described by Rourke et al. 1986, and by Tramontana and Hooper 1987).

For the second edition we have deleted the previous section on methodological issues as a topic too large to fit into a single chapter. Instead, we have tried to deal with methodological issues where appropriate to the research under discussion, and specifically in Chapter 10. We have added a chapter on normal cognitive development and a chapter focusing on newborn and infant assessment, a subject that was briefly dealt with in several different chapters of the first edition. The scope of other chapters (e.g. 14, 21, 24) has been enlarged (Chapter 14, for instance, now includes the pediatric HIV infection) and previous double-topic chapters ("Brain Injury and Focal Neurological Diseases," "Infections and Intoxication") have been divided into two. All other chapters have been rewritten and carefully updated, following new clinical and research developments. Chapter 24 has a new section on disorders of praxis and neuropsychological aspects of Tourette syndrome, and Chapter 30 has been completely revised in light of new findings on psychiatric disorders.

Throughout the text we provide brief definitions of terms that may not be readily understood by readers with little background in biology or medicine. Usually, the terms are defined the first time they are used and the page number indexed in italics. The index then can be used as a glossary to allow the reader to find the definition more readily if the term appears later in the text.

We would like to thank Dr. David Tupper for providing material for the revision of the chapter on soft signs (Chapter 22), and Drs. Tupper and Holly Tuokko for their contribution to the first edition. We are also grateful to Jeffrey House of Oxford University Press, for his encouragement and numerous valuable critical comments.

Contents

I

Early Life Neural and Cognitive Development

The normal development of the human nervous system is an orderly, sequential process. The principles governing this elaborate process are outlined in the first part of this book so that the effects of abnormal influences, to be discussed later, can be understood as deviations from the expected level of development for a particular individual at a given age.

1

Principles of Neural Development

This chapter is devoted to theoretical issues, basic principles, and approaches to the study of nervous system development. First, we discuss the role of the developmental neuropsychologist in understanding nervous system development, emphasizing difficulties that arise both in research and in practice when an attempt is made to correlate neuroanatomy and behavior. Then two basic approaches to the study of nervous system development—gross and microscopic—are presented. Finally, the role of specific neural elements in the building of the central nervous system is discussed in detail.

1.1 Problems in Correlating Anatomical and Behavioral Development

The first major difficulty in understanding the relationship between human anatomical and behavioral development arises from the variety of different approaches used to study essentially the same subject matter (Birch 1974). Research fields have tended to become isolated, each growing so highly specialized that adequate communication with other disciplines is difficult. This often happens when different species are used for research. For several good reasons, developmental neurobiologists frequently use rats in their studies, which limits generalizations to humans or other primates. We do not know, with regard to general principles, what inferences for humans can be made from animal research. Developmental sequences necessary for survival are different for other species. However, research on nonhuman primates (Rakic's work with rhesus monkeys, for example) has often confirmed and extended previous findings from studies of lower vertebrates. Until more studies along these lines are done, pediatricians, neurologists, and psychologists will have trouble applying the results of animal research to the problems of their patients.

A second major difficulty in correlating anatomical and behavioral development is the use of the term "development." The term "development" implies more of a search for relationships among processes than such other terms as "maturation" (Connolly and Prechtl 1981, Rose 1981), "growth" (Trevarthen 1980), or "ontogeny" (Goldman 1976). It also puts the focus on the search for mechanisms underlying change, rather than just a description of change over time. As an organism develops neuropsychologically, many extrinsic influences create pressures that modify, through processes of their own, the mechanisms involved in the intrinsic differentiation of a unique, complex organism. Thus, the nervous system of an infant can be seen not as immature but rather as adapted to the specific functions necessary for survival at that age. For example, rooting and sucking as well as grasping (to hold onto the mother) are primitive reflexes appropriate for the neonate; the trigeminal nerve is also well developed for the same reason. (Connolly and Prechtl 1981). At this point, however, researchers have only a glimpse of the underlying mechanisms and must rely heavily on descriptive analyses of changes over time in the nervous system and behavior (Cooke 1980). Our search for "developmental" processes in this sense has just begun.

The third major difficulty is that any behavior has multiple causes. For example, numerous causes have been linked to cognitive deficit, delayed language development, and learning disabilities. On the other hand, the same antecedent conditions and events contribute to different behavioral outcomes; in some cases, many conditions will be necessary to produce a particular outcome. Straightforward cause-effect relationships are not likely to be found with contemporary methods of developmental psychology (Baltes and Nesselroade 1970). When studying the relationship between anatomical and behavioral development we have to be aware of this complicating pitfall and recognize explicitly the many possible antecedent events ("causes") that interact as mechanisms involved in development (see also discussion by Hebb 1949).

A more theoretical caution put forth by Riesen (1971) concerns correlations between behavioral and anatomical changes. A proposed correlation, he suggests, may be misleading because, in early development, many changes are taking place in the organism that may or may not be directly related to the behavioral variable under study. Because many relatively independent processes may show a temporal relationship in a developing organism since they occur during the same short time period, it is better to use the suspected correlation as a general indicator of a relationship and to pose a new question, "What events and conditions produced the correlation?" (Riesen 1971, p. 60). For example, considerable progress has been made in specifying the conditions resulting in low birth weight, stressing such contributing factors as malnutrition, alcohol use, and smoking while distinguishing the "small for date" infant from the premature baby and the baby who is small in relation to actual gestational age.

The formation of the nervous system is presumed to be largely under genetic control. It has been estimated that approximately 30 per cent of the entire genetic information (genome) is specific to the brain and its development (Sutcliffe et al. 1984).

1.2 Gross Aspects of Neural Development

The human nervous system can be divided into two major parts: the **central nervous system** (CNS) comprising the brain, brainstem, and spinal cord and the **peripheral nervous system** comprising the sensory and motor nerves branching from the CNS. Our emphasis is on the more complex CNS. Table 1-1 presents the major divisions of the CNS and the main structures within each division. There are three major divisions of the brain: the forebrain or **prosencephalon** (Greek: pro=forward + en=in + kephalon=head), the midbrain or **mesencephalon**, and the hindbrain or **rhombencephalon**. Each of these areas is subdivided into several regions consisting primarily of either nerve cell bodies or nerve fibers. Regions that consist of cell bodies are called **gray matter** because the cells have that color, and regions that consist of nerve fibers are called **white matter** because the fatty sheath surrounding them is white. Nerve fibers that connect different divisions of the nervous system are called **projection fibers**. Those that connect opposite areas in the two hemispheres are called **commissural fibers**, and those that travel only within a single division are called **association fibers.**

Figure 1-1 diagrams, in two views, some of the major structures in the adult brain. More detailed information concerning the location of particular structures can be found in any neuroanatomy text. Cytoarchitectonics and myelogenesis are two approaches to the mapping of cerebral regions.

Cytoarchitectonics

Cytoarchitectonics refers to the arrangement of cells in a tissue and is commonly applied to studies of the location of different types of neurons in the cerebral cortex. Neurons are classified according to their structure; the classes are then charted on the brain. This classification yields a "map" of the cortex showing different zones for various structures and cell types. Figure 1-2 portrays such a cytoarchitectural map with the numbering system first developed by Brodmann and von Economo.

In the study of brain development, cytoarchitectonics has been used to establish the "birthdays" of cells in various CNS regions (Hunt 1982) and to study changes in cellular areas during development (Rabinowicz 1979). The cytoarchitectural zone designation system implies a correspondence between cellular zones in the adult and in the child; changes in cellular zones during development have not been widely studied.

Table 1-1 Major Divisions of the CNS with the Principal Structures Associated with Each Division

Major division	Neural tube derivative	Major regions and nuclei	Major fiber tracts
Forebrain Telencephalon	Lateral ventricle	Cerebral cortex (neocortex) Hippocampal formation Septal nuclei Basal ganglia (striatum)	Corpus callosum Fimbria
Diencephalon	Third ventricle	Thalamus Hypothalamus	Internal capsule Medial forebrain bundle
Eye		Neural retina Pigment epithelium	
Midbrain	Aqueduct	Tectum (superior and inferior colliculi) Red nucleus Oculomotor and trochlear nuclei	Cerebral peduncle Cerebral-rubro-thalamic tract
Hindbrain	Fourth ventricle	Cerebellum Pontine nuclei Inferior olive Dorsal column nuclei Trigeminal nucleus	Cerebellar peduncles Pyramidal tract
Spinal cord	Central canal	Dorsal and ventral horns	Dorsal columns Pyramidal tract

Source: Lund 1978.

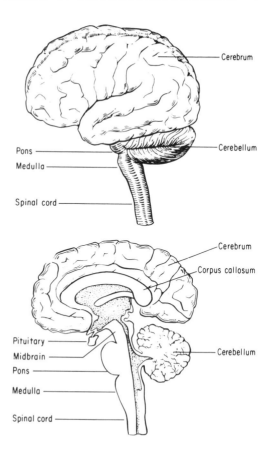

Figure 1-1. Lateral (*above*) and medial (*below*) aspects of the adult brain and their associated structures (Thompson 1967).

Myelogenesis

Myelogenesis (also "myelinogenesis") refers to the development of myelin, the fatty sheath surrounding the nerve fiber. The sequence of myelin formation in the CNS is discussed in conjunction with glial cell development (Section 1.3). It is assumed that the formation of myelin sheaths around an axon increases the conduction velocity, lowers the action potential threshold, and increases the neuron's ability to carry repetitive impulses, thus making the neuron more functionally capable and efficient.

Flechsig (1901), a pioneer researcher in the study of regions of myelin development, divided the cortex into what he termed "myelogenetic fields" and numbered them in order of their progressive myelination. His developmental sequence of myelination included three general types of fields called primordial, intermediate, and terminal zones.

Primordial, or "premature," **fields** are those that myelinate before birth and include such areas as the somesthetic cortex, primary visual cortex, and primary auditory cortex. **Intermediate**, or "postmature," **fields** myelinate during the

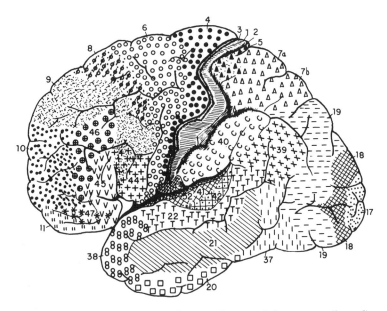

Figure 1-2. Brodmann's areas. Cytoarchitectural map of the convex (lateral) surface of the adult brain (von Economo 1929).

first 3 postnatal months. These fields are generally considered to be secondary association areas; that is, areas that surround primary sensory or motor cortices. The **terminal fields** are the last to myelinate, between the fourth postnatal month and 14 years of age. They include the classical association areas; that is, areas assumed to subserve higher cortical functions.

In defining these myelogenetic fields, Flechsig conceived of what he called the "chronogenic hierarchy of myelogenetic zones." Many other investigators have followed similar lines of investigation, attempting also to correlate myelination and behavioral development (e.g., Langworthy 1933, Yakovlev 1962, Yakovlev and Lecours 1967). Meyer (1981) reviewed Flechsig's original position in the light of more recent study and concluded that myelogenetics remains a valid approach to the study of structural neural development. Yakovlev and Lecours's (1967) work is presented in more detail when the chronology of postnatal development is discussed in Chapter 2.

1.3   Neural Development at the Microscopic Level

Light and electron microscopes are widely used in studies of the structural changes that occur in the CNS during development. These microscopic changes are often correlated with physiological changes in the developing organism. Recently, this approach has been extended to observations of biochemical and physiological changes in the microscopic structure and chemicals of the neurons during development (DiBenedetta et al. 1980). Changes at the microscopic level are almost always more difficult to correlate with specific developing behaviors, but may, as in the case of nutritional disorders, be vital to an understanding of normal and abnormal neural development.

The subject of microscopic studies by neuroscientists has typically been the nerve cell, or neuron (Figure 1-3). A **neuron** consists of a cell body, a fiber that conducts impulses away from the body (**axon**), and an area of branching **dendrites**, which conduct impulses to the cell body from other neurons. Axons and dendrites are called the processes of the neuron. There are several types of neurons of various sizes and shapes in the CNS. A major structural classification is **Golgi** type I versus Golgi type II **neurons**. The former are usually large neurons with long axons and a large dendritic "tree." They are thought to be formed prenatally and to serve as the major connections of the nervous system. They also act as part of the supporting structure of the CNS. Golgi type II

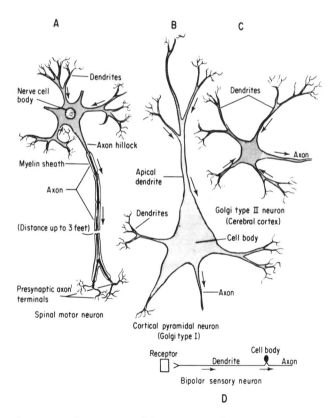

Figure 1-3. Some typical neurons and their associated structures: (a) neuron; (b) Golgi type I neuron; (c) Golgi type II neuron from cerebral cortex; (d) schematic drawing of a bipolar sensory neuron. (Thompson 1967).

neurons, also called interstitial neurons, are usually small cells with small axonal and dendritic expansions. Many of them are formed postnatally and may be important for higher cerebral functions (Courchesne 1991, Diamond 1990). The nervous system also contains non-neuronal cells, called **glial cells**, which are thought to play a primary supportive and nutrient role in the CNS (Lund 1978); glial cells also form the myelin sheaths that surround nerve fibers to aid conduction of electrical nerve potentials.

The notion of the single neuron as the significant unit of activity has been questioned recently (Douglas and Martin 1991). Every cortical neuron has a complex dendritic tree and a local network of axon collaterals that branch profusely, forming synapses with hundreds and thousands of nearby neurons. Hence, the excitatory drive for any single neuron is provided by the convergent action of hundreds of neurons. Neuronal interactions on a synapse-by-synapse basis are inadequate to explain the sophisticated operations performed by the nervous system. Instead, Douglas and Martin (1991) suggest the mechanism of "**microcircuits**." These are "large clusters of highly interconnected neurons, each performing fairly simple tasks and evolving a response over many milliseconds. The response of individual neurons then reflects not its own specific interests but rather the complex behavior of a microcircuit containing many neurons" (p. 286).

Development and Placement of Neurons

The final location of a neuron in the nervous system is the result of many factors, both intrinsic and extrinsic to the organism. These factors follow the principles of specificity and plasticity, but generally in a precise sequence (Cowan 1979). The terminology used here is that suggested by the Boulder Committee (1970).

Cell generation by **mitosis** (cell division) is called **proliferation**. Mitosis occurs inside the neural tube (in the ventricular zone). The mitotic cycle of each germinal cell follows a fixed sequence, as shown in Figure 1-4, and results in the production of **neuroblasts**, or nerve cell precursors, and **glioblasts**, or glial cell precursors. Over a period of days to weeks, cells in this area take on the highly asymmetrical shape that is characteristic of all neurons (G. Bennett 1987). **Neurogenesis** is the term used to describe nerve cell production.

The mitotic cycle begins as the nucleus of the germinal cell moves away from the ventricle, enters the S phase of the cycle, and begins to synthesize deoxyribonucleic acid (DNA). As the cell moves into the premitotic or second gap (G2) period, the nucleus returns to the ventricular surface, and the cell becomes detached from the basal surface (top of Figure 1-4). During the mitotic (M) phase, the cell splits into two daughter cells, which begin to extend their processes back to the surface before entering the presynthetic or first gap (G1) phase, prior to further DNA synthesis. The mitotic cycle varies randomly for cells throughout the ventricular zone. It is repeated many times, the population of cells doubling roughly every 8 to 24 hours (Cowan 1979), but at some point

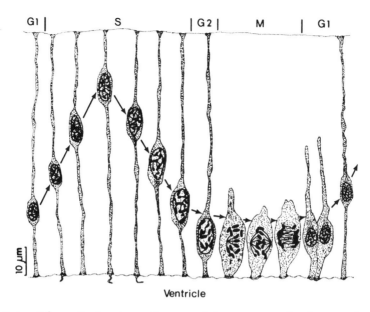

Figure 1-4.   Schematic time-lapse diagram of the mitotic cycle of a neural germinal cell in the developing neural tube (Jacobson 1978).

some of the daughter cells (those destined to become neurons) become permanently arrested in the G1 phase and never divide again.

Migration

Upon completion of the mitotic or proliferative phase of neural development but not before 6 weeks of gestation, the neuroblasts move from the proliferative zone into their permanent locations (Kolb and Fantie 1989). Rakic (1984) reviewed this process of migration in the human. **Migration** determines the ultimate destination of neurons and in so doing creates different cellular zones (Figure 1-5). We shall use the developing cortex as the primary example of migration (Berry 1974), but the process also occurs in other brain regions.

The early neural tube consists only of a ventricular (V) zone of mitotic cells and a marginal (M) zone of the cellular processes. As proliferation continues and migration begins, an intermediate (I) zone of neurons forms. By 8 to 10 weeks after conception, the intermediate zone has enlarged to form the region from which cortex develops, i.e., the initial **cortical plate** (CP) of neurons and a subventricular (S), or subependymal zone, which is a secondary zone where cell proliferation may continue for several weeks. In fact, the smaller neurons (the microneurons or Golgi type II neurons) of the brain, as well as some glial cells, are thought to be generated from this zone (Cowan 1979).

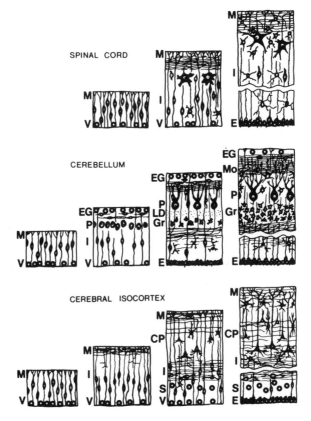

Figure 1-5. Cellular zones in the developing cerebral cortex, cerebellum, and spinal cord (Jacobson 1978). E = ependyma, EG = external granular layer, LD = lamina dissicans, P = Purkinje layer, Mo = molecular layer.

By staining with a tracer compound (e.g., thymidine with a radioactive isotope attached), it is possible to follow the migration path of cells generated at the particular time of staining. The initial formation of the cortical plate occurs by migration of cells to the deepest (sixth) layer of the cortex, and subsequent migrations follow what has been described as an **inside-out pattern** (Marin-Padilla 1978, Rakic 1979a, 1981, 1984). Thus, the next layer to be formed is the next deepest layer; the top layer is formed last by neurons that must migrate past the cells of the deeper layers, over considerable distances, at later stages of development. A second migratory wave of cells occurs at 11 to 15 weeks of gestation and greatly thickens the cortical plate (Figure 1-6).

Cell proliferation and migration vary from area to area and from stage to stage in the development of the nervous system. It seems that cell proliferation is generally complete in the human cerebral neocortex by 6 months gestational age, but that glial cells may continue to be produced in the subventricular zone beyond that time.

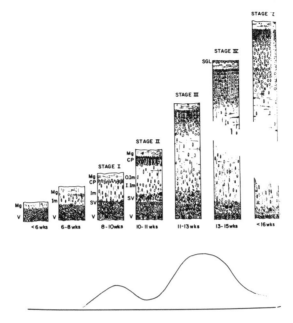

Figure 1-6. The developing cerebral cortex at various fetal ages with the two major waves of cell migration indicated by the curve below (Sidman and Rakic 1973). Im & Om = inner and outer intermediate zones, Mg = marginal zone, SGL = subpial granular layer, SV = subventricular zone, V = ventricular zone, wks = age in fetal weeks.

It is still not known exactly what factors are responsible for the migration of neurons, which has been described as "amoeboid." Two possible explanations are (1) mechanical guidance by radial fibers and (2) chemospecificity. The latter hypothesis is discussed more fully later in this chapter in the context of axonal growth. The concept of mechanical guidance by radially oriented glial fibers has gained much support from the work of Rakic (1975, 1981). Fairly early in development, when it is difficult to distinguish cell types, a group of glial cells is radially oriented from the ventricular to the basal surface and appears to guide the migration of neurons from the site of their proliferation to their final destination in the cortical plate. These cells are called **radially oriented glia**. Figure 1-7 shows a neuron (N) that is migrating along a typical radial glia fiber (RF). Eventually, these radial glia disappear, and they are transformed into astrocytes (Sidman and Rakic 1973). The discovery of radial glial as guides for migration is a major step in our understanding of the mechanisms underlying the process of neural development, but many questions still remain unanswered. Later changes in cell placement are mainly the result of the inside-out migration of other cells and are considered passive cell displacement, rather than active migration.

In contrast to the course of events in the cerebral cortex and many other areas, migration in the cerebellum occurs in an "outside-in" fashion (Figure 1-5).

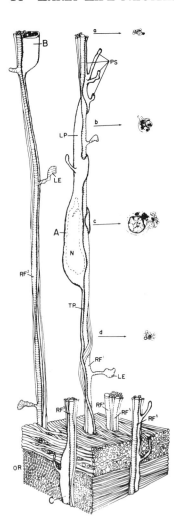

Figure 1-7. Relationship between migrating cells and radial fibers in the developing cerebral cortex of the rhesus monkey (Rakic 1972).

Between 9 and 13 weeks of gestational age, germinal cells from the ventricular zone produce neuroblasts that migrate to the outermost layer of the cerebellum, the external granule (EG) layer, and then proliferate. At the same time neurons from the ventricular zone continue to migrate into the Purkinje (P) layer where they differentiate. External granule layer cell proliferation and migration continue through gestation. In the cerebellum the gray matter ends up external to the white matter, as in the rest of the brain but not the spinal cord. Particular radial glial (**Bergmann glia**) are thought to be responsible for this final migration of the granule cells in the external granule layer to their adult position beneath the Purkinje cell layer; this migration occurs in humans in the first year after birth.

Several migratory defects, termed **neuronal heterotopias** (displacement or malpositioning), can occur in this sequence, resulting in abnormal structure and function of the neurons (Rakic 1975b). Three broad categories of defects can be distinguished: (1) complete failure of migration, (2) curtailment of migratory cells along the migratory pathway, and (3) aberrant placement of postmitotic neurons within the target structure (ectopias). Anomalies may occur during normal development, but are usually eliminated later in the process of selective cell death described below. Anomalies persisting into later development occur infrequently, though they may result in certain types of mental retardation and have been connected with structural abnormalities, dyslexia, and schizophrenia (Chapters 12, 29, and 30). A study of genetic mutations in mice by Caviness and Rakic (1978) indicates that migration errors may be under the control of a single or several genes (Nowakovski 1987).

Aggregation

During their migratory cycles, neurons selectively aggregate to form the major cellular masses, or layers, in the nervous system. This process is called **lamination** (Wolff 1978) and precedes cell differentiation into distinctive types in each region. Cowan (1979) has specified two distinguishable events in this aggregation process. First, the neurons come together and establish some form of mutual adhesion between the necessary cells; second, they align themselves preferentially with respect to their immediate neighbors. The aggregation process can be regarded as an aspect of neuronal specification or modification directed toward future functioning.

Cytodifferentiation

After aggregation, neurons begin the process of differentiation (Pease 1971). Cellular differentiation, or **cytodifferentiation**, can be subdivided into four major concurrent aspects: (1) development of the cell body or perikaryon; (2) selective cell death; (3) process formation (i.e., axonal and dendritic development); and (4) formation of synaptic connections (synaptogenesis).

DEVELOPMENT

The morphological development of the cell body is a poorly understood process. Major influences on shape and function are thought to include genetic factors and mechanical pressures during migration and aggregation. LeDouarin (1980) has described one important factor in his work on neural crest tissue. In this tissue, environmental location helps determine whether neurons will become adrenergic or cholinergic, i.e., whether upon stimulation they will release noradrenaline or acetylcholine, two important neurotransmitters. A critical period of development (Scott et al. 1974) in the production of neurotransmitters, dependent upon environmental stimulation, has therefore been postulated.

Selective Cell Death

The selective death of neurons during CNS development seems to be widespread and of sizable magnitude. It has been estimated that 40 to 75 per cent of all neurons in the nervous system of birds die during development, although precise counts are difficult to obtain. Cell death could be a major determinant of the final cell number during development (NINCDS 1979, Oppenheim 1981). First, a population of neurons is generated; then, within a few days, this number is cut drastically by cell death. This pattern has led some investigators to suspect that it is programmed to occur by genetic control, although little evidence has been found for this as yet. The most plausible hypothesis is that it occurs when synaptic contacts are made. Selective cell death may reflect the fact that only a limited number of neurons succeed in sending their axons to the correct targets and may adjust the magnitude of each neuronal population, a "fine-tuning of neural wiring" (Cowan et al. 1984, p. 1258). Selective cell death has been related to the functional maturation of individual areas of the brain and to plasticity of function before functional maturation is reached. Measurements of synaptic density and volume indicate that the total number of synapses changes at a different rate in different parts of the brain. For the frontal cortex a slow decline in neuronal density by about 35 per cent continues after the first year of life until adulthood (Huttenlocher 1984, 1990). Paradoxically, failure of cell death or synaptic loss has been viewed as contributing to developmental disorders and even schizophrenia (Feinberg 1982).

Axonal and Dendritic Development

Sperry (1968, 1971) put forth the theory of **chemospecificity**, or chemoaffinity, arguing that a biochemical specificity is programmed into each nerve cell that determines the sequence of development and the contacts made by the cell. This theory of chemospecific contact guidance suggests that a neuron, as it forms an axon and dendrites, sends out an advance spray of cellular processes, termed **microfilaments**, that seek chemical attractions (Gazzaniga et al. 1979). A chemical correspondence between the growing filament and appropriate sites for connections with other nerve cells would help determine the functional development of that neuron. A modification of the chemoaffinity theory is based on the discovery of several specific **cell adhesion molecules** (CAM) by Edelman and collaborators (Edelman 1984, Edelman et al. 1983). Edelman pointed out that the chemoaffinity model must assume an implausibly large number of cell location markers carried by genes and is essentially static. That is, once the right markers come together, no further dynamism is necessary; this static quality of markers does not allow for substitution of cells or a gradual shaping of cell structures. Instead, Edelman suggested that individual cell-to-cell recognition is not needed as long as a gradually increasing dynamic specificity is maintained. CAMs seem to serve that purpose. They are glycoproteins secreted by the ependymal gland (Oksche et al. 1993) in the circumventricular complex. Some of the glycoproteins have a tripartite structure called triskelion. N-CAMs (specific for neural cells) are present in the notochord, primary and secondary inductions, and just before the formation of germ layers; later in development, Ng-CAMs appear that seem to mediate the binding of neurons to support the glial cells.

Another hypothesis, the synaptic and dendritic growth hypothesis (Berry et al. 1980), is illustrated in Figure 1-8. It is based on the extension of processes called **growth cones** and **filopodia** (Kater and Letourneau 1985). This theory suggests that specific contacts between cells are guided to their final targets by "recognition molecules" displayed on the surface of the filipodia (Goodman and Bastiani 1987). It has been supported by research (Letourneau et al. 1991) and has been taken as a general model of process formation and elongation (Johnston and Wessells 1980).

The development of an axon begins soon after or concurrently with the differentiation and migration of the cell body. Once the axon is formed, two problems arise. The first is that the axon has to reach the proper place in relation to other cells. Under the synaptic and dendritic growth hypothesis, mechanical constraints imposed by the developing nervous system (rather than chemospecificity) guide the axon along a particular path to a particular terminal site (Cotman and Banker 1974). The length of axonal growth is presumably genetically determined. Recent research has shown that axons may grow "exuberantly," forming both divergent (innervating several cells) and convergent (several cells innervating one other cell) transient connections that are subsequently elimi-

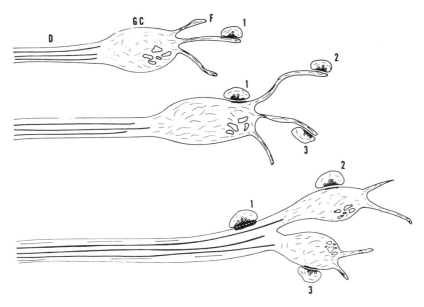

Figure 1-8. Sequence illustrating the synaptic and dendritic growth hypothesis with growth cone (GC) and filopodium (F) (Berry et al. 1980).

nated by the reorganization of axonal and dendritic trees, as well as by neuronal death (O'Leary and Stanfield 1985). The second problem is that of forming synaptic connections between axons and dendrites at specific sites. This is discussed below under synaptogenesis.

The development of dendrites has been studied extensively (Courchesne 1991). The major factor underlying dendritic growth and branching in the nervous system seems to be the presence and arrangement of the afferent (those leading to the neuron) axonal fibers. The dendrites of many types of neurons remain in a relatively primitive condition until the afferent axons arrive; many new processes then sprout, and gradually the dendritic tree is remodeled until the final form is established.

Growth of the dendritic spine is very important for both normal and aberrant neuronal development (Purpura 1975, 1977a). The **dendritic spine** is a very small appendage located on the individual dendrites of most neurons and showing a definite developmental progression. Purpura (1975) found well-developed apical dendritic spines on hippocampal pyramidal neurons at 14 weeks of gestation, whereas more basilar dendrites showed dendritic spines later, at 18 to 22 weeks of gestation. Various forms of malformations of the neural tube can be related to abnormalities in dendritic spine development (Smith 1988).

SYNAPTOGENESIS

Perhaps the most intriguing question in the study of neural development is how specific synapses are formed. Cotman and Banker (1974) emphasized that the formation of synapses in the human brain may not be under genetic control since the number of neurons and the possible combinations among them are well beyond the amount of information carried in human genes. Therefore, at least some portion of these connections must be made by mechanisms other than genetic ones.

Synaptogenesis includes the termination of axonal growth, the selection of synaptic sites, and the formation of the synapse. The appropriate formation of synaptic contacts requires that the neurons use positional and areal information to organize themselves within a topographical field (Rakic 1981) and find their way to the appropriate fields; axons and dendrites must also establish structural and functional connections with their mates. During normal nervous system development, these processes are closely related and are dependent upon intrinsic and environmental influences (Goldman and Rakic 1979). Synaptic differentiation is most extensive during fetal development, but may also continue as a modulating mechanism in response to change throughout the life-span (Cotman and Nieto-Sampedro 1984).

Synaptogenesis peaks at different times in different areas of the brain. Huttenlocher (1990, Huttenlocher et al. 1982) found that rapid dendritic and synaptic growth in the visual cortex stopped at the age of 8 months, whereas the process of subsequent synapse elimination (Purves and Lichtman 1980) may extend beyond the age of 3 years; in the frontal cortex, dendritic and synaptic density reaches its peak during infancy and early childhood and then declines between 2 and 16 years. Excess synaptic connections are eliminated during later childhood years (Huttenlocher 1990).

Glial Cell Development and Myelogenetic Cycles

Three types of glial cells are usually distinguished: (1) astrocytes, (2) oligodendrocytes, and (3) microglial cells. Timiras et al. (1968) concluded that glial cells have several functions: they respond to injury by foreign agents; they regulate neuronal metabolism, contributing to the blood-brain barrier; and they play a role, through myelination, in the electrical activity of the nervous system. Glial cells are relatively immature in the early stages of CNS development, as evidenced by the lack of a glial reaction (gliosis) to a penetrating wound in the newborn brain. The number of glial cells increases with the maturation of the CNS, and glia continue to proliferate throughout life.

The most important role of glial cells is believed to be in **myelination**, a process whereby the axon in the developing CNS becomes surrounded by a myelin sheath made of proteins and lipids. These sheaths are thought to result from the deposition of multilaminar spiral sheaths by surrounding oligodendrocytes (Figure 1-9).

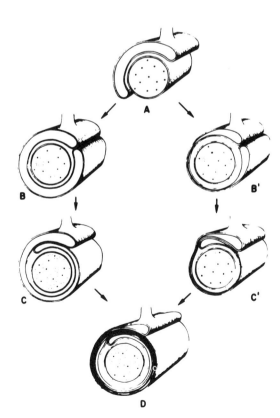

Figure 1-9. Formation of myelin in the CNS (Davison and Peters 1970).

Myelogenetic cycles may give an indication of the sequence of glial cell development in different regions of the brain. The various regions myelinate at different times in a definite sequence. Figure 1-10 presents the results of a large-scale study of myelogenetic cycles in humans (Yakovlev and Lecours 1967). In humans the myelin sheath begins to appear around many nerve fibers between the fourth month of fetal life and the end of the first year of postnatal life. Myelination starts in the spinal cord and then spreads to the medulla, pons, and midbrain and finally to the diencephalon and telencephalon. Many researchers have attempted to correlate these myelogenetic cycles with the development of specific abilities (Bjorklund and Harnishfeger 1990, Lecours 1975, Lenneberg 1967, Chapter 4). It is assumed that myelination precedes functional ability; however, functional activity may occur without myelination, and in the adult nervous system some unmyelinated nerves are fully capable of conducting impulses, though with slower conduction velocity.

Metabolic and Biochemical Aspects

Many researchers have studied in detail the relationship between nervous system development and biochemical maturation (Dodge et al. 1975, Himwich 1973, Hunt 1980, 1982, Hurley and Hunt 1980, Richter 1975). Only a brief

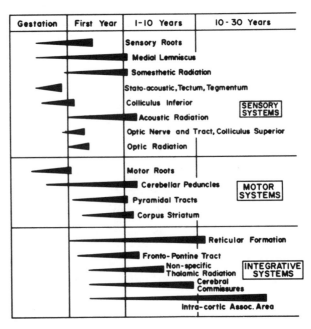

Figure 1-10. The myelogenetic cycles of regional maturation in the human brain (Yakovlev and Lecours 1967).

overview can be presented here, and it is confined to the developmental changes in four major constituents of the brain: (1) the nucleic acids, DNA and ribonucleic acid (RNA), (2) amino acids and proteins, (3) lipids (fats), and (4) neurotransmitters. Hormones, especially sex hormones and their relationship to brain development, are discussed later in the context of sex differences (Section 4.2).

The physiological properties of all brain and CNS tissue are largely determined by the set of protein molecules made by the cells in that tissue: proteins involved in neurotransmitter metabolism (neuropeptide precursors, enzymes for neurotransmitter synthesis and degradation, and transmitter uptake systems), neurotransmitter receptors and ion channels, components of cellular specialization unique to neurons (axons, dendrites, and synapses), proteins to regulate neural connectivity during development, unique glia structures (such as myelin), and molecules that may mediate higher mental processes, such as memory and learning. These properties are presumably under control of "brain-specific genes" (Milner et al. 1987) that have their specific expression in each cell type; gene expression changes in response to temporal and spatial cues. A considerable amount of research has isolated some of these molecules unique to brain tissue and their genetic message.

The total brain content of RNA and DNA is high during the early phases of brain development, but it gradually decreases. Early proliferation of cells is reflected in the synthesis of DNA. As differentiation occurs, DNA replication is followed by increased transcription (change) of DNA to RNA and then the transcription of RNA to protein. DNA levels thus decline faster than RNA levels. DNA content is considered to be a reliable indicator of cell number. In humans, two periods of cell proliferation have been detected by measuring DNA levels (Dobbing 1975). The first period begins at 15 to 20 weeks of gestation and corresponds to neuroblast proliferation. The second begins at 25 weeks and continues into the second year of postnatal life, representing the multiplication of glial cells.

Several behavioral disorders result from disturbances in nucleic acid metabolism. **Lesch-Nyhan syndrome**, for example, is a rare genetic defect in which there is a mutation of a gene that affects the enzyme involved in the making of one of the nucleotide bases of the nucleic acids.

The amino acid composition of brain proteins changes during development. Since the ratio of protein to DNA indicates cell size, an increasing ratio in development indicates protein increases. The absorption of amino acids from the blood is also much higher for newborns than adults; the rates of protein synthesis and turnover are much greater in the young organism. The rate of protein synthesis in the brain peaks during myelination since protein is also a major component of myelin.

Many inborn errors of amino acid metabolism lead to developmental defects. One major amino acidopathy, as these defects are called, is phenylketonuria, a result of the absence of the enzyme phenylalanine hydroxylase, which breaks down phenylalanine (Chapter 11). The consequent build-up of phenylalanine within the body and brain reaches toxic levels and often produces mental retardation unless an appropriate diet is started soon after birth.

A rapid increase in the lipid content of the brain begins after the peak periods for DNA and protein synthesis. In the fetal brain, little difference can be found between the composition of lipids in gray matter and the composition of those in white matter. The adult pattern is attained during myelination with increases in three major lipids—cholesterol, cerebrosides, and sphingomyelin—especially in the white matter. The increased lipid content has been ascribed to myelin sheath development (Benjamins and McKhann 1976). Two representative disorders of lipid metabolism are Tay-Sachs disease (a lipid defect, specifically ganglioside) and Niemann-Pick disease (an intracellular accumulation of sphingomyelin).

The **neurotransmitters**, which mediate transmission between neurons at synapses, include acetylcholine, dopamine, glutamate, epinephrine, and norepinephrine. Increases in their levels in the developing brain serve as developmental signals for such processes as neural tube formation, germinal cell proliferation, and neuronal and glial differentiation (Lauder 1983). A net increase in the concentration of neurotransmitters during development is accompanied by a simultaneous change in the enzymes that synthesize and degrade them (Engelsen 1986, Gupta 1984, Lanier et al. 1976). Acetylcholinesterase activity, for example, has been used as evidence for the presence of the excitatory neurotransmitter acetylcholine. Other neurotransmitters showing similar increases include the monoamines (serotonin and histamine) the catecholamines (noradrenalin [or norepinephrine] and dopamine) the prostaglandins, and the amino acids that are thought to have a modulating or inhibitory rather than a facilitating function (glycine and gamma-aminobutyric acid [GABA]).

Summary

This chapter outlined the major aspects of neural development after conception and the gradual arrangements of cells in a pattern leading up to the adult atlas of the fully myelinated adult brain. The process of generating nerve cells; their migration, aggregation, and differentiation; and the formation of connecting links with other cells by axonal and dendritic development and the formation of synapses were traced through the prenatal period. The development of supporting glial tissue and the cycles of myelination were also described.

2

Chronology of Gross Neural Development

Approximately 7 days after fertilization of the ovum by the sperm, the ovum in the **blastula** (or hollow ball) **stage** attaches itself to the uterine endometrium (mucous membrane) and becomes implanted. On day 9 the fertilized ovum is composed of two layers, a dorsal ectoderm and the inner endoderm. Later, during **gastrulation**, when the blastula invaginates (folds in), a third layer, called the mesoderm, develops between the ectoderm and the endoderm. Gastrulation is essential for **neural induction**, the ability of these early cell layers to initiate formation of the nervous system (Saxen, 1980). Neural induction takes place on day 18 of gestation. The formation of the nervous system begins at the thickened ectoderm on the dorsal surface of the embryo. For general reviews of gross neural development, see Berenberg (1977), Cowan (1979) and Kolb (1989).

Table 2-1 traces the stages of development in a chronological review of growth periods in the human. This chapter discusses two major time periods: the prenatal and the postnatal.

2.1 Prenatal

The prenatal period in the human extends from fertilization of the ovum to approximately 280 days of gestational age. The prenatal period can be subdivided into smaller segments. Table 2-2 shows the sequential development of the nervous system.

Embryo

In what is termed the **neurula stage** of the developing embryo, during the third week of gestation, a pear-shaped neural plate appears from the dorsal ectoderm. In the center of this plate the cells on the edge become narrower on their inner surface, whereas those surrounding them become narrower on their

Table 2-1 Stages of Human Growth and Development

Growth period	Approximate age
Prenatal	0 to 280 days
Ovum (pre-embryonic)	0 to 14 days
Embryo	14 days to 9 weeks
Fetus	9 weeks to birth
Premature infant	27 to 37 weeks
Birth	Average 280 days
Neonate	First 4 weeks after birth
Infancy	First year
Early childhood (preschool)	1 to 6 years
Later childhood (prepubertal)	6 to 10 years
Adolescence	Girls, 8 or 10 to 18 years / Boys, 10 or 12 to 20 years
Puberty (average)	Girls, 13 years / Boys, 15 years

Source: Adams and Victor 1981.

outer surface. These changes produce a longitudinal **neural groove**, composed of neural folds, which gradually deepens and eventually folds over onto itself. It begins to close starting at the midpoint and extending in both rostral (toward the head) and caudal (tail) directions. As it closes (Figure 2-1) there are temporarily two open ends, the anterior and posterior neuropores, which close at approximately day 25 of gestation. The resulting tube surrounding a fluid-filled central canal is called the **neural tube**, and the process of its conversion from open groove to sealed tube is termed **neurulation**. Figure 2-2 shows the formation of the neural tube in cross-sectional views.

Table 2-2 Timetable for Normal Growth and Development of the Human Nervous System

Age in days	Size (crown-rump length) in mm	Nervous system development
18	1.5	Neural groove and tube
21	3.0	Optic vesicles
26	3.0	Closure of anterior neuropore
27	3.3	Closure of posterior neuropore; ventral horn cells appear
31	4.3	Anterior and posterior roots
35	5.0	Five cerebral vesicles
42	13.0	Primordium of cerebellum
56	25.0	Differentiation of cerebral cortex and meninges
150	225.0	Primary cerebral fissures appear
180	230.0	Secondary cerebral sulci and first myelination appear in brain
>180		Further myelination and growth of brain

Source: Lowrey 1978.

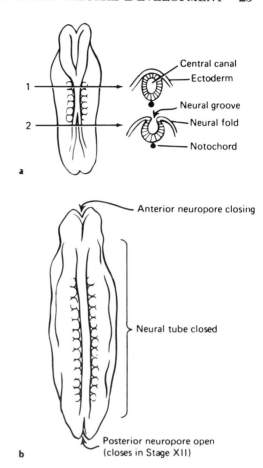

Figure 2-1. Beginning of the development of the nervous system. (a) Start of neurulation, two cross-sectional views. (b) Late stage of neurulation, showing the anterior and posterior neuropores (Lemire et al. 1975).

If neurulation is defective and the neural tube has difficulty closing, one of several possible anomalies can occur. Among these are anencephaly, in which the forebrain fails to develop properly because the anterior neuropore does not close, and spina bifida, which results from more caudal difficulties (see Chapter 12). These neural tube defects occur during the third and fourth weeks of gestation (Reinis and Goldman 1980). Intake of folate preconceptionally and during early pregnancy has been suggested as a means of reducing the incidence of failure of closure of the neural tube (Milunsky et al. 1989).

Cells adjacent to the lateral margins of closure of the neural tube are called **neural crest cells**. They are free of the overlying ectoderm and form an irregular bundle of tissue surrounding the tube (Bronner-Fraser and Cohen 1980, LeDouarin 1980). These clumps of cells migrate and differentiate to form **ganglia** (or groups of peripheral sensory cells) in other parts of the nervous system, innervating glands and smooth muscle. An important derivative of the neural crest is the dorsal, or posterior, root ganglion (Figure 2-2), a spinal ganglion

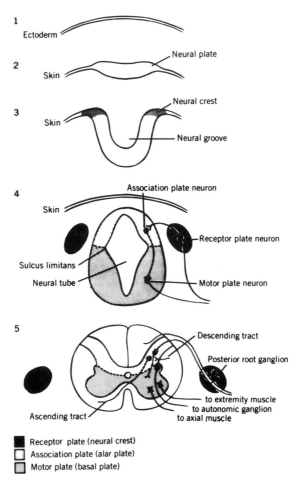

Figure 2-2. Stages in the development of a spinal cord segment. Note the development of the alar and basal plates into sensory and motor regions, respectively (Lemire et al. 1975).

whose cells become bipolar. **Bipolar cells** have only two processes, a dendritic and an axonal process. Spinal ganglion cells send dendrites to the skin and an axon back into the spinal cord, thus serving as sensory nerves.

Once the neural tube is formed, at about the fourth week of gestation, two events occur: cells in the wall of the tube begin to proliferate, and growth increases at the cranial end, where three primary vesicles, or outpouchings, appear; namely, the prosencephalic vesicle (to become the forebrain), the mesencephalic vesicle (midbrain), and the rhombencephalic vesicle (hindbrain). The caudal or tail end, comprising about 50 per cent of the tube, becomes the spinal cord, maintaining its diameter, but elongating and developing into segments, each of which is associated with the sensory and motor innervation of a small part of the body. During its development the spinal cord keeps a remnant of the neural tube as the central canal. In the developing cord itself (Figure 2-2), the neural tissue desegregates into two main bodies of neurons—the dorsal, or posterior, horns and the ventral, or anterior horns—divided by the sulcus limitans. The dorsal horns (also called the **alar plate**) receive axons from the dorsal root ganglia, the derivatives of the neural crest, and are involved in sensory events. The ventral horns (**basal plate**) contain the cell bodies of axons that innervate muscles and are considered part of the motor system.

At the cranial end of the neural tube, the brain bends ventrally during the fourth week, forming two curves, termed the midbrain or mesencephalic flexure in the neck region and the cervical flexure (Figure 2-3). These curves are followed later by a third bend in the opposite direction, the pontine flexure (Figure 2-3). Otherwise, the brain has essentially the same cross-sectional structure as the spinal cord at this time, with dorsal alar and ventral basal plates.

During the fifth week of development, however, further divisions appear in the primary vesicles. The prosencephalic vesicle divides into the telencephalon and the diencephalon, and the rhombencephalic vesicle divides into the metencephalon and the myelencephalon (see Table 1-1). Later, beginning at approximately the seventh week of gestation, the telencephalon is transformed into the cerebral hemispheres, the diencephalon into the thalamus and related structures, the metencephalon into the cerebellum and pons, and the myelen-

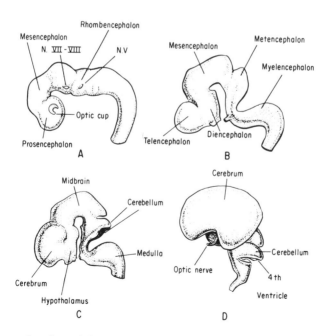

Figure 2-3 Embryological development of the human brain (Peele 1954).

cephalon into the medulla oblongata. In vestigial form, the neural tube becomes the cerebral ventricles and the cerebral aqueduct.

Fetus

This discussion of changes in the brain during the fetal period concentrates on the development of the cerebral hemispheres (telencephalon) since the higher functions are of primary interest in neuropsychology. The sensory, motor, and integrative systems are covered in Chapter 3.

The fetal period begins at about the eighth or ninth week of gestation as the embryo starts to develop into a recognizable human being. During the eighth week the head constitutes at least half of the fetus, but this ratio gradually decreases. In the fetal period there is little further differentiation of the tissues of the body, including the nervous system, and this lack of development decreases the vulnerability of the fetus to possible harmful effects of mechanical or chemical disruptions—teratogens (Langman et al. 1975). It is during this period that myelin begins to form (see Chapter 1). Brain weight rapidly increases from this stage and reaches approximately 350 g at birth. By age 2, brain weight is approximately 1300 g, close to the adult weight of 1400 to 1500 g (Figure 2-4, Dobbing and Sands 1973).

During the sixth week, the basal ganglia become visible in each hemisphere as swellings in the floor of the hemispheres. Later the internal capsule fibers from the developing cortex divide the basal ganglia into the caudate nuclei and the lentiform nuclei. The internal capsule then projects into the spinal cord as the pyramidal tract.

Microscopic studies of the developing cerebral cortex have shown that the early cortical plate forms from migrating cells during the first major wave of migration at 8 to 10 weeks of gestational age (Rakic 1984). Four layers of cortex are visible at this time: ventricular, subventricular, intermediate, and marginal. As the cortical plate thickens due to migrating neurons, more layers are formed, giving the cortex its final six-layered composition by approximately the sixth prenatal month. A columnar organization within the cortex eventually develops (Goldman and Nauta 1977). Beginning in the fifth month, the increasing number of cortical cells causes the smooth surface of the developing brain to develop the typical pattern of convolutions and sulci. Much of this growth is the consequence of glial cell proliferation and axonal and dendritic differentiation (neuron production and migration cease at about this time). The development of the cerebral hemispheres progresses rapidly during the fetal period.

The developing convolutional and sulcal patterns in the brain follow a regular sequence. The primary sulci appear first, the hippocampal sulcus at 13 to 15 weeks and the parieto-occipital, calcarine, and olfactory bulb sulci at 19 weeks. The sylvan (lateral) and Rolandic (central) sulci become visible at 24 weeks, when the calcarine and the parieto-occipital sulci join in a Y-shaped juncture. The secondary sulci, such as the first temporal sulcus and the superior frontal sulci, appear at 28 weeks (Larroche 1967) (Figure 2-5). The tertiary convolutions

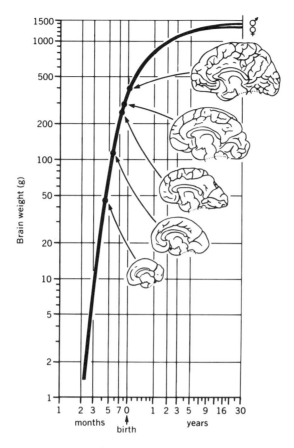

Figure 2-4   Representative growth curve of the weight of the human brain into adult life (Lemire et al. 1975).

are not formed until the third trimester of prenatal development and continue to develop after birth (Chi et al. 1977, Rabinowicz 1979). Generally, the development of the convolutions is thought to depend upon the ratio of growth of the inner and outer cortical layers since, in two malformations of cortical development, **lissencephaly** (literally, smooth brain, absence of gyri) and **microgyria** (multiple very small gyri), abnormalities in the layering pattern are also evident. The extent of convolution development is frequently used to judge the age of the fetus.

Closely related to the changes in the cerebral cortical layers during this time period are changes in the intercerebral commissures, the major connections between the hemispheres. Their growth is rather slow and related to the maturation of association cortex (Trevarthen 1974). The first commissural fibers cross in the rostral end of the forebrain at approximately day 50 of gestation, creating the anterior commissure and the hippocampal commissure. The fibers

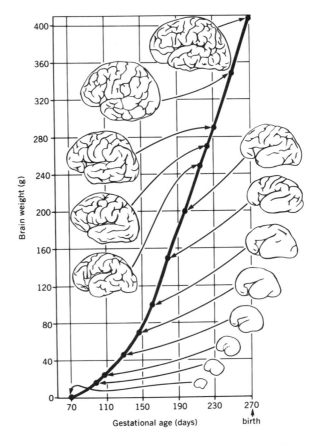

Figure 2-5 Development of the lateral cerebral sulci correlated with brain weight and gestational age (Lemire et al. 1975).

of the corpus callosum cross the midline later. Hewitt (1962) pointed out that the fibers of the corpus callosum develop in parallel with the various cerebral lobes and that this process is not complete until after birth. Failure of the commissures to cross the midline results in a variety of defects, most commonly agenesis of the corpus callosum, in which this major structure is absent. This condition is discussed in Chapter 9 in the context of disconnection syndromes.

2.2 Postnatal

Birth

At approximately 280 days of gestational age, the human fetus emerges from the womb and enters the postnatal period. The birth of even the most healthy organism can be a traumatic event. Many possible traumatic factors, such as mechanical injury, can disrupt the normal development of the nervous system. Some of these factors are discussed in Part III.

A newborn or **neonate** (terms used for the first month of life) has a characteristic set of reflexes and behaviors (Humphrey 1970) that reflect the normal functioning of its nervous system (see Chapter 8). Pediatricians often use a scoring system based upon the work of Apgar (1953, 1962) to evaluate general health after birth; the Apgar measures may have some predictive value for future development (Chapter 7).

Immediately after birth the brain weighs between 300 and 350 g and continues to grow rapidly, increasing to 80 per cent of the adult weight of 1250–1500 g in about 4 years. Much of this growth is due to an increase in the size, complexity, and myelination—rather than to an increase in number—of nerve cells after birth. Conel's (1939–1967) histological photographs of the stages of human neural development document most of these changes: development during the first month is relatively slow in comparison to the progress shown at 3 months and beyond. At birth and during the first year, primary sensory (and especially the somatosensory areas) and motor areas are most advanced, followed by the progressive development of adjacent sensory association areas, and finally the parietal and temporal association areas. The prefrontal lobes are least developed at birth and do not show marked development until after the second year. This pattern is similar to that described for myelogenetic cycles of regional maturation (see Figure 1-10). Bronson (1982) commented that this order parallels the general sequence in which information is processed in the adult neocortex.

Infancy

Infancy is the period from about 1 month to 1 year of postnatal age. As the infant becomes more mature in a variety of spheres—sensory, perceptual, motor, neurophysiological, and cognitive (Bower 1977)—more complicated and sophisticated behavioral patterns appear. The baby interacts more with the outside world through locomotion, learns how to manipulate it, and tries to make some sense out of the information that reaches its brain. As Dimond (1978) wrote, "It would be surprising if somehow this were not reflected by parallel changes in the workings and structure of the brain" (p. 115).

Along with an increase in brain size, as usually inferred from head circumference (Figure 2-6), there is taking shape a functional organization of the nervous system that reflects its increasing responsiveness to stimulation from the environment (Goldman and Rakic 1979). Details of this growing functional organization are discussed in subsequent chapters. One of the major indices of the brain's increasing responsiveness is the elaboration of association fibers and tracts (Altman and Bulut 1976). This increasing connectivity is often regarded as an indicator of information storage and processing. The plasticity to form connections in the young child's nervous system is reflected by postnatal in-

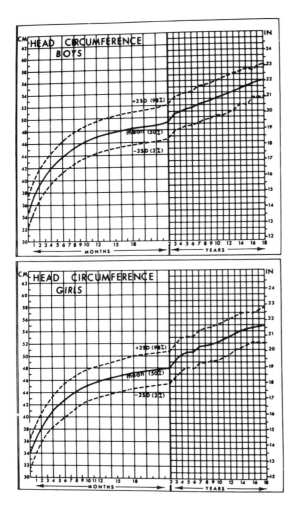

Figure 2-6. Head circumference charts, used for inferring brain maturation for both sexes (Nelhaus 1968).

creases in granule or Golgi type II cells that aid in the ability to form connections.

Neurophysiological changes are also evident during the first year of life, as reflected by changes in the **electroencephalogram** (EEG), a recording of the spontaneous electrical activity of the brain, and in sensory evoked potentials (Spehlmann 1981, Vaughan and Kurtzberg 1989). These measures, a summation of discharges from millions of neurons in many parts of the brain, give a picture of the brain's electrical activity at a given stage of maturation. Just after birth EEG potentials are present, but they are usually irregular and of low amplitude (Figure 2-7). By approximately 4 months of age the first slow rhythm (3 to 4 discharges per second) becomes evident, primarily over the occipital cortex, possibly reflecting maturation of the visual system. The frequency of EEG discharge gradually increases over time until a characteristic stable alpha rhythm

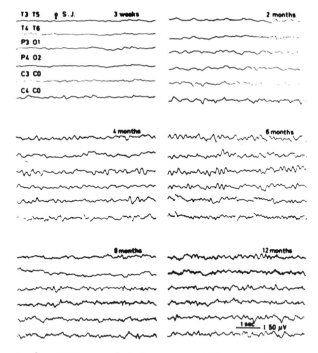

Figure 2-7. Awake EEG recorded from one child at six different ages showing changes in electrical activity. Note the appearance of a dominant frequency at 4 months (Hagne 1968).

(11 to 12 per second) is attained. Evoked potentials and nerve conduction velocity also evolve and mature with age similar to the EEG.

Early Childhood

Cellular patterning and increasing myelination in the CNS continue during early childhood, from years 1 to 6 (Dekaban 1970). Morphological and neurophysiological changes take place concurrent with the development of many abilities, such as language (Eeg-Olofsson 1970, Leary 1978). Table 2-3 summarizes some of the major postnatal changes. The biopsychology of childhood development is discussed in subsequent chapters.

Summary

This chapter reviewed the chronology of pre- and postnatal neural development in some detail. Tracing this remarkable sequence, which is almost to the day of prenatal development, leads to an appreciation of the highly specific consequences that may occur when disrupting influences affect prenatal development at a specific time.

Table 2-3 Summary of Postnatal Human Development

Age	Visual and motor function	Social and intellectual function	EEG	Average brain weight, grams	Total DNA, mg	Degree of myelination
Birth	Reflex sucking, rooting, swallowing, and Moro reflexes; infantile grasping; blinks to light	—	Asynchronous; low-voltage 3–5 Hz; period of flattening; no clear distinction awake or asleep	350	660	Motor roots + +; sensory roots + +; medial lemniscus + +; superior cerebellar peduncle + +; optic tract + +; optic radiation ±
6 weeks	Extends and turns neck when prone; regards mother's face, follows objects	Smiles when played with	Similar to birth records with slightly higher voltages; rare 14 Hz parietal spindles in sleep	410	800	Optic tract + +; optic radiation +; middle cerebral peduncle ±; pyramidal tract+
3 months	Infantile grasp and suck modified by volition; keeps head above horizontal for long periods; turns to objects presented in visual field; may respond to sound	Watches own hands	When awake, asynchronous 3–4 Hz, some 5–6 Hz; low voltages continue; sleep better organized and more synchronous; more spindles but still often asynchronous	515	860	Sensory roots + + +; optic tract and radiations + + +; pyramidal tract + +; cingulum +; frontopontine tract +; middle cerebellar peduncle +; corpus callosum ±; reticular formation ±
6 months	Grasps objects with both hands, will place weight on forearms or hands when prone; rolls supine to prone; supports almost all weight on legs for very brief periods; sits briefly	Laughs aloud and shows pleasure; primitive articulated sounds, "ga-goo"; smiles at self in mirror	More synchronous, 5–7 Hz activity frequent; many lower voltages, slower frequencies; drowsy busts can be seen; humps may first be seen in sleep	660	900	Medial lemniscus + + +; superior cerebellar peduncle + + +; middle cerebellar peduncle + +; pyramidal tract + +; corpus callosum +; reticular formation +; associational areas ±; acoustic radiation +

Table 2-3 Continued

Age	Visual and motor function	Social and intellectual function	EEG	Average brain weight, grams	Total DNA, mg	Degree of myelination
9 months	Sits well and pulls self to sitting position; thumb-forefinger grasp; crawls	Waves bye-bye, plays patty cake, uses "dada," "baba"; imitates sounds	Mild asynchrony; predominant frequencies 5–7 Hz and 2–6 Hz, especially anteriorly; drowsy burst frequent; humps and spindles seen frequently in sleep	750	~900	Cingulum + + +; fornix + +; others as previously given
12 months	Able to release objects; cruises and walks with one hand held; plantar reflex flexor in 50% of children	Two to four words with meaning; understands several proper nouns; may kiss on request	5–7 Hz in all areas, usually synchronous; some anterior 20–25 Hz, some 3–6 Hz; humps often seen in sleep and usually synchronous	925	970	Medial lemniscus + + +; pyramidal tracts + + +; frontopontine tract + + +; fornix + + +; corpus callosum +; intracortical neuropil ±; association areas ±; acoustic radiation + +
24 months	Walks up and down stairs (two feet a step); bends over and picks up objects without falling; turns knob; can partially dress self; plantar reflex flexor in 100%	Two- to three-word sentences, uses "I," "me," and "you" correctly; plays simple games; points to four to five body parts; obeys simple commands	6–8 Hz activity predominates posteriorly with some 4–6 Hz seen especially anteriorly; humps in sleep always synchronous	1065	—	Acoustic radiation + + +; corpus callosum + +; association areas +; nonspecific thalamic radiation + +

Table continued

35

Table 2-3 Continued

Age	Visual and motor function	Social and intellectual function	EEG	Average brain weight, grams	Total DNA, mg	Degree of myelination
36 months	Goes up stairs (one foot a step); pedals tricycle; dresses and undresses fully except for shoelaces, belt, and buttons; visual acuity 20/20/OU	Numerous questions; knows nursery rhymes, copies circle; plays with others	When awake, synchronous 6–9 Hz predominates posteriorly; less 4–6 Hz activity seen; in sleep, spindles usually synchronous	1140	—	Middle cerebellar peduncle + + +
5 years	Skips; ties shoelaces; copies triangle	Repeats four digits; names four colors; gives age correctly	When awake, some 9–10 Hz posteriorly; mostly 7–8 Hz with occasional 4–6 Hz; synchronous; drowsy bursts less frequent and often limited to frontoparietal	1240	—	Nonspecific thalamic radiation + + +; reticular formation + +; corpus callosum + + +; intracortical neuropil and association areas + +
Adult	—	—	When awake, synchronous 9–12 Hz posterior frequencies; rare 7–8 Hz waves; 18–25 Hz waves and low voltage fast anteriorly; with drowsiness, flattening and low voltage theta; spindles and humps in sleep as before	1400	~1500	Intracortical neuropil and association areas + + to + + +

Source: Dodge et al. 1975.

3

Development of Functional Systems

When we discuss the disorders resulting from abnormal influences on nervous system development and on neuropsychological functioning (Chapters 11 to 30), they will be seen as deviations from normal development in specific neurologically based systems of psychological functions. A **functional system** consists of those neural structures involved in the successful completion of an individual sensory, motor, or higher cognitive task, e.g., all parts of the visual system, as well as structures mediating the response to visual stimuli (Woolacott 1990).

The normal development of functional systems involves an interaction between brain development and experience. Each system is to some degree "experience-expectant" (Greenough et al. 1987) to take in and respond to the environmental information of the species, as well as "experience-dependent" to absorb and store information that is unique to the individual. Sensory deprivation experiments on animals have shown long-lasting or permanent sensory impairment, as well as changes in the associated central structures and the cortex, including reduction in synaptic density and the amount of dendrites. Rats raised in individual cages (i.e., without environmental stimulation) showed 20 to 25 per cent less synapses per neuron in the visual cortex compared to those raised in environmental cages, i.e., with numerous objects and with other animals (Turner and Greenough 1985). In addition, Tieman and Hirsch (1982) reported a change in the pattern arrangement of the visual cortex in cats reared in either a vertical or horizontal stripe environment. Studies have shown that drugs that interfere with norepinephrine action reduce or block the brain's ability to experience full environmental complexity, suggesting that this neurotransmitter as well as acetylcholine may be involved in regulating the developing sensitivity of the cortex (Mirmiran and Uylings 1983). In other studies, specific training tasks led to higher dendritic branching in the corresponding unilateral motor cortex (Greenough et al. 1985). It should be kept in mind that more subtle disturbances in functional systems can occur without measurable changes in neurological structure or function.

This chapter reviews the normal development of the functional systems that in later life regulate specific adult behaviors. Primary sensory and motor systems are discussed first and then the higher-order integrative systems. Because of the complexity of each system, only a brief description of structure and development can be provided.

3.1 Sensory Systems

Auditory System

The adult auditory system is illustrated in Figure 3-1. Briefly, the external ear canal begins with the outer ear, or **pinna**, and ends at the eardrum (**tympanic membrane**). The eardrum connects to three small, interconnected bones of the middle ear (**ossicles**) and then to a membrane covering the end of the coiled cochlea, which is part of the inner ear. Within this coiled tube lies a smaller tube, the cochlear duct, containing the **organ of Corti**, the sense organ of hearing.

Sounds, which consist of air vibrating at numerous frequencies, pass through the ear canal and cause the ossicles to vibrate. This movement is in turn transmitted to the fluid within the **cochlea**, thus producing vibratory movement of the **basilar membrane** in the inner ear. This movement bends the hair cells lying between the basilar and stiffer tectorial membrane. The particular fre-

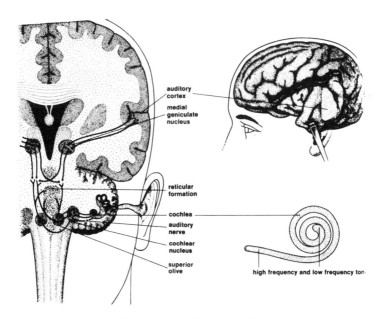

Figure 3-1. The human auditory system (Krech et al. 1969).

quency heard depends upon exactly which hair cells resting on the basilar membrane are activated. Fibers of the eighth, or auditory, nerve are stimulated by the hair cell receptors. Axons of the eighth nerve ascend into the CNS with synapses in the dorsal and ventral cochlear nuclei of the medulla. From there they are relayed through the superior olivary nucleus to the contralateral side of the brain or directly via the lateral lemniscus tract on each side of the brainstem. Auditory input is thus bilateral, with each ear transmitting impulses to both sides of the brain. The **lateral lemniscus** then synapses in the inferior colliculus of the midbrain and the medial geniculate body of the thalamus before projecting through the auditory radiation to the auditory area (transverse, or Heschl's, gyrus) of the temporal cortex. A detailed description of the central auditory system has been presented by Altschuler et al. (1991).

The embryological development of the ear (Selnes and Whitaker 1976, C.A. Smith 1975) starts at around 22 days of gestational age with the emergence of the ectodermal auditory, or **otic placodes**, the precursors of the inner ear and the vestibular system. At 4 to 5 embryonic weeks the placodes become the **otocyst**, which then divides into the cochlear and labyrinth lobes (the latter forms part of the vestibular system). By about 5 weeks the **external auditory meatus** (canal) originates from the first pharyngeal cleft by an invagination and reaches the future middle ear cavity. At 6 weeks, the cochlea appears as a short, curved tube, and the pinnae become visible and continue to grow rapidly through infancy and childhood. At about 7 weeks the middle ear ossicles appear and reach terminal size by 6 to 8 months.

The mechanical aspects of the human auditory system are therefore reasonably mature at birth. The hair cells in the organ of Corti develop at 4 to 5 months gestational age, but are not fully differentiated until later. At birth, the peripheral sensory aspects of the auditory system are functionally complete. Figure 3-2 summarizes some of these details (Clopton 1981).

The development of the eighth (auditory) nerve is also complete at birth, and it is fairly well myelinated at that time (Hecox 1975). There is some evidence that the brainstem development of the inferior colliculi and the medial geniculate nuclei is also relatively complete at birth, but the myelination of projection fibers to the cortex is sparse and continues up to at least 4 years of age. The slow myelination may explain the prolonged latency and the diminished amplitude of auditory evoked response potential (**evoked response potential, ERP**) in newborns (Ohlrich et al. 1978). ERPs are a modification of the EEG technique used for assessing the intactness of the nervous system by averaging several electrophysiological responses to time-locked physical stimuli, either visual or auditory. ERPs are averaged over many repeated presentations until a reliable waveform is obtained. As shown in Figure 3-3, two fast responses (N100, N200) and one slow wave (P300, N400) are typically seen. ERPs are indicators of the efficiency of processing in the system, as well as of differential lateralization, depending on the nature of the stimulus (Jeffrey 1980).

Within the first few days of life, auditory acuity improves as a result of the draining of amniotic fluid from the middle ear. Parts of the auditory system,

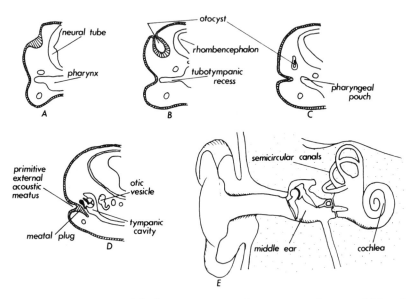

Figure 3-2. Development of the human inner ear beginning at the age of 24 embryonic days (A) to the adult age (E) (Reinis and Goldman 1980).

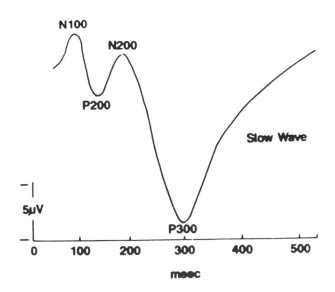

Figure 3-3. Typical evoked response potential (ERP) indicating latencies in milliseconds at peak altitudes. N = negative, P = positive response potential.

such as the external auditory meatus and the tympanic membrane, do not reach adult dimensions until about 1 year of age; this may be the cause of the relatively poor hearing sensitivity in the neonate, which is 40 to 60 db above adult thresholds for the same sounds (Hecox 1975). Sensitivity gradually increases during infancy and until about 7 to 10 years of age. Newborn infants have the basic ability to discriminate frequency and pitch (Selnes and Whitaker 1976). At birth, the auditory cortex is electrically active, although the auditory system requires a long time to reach adult capacity. Auditory localization (as indicated by head turning in the neonate) seems to be present quite early (Muir et al. 1979). A series of experiments has shown that infants as early as 2 months can accomplish temporal perception tasks and that infants 6 to 11 months of age can recognize melodic contours of three to six notes while disregarding changes in pitch and interval size (Trehub et al. 1987). This ability seems to be fundamental to the recognition of the caretaker's vocalizations and to be a precursor of the perception of speech intonation. At present, our knowledge of the physiological correlates of auditory development is still incomplete.

Visual System

The visual pathways in the human adult (Figure 3-4) are relatively simple and have been studied extensively. The visual image enters the eye via the cornea

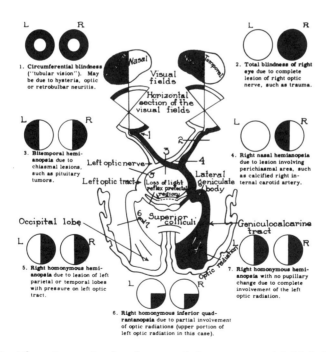

Figure 3-4. The primary visual pathways and the major visual field defects (Noback and Demerest 1981).

and lens and reaches receptors in the retina. Impulses from these receptors are then relayed through bipolar cells to ganglion cells, possibly modified on the way by two sets of interneurons (Fiorentini 1991). The axons of the ganglion cells run across the surface of the retina (light passes through the fibers to reach the receptors), leave the back of the eye through the optic disk, creating a **blind spot** in the visual field, and then become the optic (or second cranial) nerve. In higher vertebrates, including humans, where some degree of binocular vision exists, part of each optic nerve goes to each side of the brain. Optic nerve fibers from the left half of the retina (stimulated by the right half of the visual field) project to the left lateral geniculate nucleus in the thalamus, and fibers from the right half of the retina project to the right lateral geniculate nucleus. At the optic chiasm, where the two optic nerves come together, the other half of their fibers cross and project to opposite hemispheres. From the optic chiasm the fibers form the optic tracts entering the CNS and synapse at the respective lateral geniculate nuclei (Figure 3-4). Cells in these nuclei then send their axons to the middle layers of the primary visual cortex, *area 17* of the two occipital lobes. These pathways are the **primary visual projections**. Another visual pathway, usually termed the **second visual system**, projects from the retina to the superior colliculus (Stein and Gordon 1981) and thence to the pulvinar nuclei in the thalamus. These nuclei in turn project to secondary visual areas in the cortex (see Chapter 25).

The eye begins to develop, as the optic vesicle, about 30 days after fertilization (Figure 3-5). Between the second and fourth months of gestation the visual system, especially the retina, develops rapidly (Rakic 1979a). The retina differentiates gradually, the ganglion cells appearing first and the rods and cones (the receptor cells, see Chapter 25) last. In the sixth month the eyelids can open, and the **fovea** (the central area of greatest acuity) begins to form, although it is not completely developed until after birth. The level of visual acuity during the first month is 20 to 30 times lower than in the adult (Atkinson and Braddick 1982). The eye remains at a relatively fixed focus of about 30 cm. The laminated structure of the lateral geniculate nucleus also appears early in the prenatal period, although some relay interneurons may not develop until after birth (Rakic 1979b). Hickey (1977) demonstrated that the geniculate cells increase rapidly in size during the first 6 to 12 months of postnatal life, suggesting a specific growth spurt for the development of this part of the visual system. Related to this rapid growth is the development of the visual cortex (Movshon and Van Sluyters 1981), which, as discussed in Chapter 1, develops in an inside-out pattern. Other cortical development also occurs after birth, including increases in the thickness of the visual cortex; in the number of glial cells, interneurons, and dendritic spines; and in the amount of myelination. These changes are related to the development of functional connectivity and depend to some extent on visual experience. The development of visually guided skilled motor behavior later in the life of the infant has also been related to interactions with visual experience. A more detailed discussion of the role of early experience on sensory development is presented in Chapter 8.

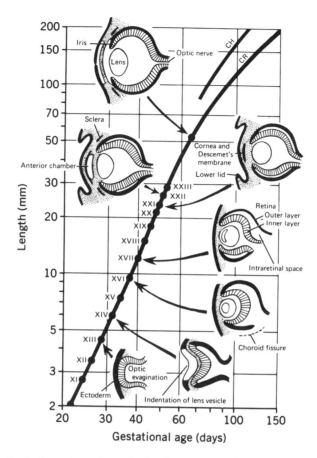

Figure 3-5. Sagittal sections through the human eye during embryonic and fetal periods (Lemire et al. 1975).

Although most senses are at least minimally functional at birth, visual perception in early life relies on more than the primary visual system. Bronson (1974) proposed that early visual perception is mediated by components of the phylogenetically older second visual system, which develops earlier since it is primarily subcortical. At its receiving end, the second visual system involves mainly the more peripheral areas of the retina. It transmits information regarding the location and orientation of visual stimuli, rather than highly resolved details, and relays this information via subcortical structures to different areas of the occipital lobes. Visual reactions to more complex visual information appear during the second and third postnatal months, although some activity can be deduced from head turning after foveal visual fixation in neonates (Lewis et al. 1978) and visual evoked potentials at birth in full-term, but not in preterm babies. Bronson (1994) suggested that this activity is a reflection of increasing participation by the primary visual system in the processing of visual input. The phylogenetically more recent primary system is concerned with the analysis and encoding of complex stimuli. Therefore, postnatal development of the visual system can be viewed as a progressive encoding of increasingly more complex aspects of visual information, calling upon different components of the visual network.

Many visual abilities increase during the infancy period. Binocular vision appears at about 6 weeks and is well established by about 4 months. Conjugate eye movements, necessary in binocular vision to prevent strabismus, are present at birth and usually stable by 6 months. Color vision also develops in this period. Although all these functions are "wired in" prenatally, their development, refinement, and stabilization in terms of synaptic connectivity depend on information from patterned stimuli, which cannot be experienced until after birth (Atkinson and Braddick 1989, Held 1989, Johnson 1990).

Chemical Senses

Taste relies on **taste receptor cells** grouped into taste buds for sweet, salty, sour, and bitter, although each receptor can be responsive to a wide diversity of tastes beyond these four basic ones. These receptor cells are innervated by specific branches of three cranial nerves: the facial (VII) for the anterior two-thirds of the tongue, the glossopharyngeal (IX) for the posterior third, and the vagus (X) that innervates the pharynx. The nerves meet in the solitary nuclear complex in the medulla and synapse via the ventral posterior medial nucleus to the postcentral gyrus and the insula.

Taste receptors are mature by approximately 12 weeks of gestation (Bradley and Mistretta 1975) and seem to be functional before birth. Reinis and Goldman (1980) report an increase in fetal swallowing after the intra-amniotic injection of saccharine. After birth, very small volumes of salt solution decreased non-nutritive sucking by an amount that increased with the concentration.

Olfactory receptor cells are embedded deeply in the nasal cavity and connect to the olfactory bulbs and form the olfactory (I) cranial nerve. The first nerve does not synapse in the thalamus, but branches on into limbic system structures, including the amygdala and the entorhinal cortex, while another branch goes to the orbitofrontal cortex. The first branch is considered to evoke emotional components of smell, whereas the second is involved in the conscious perception of smell.

Odor preferences and aversions are present very early in life, indicating that the sense of smell is developed at birth. One to 2-day-old neonates turn away from a drop of ammonium on a cotton swab and produce an accepting expression at the smell of fruit odors (Steiner 1979). MacFarlane (1975) found even more striking olfactory abilities in 6- to 10-day-old infants: they oriented toward their mother's breast pad in preference not only to an unused breast pad but also to breast pads of an unfamiliar nursing mother. Such complex sensory discriminations among human individuals have been found not only in olfaction but also, a few weeks later, in vision (Bushnell 1980) and hearing (Mills and Melhuish 1974).

Somesthetic System

The **somesthetic** (or somatosensory) **system** relays thermal, tactile, and positional information to the brain. The system is not only crucial for the infant's early exploration of the world by touch but also interacts with the visual, motor, and other systems in the development of active tactile exploration, visually guided motor behavior, body movement, posture, walking, and many other activities of the developing organism (Urban 1994). Generally, two subsystems are distinguished: (1) the **lemniscal system**, which is involved in the transmission of light touch and pressure stimuli, and (2) the **spinothalamic system**, which carries diffuse touch, pain, and temperature information.

The lemniscal system represents the more prominent cutaneous sensitivity. The lemniscal pathway of the adult begins as a peripheral process of the dorsal root ganglion, which sends axons into the spinal cord. The axons either end in the dorsal horns of the cord at the level of entry or run up the spinal cord in the white matter (the dorsal columns) and end in the dorsal column nuclei of the medulla. Fibers from these nuclei then cross and ascend in a tract called the medial lemniscus to synapse in the ventral posterior nucleus of the thalamus. From there, axons project through the internal capsule into the somatosensory areas of the postcentral gyrus in the parietal lobe. This major pathway is contralateral, left body surface to right hemisphere, since it crosses (decussates) in the brainstem.

Fibers entering the spinal cord from the spinothalamic receptors form synapses in the spinal cord with the dorsal horn cells. They then cross and ascend the spinal cord in spinothalamic tracts, relaying fibers to the reticular formation and synapsing again in the ventral nuclei of the thalamus before ascending to the somatosensory areas of the cortex. There is some evidence that this tract has some ipsilateral as well as contralateral connections.

The development of the somatosensory systems in humans has been described by Woolsey et al. (1981) and Rowe and Willis (1985). Early development of one spinal cord segment, the sensory ganglia, is discussed in Section 2.1. The sensory nerves approach the skin of the fetus in the eighth week and make contact by the ninth week. However, no receptors have been described at this early stage.

Myelination of the tracts in the spinal cord begins by midgestation and continues until birth for the sensory roots and until 1 year after birth for the medial lemniscus (Yakovlev and Lecours 1967). Recent evidence suggests that somatosensory cortical maps are maintained and are alterable by experience throughout life (Merzenich 1992).

3.2 Motor Systems

Two systems, operating semi-independently, are involved in human motor activity. The **pyramidal system** is responsible for the initiation of voluntary, skilled movements involving rapid and precise control of the extremities. It is therefore regarded as the "executive" system concerned with motor control (Figure 3-6). The **extrapyramidal system** is more concerned with alterations and adjustments in posture and with modification and coordination of movements initiated by the pyramidal system. These two systems allow the developing organism to move around and, in humans and higher animals, to manipulate the environment directly. Any response of the organism, even if it is just a reflexive response to stimulation, involves the participation of some segment of the motor system.

Motor activity develops early during gestation. In 1885, Preyer (summarized by Espenschade and Eckert 1980) established the developmental primacy of the motor system over the sensory systems; the embryo is capable of movement early in the second trimester, before responses to sensory stimulation can be demonstrated. Early motor behavior is generated spontaneously within the organism. As Humphrey (1970) suggested, such early movements may be necessary for the normal development of motility and leg structure. Reflexes also appear before regulated patterned movement and skills (Brandt 1979, Bullock and Grossberg 1989). In fact, most of the motor responses of the neonate can plausibly be related to subcortical processes. Prenatal and early postnatal activity may then lead to neonatal movement representing the integration of earlier reflexes with responses to environmental demands.

Development of the milestones of motor abilities is sequential in most children, although there is much variability among individuals. The infant generally progresses from the ability to lift the chin up when lying on the stomach at 1 to 2 months of age to sitting at 7 to 8 months, creeping and crawling at 9 to 10 months, and standing and walking at about 1 year. The span for developing the ability to walk without assistance varies from 8 to 18 months.

Manipulatory abilities increase continually during infancy. After the first 2 or 3 months the primitive grasp reflex disappears, and by 12 weeks voluntary grasping has begun. Reaching and grasping improve up to 20 weeks of age, and at 24 weeks the child may be quite competent at eating dry food.

Throughout early childhood the locomotor and manipulative abilities continue to improve steadily. By the age of 2 to 3 years, a child usually can dress and feed him- or herself, has voluntary sphincter control, and can walk without assistance. The development of the two interacting motor systems forms the basis for these increasing abilities.

Pyramidal System

The two motor systems "begin" at a different CNS level than sensory systems, and neural signals move in the opposite direction. Sensory systems relay infor-

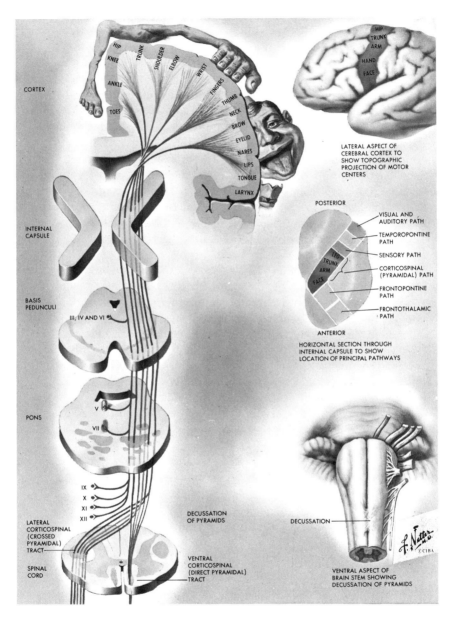

Figure 3-6. The pyramidal system (Netter 1962).

47

mation up the spinal cord to the brain, and motor systems send information and instructions from the brain down the cord and out to the muscles involved.

The pyramidal tract begins in the cerebral cortex, in the area known as the motor cortex of the **precentral gyrus**, Brodmann's area 4 (see Figure 1-2). The neurons at the beginning of this tract, in layer 5 of the cortex, are called giant pyramidal cells (hence, the name pyramidal tract) or, after their discoverer, **Betz cells**. The giant cells send their axons into the internal capsule forming the pyramidal tract and through the cerebral peduncles of the midbrain. At the level of the medulla, 80 per cent of the fibers cross to the other side. This decussation is responsible for the predominantly contralateral representation of the motor system from brain to body. The crossed fibers descend through the **lateral corticospinal tract** to their respective spinal cord level and synapse with large anteriorly located motor neurons. Uncrossed fibers (about 20 per cent) descend in the **anterior corticospinal tract** to their appropriate levels. The anterior motor neurons, located in the anterior horns, send axons out of the cord through motor nerves to innervate their respective muscles or muscle groups (see also Figure 3-6).

Development of the pyramidal system and spinal cord is perhaps the most thoroughly studied aspect of CNS development. The neural elements of the pyramidal system develop from embryonic ectoderm, and the effector (muscle) elements are derived from the embryonic mesoderm. During early prenatal development these two types of tissue are in contact with each other (Hollyday 1980). The basal plate of the developing neural tube is the precursor of the developing pyramidal system; the system differentiates fully before birth. Myelination of the pyramidal tracts by Schwann cells in the spinal cord, however, occurs only later—in the first postnatal year (Yakovlev and Lecours 1967). The late myelination is often associated with the onset of walking. The cortical connections of this tract also begin to develop early, but further maturation and differentiation of tissues and cells continue into early childhood. Maturation of corticospinal connections is thought to underlie the emergence and improvement of motor skills during normal development.

Extrapyramidal System

Certain motor projections from several cortical areas are not part of the pyramidal tract. These projections have been called the "extrapyramidal" system, although the term has been criticized as inadequate. The pyramidal system proper and the spinal motor neurons are excluded from this system, but parts of the cerebellum, the basal ganglia, and some brainstem areas, such as the red nucleus and the substantia nigra, are generally included. Developmental data for extrapyramidal structures are scanty and are concentrated on the basal ganglia and the cerebellum.

At 3 to 8 weeks of gestational age, the human cerebellum has three primary layers: the ventricular (V), intermediate (I), and marginal (M) layers (Figure 3-7). At about 13 weeks, some neuroblasts migrate to the surface of the cerebellum to form the cerebellar cortex, whereas others remain in place to form the deep

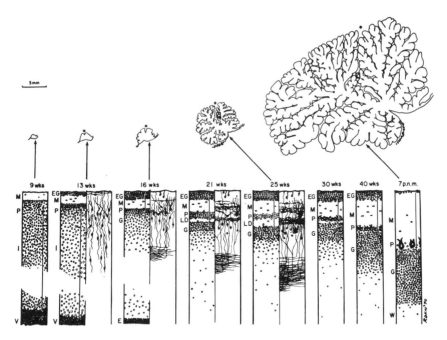

Figure 3-7. Development of the cerebellar cortex in the human from 9 weeks prenatal to 7 months postnatal (Sidman and Rakic 1973). E = ependyma, EG = external granular layer, G = granular layer, I = intermediate layer, LD = lamina dissecans, M = molecular layer, P = Purkinje layer, V = ventricular zone, W = white matter.

cerebellar nuclei. Cells proliferate from two zones in the developing cerebellum: the ventricular and the external granular (EG) zones. Purkinje cells (P), which are derived from the ventricular zone, migrate outward using the Bergmann glia as guides and eventually form a middle layer between these two zones. The small, spherical granule cells (G) originate in the external granular layer and migrate internally. In humans the number of granule cells at birth is only about 17 per cent of the final number; extensive neurogenesis occurs postnatally. In fact, the germinating external granular layer is present until about 18 months after birth. The importance of granule cells for later-developing cerebellar motor functions was shown by Brunner and Altman (1974), who reported locomotor deficits in rats after the postnatal irradiation of cerebellar granule cells decreased their number. Balazs (1979) also stressed the sensitivity of postnatal granule cell generation to certain metabolic disturbances, suggesting that the "clumsy child" may be suffering from the persisting consequences of such insults.

Development of the basal ganglia (caudate nucleus and putamen) begins in the sixth week of embryonic life when a prominent swelling called the ganglionic eminence develops along the floor of the lateral ventricles. However, the globus pallidus, a wedge-shaped structure at the side and near the end of the internal capsule, seems to develop in the diencephalon, rather than the telencephalon, and originates in a proliferative zone of the third ventricle before being displaced to the telencephalon.

3.3   Integrative Systems

Integrative systems of the brain oversee and coordinate several lower-order psychological and behavioral functions and are involved in such higher-order functions as learning, memory, attention, emotion, cognition, and language. The repertory of spatially directed responses has generated several studies, which were reviewed by McDonnell (1979). The newborn seems to reach for nearby visual objects frequently and in the correct direction, suggesting to some authors the notion of a central representation of space interlinking with different sensory modalities and different motor acts (Atkinson and Braddick 1982). Since integrative systems have such wide-ranging and complex functions, they necessarily draw on large areas of the brain. It is generally agreed that their anatomical basis includes association areas of the cortex, the reticular formation and brainstem pathways, commissural connections between hemispheres, the limbic system, and language areas of the cortex.

Association Areas

Association areas are regions in the cortex where the information of various other parts is thought to be integrated. They are often referred to as silent areas of the brain because they do not show sensory-evoked responses. They have also been called tertiary areas (Flechsig 1901) because they are the last to develop and myelinate. They are also the most sensitive to environmental influences (Goldman and Lewis 1978, Goldman and Rakic 1979). Several association areas of the cortex have been identified, specifically the parietal, temporal, and prefrontal areas. The prefrontal cortical association area has attracted much recent developmental research and is used as an example here.

As with all other cortical areas, the prefrontal cortex forms in an inside-out pattern of cellular layering, the neurons migrating through earlier layers to form new ones (Sidman and Rakic 1973). Goldman-Rakic (1984) demonstrated that contralateral callosal fibers interdigitate in an intricate pattern of compartmentalization with ipsilateral associational fibers at several levels, suggesting a novel basis for interhemispheric integration. In her view the association cortex, "the machinery that allows for separation of higher order inputs, could also permit combinations and recombinations among these inputs that would constitute a highly adaptive and plastic mechanism for information processing" (p. 424). A distinguishing feature of the prefrontal cortex is the presence of many granule cells that develop postnatally. For this reason the area has also been called the **frontal granular cortex**. No specific projection fibers to other systems have been found. The axons within and leaving this area myelinate in the human from the sixth month after birth up to as late as the third decade of life (Flechsig

1901, Yakovlev and Lecours 1967). Passler et al. (1985) suggested that this development is dynamic, occurs in stages, and reaches functional maturity at age 12. The late development supports the notion that higher, later-maturing functions are involved.

The developmental studies of the prefrontal cortex by Goldman-Rakic (Goldman 1972, 1974, Goldman-Rakic 1984) have underlined the importance not only of the age of the organism in the normal and abnormal development of functional connections in the prefrontal regions, but also of other variables, such as sex, and the interaction of these variables (Goldman 1975). Goldman-Rakic's work with monkeys indicates that the functional maturation of the dorsolateral prefrontal cortex extends over several years of postnatal life.

Various regions of the dorsolateral frontal cortex mature at different rates (Alexander and Goldman 1978). With the help of newer prenatal neurosurgical techniques in monkeys, Goldman-Rakic has been able to demonstrate that the effects of prenatal lesions in these areas differ depending on the rate of maturation. The major implication of this work is that, if disruptive influences impinge upon the primate brain before full functional maturation of a specific region (here, association cortex), they have little immediate impact on the development of the function subserved by that region. This body of research is discussed further in relation to plasticity (Chapter 8) and sex differences (Chapter 6).

Reticular Formation and Brainstem Chemical Pathways

The reticular formation or, more specifically, the **reticular activating system**, consists of several nuclei and neuronal groups that form a ventral core of tissue in the brainstem ranging from the medulla to the midbrain. The name refers to the core network, or reticulum, of intermingled cell bodies and fibers surrounded by the ascending sensory and descending motor pathways. The importance of the reticular formation became clear in the late 1940s and early 1950s when a relationship between arousal and reticular formation activity was discovered (Moruzzi and Magoun 1949). Much interest revolves around the role of the reticular formation in such processes as attention, alertness, habituation, and consciousness (Cohen 1993).

The reticular formation nuclei arise from the dorsal plate of the developing brainstem and are among the first nuclei of the brain to form and differentiate. The individual nuclei of the reticular formation have not been studied in detail in humans, but are known to consist primarily of four populations of neurons containing specific monoaminergic neurotransmitters: dopamine, norepinephrine, epinephrine, and serotonin. The dopamine system is located in the **substantia nigra**, norepinephrine and epinephrine in the **locus ceruleus** in the dorsal pons, and serotonin in the **midline nuclei** of the midbrain. In the human brain, most of the monoaminergic pathways extending from these neuron populations develop by 10 weeks of gestational age. Generally, the development of serotonin-containing cells precedes that of the other monoaminergic neuron groups, but all have been identified by 23 weeks of age. Since these neuron groups, especially the norepinephrine and serotonin systems, have widespread projections to many other areas in the nervous system, they may "modulate the cortical tone" by exerting a general activational role or coordinate other areas, especially the frontal lobes (Luria 1973). This action is in accord with their presumed role in attentional mechanisms and alertness (Cohen 1993).

Other studies have investigated prenatal autonomic functions, such as heart rate and heart rate during labor, for their importance for the later development of attention, arousal, and other outcome variables in infancy (Emory and Noonan 1984; Emory et al. 1982). The authors found that deceleratory patterns during birth were associated with lower birth weight, prematurity, and abnormal reflexes as scored on the Brazelton Newborn Behavior Assessment Scale. Recent research distinguishes between early (Type 1) and late (Type 2) deceleration of heart rate. Type 1 deceleration appears to be of little significance, but Type 2, particularly when associated with loss of beat or beat variations is more ominous, although interrater agreement for the interpretation of traces is poor (Behrman, 1992, Paneth et al. 1992, Paul, 1992). Another area of interest that is under autonomic control is the development of the sleep-wake cycle and the amount of rapid-eye-movement sleep. Both types of sleep gradually become less in infancy and childhood, as well as during the remainder of the life-span (Berg and Berg 1979).

Commissural-Interhemispheric Pathways

The **interhemispheric** (or neocortical) **commissures** are large fiber bundles connecting the major portions of the cortex of the two hemispheres. Although these fibers reach their greatest relative size in humans, little is known about their direct function. The largest commissure is the **corpus callosum**, which connects most cortical areas of the two hemispheres. The smaller **anterior commissure** connects primarily the anterior temporal lobes. The neocortical commissures are thought to transmit highly refined information from one side of the brain to the other and to serve an integrating function for the two sides of the body and perceptual space (Gazzaniga 1970).

The cerebral commissures do not myelinate fully until late in postnatal development. The corpus callosum in particular matures concurrently with other cortical association areas and is therefore one of the last components of the CNS to begin and complete myelination (Hewitt 1962). Kucharski and Hall (1988) report that in 6-day-old rat pups learned odor preference trained to one side can remain unilateral, but only for the first postnatal week, after which commissural fibers become effective; sectioning of commissural fibers in older pups reintroduces the possibility of training unilateral preferences. Berman and Payne (1988) review how the interhemispheric connections of the visual (striate) cortex can be altered by visual experience (e.g., monocular deprivation) in cats.

A behavioral maturation of interhemispheric functions has also been proposed. Children aged 1 to 3 years act in a "functional split-brain" fashion, i.e., as if they were unable to transfer sensory or motor information from one hemisphere to the other (Gazzaniga 1970). Presumably, the efficiency of this transfer increases with anatomical maturation of the commissures. In a study of 3- to 5-year-old children performing right-hand—left-hand tactile matching task, Galin and colleagues (1979) showed that 5-year-olds are better able to transfer information between hemispheres. However, Tupper (1982) was unable to replicate this finding. He stressed that intra- and cross-hemispheric functioning are so intimately related that they are difficult to separate and quantify in young children. Another study (DeSchonen and Bry 1987) used visual discrimination learning of stimuli similar to human faces that were presented to the right or the left visual field. A transfer test, presenting the stimuli learned in the left visual field to the right field, showed a clear gain in learning, presumably due to interhemispheric transfer, only in infants 19 to 26 weeks of age, but not in younger infants. The authors suggested that interhemispheric, or possibly subcortical, pathways, though poorly myelinated at that age, become functional for this type of transfer around 19 weeks. Visual attention and memory at birth were also reviewed by Slater and Morrison (1991) and by Weiss and Zelazo (1991).

Finally, Strauss et al. (1994) found a positive relationship between the size of the posterior area (splenium) of the corpus callosum and measured IQ in adults. They suggest that the size of this area may reflect the number of cortical neurons and interconnections between brain areas that are important for processing the kind of information measured on intelligence tests.

Limbic System

The **limbic system** is a ring of structures on the medial surface of and between the hemispheres (Figure 3-8). It includes the amygdala, the septal nuclei, the anterior thalamus, the cingulate gyrus, the fornix, and the hippocampus and dentate gyrus (Kappers 1971). Since the writings of Papez in the 1930s, the limbic system has been regarded as the morphological substrate of emotional behavior. More recently, it has been described as having modulatory and attentional functions (Tucker 1990) or a role in memory, especially recent memory. The hippocampus and the related dentate gyrus have been extensively studied from a developmental perspective.

During the third and fourth months of fetal development the major nuclear groups of the limbic system form on the ventral aspect of the temporal lobe. The basal part of the temporal lobe differentiates into the periamygdaloid area, the hippocampal area, and the fornix. After the fourth month, the hippocampal area begins to differentiate into the hippocampus proper and the dentate gyrus (Cowan et al. 1980, Gall and Lynch 1980). The **hippocampus** becomes a rolled structure inside the temporal lobe, surrounding the dentate gyrus. The overall shape of the hippocampus resembles a curve from which it gets its name, which means seahorse.

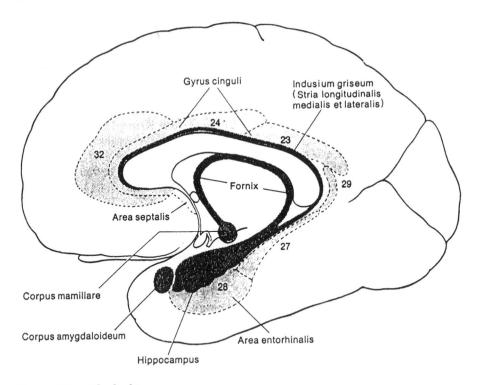

Figure 3-8. The limbic system.

Neurogenesis occurs postnatally in the dentate gyrus region (Wallace et al. 1977). Some researchers, such as Altman and co-workers (1973), have postulated that the behavioral maturation of hippocampal functions also occurs postnatally. This interpretation is consistent with the proposed functions for this part of the limbic system, which are higher-order ones, such as memory. The prolonged postnatal hippocampal development makes the structure maximally sensitive to environmental events (Altman et al. 1973).

Language Areas

Communication with others through speech and language is the most complex ability of humans. Speech requires the participation of many neurological and other structures (e.g., pharynx, larynx) and fully developed psychological abilities, as well as the opportunity to learn how to use words.

The neurological mechanisms underlying speech and language abilities in the adult are fairly well understood because damage in specific brain regions produces such disabilities as **aphasia**, a loss or disruption of the ability to produce, retrieve, and/or understand language; **alexia**, the inability to read; and **agraphia**, the inability to write. CNS structures thought to play a role in speech and language include Heschl's gyrus, the **primary auditory area** (Brodmann's area 41) of the temporal lobe. **Wernicke's area**, which is located in the posterior part of the superior temporal gyrus, is thought to be responsible for the analysis and comprehension of spoken language. **Broca's area**, (area 44) which is in the posterior part of the inferior frontal gyrus, is responsible for the motor output or expressive aspects of speech. Adequate written language requires good visuospatial and manipulative abilities that involve other CNS regions, especially the third left frontal convolution. Reading also requires the participation of additional areas and abilities, notably visual abilities and correct perceptual analysis. The left angular gyrus of the parietal lobe has been singled out as particularly important for reading (Chapter 29).

These many regions and their connections undergo extensive changes during development. Growth and adaptation of the motor speech apparatus of the pharynx, larynx, and mouth continue through puberty. Many of the changes consist of an enlargement of the various chambers, which affects the speech sounds since the anatomical structures put certain physical limitations on sounds. The sensory pathways (visual and auditory) necessary for speech mature relatively early in infancy. However, the maturation of the more specialized speech areas of the brain can be related to specific milestones in the development of language. For example, Lecours (1975) suggests that **babbling**, a phase of spontaneous production of sounds usually seen in 2- to 3-month old infants, may be governed only by subcortical CNS structures because the connections between the cortex and the subcortical structures that carry sensory stimulation develop later in infancy. **Echolalia** (direct repetition of speech sounds) in the 4- to 7-month-old infant is seen as an imitative response to specific acoustic stimuli that is possible when the cortical connections of the auditory system become more active. Learning articulated systems of speech begins at 18 to 24 months and lasts until the age of 5 to 6 years.

In a review, Joseph (1982) argued for early "neurodynamic" influences of the limbic system on emotional speech, thought, and imagery. He proposed that the left hemisphere develops earlier than the right and "gains a competitive advantage in the acquisition of motor representation," whereas the later maturing right hemisphere is assumed to have "an advantage in the establishment of sensory-affective synaptic representation, including that of limbic mediation" (p. 4).

Summary

This chapter focused on the development of the major functional systems that are crucial for the psychological development of the child. The motor system is one of the first to reach functional maturity and myelinates early. Similarly, the sensory systems for hearing, vision, and somesthetic experience form quite early in life, whereas the development of integrative systems—the areas of the brain that form intracortical associations—occurs later and does not begin myelination until after birth. The myelination of these areas continues well into late adolescence and adulthood. A similarly late development characterizes the language areas and the commissural (interhemispheric) pathways.

4

Cognitive Development in Relation to the Development of the Nervous System

Although the morphological and functional development of the nervous system described in the previous chapters shows some gross correlations with motor and sensory development in the newborn and infant, cognitive development has less clear-cut relationships. In fact, studies of cognitive and brain development have proceeded largely independently of each other, and only recently have investigators tried to establish some tenuous relations between them. In this chapter, we describe briefly some of the current models of cognitive development in infancy and early childhood as a basis for the later discussion of cognitive (Chapter 28) and other defects and attempt to outline relations between brain and cognitive development. Since many of the topics in this field have yet to be investigated in a neuropsychological context, and others are discussed separately in this book (e.g., sensation and perception in Chapters 3, 25 and 26 and language in Chapter 27), the present discussion focuses on elements of cognitive development of interest to neuropsychologists.

4.1 General Cognitive Development

The term "**cognition**" broadly refers to "knowing" or "thinking" and is now preferred over narrower terms, such as intelligence since it allows for the inclusion of a broad range of human abilities, such as memory, perception, attention, and problem solving, and such diverse topics as appreciating humor, learning distinctive features of letters, and the perception of another person's unconscious motivation. Cognitive psychologists view development in terms of the gradual acquisition of a widening range of abilities, rather than the quantitative increments traditionally associated with the term "intelligence." Impinging upon the newborn are numerous stimuli that may or may not be forms of information. The newborn or infant learns to discriminate these stimuli as "representations" of the environment or as "external codes" that must be stored and processed in the form of "mental codes." Crying, smiling, eye contact, gaze aversion, and vocalizing are all responses that indirectly modify parental care-taking behavior (feeding, bodily contact) and elicit anticipatory milk letdown and increased breast temperature in the lactating mother (Bernal 1972). The infant "learns" environmental regularities in terms of frequency and temporal information, the "when and where" of making a response, probably in a classical conditioning paradigm (Rovee-Collier and Lipsitt 1982). Little's (1970) study demonstrated the rapidly increasing ability of the newborn to learn defensive reactions (eyeblinks) to air puffs following a 1000-Hz warning tone at 10, 20, and 30 days of age, and the gain in learned responses after an interval of 10 days, indicating clearly that the information learned during the first session was retained (Figure 4-1). At this age, longer inter-stimulus intervals (ISI) were clearly more effective. Instrumental conditioning has also been investigated in several studies, e.g., increasing the duration of music by prolonged bursts of sucking (Cairns and Butterfield 1975). Habituation and dishabituation to visual stimuli have been explored in several studies, and a shorter duration of peak fixation to a face stimulus has been found to predict poorer preschool intelli-gence test results and even lower IQ scores at the age of 8 years (Colombo et al. 1987). Such experimental findings have been stimulated in part by and integrated into some of the major theories of cognitive development described below.

In line with the Gestalt views of Lewin (1935) and Werner (1953), Piaget (1928, 1952) developed a theory of stages of cognitive development that has been influential in many studies of this topic. He proposed that the infant, during the first 18 months, is in the **sensorimotor stage** when thinking inde-pendent of overt behavior is not yet developed; all reactions of the infant take the form of sensorimotor schemes, such as grasping, reaching, pushing, or vo-calizing. Thinking is present only in the form of actions and is characterized by egocentrism. Piaget distinguished six phases during this stage, ranging from "reflex schemes" to "tertiary circular reactions" in which the infant begins to develop higher-order forms of cognition. Sensorimotor schemes are gradually internalized to become the basis of cognition during the subsequent stages of development. The second stage, called the **preoperational stage**, extends through the childhood period; cognitive schemes for solving problems develop, but are relatively unorganized. The behavior of the child may be relatively stable and consistent in some situations, but does not conform to rules and logic as-sociated with integrated conceptual thought processes. The next stage, called the **concrete operations stage**, is prevalent during the elementary school years, when an understanding of numbers, classes, relations, and other aspects of the physical world develops. The final stage, called the **formal operations stage**, is characterized by thinking that is no longer limited to concrete events; this stage is usually not attained until the child reaches the adolescent and adult years.

Following some of Piaget's theories, Bruner (Bruner 1968) suggested that the earliest form of representation is "enactive": an object or event is understood,

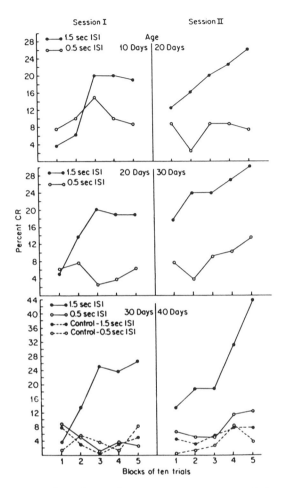

Figure 4-1. Percentage of conditioned responses on CS-US trials by infants trained at 10, 20, or 30 days of age (left side of each panel) and retrained in a second session 10 days later (right side). Infants received either a 1500-msec or 500-msec ISI. Bottom panel shows the performance of a control group (Little 1970).

known, or represented by the actions that are performed on it. That is, the infant responds by pushing, sucking, closing the eyes, or moving the head. This form of representation is not limited to the early developmental period, but is retained in such activities as walking, cycling, and other coordinated motor activities that need no other form of mental coding. The next form of representation that emerges in late infancy or early childhood has been labeled "ikonic" by Bruner and involves a form of imaginistic or configurational coding; the term refers to the formation of mental images associated with referent objects or events. Although the ikonic representation may be only a temporary step in the development of cognition in the child (as witnessed by the relatively poor "eidetic imagery" of adults as compared to children), ikonic coding remains part of the representational inventory of the growing individual: older children and adults frequently retain strong visual or emotional associations with certain smells, tastes, or colors.

The third form of representation is called "symbolic" and consists of linguistic or ever more abstract codes. It begins to develop in the child at the end of the first year and continues growing throughout the developmental period. In this case, the representation bears little if any resemblance to the actual object or event. The word or sound, or the graphic symbol in reading or mathematics, provides the code for a single object or event or for a whole sequence of representations as, for example, in solving an advanced chess problem. Luria (1966) has called attention to the fact that the acquisition of language is often facilitated by the use of enactive codes; the child frequently learns a symbolic code by accompanying motor movements, e.g., by tapping or singing of alphabet rhymes or by moving the hand with the verbal commands "up" and "down."

More specific developmental stages have been described by Kagan and Moss (1983). During the initial stage, the infant demonstrates the capacity of memory for past experiences, as shown by the ability of the 8-month-old to retrieve hidden objects while previously such objects seemed to be "out of sight, out of mind." The second stage provides the formation of active memory, as shown by acceleration of the heart rate when crawling toward an apparent visual cliff after the age of 10 months and by indications of separation anxiety when the mother leaves the room. During the third and fourth stages, a symbolic framework takes shape in the mind of the 17- to 24-month-old child, and causality can be inferred: the child shows anxiety in relation to failure, can experience empathy, and appreciates right versus wrong. Finally, the child develops self-awareness and is able to inhibit his or her own fears and separation anxiety during the period of 1 to 3 years.

Another approach to cognitive development comes from information processing theory (Kail and Bisanz 1982): an environmental event is viewed as impinging upon a "sensory register" of increasing discriminatory capacity. The child also develops a very short-term "buffer" that allows one part of the signal to be processed, after which a second competing signal may still be retrieved and processed. The event or object is then entered into the working memory or stored in the permanent memory. Cognition proceeds to the "central processor" and frequently leads to a response through the response system as shown in the simplified flow-chart in Figure 4-2:

More complex models on how the brain builds a cognitive code have borrowed liberally from computer terminology and attempt to account for such factors as attention, rehearsal processes, queuing of plans, retrieval of stored information, etc. "The functional unit of cognitive coding is seen as adaptive resonance, or amplification and prolongation of neural activity, that occurs when afferent data and efferent expectancies reach consensus through a matching process" (Grossberg 1980, p. 1). All parts of the information processing system are presumably in place in the newborn: it is the refinement of the capacity of

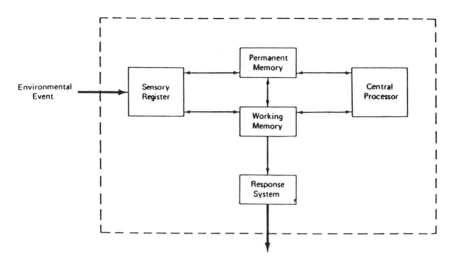

Figure 4-2.   Simplified model of an information processing system.

each part that grows with maturation. However, biological (intrinsic) maturation cannot proceed without environmental (extrinsic) stimulation or experience that forces the organism to develop, sharpen, or modify its processing ability. In fact, as Piaget already pointed out, the timing, sequence, and nature of the environmental "input" are crucial for cognitive development; they serve to reshape cognitive schemes developed earlier by both "accommodation" and "assimilation." **Accommodation** is the acquisition of new responses to such input while in **assimilation** input is understood within the context of an existing response schema.

4.2   Cognitive and Brain Development

Theories or models of cognitive development, as they have been briefly outlined above, are based on behavioral observations and their presumed underlying organization. They still form a "patchwork quilt of theories" (Gibson and Petersen 1991) that stress different aspects of behavioral development, complementing rather than contradicting each other. They are hypothetical constructs that have little, if anything, to do with the actual development or specific parts of the central nervous system. Although the formation of neural pathways, synaptogenesis, myelination, and transmitter substances, as well as specific locations relating to specific behavior, are known and were described in previous chapters, they do not correspond directly to cognitive models. Attempts to relate the two sides of the equation have had only limited success until recently (Diamond 1990, 1991). For example, the development of concrete and formal operations may, in a general way, be related to the late maturation of the frontal lobes, but such a statement leaves out the many interactions with sensory, motor, and other brain areas, nor does it provide explanations for some of the detailed findings of research in cognitive development (Scarr 1991). Bjorklund and Harnishfeger (1990) related the slow maturation of the association areas to the speed of information processing: "the slower processing of poorly myelinated nerves affords younger children less time to process information" (p. 61). The limited resources of the younger child makes their processing more effortful; in comparison, much of adults' cognitive processing is automatic, without conscious awareness, and requires little of the adult capacity (Bjorklund and Green 1992). Speech perception, as another example, requires not only acoustical perception and analysis but also phonological and linguistic processing, arousal, and attention, among other functions; these functions relate to many regions of the brain, including the lower brainstem, reticular formation, thalamus, and various cortical areas. To "localize" such functions in a single area would be naive. Similarly, although brain lesions in some specific structures are known to affect memory, such information does not explain the many detailed findings of cognitive research on the development of memory function. Majowski (1989) pointed out that coincident with the development of self-awareness between 15 and 24 months all six layers of the cortex have achieved maturation and that the developmental of memory and self-awareness requires functioning of the hippocampus and the thalamocortical projection system. Berman and Payne (1988) also stressed the importance of the commissures, relatively late-developing structures, for cognitive functions; these structures "make possible the autonomy and competition between hemispheres" (Galin 1977, p. 408). Even psychoanalysts (Levon 1990) are looking for the substrates of ego development and "archaic memory" in the changing organization of the brain in early childhood; the development of functional interhemispheric blocking is seen as an early substrate of psychological defense mechanisms and repression.

A major attempt to develop a "cognitive neuroscience," which integrates information processing models of cognitive processing and models of brain functioning, was made by Fodor (1983) and Zaidel (Zaidel et al. 1990). Other similar models have been presented by Marr (1982) and Tulving (1983). Building on knowledge about hemispheric independence gained from commissurotomy and other brain research, Fodor proposed that components of the cognitive system—"modules"—are domain specific, innately specified and not assembled from more basic elements, hard-wired, computationally autonomous (i.e., not sharing attention, memory, or other general purpose processes with other modules), are informationally encapsulated (i.e., have restricted access to information in the rest of the system) and have a characteristic pattern of development.

Zaidel modified Fodor's modularity concept by introducing the notion that all characteristics are not absolutes, but are expressed as a matter of degree: cognitive brain functions, especially those of the two hemispheres, are "dynamically modular," changing in their degree of functional independence. They are also "process-interactive," i.e., each hemisphere contributes to a different stage of processing as in the Goldberg and Costa (1981) theory that the right hemisphere is involved in the processing of novel, unfamiliar stimuli and the left hemisphere deals with the same material during later, routine stages. Zaidel also proposed that one hemisphere can function as a monitor for the other and that these modules can proceed in parallel.

A considerable amount of experimental work supports this model of brain functioning, but cannot be described here in detail. The developmental aspects of the model, however, have barely been touched upon, and for this reason the significance of the modular approach to brain and cognition to developmental neuropsychology remains to be determined in the future.

The question whether cognitive and/or brain development proceeds in steps ("discontinuity theory") or as a continuous process ("continuity theory") is still debated hotly (Bornstein and Lamb 1992, Bornstein and Sigman 1987, Fischer 1987, Prechtl 1984) and will be discussed below.

Biological Pre-Programming of the Newborn

A multitude of reflexive activities and limitations of sensory and motor abilities have been investigated since the early animal studies by Lorenz (1935) and Tinbergen (1951). To provide but one example, Meltzoff and Moore (1977) demonstrated that newborns only 1 hour after birth were able to imitate facial gestures of the caretaker, such as tongue protrusion, mouth opening, and lip protrusion (Figure 4-3), even if parent-infant interaction remained strictly controlled. This suggested that the neonate has the innate capacity to represent visually and proprioceptively perceived information in a form common to both modalities. "The infant could thus compare sensory information from his own unseen motor behavior to a 'supramodal' representation of the visually perceived gesture and construct the match required" (Meltzoff and Moore, 1977, p. 78). Studies of mother-infant gaze patterns during the subsequent months of development have shown that emotional expression can be considered part of the "language of infancy" (Slee 1984); looking time decreased at 6 to 8 months as the child's gaze extended more to other parts of the environment, although the gaze interaction remained active beyond that time.

The notion of innate pre-programming for specific external stimuli has, however, been extended by some authors far beyond reasonable limits to notions of "bonding" and "imprinting" in the neonate complete with applications to the practice of infant care. In a critical evaluation, Stratton (1984) concluded that the perceptual and cognitive systems of the neonate are specified at various levels to maximize certain kinds of contact. For example, the focus of the eye is relatively fixed at 30 to 40 cm, a typical distance from the infant to the face of the mother when breast feeding. In a natural situation, the infant looks at faces more than at other stimuli. Since the infant in particularly sensitive to events or percepts that are contingent on his or her own well-being (providing relief from pain and satisfaction of primary drives), such contingencies will be associated with the responses of care giving adults. This natural development makes theories about genetically pre-programmed bonding unnecessary, and

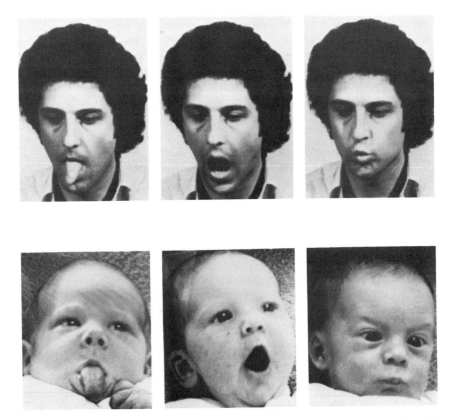

Figure 4-3. Imitation of facial gestures—tongue protrusion, mouth opening, and lip protrusion (Meltzoff and Moore 1977).

discredits the notion that disruption of bonding will necessarily lead to permanent psychological damage.

Rhythms

The correspondence between brain and cognitive development has become more obvious in the areas of sensation and perception (Johnson 1990, see Chapter 3) and has been studied in detail by Lenneberg and co-workers in the area of language development (Chapter 27). Wolff (1966) and Stratton (1982) called attention to the importance of rhythmic functions, present in the newborn, for learning and interaction with the environment. The presence of (1) biological rhythms, such as cardiac, respiratory, brain, oral, and vocal (sucking and crying); (2) circadian rhythms (day-night, sleep-wake); and (3) even rhythms in spontaneous behavior (mouthing, rocking, spontaneous startles), rather than the maintenance of a fixed level of activity, facilitates the "tuning" of neonates to environmental rhythms, their adaptation to the environment, and their inter-action with caretakers. Kaye (1977) even related sucking rhythms to early infant-mother dialogue. The changes in frequency and amplitude of such rhythms as sucking (high-amplitude sucking) have also been used successfully to measure the infant's attention to novel stimuli (see Chapter 5). However, Stratton ad-mitted that very few models have been formulated that would provide insight into the practical significance of rhythmic tendencies.

Growth Spurts

A major conceptual development that bears on the relationship between brain and cognitive development is that of **growth spurts**. In studies of nutritional deprivation and brain development, Dobbing and his colleagues (Dobbing 1975, Dobbing and Sands 1973, Dobbing and Smart 1974) found that there are pe-riods of development "when the brain is increasing its weight particularly rap-idly" (Dobbing and Smart 1974, p. 164). The neural growth spurt does not begin until the number of neurons in the developing brain reaches the adult level. At that time (about 30 weeks of gestation) an enormous proliferation of glial cells occurs, which marks the first growth spurt. The second growth spurt involves rapid myelination in the second postnatal year and continues well into the third and fourth years.

A more specific theory about the relationship between cognitive and brain development has been presented earlier by Hebb (1949), who proposed that the greater the ratio of "associative tissue" to sensorimotor tissue in the brain the greater the potential for cognitive complexity in the individual. Hebb noted that the first 24 months of life constitute the crucial period for the growth of associative tissue. This period coincides with Piaget's "sensorimotor stage," which, in his view, provides the experiential foundation for the establishment of more complex cognitive activity and coincides with Dobbing's hypothesis de-scribed above. The importance of this time span is also supported by studies of severe malnutrition in the first year (Chapter 16) that indicate that few of these children regain their cognitive potential even if adequate nutrition is available after this period of development.

Phrenoblysis

Epstein's (1978) idea of correlated brain-mind growth spurts, called "**phren-oblysis**," was intended as an explanatory principle for specific sensitive stages of normal development in later childhood. He found that head circumference and brain weight relative to the weight of other organs were related to mental growth. Several studies suggest that peaks and troughs occur at similar times in all these measures, although reanalyses of the data have questioned these con-clusions (Marsh 1985). Epstein's latest review (1986) indicated peak growth also for cortical thickness and increased arborization of neurons for the periods between the ages of 6 to 8, 10 to 12, and 14 to 16 years (and possibly also around 3 years). Epstein found the peak for head growth was statistically significant only for females, although other data were significant also for males. The peak at age 15 was significant for males only—he referred to this finding as an expression of sexual dimorphism.

If such stages of brain development can be viewed as reflecting periods of accelerated cognitive growth, important implications for child-rearing and education practices would arise. If there is a trough of mind-brain growth at age 4 to 6 years, as Epstein (1978) claimed, then additional stimulation during those years might have little or no effect on the individual's cognitive development. Even though Epstein's findings have been criticized by other researchers who prefer to view development as relatively continuous, Epstein suggested that the "slow" stage may at least in part account for some of the reported failures of the Head Start program in the United States aimed at preschool children. Epstein (1978) and other authors (Thornburg 1982, Toepfer 1980) have, perhaps somewhat prematurely, also attempted to relate the findings to Piagetian stages of development and educational issues.

Unfavorable conditions during growth spurt periods can be expected to retard development, possibly producing such lasting effects as small brain size, fewer cerebral cells, and lower brain lipid content. Disturbances during the growth spurt presumably could reduce the extent of many, if not all, brain growth processes. A discussion of sensitive periods and nutrition deals with this issue in detail (Chapter 8).

4.3   Executive Functions

The relatively recent term "**executive functions**" has been used to single out several higher cognitive activities in an information processing model, such as strategic planning, impulse control, organized search, and flexibility of thought and action and self-monitoring of one's behavior—activities that help maintain an appropriate mental set in order to achieve a future goal (Borkowski 1985, Luria 1966, Shallice 1982). Evidence from studies of patients with lesions of the prefrontal cortex have for some time pointed to the localization of such functions in these areas, and such terms as "categorical behavior" (Goldstein 1944), "biological intelligence" (Halstead 1947), and "fluid intelligence" (Cattell 1963) have been used to describe similar aspects of intellectual activity. Behavioral functions per se cannot be localized in the frontal areas; rather, the frontal lobes seem to be essential for the control of "organized, integrated, fixed functional systems" (Stuss and Benson 1986, p. 229). The development of these functions in childhood from a neuropsychological point of view has been the subject of earlier descriptive studies by Luria, but only recently has it become the subject of empirical investigations.

The crucial role of the prefrontal cortex is based on its neuroanatomical linkage with both the limbic (motivational) and the reticular activating (arousal) systems, as well as with other cortical regions (the motor areas of the frontal lobe and the posterior association cortex). This "bi-directional" linkage allows regulatory control both over the perceptual codings mediated by the posterior cortex, as well as over the attentional functions of the subcortical structures (Pribram and Luria 1973, Trevarthen 1990). As described in Chapter 3, these integrative systems, although functioning in a rudimentary fashion at an early age, are slower in maturation than any other structure in the human brain (Figure 1-10).

As mentioned briefly in Chapter 3, the results obtained with ablation of the prefrontal motor association areas in monkeys provide a direct paradigm for comparisons between animal and human development, as well as a direct neurological validation of theories of human development. If monkeys and human infants display the same behavior on a task, and if lesions of specific areas of the frontal lobes disrupt this behavior in infant monkeys, then it may be inferred that the same brain areas are responsible for the same behavior in human infants.

A major research advance into the parallels between cognitive and brain development comes from Goldman-Rakic's (1987) experiments with rhesus monkeys on the development of prefrontal lobe functions in relation to one specific cognitive activity—object permanence or the emergence of representational working memory—and comparing it to similar developments in humans. Object permanence, the recognition that an object has continuity in time and space even when not in view, was measured with delayed-response trials in which an object (peanut) was placed in one of two food wells, which were then covered by an opaque screen. After delays from 0 to 10 seconds, the animal was allowed to select one of the two locations. Another variation of the delayed response experiment calls for alternation between right and left food well as the correct choice. Clearly, the response must be guided by internalized knowledge of what happened at the previous trial. Subjects with lesions in the sulcus principales (prefrontal) cortex exhibited deficits mainly in the spatial delayed response task, but retained memory for the features of objects; in contrast, subjects with lesions of the inferior convexity cortex showed deficits on tasks requiring working memory for visual features (color, shape), rather than location.

Goldman-Rakic noted that working memory with a 2- to 5-second time base, "a cornerstone of cognitive development" (p. 615), is clearly demonstrated in 2- to 4-month-old monkeys and that this time coincides with the period of excess synaptic density (which decreases after this time) in the prefrontal cortex. The same period of synaptic density in the human infant begins at 8 months and peaks at 2 years of age (Huttenlocher 1990), a time when similar delayed response tasks can be mastered by the child, i.e., the capacity to guide behavior by stored information has matured.

Goldman-Rakic proposed a simple model for studying the relation between brain and cognitive development. In this model the first words uttered by the child signal the period of excess synaptic density in Broca's area of the frontal lobe; the appearance of visual tracking in the child indicates the maturation of the visual occipital cortex, etc. The further development of each of these functions depends upon a fine-tuning of the respective function, related to the phe-nomenon of synapse elimination, which continues at a reduced rate into adult-hood to reach an optimal level of 15–20 synapses per 100 square micrometers (Rakic et al. 1986).

The findings by Harlow et al. (1970) indicated that sparing of function was directly related to size of the lesion and age of the animal at the time of the surgery, although compensation for a deficit of function was not found in animals older than 12 months. Goldman et al. (1970) introduced a distinction between the role of the dorsolateral and orbital prefrontal cortex and suggested that the recovery of function after early lesions depends on the maturation sequence of that structure. The dorsolateral cortex becomes functional only later in infancy. Since it seems to be "uncommitted" earlier, it possesses the capacity to com-pensate for orbital lesions within certain age limits. In contrast, the orbital region cannot compensate for dorsolateral ablations even if such lesions are made as early as 1 month because it matures earlier. If both areas are ablated, no re-covery of function can occur. The studies involved the learing of alternating and delayed responses on object search and retrieval, relatively complex behaviors involving the frontal as well as association and visual cortex.

In Diamond's studies of object retrieval, the subject was able to reach a goal only by making a detour around a barrier: the goal object is seen in a plexiglass box, but can be reached only if (1) the subject inhibits the direct reach along the line of sight, and (2) a new plan is developed to reach the object by finding an opening along the side of the box. Hence, both self-control and planning are needed. Diamond's experiments (1990) showed that 6½- to 7-month-old human infants cannot inhibit the direct reach and that the successful execution of the task is not possible until 11 to 12 months of age. The comparable ages in infant monkeys without frontal lesions were 1½ to 2 months and 4 months, respec-tively. In a later evaluation of her work, Goldman-Rakic (1988) suggested that subdivisions of the prefrontal cortex represent parallel systems of neural net-works that play a cooperative rather than pre-eminent role in cognitive opera-tions; each subdivision performs similar operations, and differences between areas lie mainly in the nature of information on which the operations are per-formed. The prefrontal cortex, according to Goldman-Rakic, is necessary for regulating behavior guided by internalized models of reality, but is not required for behavior guided by external stimuli.

Similar comparisons between monkeys and infants were made for a delayed response and a memory-for-location task. Lee et al. (1983) hid food (a raisin) under one of three cups placed on the table; the hiding place was varied ran-domly across trials. The child was allowed to look for the reward only after a delay of 20 to 30 seconds. Toddlers performed this experiment successfully only when they reached the age of 18 to 30 months. Diamond and Goldman-Rakic's experiments showed that a similar stage in monkeys is not reached until they are 5 months old.

Both tasks require the ability to maintain a set over varying periods of time and response inhibition. Even in young toddlers rudimentary mnemonic behavior, such as verbalizing about the object, looking toward the hiding place, pointing and approaching the location, was observed (DeLoache et al. 1985).

Gradually, the child acquires executive strategies that require increasingly more complex mental sets about the rules of a dynamic physical world. Increasingly advanced problem-solving sets, involving more than one dimension of information, are developed by school-aged children. For example, the development of self-monitoring ("How good am I at this kind of activity? How am I doing right now on this task?"), also described as metacognitive awareness (Flavell and Wellman 1977), has been studied in detail. Passler et al. (1985) concluded from a cross-sectional study of proactive and retroactive inhibition in 6- to 12-year-old children that a multistage developmental model is appropriate, with the major development occurring between age 6 and 8; the development was fairly complete by age 10, and mastery was reached by age 12.

Executive-type cognitive skills have been shown to be relatively independent of IQ-measured intelligence, presumably because most intelligence tests rely heavily on measures of "crystallized intelligence," i.e., of overlearned information or established cognitive sets, rather than on the generation of novel problem-solving strategies, maintaining sets over time, or the ability to manipulate a set flexibly as circumstances change.

A series of experiments by Segalowitz et al. (1992) attempted to relate psychophysiological measures to frontal lobe development. The authors used the contingent negative variation (CNV) of the P300 visually evoked potential with bright children in enrichment classes and with average learners and compared them to adult controls; this measure has been related to activity in the dorsolateral prefrontal area. Various intelligence tests, presumed to be related to frontal lobe function, were also administered to the groups of children. The CNV was more pronounced in the average learner than in the enrichment class group, but less than in the adult group. The authors interpret the lower CNV in bright children as evidence that these children need less prefrontal activity for this task because of their advanced maturation. The difference with adult responses, however, was seen as "consistent with the notion that the prefrontal lobe is not functionally mature until young adulthood, whereas posterior systems are mature in middle childhood" (p. 295).

Welsh and Pennington (1988) pointed out how the relationship between frontal lobe and executive functioning may also be studied further by focusing on groups of children with specific disorders affecting such functions, e.g., PKU (see Chapter 15).

4.4   Spatial Cognition and Memory

Spatial cognition is another term that is frequently used in an oversimplified fashion. As described above, it is often applied to any cognitive activity that is not readily coded linguistically, although some use it specifically for tasks that involve auditory, visual, or tactile stimuli that require their perception and mental manipulation in Euclidean space. Based on studies of brain-damaged patients, the right hemisphere has been viewed as the primary substrate of spatial functions, such as recognition of shapes, mental rotation of objects, face perception, and sense of direction and spatial orientation; however, the list of right hemisphere functions also includes the perception of music and of the prosodic aspects of speech and the expression of emotion (De Renzi 1982, Heilman and Valenstein 1984). Yet, some tasks with apparent spatial components—for example, personal (as opposed to extrapersonal) space disorders (Ratcliff 1982)—have been found to be more impaired after left hemisphere lesions. Witelson and Swallow (1988) proposed that right hemisphere specialization depends on task demands in such a way that the right hemisphere processes primarily stimuli that must be "synthesized and sustained to form a unified configuration in which any temporal aspects of the stimuli are superseded" (p. 376); the temporal aspects would be processed primarily by the left hemisphere.

Developmentally, both right and left hemisphere specialization have been demonstrated to exist within the first few postnatal months if not from birth (see Chapter 2). However, studies of brain-damaged children have not yet provided detailed information about specific areas of the right hemisphere involved in specific functions or about the developmental progression of their involvement (Witelson 1985). Studies of right hemispherectomy have shown that a fair amount of transfer of spatial functions to the remaining left hemisphere is possible even in children as old as 12 years of age; some late-developing skills, such as map reading and mazes, remained impaired (Kohn and Dennis 1974). In a discussion of the critical period for spatial functions, Witelson argued that the right hemisphere may develop later and may retain greater plasticity since verbal abilities show more "sparing" after hemispherectomy than spatial functions (see Chapter 21). However, Styles-Davis (1988) reported subtle deficits in spatial cognition for right hemisphere brain-damaged children even if the injury was acquired at a very early age. Another example of a specific disorder of spatial cognition studied in recent years is **Williams syndrome** (infantile hypercalcemia), a genetic disorder of metabolism showing stenosis (or narrowing) of the aorta above the cardiac valves in association with mental retardation and a peculiar facial appearance (medial eyebrow flare, depressed nasal bridge, and thick lips with an open mouth posture, mild microcephaly, and hoarse voice). In this syndrome, linguistic capacities are remarkably spared in children with general mental handicap, and spatial functions are specifically impaired (Bellugi et al. 1988).

In very young normal children, the study of the development of spatial skills is hampered by their limited behavioral repertoire. However, from age 3 on, right hemisphere specialization for dichhaptic tasks (left hand superiority) for the perception of familiar faces, dots, and human figures (left visual field superiority) has been shown to be invariant during development into post-puberty. Strikingly, the perception of unfamiliar faces does not show left field superiority until age 10 (Levine 1985, Reynolds and Jeeves 1978), suggesting that the cognitive strategy for such tasks changes over time although hemispheric specialization may not.

Witelson and Swallow (1988) pointed out that the age of 10 may be an important "breaking point" in child development since such abilities as the visual recognition of spatial patterns, naming and discrimination of Braille, and map reading have been shown to develop and lateralize after this age. Clark and Klonoff (1990) also pointed out that right-left orientation does not show linear development; based on a study of 350 5- to 13-year-old children they proposed a three-stage multimodal model of development: (1) no understanding of right /left (age 5); (2) personal or egocentric understanding of right/left (age 6, 7, and 8); and (3) generalization of right/left to external objects (age 8 and older). No differences between boys and girls were observed. They relate this development to the myelination of the reticular formation, the cerebral commissures, and intracortical association areas.

Memory and Learning

Memory and learning, although often treated as separate human abilities, are an integral part of cognitive activity and have been touched upon in several parts of this chapter. Numerous speculations about the basic neural foundation of memory have been presented, but need not be repeated here. It has been known for some time that the hippocampal formation plays an important part in long-term retention. Pfenninger (1986) pointed out the importance of nerve growth cones for the biochemical events associated with long-term potentiation as a model for memory. A review by Greenough (1986) stressed the importance of synaptogenesis triggered by neural activity or some other neural signal in the development of information storage in animals.

Hebb (1949) and Ellis (1963) proposed the concept of "**stimulus trace**" as a model for the acquisition of memory. In Hebb's terms, this trace is a reverberatory electrophysiological circuit in the brain that is triggered by the stimulus. It ordinarily decays quickly, but, particularly if repeated or if it finds a match with already existing memory traces, it is responsible for the laying down of new memory in the brain. Pribram's (1963) holographic model first drew attention to the fact that many, if not all, parts of the brain are involved in the deposit of memory traces. Jenkins (1979) presented a tetrahedral model of memory that emphasizes the interaction of learning activities with the characteristics of the learner, the type of task, and the stimulus material.

As the child develops, it is not so much the capacity for memory that grows, but the strategies of learning and retrieving and, ultimately, the capacity for **metamemory**—knowing about knowing. Different memory tasks correlate poorly in 5-year-olds (Boyd 1988). The use of strategies, of mediation, and of semantic (rather than episodic) information during storage and retrieval all contributes to the gradual improvement of memory in the child (Rosenfield 1988). Clearly, it is the growth of cognitive abilities in general rather than of the neural capacity for storage that develops in the child and enables increasingly more accurate recall.

Memory and learning in children are affected by a variety of disorders in children as described in the following chapters. The term "learning disability" usually is restricted to deficiencies in school learning as described in Chapter 29.

4.5   Theories of The Development of Brain and Cognition

Several theories of the development of cerebral organization have been artic-ulated. One derives from some of Luria's (1966, 1973) ideas about the onto-genesis of certain functional systems in the brain. Another focuses on the topic of lateralization during cognitive development. A third, expanded by MacLean (1970), provides an evolutionary perspective based on comparative anatomy.

Luria's Theory of the Development of Functional Systems

Alexander Luria, a Russian neuropsychologist whose concepts and methods have had a great influence on contemporary neuropsychology, developed the major theoretical view of the brain's "functional systems" (Luria 1966). By this he meant those interacting areas of the brain that mediate a given behavior. Luria's view differed from the other neurobehavioral theories—localizationism and equipotentiality—in its emphasis that no single area of the brain can be con-sidered responsible for any particular behavior, nor do all areas of the brain contribute equally to all behaviors. In Luria's view, several brain regions are involved in a functional system for a given behavior. A corollary concept is **pluripotentiality**, which suggests that any specific area of the brain can partici-pate in a variety of functional systems. Luria also held that functional systems are not unique; different systems may be responsible for any given behavior, depending upon the availability of alternate systems.

As a didactic tool in understanding functional systems, Luria (1973) presented a model of functional units within the brain. In this model, all functional systems must involve three basic units of the brain because they all represent interac-tions of several areas (Table 4-1). These units are (1) the **arousal unit**, consist-ing of the reticular formation and related structures that effect cortical arousal and modulates input; (2) the **sensory input unit**, which consists of the posterior portions of the hemispheres and is responsible for the analysis of sensory input and cross-modal integration; and (3) the **output/planning unit** (mainly the frontal lobes), the highest functional level of the brain, which is responsible for planning and carrying out behavior. The sensory input and output/planning units can be further divided into primary, secondary, and tertiary areas, which rep-resent increasing levels of complexity and integration in information processing.

Luria (1973) also related his theory to the ontogenetic development of brain-behavior relations. In his "law of the hierarchical structure of cortical zones," he described how the relationships among primary, secondary, and tertiary cor-tical zones change in the course of development. "In the young child, the for-mation of properly working secondary zones could not take place without the

Table 4-1 Luria's Theory of Functional System Development

Stage	Functional system involved	Brain area involved	Ages of development
1	Arousal unit	Reticular system and related structures	Birth to 12 months
2	Primary motor and sensory areas	Visual, auditory, somatosensory, and motor regions (calcarine, superior temporal, pre- and postcentral gyri)	Birth to 12 months
3	Secondary sensory and motor areas	Secondary sensory and motor regions (peristriate, parietal, temporal, and premotor regions)	Birth to 5 years
4	Tertiary sensory input area	Parietal lobes	5 to 8 years
5	Tertiary output/planning unit	Prefrontal lobes	12 to 24 years

Source: Golden 1981, p. 289.

integrity of the primary zones" (1973 p. 74). Only after the development of the secondary ("gnostic") zones, can the "creation of major cognitive synthesis" (i.e., the full development of the higher cortical zones) take place. These tertiary zones assume the dominant role in the adult. Luria's developmental notions are based in part on theories first expressed by Hughlings Jackson in 1869 (1958) who proposed that development proceeds along the y-axis, upward along the neuraxis from spinal cord to neocortex, as well as along the z-axis, the anterior-posterior dimension, and the x-axis, the lateral dimension that shows progressive lateralization.

The development from a "maximal modal" specificity of the primary zones to the "supramodal" organizational and interpretive function of the tertiary zones parallels the hierarchical development of the three zones. In addition, development in Luria's theory includes a "progressive lateralization of function": although the right and left primary zones have "identical roles" in the functioning of the individual, handedness and the development of speech require a functional organization and specificity that take place together with the development of the secondary and tertiary zones and "differ radically" between right and left side.

The quality of the performance in any one stage does not predict the quality of performance in subsequent stages. Because psychological functions dependent upon tertiary areas of the input or output units do not develop until later in childhood or adolescence, obvious differences between the child and the adult in these skills are predicted.

Luria elaborated in particular the increasing regulatory role of language in the development of the child. Although the young infant has only a basic capacity to express him- or herself by motor movements, crying, and facial expressions ("**first signal system**"), the young child begins to accompany actions with verbal expressions, gradually developing a "**second signal system**." As the tertiary zones of the brain mature, language becomes more developed, and accompanying motor actions are no longer necessary. Language also need no longer be expressed, but becomes internalized; it mediates and regulates human behavior. Luria places the beginning of this third, mature stage at the approximate age of 6 years.

Das and Varnhagen (1986) made an attempt to relate child development to Luria's (1973) functional systems of the brain in more detail. They showed how Luria's notions of cognitive functions as "organized in systems of concertedly working zones, each of which performs its role in complex functional systems which may be localized in completely different and often distant areas of the brain" (p. 131) can be applied to the child. Using the example of a child learning to add two numbers, Das described how in the process of acquiring this skill the child may require the aid of actual physical objects, counting the objects corresponding to the first number, setting the sum aside, counting the second set, combining the two sets of objects, and counting the total number to arrive at a solution. All these actions require goal setting, concentration, and considerable mental and physical activity. After practice, the process becomes internalized, and the child is able to immediately visualize the results without performing the component activities required during the initial stage of learning the task. Many areas involved in learning the addition task are no longer necessary for adult performance, whereas others become increasingly more critical to the functional system.

Based on some of Luria's theories, Das et al. (1979) developed an information processing model that emphasized two types of processing, simultaneous and successive. **Simultaneous processing** "synthesizes separate units of information into a quasi-spatial, relational organization. **Successive processing** synthesizes units of information into a temporally organized sequence" (Das 1986, p. 126). Numerous factor-analytic studies from Das's laboratory have related suitable tasks to each of the two processing modes and confirmed their existence in various populations. Other studies attempted to relate the model to reading, linguistic functions, and to Piagetian theories of child development, suggesting that successive processing is the main factor involved in tasks of concrete operational thought. Das referred to simultaneous processing as being related to the parietal-occipital and successive processing to the fronto-temporal areas of the brain.

Unfortunately, Das's work, which started with Luria's model and was developed mainly on the basis of neuropsychological studies with brain-damaged patients, remains ultimately, like Luria's, a didactic model of cognitive processing. Although it frequently points to the potential neurological basis of cognition, the brain-cognition relationship is inferential, and the direct link between actual brain functioning and specific cognitive processes is not made. Unlike other theories of cognitive development in the child, Das's work does, however, offer suggestions for future research in this difficult area. It also directs the researcher away from simplistic localizationist notions about the neural basis of cognitive processing by pointing out the numerous factors and presumed areas of the brain involved in each cognitive activity and the changing nature of such activities during child development.

Lateralization and Cognitive Development

The Luria-Das model of successive and simultaneous processing has even been adapted to develop an intelligence test for children (Kaufman and Kaufman 1983), presumably measuring these functions, but deviating from Das by ascribing notions of adult lateralization of cognitive functions (sequential - left, simultaneous - right hemisphere) to the model. Numerous other models of hemispheric asymmetries based on the study of adult brain function (for example, analytic-wholistic, linguistic-spatial) have been developed (Springer and Deutsch 1989), although the uncritical use of such dichotomous assignments and their application to describe "cognitive styles" have been severely criticized (Efron 1990). As Hiscock and Kinsbourne (1987) pointed out in their review of such theories, "left- and right-hemisphere cognitive styles are metaphors without neurological substance" (p. 130).

Adopting any of these adult models for the description of cognitive development, however, assumes that the lateralization of cognitive functions remains stable during childhood and is similar to that used by the adult. The development of lateral asymmetries and associated motoric and cognitive asymmetries was already reviewed in Chapter 2. Although specific brain areas are undoubtedly genetically predetermined for the development of specific functions, such as linguistic functions (Piacentini and Hynd 1988), it is clear that complex cognitive activities must change gradually over time as individual areas of the brain mature at different times.

Cognition in childhood must be seen as a developing process that cannot be assumed to be firmly lateralized. One theory by Goldberg and Costa (1981) specifically proposed that the hemispheres differ in the extent to which they can process routinized versus novel material; the left hemisphere is better at tasks that involve well-routinized codes, whereas the right hemisphere is better at tasks for which no readily apparent code is available. A fair amount of evidence has been produced supporting the Goldberg-Costa theory. If we apply this theory to cognitive child development, it would follow that most tasks, whatever their nature, are at first best solved with a right hemisphere strategy, but gradually become transferred to a left hemisphere strategy as routinized codes become available. This theory would also be supported by the finding that the right hemisphere develops earlier than the left (Bracco et al. 1984, see Chapter 5). Explicit studies of the model in a developmental context would be a welcome addition to our knowledge of the relation between the development of the brain and cognition.

The Triune Brain: An Evolutionary Perspective

Drawing on comparative anatomy, neuroanatomy, neurochemistry, and evolutionary theory, MacLean (1970, 1990) proposed that the mammalian brain can be divided anatomically as well as conceptually into three hierarchical systems: a protoreptilian brain, a paleomammalian brain, and a neomammalian brain. Together, they form the **triune brain**.

The **protoreptilian brain** system is, in an evolutionary sense, the oldest; it consists of regions in the upper spinal cord, the midbrain, the diencephalon, and the basal ganglia. It plays a crucial role in many instinctive activities necessary for survival of the individual and species. The **paleomammalian brain** system represents the next evolutionary step in that it has a role in the integration of emotional expression and self-awareness. It has the ability to override and suppress the more primitive protoreptilian brain. The limbic system is the primary neural system corresponding to the paleomammalian brain (Isaacson 1975). The **neomammalian brain** is represented by the neocortex. MacLean views the cortex as responsible for the nonemotional, integrative, fine-grain analysis of the external environment. In the highly developed left hemisphere of humans, this characteristic is represented by language, which gives humans the ability to reason and to think about future prospects. The neomammalian brain is able to override the other two systems.

Van der Vlugt (1979) elaborated the triune brain concept from the viewpoint of developmental neuropsychology (Table 4-2). He cited historical precedents of similar conceptualization of the nervous system and suggested, as did

Table 4-2   Evolutionary Concepts of the Organization, Function, and Development of the Brain

Pavlov (1955)	Yakovlev and Lecours (1967)	Luria (1973)	MacLean (1970)	Isaacson (1974)	Van der Vlugt (1979)
Second signal system	Supralimbic zone	Programming, regulating, verifying mental activity	Neomammalian brain	Guru	Level III
Conditioned reflex	Paramedian or limbic zone	Obtaining, processing, storing information	Paleomammalian brain	Lethe	Level II
Unconditioned reflex	Median zone	Regulating tone or waking	Protoreptilian brain	Graven image	Level I

Source: van der Vlugt, 1979.

MacLean, that the triune brain can be a reasonable representation not only of the evolutionary but also of the ontogenetic development of the nervous system. He assumed that each developmental step depends on earlier steps and that later-developing structures subserve more refined and complex adaptive and integrative functions than earlier structures. With regard to abnormal influences on the development of the nervous system, Van der Vlugt suggested that different patterns of behavioral deficits are seen depending upon which level of the triune brain is affected.

Summary

This chapter reviewed the normal cognitive development of the child and its relationship to brain development. In particular, the biological pre-programming of the newborn, the development of executive functions, spatial cognition, and memory were related to neuropsychology. Theories that attempt to relate general stages of brain maturation to the development of the child and to lateralization were discussed. Both McLean's and Luria's theories are influenced by the stages of phylogenetic development. Both attempt to predict changes in the nervous system as related to behavior in the early years of life. Further elaboration of such theories may be helpful as research provides more insight into stages of brain development in the child. For a fully articulated theory, more specific concepts, such as those discussed under the topics of growth spurts, sex differences, and lateralization, should be included.

II
Issues in Developmental Neuropsychology

5

Cerebral Lateralization

This chapter deals with one of the central issues of developmental neuropsychology: differential lateralization of behavioral functions between hemispheres. This topic has generated considerable dispute and mutually contradictory theories. A recent critique of the research on hemispheric specialization (Efron 1990) points out that the initial studies using patients with lateralized lesions should be treated with caution because a functional deficit after such a lesion indicates that the damaged area "supports" the disturbed function, but does not necessarily imply that this function is "localized" in that area or even in that hemisphere. Efron warns that research with normal subjects, now opening a floodgate for new evidence, requires even more caution because the finding that a certain function, such as dichotic listening with verbal material, is performed better on the right side does not imply that the respective (in this case the left) hemisphere is specialized for this function; it shows merely a correlational advantage. The neural substrate remains unknown.

5.1   Lateralization in Infancy

Few neuropsychological topics have stimulated as much interest as lateralization of hemispheric functioning (Hahn 1987). Lateralized adult "cortical control" over handedness, language, and other less easily conceptualized behaviors, such as visuoperceptual ability, raise some important developmental questions. Does hemispheric control over these functions develop with age, or is it established at birth? What determines it? What purpose does it serve? What is the ontogenetic course of lateralization? When is development most rapid, and when does it level off?

Conceptual and methodological difficulties limit the research that can be conducted during the periods of infancy and childhood. It is difficult enough to examine a given behavior in early life, let alone consider its possible lateralized organization. However, an increasing number of recent studies of lateralization during the first 2 years of life testify to the importance of the topic and have culminated in several books on the subject (Best 1985, Bradshaw and Nettleton 1983, Corballis 1983, Herron 1980, Molfese and Segalowitz 1988, Young et al. 1983) and even in detailed investigations of lateralization in nonhuman species (Glick 1985). It has been speculated that lateral asymmetry became advantageous and even necessary during the evolution of humans in order to eliminate incompatibility between two very different forms of cognitive processing (Levy 1969).

The neuropsychological findings in adults from which current developmental concerns arise were first derived from the clinicopathological cases of Broca, Wernicke, and others in the nineteenth century. This work provided invaluable information leading to hypotheses about the relationship between language functioning and the left hemisphere of the brain and numerous other aspects of brain-behavior relations. Contemporary research on laterality was stimulated by Sperry's examination of patients undergoing split-brain surgery (commissurotomy) for the control of intractable seizures, which revealed stunning hemispheric differences not readily apparent in everyday activity (Sperry 1970, Sperry et al. 1969). Sperry's methods of examination included the selective tachistoscopic stimulation of one portion of the visual field to project to one or the other occipital cortex. This approach, together with Kimura's (1967) modification of the dichotic listening techniques, soon became the cornerstone of lateralization methodology and suggested left hemispheric specialization for the recognition of speech and right hemispheric specialization for nonspeech sounds. The adult dichotic listening paradigm uses ear channels to deal with lateralized cortical processing as each ear predominantly, but not solely, sends sensory information to the contralateral hemisphere. Therefore, the left ear channel is assumed to relate to right hemisphere functioning, and the right ear channel is assumed to relate to left hemisphere functioning.

If the cerebral hemispheres of the brain are so divergent in function, the important question arises as to how this hemispheric specialization reaches normal adult levels. Developmental interest in lateralization was also stimulated by turn-of-the-century educational speculations about difficulties attributable to left-handedness and interventive strategies to correct a student's handedness "problem." Orton's (1925) ideas about the relationship between learning disabilities and poorly developed lateralization and left-handedness marked the onset of systematic work on this question, which has yet to find a definitive answer (Porac and Coren, 1981).

Two theoretical positions dominate contemporary thought on the ontogeny of lateralized functioning. The first views lateralized functioning as a phenomenon that develops progressively during childhood, and the second sees it as an inherent property of brain-behavior relations present at birth. These two broad positions have been best articulated by Lenneberg and Kinsbourne.

Based on clinical data concerning recovery from acquired aphasia in childhood (e.g., Basser 1962), Lenneberg (1967) proposed that the cerebral hemispheres of infants from birth until 2 years of age have an equal potential for serving as the substrate for language functioning or other lateralized functions. From 2 years of age until the onset of puberty, the left hemisphere assumes increasing importance as the substrate for language. As the right hemisphere loses its ability to subserve language functioning to the increasingly more specialized left hemisphere, cortical plasticity for recovery of function after brain damage decreases. After puberty and throughout adulthood, the lateralization of language control in the left hemisphere remains relatively inflexible.

The second theory, nurtured by empirical data on early-life behavioral and anatomical asymmetries, holds that lateralized functioning "does not develop. It is there from the start" (Kinsbourne 1976, p. 189). The cerebral hemispheres are programmed at the time of birth to function asymmetrically; the left hemisphere mediates language and motor function for the majority of the population. In a similar vein, Witelson (1985, 1987) maintained that hemisphere specialization exists from birth onward and does not further change in nature or degree.

Because laterality can be observed very early in life, the notion of true equipotentiality of hemispheric function in early life has been generally rejected. In addition, cortical asymmetry has been found in human fetal brains regardless of the age of the fetus (de Lacoste et al. 1991). However, this finding does not rule out the notion of progressive lateralization. Reviews by Satz and Bullard-Bates (1981) and Satz et al. (1990) stressed that the risk of aphasia after left hemisphere damage in children is the same as in adults, at least after infancy. The latter authors view progressive lateralization as "a dynamic process of increasing cortical specialization . . . that develops within the hemisphere in a vertical (subcortical-cortical) and horizontal (anterior-posterior) progression during infancy and childhood" (Satz et al. 1990, p. 611). Segalowitz and Gruber (1977) and Bryden (1982) provide a detailed examination of the key issues concerning lateralization through puberty. The various types of evidence are summarized by Lebrun and Zangwill (1981). The remainder of this section describes the major investigations of early-life lateralization with emphasis on the first years, as summarized in Table 5-1. Lateralization in neuroanatomical structure, speech perception, motor behavior, and electrophysiology is examined in turn.

5.2 Neuroanatomical Asymmetries

Normal brain structures show some degree of variability in gross appearance among individuals, but the relationship of structures to one another remains relatively constant. Morphological examination of the brain to determine reliable differences between left and right hemispheres in weight, size, and density has a long history. Gall had already suggested that the brain is not symmetrical when Cunningham examined infant brains for differences in the length of left and right Sylvian fissures in 1892. However, most researchers felt that the observed anatomical differences were too small to explain the differences in hemispheric

Table 5-1   Age of Asymmetry for Different Behaviors

System	Age	Dominance	Reference
Auditory			
Speech syllables	Preterm	Right ear	Molfese & Molfese 1979
Music	22–140 days	Left ear	Entus 1977
Phonemes	22–140 days	Right ear	Entus 1977
Words	4 years	Right ear	Kimura 1963
Environmental sounds	5–8 years	Left ear	Knox & Kimura 1970
Visual			
Rhythmic visual			
stimuli	Newborn	Right field	Crowell et al. 1973
Face recognition	7–9 years	Left field	Marcel & Rajan 1975
	6–13 years	Left field	Witelson 1977a and b
	9–10 years	None	Diamond & Carey 1977
Somatosensory			
Dichhaptic recognition	All ages	Left hand	Witelson 1977a and b
Motor			
Stepping	<3 months	Right	Peters & Petrie 1979
Head turning	Neonate	Right	Turkewitz 1977
Grasp duration	1–4 months	Right	Caplan & Kinsbourne 1976
Finger tapping	3–5 years	Right	Ingram 1975
Grip strength	3–5 years	Right	Ingram 1975
Gesturing	3–5 years	Right	Ingram 1975
Head orientation	Neonate	Right	Michel 1981

Source: Modified from Kolb and Fantie 1989.

function, e.g., von Bonin (1962). Nonetheless, Geschwind and Levitsky's (1968) report that the left planum temporale (Figure 5-1) was larger than the right in 65 per cent of their series of adult brains reawakened interest in the anatomical correlates of lateralized control over various functions.

Chi et al. (1977) studied several hundred sectioned fetal brains to establish the timing of gyral and sulcal development during fetal life. In some cases, gyri and sulci developed sooner in the right than in the left hemisphere. In two-thirds of the series, the transverse temporal gyrus (Heschl's gyrus), known as an essential region for language decoding and comprehension, was found to develop in the right hemisphere at 31 weeks of gestational age, 1 to 2 weeks before it developed in the left hemisphere. The calcarine fissure of the occipital lobe, the superior frontal gyrus, the angular gyrus, and the superior temporal fissure all developed earlier in the right than in the left hemisphere in most cases.

Despite the consistent reports of earlier development of right hemisphere areas, three studies of early-life neuroanatomical asymmetries indicated that, even in fetuses as young as 29 gestational weeks, the left planum temporale is usually larger than the right. Roughly 90 per cent of the 100 fetal, neonatal,

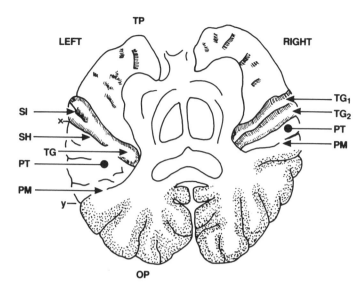

Figure 5-1. Upper surfaces of human temporal lobes exposed by a cut on each side in the plane of the Sylvian fissure. Anatomical landmarks and typical left-right differences are shown. The posterior margin (PM) of the planum temporale (PT) slopes backward more sharply on the left than on the right, so that end *y* of the left Sylvian fissure lies posterior to the corresponding point on the right. The anterior margin of the planum formed by the sulcus of Heschl (SH) slopes forward more sharply on the left. In this brain there is a single transverse gyrus of Heschl (TG) on the left, but two on the right (TG1, TG2). Other parts shown are temporal pole (TP), occipital pole (OP), and sulcus intermedius of Beck (SI) (Geschwind and Levitsky 1968).

and infant brains examined by Wada et al. (1975) had a larger left planum temporale. A less consistent anatomical asymmetry in the **frontal operculum**, the anterior region containing Broca's area of speech production, was also reported: the right frontal operculum was generally larger than the left. Witelson and Pallie (1973), examining 14 neonatal and infant brains, reported a larger left planum temporale in 75 per cent of their cases. Teszner et al. (1972) reported a larger left planum temporale in six of eight fetal brains, and LeMay and Culebras (1972) found higher height in the right Sylvian points in all 10 fetuses. Interestingly, Cunningham had already determined in 1892 that the Sylvian fissure was generally larger in the left than in the right hemisphere, suggesting larger left temporal regions. In addition, a study by Kooistra and Heilman (1988) reported that the right half of the globus pallidus was larger than the left in 16 out of 18 brains; the authors view this asymmetry as a reflection of axial (whole body rotations) or limb motor dominance in humans and refer to animal studies with similar results.

The results admittedly deal only with gross aspects of the brain. More sophisticated morphological techniques, such as the cytoarchitectonic analyses by

Galaburda et al. (1978) of adult brains, have yet to be used in developmental studies. Galaburda et al. (1990) reviewed the variability in brain morphology at the level of gross anatomy, cytoarchitecture, and callosal connectivity in humans and other animals and concluded that networks of neurons emerge as a result of greater or lesser development of cortical asymmetry and differ in the number of cells and connections comprising them. They interpreted this finding as the basis for individual variability in behavioral capacities and cognitive styles, as well as lateralization. Taylor (1982, personal communication) reported that, based on sodium amytal tests (injected to obtain a temporary anesthesia in the ipsilateral hemisphere), left-hemisphere-damaged children under 2 years of age showed a change of speech lateralization to the right hemisphere; between 2 and 6 years such children showed evidence of bilateral speech representation, and above 6 years of age most had a permanent deficit consistent with speech lateralization in adults. The continued refinement of new imaging techniques, such as positron emission tomography (PET) and magnetic resonance imaging (MRI), has provided additional direct evidence of the correlation between anatomical and functional asymmetries to be discussed below.

The mechanism creating lateral asymmetries in brain development has been the subject of considerable speculation. Morgan (1977) proposed that lateralization depends solely on the orientation of the cytoplasm in the ovum. If this hypothesis is true, lateralization would ultimately depend on genetic factors of the mother, but not the father. In contrast, Annett (1970) proposed the action of a single "right-shift" gene that is responsible for lateralization; the action of this gene, however, would be modified by environmental factors to account for the variability found in the general population. Levy and Nagylaki (1972) proposed a two-gene model, each with two alleles, allowing for different variations in brain lateralization for speech and handedness. Finally, polygenetic models have also been considered (Porac and Coren 1981). None of the models has found general acceptance, nor do they explain published statistics on behavioral lateralization to everybody's satisfaction. Geschwind and Behan's (1982) work went beyond genetic theories and addressed the actual mechanism of lateralization; this work is discussed at the end of this section.

5.3 Perceptual Asymmetries

Examination of the functional lateralization of a given perceptual ability presupposes that the ability itself does exist in the organisms' repertoire and that it can be measured adequately. The abilities currently attributed to the infant are much more numerous, active, and nonreflexive than those listed 25 years ago. Since then, data on adultlike linguistic perception in the infant have accumulated almost concurrently with data on lateralization in adults (see review by Eimas 1986).

The prime finding of this linguistic research is that the infant seems to be able to discriminate phonemic differences (e.g., /pa/ as opposed to /ba/) in the same categorical fashion as adults (Eimas et al., 1971). That is, when a speaker says /pa/ and then says /ba/, the difference between the two utterances crosses a phonemic boundary and therefore can be considered of linguistic importance. If two different speakers each say /pa/, the difference between the two utterances does not cross a phonemic boundary and is of acoustic, rather than linguistic, importance. If an individual can reliably discriminate changes in linguistically relevant utterances that cross phonemic boundaries, then he or she is able to make a categorical discrimination and identify phonemic utterances in their proper linguistic categories. Since this basic linguistic ability is similar in infants and adults, it is plausible to look for similarities in cortical substrate between infants and adults. Although it is usually easy for adults to respond verbally to such tasks, such responses are not possible for infants. Special procedures have been developed to test infant speech perception so that comparisons across age can be attempted. Similarity in discriminative ability, however, does not necessarily imply the existence of similar cortical mechanisms in infants and adults. In fact, categorical discriminations similar to those made by human adults have also been reported in chinchillas (Kuhl and Miller 1975).

The procedure used most widely in examinations of speech perception by infants is the habituation and dishabituation of high-amplitude sucking (HAS) in response to linguistic stimuli. A particular language stimulus (e.g., the syllable /pa/), when presented to the infant, evokes a high frequency of strong sucking on a pacifier modified to serve as a recording instrument. Repeated presentation of the stimulus results in a gradual decrease in the intensity of sucking. When such habituation has occurred, a new speech stimulus that differs from the original one along a dimension that may or not be of linguistic relevance is presented. If the across-boundary (linguistically relevant) change elicits a dishabituation of the sucking response but the linguistically irrelevant (acoustic) change does not, one can infer that the infant has discriminated speech sounds in an adultlike, categorical fashion. Another technique uses preferential looking (head movement): the infant attends to a toy held by the experimenter when habituation to a repeated stimulus occurs, but turns to the loudspeaker when a linguistically relevant novel stimulus is presented; the head turning at such a time is rewarded by the appearance of a toy rabbit next to the loudspeaker.

In general, results of perceptual studies do indicate that young infants can distinguish linguistically relevant stimuli categorically along such basic dimensions as voice onset time and the transition of parts of the acoustical spectrum (formants) of a sequence of speech sounds. Discrimination in infants is much the same as in adults and seems to rely on an innate mechanism (Eimas 1986). However, serious technical and interpretation questions have been raised about linguistic studies employing both the HAS and preferential looking techniques, as discussed by Pisoni (1977) and Trehub (1979). For example, performance on an HAS task seems to require both memory and linguistic ability, possibly confounding the interpretation of findings: the infant needs to remember the previous stimulus in order to be able to respond to the novelty of the current stimulus (Trehub 1979).

The habituation-dishabituation procedure has been adapted by neuropsy-chologists to examine hemispheric specialization in infants. The dichotic listen-ing adaptation (Figure 5-2) for examination of the lateralization of categorical discrimination involves the use of two independent stimulus channels, one di-rected into the left ear and the other into the right ear. Stimuli are presented by headsets that allow projection of sound to a single ear. After the response (e.g., sucking) has habituated, a new stimulus is presented to one ear while the other continues to receive the original stimulus. If dishabituation occurs more readily in one ear than in the other, then inferences about the brain lateralization of that ability can be made.

Three different methods to study the lateralization of categorical perception in infants have contributed to our understanding of the subject. Glanville et al. (1977) used a dichotic task to examine dishabituation of a heart rate (rather than sucking) response to auditory stimulation. Twelve infants ranging in age from 3 to 4 months were tested under four conditions: verbal or musical pre-sentation with the stimulus change in the right or left ear. Eight of the infants showed more rapid heart rate dishabituation to verbal stimuli when the stimulus change was presented to the right ear. Ten of the infants showed greater dis-habituation to changes in musical stimuli when the change was in the left ear

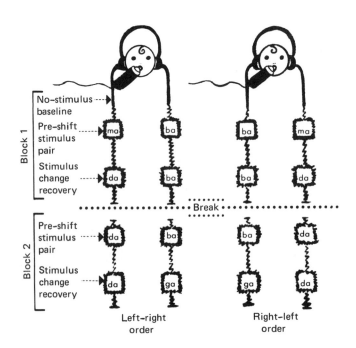

Figure 5-2. The experimental procedure showing stimulus sequence and ear order for the dichotic listening adaptation of the habituation-dishabituation paradigm with high-amplitude sucking response in infants (Entus 1977).

channel, though both ears showed some dishabituation to musical stimulus change.

Both Entus (1977) and Vargha-Khadem and Corballis (1979) have used a dichotic task in conjunction with habituation-dishabituation of the HAS response; however, their results conflict with one another. Entus examined dishabituation of HAS to verbal and musical stimulus changes as a function of ear channel in infants under 4 months of age. She found that 34 of 48 infants showed greater dishabituation to a change in verbal stimulation when the change was in the right ear channel; 38 of the 48 infants showed greater dishabituation to a change in musical stimuli when the change was in the left ear channel. Her results, along with those of Glanville et al. (1977), are strikingly similar to the adult right-ear advantage for verbal stimuli and left-ear advantage for nonverbal stimuli. Vargha-Khadem and Corballis failed to replicate Entus' verbal-stimulus finding. Using a modified procedure to reduce possible experimenter bias, which they felt was present in Entus' original design, they interpreted her results as reflecting experimenter bias.

The finding of asymmetries in the perception of speechlike auditory stimuli in infants similar to those demonstrated in adults is striking. However, as the failure to replicate Entus' results suggests, the studies are fragile, exploratory efforts to examine lateralization of functions in the infant's repertoire of abilities.

Rose (1984) investigated hemispheric specialization for tactual processing in 1-, 2-, and 3-year-old children. The children palpated six nonsense three-dimensional shapes with either the right or the left hand for 25 seconds and then viewed a familiar and a novel shape in a 10-second test of visual recognition. Although the novel stimulus generally elicited more visual fixation regardless of the hand used for palpation, 2- and 3-year-olds showed more fixation after palpation with the left as compared to the right hand. The author interpreted the finding as evidence for the development of right hemisphere superiority for tactile information processing and/or interhemispheric transfer.

The dichotic listening task, designed for adults, has been widely used throughout childhood. A relatively consistent right-ear advantage (REA) for verbal stimulation has been reported by most investigators from young childhood to adult age. Although some argue that the strength of the REA shows progressive lateralization, some studies failed to find such an age effect (Bryden and Allard 1981, Hynd et al. 1979, Kinsbourne and Hiscock 1977). As an explanation for the failure to find progressive lateralization, Van Duyne (1982) and Kinsbourne and Hiscock (1977) pointed out that dichotic listening is related to verbal and cognitive development and is dependent on the task demands, not lateralization alone. However, a study by Larsen (1984) found progressive lateralization when right-handers were separated from left-handers; pronounced right-ear advantage ranged from 65 per cent of 9-year-olds to 94 per cent of 14- to 15-year-olds while the degree of ear asymmetry decreased; left-handers did not show progressive lateralization. The author related the finding to the progressive myelination of interhemispheric fiber connections and argued that delayed interhemispheric transmission "is a necessary precondition of hemispheric specialization because a relative separation might facilitate independent and different functions in early childhood" (p. 14). The lack of progressive lateralization in left-handers was attributed to the nonhomogeneity of lateralization in this group. Kraft (1981) found that laterality effects in verbal and nonverbal dichotic listening tasks were related to the family history of handedness regardless of the age and handedness of the subject, thus confirming the effect of genetic factors in lateralization; specifically, familial sinistrality was associated with lower REA for verbal material and poorer nonverbal accuracy scores compared to familial dextral subjects.

Another perceptual asymmetry found in infants as early as 3 months of age is the processing and recognition of physiognomies. De Schonen and Mathivet (1989) reviewed the evidence pointing to a definite advantage of the right hemisphere (left visual field) for the recognition of faces in humans, primates, and other mammalian species. They pointed out that this region of the brain does mature more rapidly than its left counterpart and that interhemispheric connections are not yet functional at this stage of development. Although the right hemisphere advantage is maintained in adults (Sergent 1986), De Schonen and Mathivet argue that physiognomy processing and recognition are organized very differently from that in adulthood because of the limitations of visual sensitivity in infants.

5.4   Motoric Asymmetries

Studies of laterality in motor performance and manual preference have a long history in neuropsychology. Two related aspects of infancy have been studied: the appearance of neonatal postural asymmetries, such as head position, and the development of handedness. The relationship between these two aspects of motor asymmetry has also been addressed (Michel 1981).

Head Position

It has been a common observation by pediatricians, maternity ward nursing staff, and parents that when newborn babies lie on their back their head usually remains turned in one direction. Because it can be observed easily, the direction of the neonate's head posture has been the most frequently examined aspect of neonatal lateralization. The results indicate two types of predominantly rightward lateral head position in the normal newborn: (1) an asymmetry in the attainment and maintenance of a rightward head posture and (2) a greater right-sided ipsilateral responsiveness to stimulation (Figure 5-3).

Turkewitz and his co-workers (e.g., Turkewitz and Birch 1971, Turkewitz and Kenny 1982) observed spontaneous behavior and behavior subsequent to holding the baby's head in the neutral, body-midline axis position for a period of time. Similar studies have been done in a variety of hospitals with different patterns of early infant care (Cioni and Pellegrinetti 1982, Michel and Goodwin

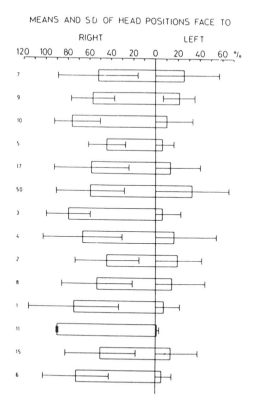

MEANS AND SD OF HEAD POSITIONS FACE TO

Figure 5-3.   Preferences of head position. Mean and SD of minutes from all observations in which each of 14 children had face to the right or left side (Prechtl 1979).

1979, Risser et al. 1985). They indicate that, even when the baby's head is held in the midline position for as long as 15 minutes to minimize any asymmetric motor tone, most infants show a rightward preference in head positioning. This preference shows a very rapid development: neonates under 12 hours of age are likely to turn right as often as left, whereas infants over 12 hours of age are much more likely to turn right. With few exceptions, full-term newborns maintain a strongly prevalent lateral head position soon after birth, which is rightward for most and leftward for some. Rightward ipsilateral responsiveness to lateral stimulation has also been observed in newborns. The baby's head is held in the neutral midline position, and one or the other side of the face is quickly stimulated by touch. The neonate responds to right-sided stimulation with a rightward head turn much more frequently than to left-sided stimulation with a leftward turn.

The underlying mechanisms for these two very early lateralized behaviors remain obscure. There is some evidence that the first-appearing type of laterality, the spontaneous tendency toward positioning of the head to the right, contributes to the development of the second, stronger responsiveness to stimulation from the right side. There is also some evidence that the forced head position of the fetus as it grows in the uterus may contribute to the lateralized behavior after birth (Michel and Goodwin 1979); however, a study by van Gelder et al. (1989) found that head position determined by ultrasound at age 16 and 24 weeks was along the midline in 60 per cent of the scans and deviations to the right and left were of equal frequency. The study leaves open the possibility that right-sided head orientation may occur during the third trimester of pregnancy. In contrast, Kinsbourne (1976) and Liederman and Coryell (1982) attributed the lateralized response to stimulation directly to programmed asymmetrical cortical control of motor behavior. This interpretation is strengthened by findings of an asymmetry of the stepping reflex in newborns (Melekian 1981). Turkewitz (1991) views the head turning preference in the context of a model of preferential attention to processing of unfamiliar stimuli by the right hemisphere which has its origin in the pre- and perinatal period.

Lateral head positioning has also been examined in relation to the development of handedness (Coryell and Michel 1978, Gesell and Ames 1947, Michel 1980). Michel tested babies at several points during the first 22 weeks of life with a task to elicit reaching by visual stimulation. Those who showed left-sided biases in neonatal head position used their left hands more than their right, and those who showed right-sided neonatal position preference reached with their right hand more than with their left. It must be remembered that head turning preference allows the infant to see the ipsilateral hand more often. Whether or not the experience of viewing the hand on the side of the neonate's head preference contributes to later handedness has been debated. It is plausible that "headedness" (i.e., the preferred side toward which the head is pointed) may represent the handedness of early life; alternatively, headedness may be the early-life manifestation of the same mechanism(s) that, in later life, leads to manual preference.

It has been pointed out that postural asymmetries in newborns may be relatively weak. Trehub et al. (1983) elicited head turning in 20 children across 12 trials. Individual children did not necessarily show consistent direction of head turning across trials. When all the turns were added together across children, there was only a weak trend for right-sided bias. As Trehub et al. (1983) pointed out, stronger postural asymmetries in normal infants would contradict conventional teaching in pediatric neurology where motor asymmetries in neonates are regarded as indicative of neurological dysfunction (Prechtl 1977).

Premature infants and infants with low Apgar scores fail to show these lateralities in head positioning (Lewkowicz et al. 1979, Turkewitz et al. 1968). In addition, Liederman and Coryell (1982) reported that 6-week-old infants with a history of perinatal complications lacked the rightward head-turning bias of infants without a history of perinatal trauma. The former also remained in the same posture longer than normal children after the tonic neck reflex had been elicited and showed less asymmetry of the reflex itself.

MANUAL PREFERENCE

Because of the importance of handedness in adult neuropsychology, the origin and the development of preferences and consistencies of hand use and manual skills in infants have been examined in a number of recent studies. Historically, developmental research has focused on the observed types of manual skills per se, rather than on their lateralization (Young 1977). Whether handedness is inherited has been an issue of lively debate. Annett's (1970) right-shift gene hypothesis has found tentative acceptance by many researchers in the field; this dominant gene (rs+) also determines left hemisphere language lateralization. Since the sensorimotor areas are situated closely to the manual and language areas, these areas develop more actively and possibly earlier on the left than the right hemisphere. Girls often are homozygotic (rs++) for the gene, which in turn leads to fewer left-handed females (as well as earlier language development). If the right-shift gene is heterozygous (rs+−) less marked asymmetry of motor functions would be expected; if the gene is negative (rs− or rs−−) lateral preference may be due to environmental factors. One corrolary of the right-shift gene hypothesis is that in strongly right-handed individuals mathematical ability may be underdeveloped; a large-scale British study (Whittington and Richards 1991) found only marginal and nonsignificant support for this hypothesis.

The development of handedness has also been related to coding in the cytoplasm in the ovum, rather than the gene (Corballis and Morgan 1978) and to fetal head position in utero, although the correlation is weak (Churchill et al. 1962). In contrast, Bakan (1990) claimed that left-handedness occurs only as the result of birth stress, which is related to oxygen deprivation during difficult births and to birth order (first and fourth and later births are more stressful) that affect primarily left hemisphere structures. The notion has been partially supported by Coren and Porac (1980), but refuted in studies by Hicks et al. (1979), Nachshon and Denno (1986), Schwartz (1988), and van Strien et al. (1987). Coren and Halpern (1991) also claimed that left-handers have a shorter lifespan, a finding that they linked to Geschwind and Galaburda's hormonal theory (discussed below). However, a careful review of the evidence by Harris (1993) found many contradictory studies and rejects the notion of a shortened lifespan in left-handers as the result of a modification effect: older cohorts may show fewer left-handers because a number of activities have switched from left to right hand as a result of environmental demands.

Increased numbers of minor physical anomalies have also been found in left-handers (see Chapter 12). Witelson (1985, 1990) interpreted the finding of more left-handedness in prematurely born males to the onset of axon loss in the corpus callosum. This naturally occurring loss may be the basis of the embryological development of handedness and of hemispheric anatomical and functional asymmetries in males, which are genetically programmed; premature birth may change the course of such axon loss, modifying prenatal and postnatal events.

Satz (1972) allowed for both genetic and pathological factors in his theory of **pathological left-handedness**. His theory makes the assumption that prenatal or perinatal stress affects an equal proportion of between 5 and 20 per cent of both genetic right-handers and left-handers and affects the left or the right side of the brain with equal frequency; however, because of the preponderance of genetic right-handers in the population, a shift toward pathological left- or ambiguous handedness is much more frequent than a shift toward pathological right-handedness (Figure 5-4). As might be expected from this model, the majority of left- and right-handers show normal developmental progression.

Tan (1985) found no evidence of "pathological" motor development in left-handers: there was no difference between right- and left-handed 4-year-olds on the McCarthy Motor Scale and on a series of fine motor tasks, but the group lacking definite hand preference performed significantly more poorly, regardless of gender. However, a recent study of 31 congenitally hemiplegic children, using a variety of measures including dichotic listening (Carlsson et al. 1992), lends support to the hypothesis. Much remains to be clarified on this topic. Harris and Carlson (1989) pointed out in a recent review, "We are still in the dark with respect to neurological loci that might set a bias towards left- or right-handedness in the normal individual. . . . Until we do, we shall not understand anomalous handedness either" (p. 358).

Lateralized hand preference and efficiency in infancy and childhood are variable at first. Gesell and Ames (1947) concluded that, at different times during normal development, a child may show right-hand preference, left-hand preference, or apparent bilaterality. Gesell and Ames' studies agreed well with clinical thought at the time. Several studies since then have examined lateralization of gross movement, grasping, or reaching behaviors but, as was the earlier research, are methodologically unsatisfactory. Caplan and Kinsbourne (1976) examined lateral consistencies in the grasping behavior of infants and reported a possible asymmetry in holding an object with the hand. The results suggested longer grasping with the right hand, but were ambiguous in that this finding might be interpreted either as an indication of hand preference or as evidence that the hand that grasps for a shorter time is dominant because it remains ready for active manipulation. Strauss (1982) failed to replicate the reported differences in grasping time.

A more recent study (Ramsay 1985) investigated hand contact with ten toys in 6-month-old infants, after the onset of duplicated syllable babbling, over a 14-week period. The author found that right-hand preference fluctuated with ambilaterality, with troughs in preferred hand performance at 4 and 8 weeks after the onset of babbling. The author concluded that Gesell and Ames' notion of fluctuation can be confirmed and that the alternations may indicate successive reorganizations in hemispheric specialization or asymmetrical brain organization for motor control.

Gottfried and Bathurst (1983) investigated consistency in hand preference (hand use on drawing items from the Bayley and McArthur Scales) in a longitudinal study of 130 children on five occasions, beginning at the age of 12 months. The study found consistency (same hand preferred on all occasions) to be related to intellectual precociousness in infant and preschool females, but not in males. Using a dual-task paradigm (finger tapping while reciting nursery rhymes), Kee et al. (1987) tested the same children at age 5; it is assumed that

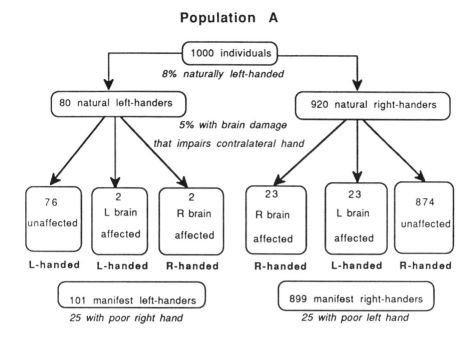

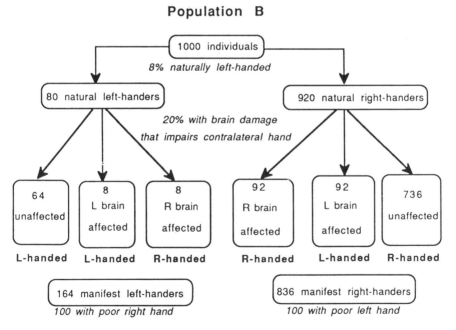

Figure 5-4. Model of pathological handedness (Bishop 1990b).

interference is asymmetrical, i.e., that tapping and/or verbal performance decreases if the right hand is used because both tasks require left hemisphere activity. The authors found the expected asymmetry only in hand-consistent females, whereas both consistent and inconsistent males showed asymmetrical interference. The results seem to confirm sex differences in interhemispheric functional organization discussed in the subsequent section.

5.5   Electrophysiological Cortical Asymmetries

Electrophysiological recording methods have been used to study lateral hemispheric responsiveness to a variety of stimuli in early life. The techniques are described briefly in Chapter 1. One advantage of their use with young infants is that the infant need not be an active and attentive participant in the experiment, an advantage that very few behavioral techniques for the study of developmental laterality offer. However, the frequency of recording artifacts from the infant's movements, as well as the maturational changes observed in both the EEG and evoked potentials, seems to cancel out these advantages.

Davis and Wada (1977) examined the evoked responses of infant's brains by recording auditory evoked responses (AERs) to click stimuli, visual evoked responses (VERs) to flash stimuli, and power spectral transformations (a computer analysis of certain frequencies of the electrical recording) of both AERs and VERs (see Chapter 3). To study specific hemispheric contributions, recordings were made from right and left occipital and temporal scalp locations (01, 02, T3, T4 in the standard system). The results indicated a center of high-amplitude activity in the left temporal lobe for the auditory click stimuli and a center of high-amplitude activity in the right occipital lobe for visual flash stimuli. Thus, even in infants, lateralization of cortical activity in response to different types of stimulation is discernible.

Molfese and co-workers (Molfese 1977, Molfese and Molfese 1979b, Molfese et al. 1976) have used electrophysiological recording techniques to examine language-related cortical mechanisms and their possible lateral asymmetry in a cross-sectional study of neonates, infants, adolescents, and adults. The general format was to record cortical responses over both the left and right temporal regions of the scalp (i.e., recording areas T3 and T4) evoked by a variety of auditory stimuli that either were or were not speech-like. In an initial study, Molfese (1977) examined hemisphere-specific AERs to four speech stimuli, noise, and a C-major piano chord in small groups of infants, children, and adults. Most subjects of all ages showed a greater amplitude in the left-hemisphere AER to speech sounds and a greater right-hemisphere AER amplitude for music and noise. It is tempting to interpret this cross-sectional analysis of the AER as indicating a consistent electrophysiological asymmetry from infancy through adulthood. Later work by Molfese (1979b), however, suggested that neonates were relying on acoustic rather than linguistically relevant phonetic cues when the AERs were recorded, whereas adult AERs were more cued by phonetic aspects of the stimuli. Indirect confirmation of this interpretation came from a study by Dillon et al. (1989) in which brainstem auditory evoked potentials in response to click stimuli in newborns were consistently faster for the right ear compared to the left, suggesting a more general superiority of right ear pathways, rather than one that is specific to linguistic stimuli.

A factor analysis of neonatal AERs to speech and nonspeech sounds yielded four factors (Molfese et al. 1976): a sex effect in the initial part of the AER (females showed a greater response amplitude), stimulus bandwidth, a greater amplitude for a specific stimulus, and a general hemispheric response difference across all stimuli. The absence of an interaction between hemispheric response and either stimulus transition or bandwidth suggested that no specific acoustic function was responsible for the differential hemispheric responsiveness reflected by this fourth factor.

Molfese (1979b) described the AER habituation to repetitive stimulation for a small group of neonates and a small group of adults. The dishabituation stimulus sound differed from the original stimulus either across a linguistically relevant phoneme boundary or within a phoneme boundary (not linguistically relevant). The left hemisphere AER in five of the six adults showed an increase in amplitude, whereas the right hemisphere AER continued to habituate in the presence of linguistically meaningful changes of the stimulus. With the linguistically irrelevant stimulus changes, AERs of both hemispheres continued to decrease in amplitude. This finding was interpreted as evidence of left hemisphere perception of linguistically relevant stimuli. In contrast, the neonates did not show differential hemispheric AERs: across-boundary dishabituation resulted in an increment in response in both hemispheres, and within-boundary dishabituation resulted in the continued decrease of amplitude in both the right and left hemispheres.

Hence, the neonates showed adultlike perception of the across-boundary changes. However, responses were bi-hemispheric rather than lateralized in the infant group, indicating that, when infant's lateralized AERs to speech-like stimuli are recorded, the responses are to acoustic rather than phonetically meaningful cues. It is these non-linguistic, acoustic mechanisms that are lateralized in the neonate.

In a later study, Molfese and Molfese (1979a) reported differential hemispheric AER responses to voice-onset time changes in neonates without the categorical discrimination across phoneme boundaries seen in adults and even in older infants. The older infants showed two specific components in the AER: a first factor representing variables of the right hemisphere response to phonemic categories that had to be discriminated and a second factor common to both hemispheres representing the ability to discriminate phonemic categories. Only the first component was observed in the neonates.

Molfese and Molfese (1979b) attempted to identify acoustic cues responsible for differential hemispheric responsiveness in early infancy. They found a left hemisphere ability to distinguish consonants differing in second-formant transitions containing normal formant structure. A later-appearing AER component, reflecting the same ability but bihemispheric, was also noted.

In sum, the Molfeses have demonstrated that the newborn's and young infant's brain responds electrophysiologically to differences in speech stimuli and that there is some evidence of lateralization in cortical response. They have shown that newborns have a limited ability to discriminate acoustic cues and that the older infant has an adultlike ability to utilize phonemically relevant cues categorically. The Molfeses' studies of differential hemispheric AER patterns with systematic variations in the linguistic and acoustic nature of auditory stimuli provide the most direct evidence to date of some form of hemispheric specialization in language ability very early in infancy.

5.6   A Hormonal Theory of Lateralization

In a more inclusive theory of development, Geschwind and colleagues (Geschwind and Behan 1982, Geschwind and Galaburda 1987) described neuroanatomical differences found in the left hemisphere temporal cortex (planum temporale) in several learning disabled males, which they attributed to increased in utero levels of testosterone or an abnormal sensitivity to it. **Testosterone** is produced from the maternal ovaries, adrenal glands, and other tissues, such as fat; in males, testosterone is produced by the fetus's own developing testes. The authors postulated that this hormone controls neuronal migration to the cortex. Its increased production may result in differences in cortical lamination and delayed development, especially in the left hemisphere language region (Galaburda and Kemper 1979), whereas the right hemisphere develops in a more pronounced fashion. Females, in contrast, develop both hemispheres in a similar pattern (Bradshaw and Nettleton 1983). Geschwind and Galaburda (1987) claimed that, in addition to a learning disability, increased testosterone levels predispose the individual to immune dysfunction (asthma, allergies, migraine headaches etc.) because such an increase also delays the development of the thymus gland that controls the immune system. Because of the unequal exposure to testosterone, all of these disorders are more frequent in males. Within the normal range of variability, testosterone produces more male characteristics; these include higher skills in mathematics and visuo-spatial skills (Marsh 1989).

Because of its wide-ranging implications, the Geschwind theory has been critically reviewed by McManus and Bryden (1991), who called it a "grand" theoretical model that contains no less than 30 postulates, some of which are illustrated in Figure 5-5. In addition to the theories about brain asymmetry (anomalous dominance), lateralization, and immune deficiency disorders, the postulates include claims that increased concentrations or abnormal sensitivity to testosterone is involved in homosexuality, masculinization in females, altered metabolism leading to adverse drug reactions, birth complications and birth stress, decreased rates of cancer, susceptibility to infections, AIDS, and lymphoid malignancies and that testosterone adversely affects the development of

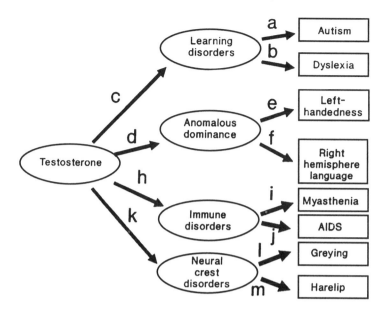

Figure 5-5. A formal path model for a reduced version of several components of the Geschwind model (McManus and Bryden 1991).

the neural crest, resulting in minor and major structural abnormalities, e.g., facial abnormalities (see Section 12). Geschwind and Galaburda also claimed that such hormonal effects are particularly important for the origin of dyslexia and autism and, because they favor right hemisphere development, for gifted-ness in athletic, dancing, and other motor skills, as well as music, mathematics, and artistic and spatial abilities. As McManus and Bryden pointed out, the the-ory is overinclusive in two ways. First, it posits that not only left-handers but also those with weak lateralization are part of the abnormal dominance popu-lation; they may include as many as 60 to 70 per cent of the general population. "A criterion of 'anomalous' which runs the risk that a substantial majority of the population will be included does not seem pragmatically useful or biologically realistic" (p. 249). Second, the theory attempts to explain a vast array of physical and psychological characteristics based mainly on a weak or questionable asso-ciation with handedness while the relationship with testosterone levels remains only hypothetical (Spreen 1989a and b). Every link in this hypothetical chain needs to be tested; the results of such testing have not been fully supportive.

Geschwind and Galaburda ascribed the varying affects of increased testoster-one on different individuals to differences in the timing of the increase. Al-though this is "a theoretical certainty, the precise timings . . . are not stated and are, we suspect, unknowable within the current status of the theory and within the current limits of experimental embryology" (McManus and Bryden, 1991 p. 30). Bakan (1990) raised other questions: What is it that causes excess testosterone production, or could prenatal stress be the cause rather than the result of that increased production? Bakan noted that prenatal stress has been related to dopamine asymmetries (Fride and Weinstock 1989). Is testosterone the only agent that causes anomalous development? Satz and Soper (1986) questioned the validity of some of Geschwind's studies relating left-handedness, dyslexia, and autoimmune disorders. For example, van Strien and co-workers (1987) failed to find any association between left-handedness and autoimmune disorders. Another study by Hansen et al. (1986, 1987) provided somewhat paradoxical results: nondiabetic relatives of children with diabetes mellitus (considered here an immunological disorder) showed a higher rate of dyslexia than the children themselves, suggesting a negative association between immunological disease and dyslexia; the results were confirmed recently by Kaplan and Field (personal communication, 1990). Wiley and Goldstein (1991), however, failed to find a higher incidence of left-handedness or of allergies among 96 gifted seventh-graders. McCardle and Wilson (1990) examined language functions in 32 5- to 12-year-old children with accelerated maturation caused by conditions that elevated sex hormone levels. Estrogen-exposed children showed better language performance than androgen-exposed subjects, regardless of genetic sex or diagnosis. The authors viewed this as supporting Geschwind and Galaburda's multifactorial theory for the origin of sex differences in language development. A large-scale follow-up study of 1603 children who had been exposed in utero to estrogen or placebo for the treatment of at-risk pregnancies during 1950–1952, in contrast, showed no effect of estrogen on college entrance examination scores in females and only a marginal effect in males (Wilcox et al. 1992). A review of 19 similar studies on the behavioral effects of prenatal exposure to hormones (Reinisch et al. 1991a, b) concluded that overall androgen-based exposure had a masculinizing or defeminizing influence on behavioral development, particularly on female children, whereas estrogen exposure had a feminizing and/or demasculinizing influence on boys; some studies suggested also that estrogen-exposed female subjects were masculinized. Such results suggest that the relationships postulated by Geschwind and Galaburda may be more complex and may include both negative and positive associations. In a detailed review of handedness and developmental disorders, Bishop (1990a) pointed out the highly selective citation of evidence by Geschwind and Galaburda: "small-scale studies and even anecdotal reports are given prominence, while substantial bodies of contrary work are ignored" (p. 162).

Geschwind and Galaburda developed what has quickly become one of the most influential neuropsychological theories about sexual dimorphism and laterality, as well as many other topics of neuropsychological study. However, the evidence supporting this "grand" theory remains weak; McManis and Bryden (1991) concluded that the concept of anomalous dominance at present "does not provide sufficient additional theoretical advantage to be a useful addition to the measurement tools available to neuropsychology" (p. 250).

Summary

Evidence has accumulated from several different lines of investigation that even the newborn infant's nervous system has anatomical asymmetries similar to those of adults and that it shows clear lateralization of function. How the different pieces of evidence fit together and how well they correlate with adult patterns of lateralized neuropsychological organization are two important questions. The two basic theoretical positions find partial support: the young infant does have lateralized brain structure and function, and as the infant develops, there is further progressive lateralization through childhood until adulthood.

6

Sex Differences

6.1 Sex Differences

As with lateralization, the investigation of sex differences is plagued with problems of understanding and presents many unanswered questions. Is sex a categorical variable with mutually exclusive categories? Have any sex differences in the underlying neural substrate been found? Have neural sex differences in any way been related to psychological (dis)abilities, and how? Finally, how do neural and behavioral sex-related differences arise in development?

Sex-related differences that change during development have to be discriminated from more static sex-related differences in the adult. Reviews by Bradshaw and Nettleton (1983), Bryden (1982), Kimura (1987), Kolb and Wishaw (1990), and McGlone (1980) present the current understanding of sex differences in the neuropsychological abilities of the adult and child. This section is concerned only with sex differences as they arise in early pre- and postnatal development; sex-related changes that occur during or after puberty are not discussed.

At first glance neuropsychological differences between the sexes during development seem easy and convenient to study: groups of subjects of each sex can be compared by looking at their chromosomes, their brains, and their performance on specific behavioral tasks. However, such a comparative approach, although sometimes valuable, tends to focus attention away from determining the mechanisms for these differences. It must be kept in mind that there is typically more individual variation within a sex than between sexes.

Mechanisms of neuropsychological sex differences in development may range from genetic, hormonal, neural, and behavioral factors to differential socialization practices and sex roles. Although each of these factors has been suggested as a "cause" of sex differences, none of them alone can fully explain the findings. For these reasons, the study of sex differences in development has been confusing and perhaps misleading at times. The inclusion of a sex factor in many behavioral studies has to be weighed carefully.

Sex Differences in Neural Development

Sex can be defined at two basic levels: that of the chromosomes (**genetic differentiation**) and that of the sex organs and sexual characteristics (**gonadal differentiation**). Sex can be identified prenatally by examining the chromosomes; a karyotype displays the genes and indicates whether the embryo is male or female. Of the 23 pairs of chromosomes in humans, one pair (the **gonosomes**) specifies the sex of the individual; XX is the female, XY the male pattern. Sex is determined at fertilization since the ovum and sperm each carry half of the genetic material. The sex of the child depends upon the sex of the sperm since approximately half the time the sperm carries the X sex chromosome and half the time it carries the Y chromosome, whereas the ovum always contributes an X chromosome. At subsequent cell divisions, either the male (XY) or female (XX) pattern is passed on to all cells. At conception, the male/female ratio has been estimated as between 1.6 to 1.22/1 and at birth as 1.05/1 (Mosley and Stan 1984), suggesting a poorer survival rate during pregnancy for the male fetus; this may be due in part to the production of antigens by the male fetus and the response by the mother of production of potentially harmful immunoglobulin antibodies.

Up until about 7 to 8 weeks after fertilization, the gonads remain undifferentiated. The genetic male and the genetic female look alike. At this time, the male gonad becomes recognizable as testes; the female gonad does not differentiate into ovaries until about 10 weeks after fertilization. Thereafter, the sex chromosomes have no known direct influence on subsequent sexual differentiation. External genitalia begin to develop during the ninth week as the testes begin to secrete testosterone (MacKinnon 1979). Under this hormone's influence the external genitalia differentiate to form a penis and a scrotum. In contrast, the development of the female reproductive tract does not require hormonal stimulation. In the absence of testosterone, the external genitalia differentiate into those of the female. Female ovarian hormones (estrogen, for example) seem to have no effect at the early stage.

Several abnormalities are related to disorders in fetal sex differentiation. One has been studied extensively and is called the adrenogenital syndrome or **congenital adrenal hyperplasia** (CAH). The condition is transmitted in the autosomal recessive mode; both parents have to be carriers to produce the condition, in which an excessive amount of androgen is produced. In a genetic female with the adrenogenital syndrome, there is a masculinization of the external genitalia while the internal reproductive organs remain female (Ehrhardt and Baker 1974, Money and Ehrhardt 1972). Nass et al. (1987) found a strong bias toward left-handedness in this population as compared to their normal sisters. Treatment usually involves lifelong hormonal control and early surgical feminization of the external genitalia. A variant of this syndrome occurs in genetic males with no noticeable effect on the genitalia; no left-handedness bias was found for these boys. With early hormonal treatment, they appear normal; without treatment they experience premature pubertal development.

In another disorder, the testicular feminization or **androgen-insensitivity syndrome**, genetic males cannot appropriately use androgen. This defect results in a discrepancy between genetic and gonadal sex (XY) on the one hand and the external morphological sex appearance (female) on the other.

In Turner syndrome (XO), children are not exposed to any gonadal hormones during the early critical period (see Chapter 11). One of the sex chromosomes is missing, and the individuals develop morphologically as a female.

As this brief introduction shows, fetal sex hormones have a profound effect on the development of sex-related characteristics. The next question is whether or not sex hormones also have an effect on neural development. The term used for the development of two forms of a structure from an undifferentiated precursor is **dimorphism**. The question to be addressed is therefore: Is there a structural-chemical dimorphism in the brain?

Hormones and Neuronal Development

Because sex differences have traditionally been set as dichotomous and absolute, it was assumed that females produce only estrogens and males produce only testosterone. In actual fact, there is overlap, and the hormones of both sexes are present in both men and women. Thus, the hormonal difference between the sexes has to do with the relative proportions of both hormones as long as they both are present.

Hormones have been known to influence the nervous system and its development for some time (Reinisch 1974). Theoretically, they have two possible functions: (1) to act locally to activate a particular structure by influencing some of the functional properties of the neurons and (2) to help differentiate and organize the nervous system as a whole early in development by influencing nerve growth, neuronal circuitry, and brain architecture. These have been described as the activational and the organizational hypotheses (Arnold 1980, Goy and McEwen 1981, Harlan et al. 1979). From an evolutionary point of view, differentiating peripheral organs, such as the testes or ovaries, is of little interest unless there are differences in function and neural control as well, i.e., unless there are different functions for each of the gonads and also different neural centers controlling them.

> Normal differentiation of genital morphology entails a dimorphic sex difference in the arrangement of peripheral nerves of sex which, in turn, entails some degree of dimorphism in the representation of the periphery at the centrum of the central nervous system, that is to say, in the structures and pathways of the brain (Money and Ehrhardt 1972, p. 8).

Evidence for the organizational hypothesis came primarily from animal research. Hormonal messages governing the functions of the gonads are sent from the pituitary gland, which secretes hormones called **gonadotropins**. These hormones stimulate the ovaries to operate cyclically (the menstrual cycle). The pituitary gland is controlled by portions of the "sexually dimorphic" nucleus of the hypothalamus, specifically the anterior and preoptic regions. The sexual dimorphism of these regions can be attributed to the prenatal masculinizing effect of androgen, which alters cell structure and function (Janowsky 1989, MacKinnon 1979). Without androgen, these regions differentiate functionally as female. Thus, it is the male organism, again, that is changed.

One often overlooked interaction in studies of neural sex differences is that between sex hormone levels in the body and the number of sex hormone receptors available. There seem to be individual differences in both the number and the sensitivity of sex hormone receptors in the brain and in peripheral organs. These differences may cloud any relationship between the level of sex hormone and the functional activity of the brain.

With regard to brain structure, evidence for sex differences in human neuronal circuitry or architecture has been slowly accumulating, although it has been known for some time that at all ages the average brain weight of males is about 10 per cent greater than that of females. The sex difference in brain weight probably reflects a sex difference in neuronal size, rather than neuronal number, and therefore does not imply any sex differences in performance.

In a study of rhesus monkeys, Goldman and colleagues (1974) were able to show sex-dependent behavioral effects of cerebral cortical lesions during development. They found that male rhesus monkeys with orbital prefrontal lesions were impaired on behavioral tasks at 10 weeks of age, but similar deficits were not detected in females until 15 to 18 months of age. The results indicate earlier maturation of the orbital prefrontal areas in male monkeys, a sexual dimorphism in neural development. Ayoubet et al. (1983) also found more dendritic bifurcations and a higher frequency of dendritic spines in the preoptic area in male as compared to female prepubertal macaques, suggesting a structural difference without differences in gross measurements of these areas.

Diamond et al. (1981) found that, in male rats, the right cerebral cortex was thicker than the left from birth to old age; in female rats at the age of 90 days, the left cortex was thicker than the right, although this difference was not significant. Females whose ovaries were removed at birth developed a male pattern of hemispheric asymmetry.

Recent studies (de Lacoste et al. 1991), using sophisticated volumetric analyses rather than linear measurements, did indeed report asymmetries in 21 fetal brains favoring the right hemisphere in males, whereas female brains were of the same size or showed a slightly larger left hemisphere (Figure 6-1). These differences were found mainly in the prefrontal and the striate-extrastriate region. De Lacoste interprets these findings as supporting the Geschwind and Galaburda (1987) theory that asymmetries begin as early as the period of neural induction and that sex differences are due to the effects of circulating testosterone in utero.

Peters (1988) found no sex differences in the size of the corpus callosum, but de Lacoste et al. (1986, 1991) found that the posterior part of the corpus callosum is larger in females than in males. A morphometric analysis by Clarke et

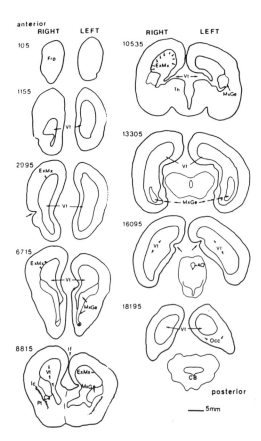

Figure 6-1. Male brain at 15 weeks gestational age. The right hemisphere is visibly larger than the left counterpart (de Lacoste et al. 1991).

al. (1989) showed a smaller cross-sectional callosal area with a larger fraction in the posterior fifth of the corpus callosum and more bulbous splenia in females; fetal brain measurements revealed similar dimorphisms in the early, but not the later prenatal period, with a recurrence of the differences postnatally. The authors speculated that axonal elimination may be the reason for the prenatal pause of growth in the cross-sectional callosal area and the concomitant changes in callosal shape. These findings have been interpreted as the basis for more interhemispheric interaction in females (Kimura 1987). Gender differences in behavioral susceptibility to teratogens have also been reported (Riese 1989).

Earlier findings by Wada and colleagues (Wada 1976, Wada et al. 1975) showed a trend for the left planum temporale to be larger in male adults than in females, whereas a reversed pattern of asymmetry was more often found in male than in female infants. The frontal operculum was also larger in infant females than in infant males, and male infants had a larger planum temporale on both sides. However, Witelson and Pallie (1973) demonstrated less asymmetry in female than in male infants. Hence, there is a suggestion that asymmetry of the superior part of the temporal lobe increases with age, and more so for males than for females. However, the actual frequencies (in infants 56 left, 12 right) of such differences observed by Wada do not approach the proportions reported for functional hemispheric specialization for speech in adults. In cerebral blood flow studies Gur (1982) also found more activation of the whole brain at rest in females than in males. Finally, in a study of electrophysiological responses evoked by binocular pattern reversal, Cohn et al. (1985) failed to find lateral differences in 5- to 14-year-old boys and girls, although the amplitude of the response was higher for younger girls; this sex difference gradually decreased toward adolescence.

6.2 Sex Differences in Behavior

The differences in behavior demonstrated between the sexes have been reviewed by Maccoby and Jacklin (1974). We present a short summary here before considering the often conflicting evidence for theories of cerebral organization in relation to sex differences.

It is fairly well agreed that there are few, if any, sex differences in the early development of activity level, vocalization, oral behaviors, auditory receptivity, and visual tracking (Korner 1973). However, female infants have been shown to be more sensitive to auditory, photic, and tactile stimulation; they gaze at a silent face or photographs longer than do male infants. They also show more mouthing and increased responsiveness to sweetness. Male infants showed more spontaneous startle during sleep, which may be related to the development of physical strength or vigor. Reviewing data of developmental milestones (e.g., sitting, crawling, walking) for a cohort of 4653 infants, Reinisch et al. (1991a) reported that boys reached three milestones significantly earlier than girls, whereas none of the milestones appeared earlier in girls than in boys. The authors interpret this finding as evidence for a biologically based sexual dimorphism.

General intellectual functioning as measured by IQ usually fails to show sex differences, although two reports stimulated renewed interest in this issue (Kaufman and Doppelt 1976, Wersh and Briere 1981). Studies of IQ differences in children, if they exist, are further obscured by the fact that the WISC-R, the most commonly used intelligence test, was deliberately constructed to avoid sex differences.

Sex-related differences in cognitive abilities appear most frequently and most consistently in the linguistic and spatial domains (Maccoby and Jacklin 1974, Ray et al. 1981). Specifically, girls tend to achieve higher scores than boys on tests of verbal abilities, and boys tend to achieve higher scores on tests of spatial abilities. The consistency of these findings, however, depends upon the ages studied. In the age range from 8 to 11 years, no consistent sex differences in verbal abilities can be demonstrated, but before age 8 and after adolescence girls generally seem to outperform boys in measures of verbal skills (Burstein et al. 1980, Gaddes and Crockett 1975), although in recent studies these differences seem to be quite small (Marsh 1989). Speed of color naming in pre-readers seems to be a forerunner of this trend (Jaffe et al. 1985). The male superiority in tests of spatial ability, however, seems to show up in the age range from 6 years to adolescence (Kirk 1992, McGee 1979) and in one study with 4- and 5-year-olds (McGuinness and Morley 1991). Hassler (1991) related spatial skill to maturation in 9- to 14-year-old boys (mutation) and girls (menarche); the testosterone level in the saliva was related to cognitive performance in boys and to musical talent in girls, although this difference did not emerge until a mean age of 15.5 years.

Although seriously questioned in a recent critique (Caplan et al. 1985), numerous studies have confirmed the sex difference in spatial ability, despite the fact that the concept is not unitary and deserves further clarification. Studies of sex differences have usually disregarded the two-factor theory of McGee (1979), which separated spatial visualization and spatial orientation, and have instead focused on specific tasks of spatial ability. Harshman et al. (1983) found that female children excel at perceptual speed and visual memory, whereas males are better at perceptual closure and disembedding of complex visual arrays. A recent study (Alyman 1991) yielded no support for the notion of sex differences in 7- to 9-year-old children, 15- to 19-year-old adolescents, or adults for a series of regular spatial tasks with familiar objects, but Alyman conceded that sex differences can be shown with more intricate visual processing tasks, such as spatial rotation.

Kimura's (1987, Kimura and Harshman 1984) detailed studies confirm some of these asymmetries in brain-damaged patients. She pointed out that constructional and manual apraxia occurs in women primarily after right anterior lesions, whereas in males lesions causing these deficits are widely distributed over the right hemisphere. Verbal functions are less asymmetrically organized in women than in men, but again are more dependent on the anterior left hemisphere than in men. In support of this thesis, Lewis and Christiansen (1989) found greater interference in women during dual task performance (finger tapping while reading aloud). Finally, Mateer et al. (1982) supplied further confirmation based on direct brain stimulation during surgery, which showed interference of naming in males after anterior and posterior stimulation, whereas such interference occurred only after anterior stimulation in women.

These gender differences are of course group differences. The distributions of the two sexes on measures of verbal and spatial ability overlap greatly.

6.3 Sex Differences in Cerebral Functional Organization

The question whether there are sex-related differences in the degree and development of cerebral lateralization of cognitive functions has stirred considerable interest over the past decade. A critical look reveals much confusion and contradiction in this area.

Several researchers have proposed that there are sex differences in the development of cerebral lateralization and that they relate to differing behavioral capacities of the sexes. Buffery and Gray (1972, also Buffery 1976) argued that both speech and spatial skills become completely lateralized in females, but remain more bilateral in males since developmental studies indicate an earlier acquisition of language function in females. The underlying assumption is that, for optimal achievement to develop, it is better to have language represented in one hemisphere and spatial skills in both hemispheres. Hence, males are better at spatial skills, and females are better at linguistic skills.

Essentially the opposite developmental pattern has been suggested by Levy and Reid (1978), who asserted that males are more strongly lateralized for both spatial and verbal functions than females and that bilateral language representation is conducive to higher verbal ability. Carter-Saltzman (1979), Waber (1977, 1979a), and Witelson (1977) have presented similar theories. Waber assumed that early sexual maturation (the female pattern) is associated with weaker lateralization of functions and that late maturation (the male pattern) is associated with greater lateralization. Weak lateralization then would lead to greater verbal ability and stronger lateralization to greater spatial ability, consistent with the findings in our own current review. Using a dichaptic task (which requires tactile recognition of two different shapes or objects simultaneously with each hand) in children, Witelson (1976b, 1977b) found that males showed a right-hand channel superiority for tactile matching at least at the age of 6 years, but females did not show this superiority even at the age of 13 years. From this finding she concluded that there is an early right hemisphere specialization for spatial ability in males, but females retain bilateral representation during development.

Perhaps these two lateralization theories are contradictory partly because of the variety of laterality and cerebral organization measures used (Bryden 1979, 1982). Several other theories on sex differences in brain development tend to de-emphasize the role of lateralization and to stress the importance of differential maturation rates between the sexes. Ounsted and Taylor (1972), for example, hypothesized that the Y chromosome slows the rate of maturation of the male and permits more exposure to the environment and a fuller expression of the genetic material (the polygenic multiple-threshold model), which eventually leads to sex-related differences in higher cortical functioning. A corollary of this hypothesis is that males are more likely to be exposed to noxious stimuli over a prolonged period of time, whereas girls have less exposure; as a result, Ounsted and Taylor (1972) proposed that if developmental disorders occur, they should be more severe in boys than in girls. Zaide (1982) provided support for this notion in a study of learning disabled children; in a review of the literature on autism, mental retardation, learning disability, conduct disorder, and attention-deficit-hyperactivity disorder, Eme (1992) found only modest support for this model.

As mentioned above, Waber proposed that the sex-related differences in higher cortical functioning, expressed behaviorally as the sex differences in verbal and spatial ability, are due to differences in the physical maturation rate. On the basis of this theory, she postulated that, regardless of sex, early maturers would do better on tests of verbal ability, and late maturers would do better on tests of spatial ability. Her study did show that late-maturing individuals (based on Tannard scale ratings) of both sexes performed better than early maturers on tests of spatial ability, but the groups did not differ on tests of verbal ability. A crucial assumption, only indirectly addressed by Waber, is whether the earlier physical maturation of girls is related to earlier mental development. In support of Waber's findings, Gordon (1983) presented dichotic listening data that showed decreasing left hemisphere specialization by late childhood in females, but not in males.

Further support was presented by Kimura and Carson (1993) who found a higher finger-ridge count in males (as well as a higher ridge count in the right compared to the left hand). Dermal ridges are formed early in fetal life and remain unchanged throughout the lifespan. Both male and female subjects with a higher ridge count on the right hand performed better on "masculine" tests (e.g., spatial and mathe-matical tasks). Hall and Kimura (1993) also found higher left-hand ridge counts in homosexual men, as well as a lower right-ear effect in dichotic listening compared to heterosexuals, suggesting a "relationship between an aspect of physical asym-metry, functional brain asymmetry, and sexual orientation."

Yet another feature of sex differences in perceptual asymmetry in a fused dichotic listening test was reported by Wexler and Lipman (1988). The authors found a right ear advantage in males during the first 60 trials, which then de-creased over the next 60 trials; females showed less right ear advantage initially, which then increased. The asymmetry during the last 60 trials was the same for males and females. The authors suggest that males respond more to the novelty of the task with relative left hemisphere activation, whereas females respond with right hemisphere activation.

McGuinness and Pribam (1979, see also Goleman 1978) presented another neurobehavioral theory relating cerebral functional organization to differing abilities of the sexes. They suggested that there are sex differences in brain structure that arise when different levels of sex hormones act on the structures that underlie behavioral sex differences. Sex differences are evident in the arousal (amygdala-frontal lobe) and readiness (basal ganglia) systems of the brain. According to this theory, males, who are considered to be more manip-ulative, would have a spatial-mechanical aptitude through the readiness system. Females, considered to be more communicative, would have an auditory-verbal aptitude and would show greater flexibility in the control of hemispheric func-tions through the arousal system. Eaton and Yu (1989) found that in 5- to 8-year-old children girls were advanced in relative maturity (percentage of estimated adult height attained) and less motorically active than boys. Maturity level and activity level were negatively related. Smoll and Schutz (1990), on the other hand, argued that 50 per cent of the variance in the gender differences on motor performance is accounted for by adiposity. In this study with over 2000 children between 9 and 17 years, the effect of anthropomorphic measurements decreased with age; the authors concluded that with increasing age gender differences become more a function of environmental factors.

In addition to these general theories of neurobehavioral sex differences, there have been numerous reports of developmental sex differences in relation to cerebral organization. Research with identical and fraternal twins has indicated that spatial ability has a genetic component. Identical twins are significantly more similar than fraternal twins on tests of spatial ability (Vandenberg and Kuse 1979), which therefore seems to be linked to the X chromosome. The theory has been called the "sex-linked major gene hypothesis." However, a critique by Boles (1980) showed that severe methodological difficulties in many of the studies render the hypothesis unsatisfactory.

In other studies (Shucard et al. 1981), significant sex-dependent AER asymmetries in 3-month-old infants presented with verbal and nonverbal auditory stimulation were found. Females showed greater AERs from the left hemisphere, and males produced greater right hemisphere responses during both the verbal and the nonverbal presentations. The authors suggested that their results support the behavioral data on the presence of sex differences in cognitive functioning at an early age: the left hemisphere in female infants is more receptive to complex sensory input and hence is predisposed for language-related functions, whereas in male infants the right hemisphere is more receptive, which may be related to the earlier development of spatial functions. Their results need to be replicated and extended to other responses, since at least one study (Yamamoto 1990) did not find a gender difference in language development in 3½- to 6-year-old Japanese children.

The topic of sex differences in behavior during development and at the adult level has raised considerable interest over several decades. More recently, attempts have been made to relate these differences to differences in the structure and function of the brain. The results of these efforts provide a limited amount of factual information relating to brain function and a considerable amount of often contradictory theories. Although differences in the development of lateralization (which presumably become permanent functional differences of brain organization) remain mainly conjecture, proposed sex differences in the rate of maturation find at least some indirect support in evidence of differential physical maturation and in the ablation studies with rhesus monkeys described earlier. One is likely to agree with Burstein et al. (1980) that there are several demonstrated sex differences in cognitive and other behavioral functions, but few "hard" explanations as to why they occur.

Reinish (1991) extended the search for hormonal-based sex differences to the area of social and personality development. Girls tend to play out "homespun dramas," whereas boys tend to play more competitive games. She relates testosterone level to aggressiveness, ambition, and violence. In infancy, boys tend to persist and pull hard when faced with photographs that can be changed with a string pull, whereas girls tend to give up, cry, or get cranky in the same situation (Lewis et al. 1985, 1986). The author sees more competitiveness, but also more inflexibility in boys.

6.4   Developmental Disabilities and Sex Differences

Further understanding of sex-related differences in brain and behavior may be gained from research on sex differences in neuropsychological disabilities as related to specific developmental mechanisms. One of the most frequently studied disabilities now known to show a sex difference is developmental dyslexia, a disorder in acquiring the ability to read (Chapter 29). In a critical review, Finucci and Childs (1981) reached the conclusion that epidemiological evidence confirms that there really are more dyslexic boys than girls, as clinical observations have indicated for many years. They concluded that the mean boy/girl ratio is 5.1/1, although it is partly related to the age of the subjects. The boys in their own study not only showed more severe disability but also tended to be slightly older than the dyslexic girls. When Finucci and Childs began to explore the sex differences, however, they found that females seemed to function better in the presence of a dyslexic deficit than males. Witelson (1977b) agreed that females show more plasticity in development. When severity was included as a factor, the sex difference decreased to a male/female ratio of 2/1.

Other developmental disabilities also show an increased prevalence in males: mental retardation (the sex ratios differ for particular forms, but males are almost always over-represented); hyperactivity; X-linked disorders, such as Lesch-Nyhan syndrome (an inability to metabolize nucleic acids in food because of an enzyme deficiency); agenesis of the corpus callosum; and epilepsy (Mosley and Stan 1982, 1984). The male predominance in all of these disorders led Mosley and Stan to develop further a general theory, already put forth by Taylor (1976), that during the early embryological phase of human sexual dimorphism the male is exposed to greater risk. Females have less range of variability in genetic expression than males because the hemizygous nature of the male sex chromosome pair (XY) increases genetic variability. Therefore, the male is represented with greater frequency among both the positive and the negative extremes of behavior, including intellectual functioning. Mosley and Stan's theory seems to contradict some of the evidence just presented and suggests that there are sex differences not only in the quantity but also in the quality of cognitive abilities. A recent study (Rudolf and Hochberg 1990) reported also that boys show more psychosocial growth retardation and nonorganic failure to thrive.

Summary

Few definite conclusions about the relation between sex and neurobehavioral function can be drawn, as few studies have actually demonstrated interdependence between the two. Perhaps the most encouraging development is the increasing recognition that a wide variety of factors influence neuropsychological functioning. Petersen (1981) has constructed a "biopsychosocial" model including genetic, hormonal, psychological, and sociocultural influences that can be applied throughout the life-span. Such interactive models are necessary to understand even a "simple" dichotomy, such as sex.

7

Newborn and Infant Assessment

In clinical settings, assessment of the infant contributes information for the early diagnosis of developmental problems and the treatment of young children. The findings also increase our understanding of the variety of treatments and environments that support or impede development and the degree to which individual abilities are able to tolerate changes in environmental experience. This field has expanded rapidly in the last 30 years and has emerged as an important subdiscipline in its own right. This expansion has been facilitated by innovative research techniques, improved technology, and the realization that infants are more responsive to environmental stimulation and are more able to process certain types of perceptual information than previously assumed (Lamb and Bornstein 1987).

7.1 Historical Perspective

Biographical accounts of infants in their natural settings by their parents are an example of one of the earliest methods of infant assessment. Biographical sketches of their infant children were provided by Tiedemann in 1787, Taine in 1869 (Lamb and Bornstein 1982), and Darwin in 1877. In the United States, G. Stanley Hall (1904) is credited with initiating the normative study of child development, which formed the basis for **norm-referenced assessment** (scores based on norms derived from a representative part of the age group for whom the test is designed). He believed that an understanding of child development could help clarify the evolutionary development of the human species. About the same time in France, interest in the educability of the mentally retarded led Esquirol and Seguin to develop a reliable and valid diagnostic procedure to delineate mental deficiency and insanity. Infants were included in their studies because the profoundly retarded were thought to exhibit the mental abilities of 2-year-olds (Brooks and Weintraub 1976). Soon after, Binet and

113

Simon (Binet 1905, Binet and Simon 1908) developed a test to identify children in the Paris school system who were mentally retarded and in need of special education. Their 30-item intelligence scale, later revised by Terman at Stanford University, led to the **Stanford-Binet Intelligence Scale** (Terman and Merill 1937), which provided an estimate of ability expressed as a global test score with mental age equivalents, and it established the importance of standardization procedures. During the 1920s the demand for tests, primarily for diagnostic purposes and for adoption agencies, led to the development of several infant scales. Arnold Gesell at the Yale Clinic of Child Development produced the Gesell Developmental Schedules (Gesell and Amatruda 1954, Gesell and Thompson 1934). In Vienna, Charlotte Buehler developed the Buehler Baby Tests (Buehler and Hetzer 1935). An infant test was also developed by Mary Shirley in Minnesota (Shirley 1933). Nancy Bayley produced the California First Year Mental Scale, later revised and renamed the Bayley Scales of Infant Development (Bayley 1933, 1969). Few new tests were introduced until the appearance in the 1940s of the Cattell Infant Intelligence Scale (1940); the Griffiths' Mental Development Scale (1954) and the Neurobehavioral Maturity Assessment (Korner et al. 1989, 1991). Freud (1940), Erikson (1963), Bowlby (1969/1982), Ainsworth (Ainsworth et al. 1978), and more recently Teti and Nakagawa (1990) established a conceptual basis for assessing infant attachment. Piaget's descriptions of infant cognitive development led to methods for testing children's understanding of such concepts as conservation and classification (Uzgiris and Hunt 1975).

Tests developed in the last 25 years have been designed to assess specific aspects of mental development in infancy. Some of the more specialized tests focus, for example, on neonatal assessment, sensorimotor development, and early language development. In the 1970s, renewed interest in the social development of the infant spurred research on mother-infant dyads and early social and cognitive development (Ainsworth et al. 1978, Clarke-Stewart 1973, Edgell 1979). An understanding of individual differences in infant temperament and how these differences influence the quality of relationships with caregivers led to the development of measures to assess infant temperament (Thomas et al. 1968, Williamson and Zeitlin 1990). Current views hold that since development proceeds within a social-emotional context, and there are wide-ranging and bidirectional effects between the environment and the child, infant abilities cannot be described using single tests. Such complex variables as socioeconomic status, parental education, parenting styles, and quality of the home environment interact (Sameroff and Chandler 1975), and a complete picture of the status of the infant needs to consider the total infant milieu.

Infant assessment has also played a role in research related to socially disadvantaged children. Educational enrichment programs, such as Head Start, and techniques for measuring their effectiveness stimulated interest in infant measurement. A series of federal laws in the United States on the care of handicapped children enacted during the past 30 years also increased the need for early and periodic assessment, diagnosis, and treatment. More recently, infant assessment techniques have been used to measure the impact of day-care experiences on child development, with some results suggesting that they disrupt the development of secure attachments between parent and child (Belsky and Isabella 1988), and other researchers asserting that such an impact must be interpreted in terms of the quality of day care (Phillips et al. 1987, Teti and Gibbs 1990). Infant assessment has extended its influence into the field of the assessment of children with special needs including the motorically handicapped, the visually impaired, the hearing impaired, and the language-delayed child. Assessment of the child's milieu has brought into focus family systems and cultural factors. Social and emotional aspects, including children's play, have become important parts of the evaluation of young children (Bond et al. 1990, Murphy 1972).

7.2   Current Perspectives

Assessment in infancy is particularly important in populations at risk. Established risk refers to risk from a known etiology, such as Down syndrome. Environmental risk considers such factors as the quality of infant-mother interaction and opportunities for infant stimulation. Biological risk refers to infants exposed to potentially noxious events (Tjossem 1976).

Typically the results from infant assessments are used for screening, diagnosis, and prescriptive purposes. Screening, diagnostic, and prescriptive tests are not mutually exclusive, and infant assessment frequently involves a variety of test instruments and procedures.

Screening Tests

Screening assessments are brief and easy to administer. Quantitative scores can be used to determine the need for interventions and should minimize false-positive identification (Gibbs 1990). The **Apgar test** is a quick and easy screening device used to describe newborn status. Infants can be rated at 1, 3, 5, and 10 minutes after birth on five signs (Table 7-1). A score of 0 to 2 suggests severe hypoxia or depression, a score of 3 to 6 suggests moderate hypoxia or depression, and 7 to 10 indicates a normal infant.

The Brief Infant Neurobehavioral Optimality Scale (Aylward et al. 1985), a shortened version of the Prechtl Neurological Examination (Table 7-2), is a brief screening measure to assess CNS intactness at 12 months of age based on muscle tone, tendon reflexes, spontaneous activity, and selected primitive reflexes. The Denver Developmental Screening Test (DDST, Frankenburg and Dodds 1967, Frankenberg et al. 1975) is used by many pediatricians in the early identification of delayed development or for ongoing assessment in young children from birth to 6 years. It is norm-referenced and covers the formative years of development in personal/social, fine motor/adaptive, language, and gross motor domains. However, recent validity studies, together with the recognition of the

Table 7-1.   Apgar Test

Sign	Score 0	Score 1	Score 2
A. Appearance (color)	Blue, pale	Body pink, limbs blue	All pink
P. Pulse (heart rate)	Absent	<100	>100
G. Grimace (irritability)	None	Grimace	Cry
A. Activity (muscle tone)	Limp	Some flexion of limbs	Active movement
R. Respiratory effort	None	Slow, irregular	Good strong cry

Source: Black 1972.

limited language item content at the upper age levels, raise questions about its utility as a screening test. Although the DDST is useful in identifying mental retardation, it is not recommended for preschool children with lesser degrees of delay or specific developmental disabilities (Ireton 1990). A widely used screening measure based on parental report is the Minnesota Child Developmental Inventory (MCDI, Ireton and Thwing 1974). This is a standardized inventory consisting of 320 statements that describe the developmental behaviors of children from birth to 6 years. The MCDI profile provides a graphic layout of development in eight domains. Briefer parent screening measures have been derived from these scales, including the Preschool Developmental Inventory for 3- to 6-year-olds (Ireton 1984) and the Early Childhood Developmental Inventory for 1- to 3-year-olds (Ireton 1988).

Diagnostic Tests

The more widely used traditional infant assessment tests are diagnostic tests that provide detailed information about developmental status. Diagnostic tests are norm-referenced and can provide serial test data over a period of time to monitor a child's progress. The traditional scales of infant assessment were developed by Gesell and Amatruda (1954), Cattell (1940), and Bayley (1969, 1970). Gesell and Amatruda, both physicians, were interested in measuring the overall developmental status of the infant. In contrast, Cattell and Bayley focused on measuring infant intelligence and determining which behavior would predict later intelligence. Although traditional infant tests are norm-referenced, some are not based on a unified theory of development. For example, a review of factor analytic studies of the Bayley Scales of Infant Development (Yarrow and Pederson 1976) identified eight clusters of behavior: goal directedness, visually

Table 7-2. Early Neuropsychological Optimality Rating Scales at 12 months

		Classification	Optimal	Non-optimal
I.		Basic reflexes		
		Persistence of primitive reflexes (Moro, asymmetric tonic neck, palmar/plantar, etc.)	No	Yes
		Asymmetries/marked L-R discrepancy (mirroring, obvious hand preference)	No	Yes
		Presence of protective reactions (parachute reactions)	Yes	No
		Good head control	Yes	No
		Hypotonia/hypertonia—extremities	No	Yes
		Absence of stereotyped, repetitive movements and/or cortical thumb sign	Yes	No
II.		Receptive functions		
		Appropriate responses to auditory stimuli (orients, turns head)	Yes	No
		Appropriate responses to visual stimuli (tracking, lack of nystagmus)	Yes	No
		Follows simple commands	Yes	No
III.		Expressive functions		
	A.	Fine motor/oral motor		
		Neat pincer grasp	Yes	No
		Presence of midline behaviors (hands together, holds two objects simultaneously)	Yes	No
		Radial-digital grasp	Yes	No
		Babbles/appropriate sounds for age	Yes	No
		Good eye-hand coordination	Yes	No
	B.	Gross motor		
		Age-appropriate gait/ambulation (no tip-toe walking, no dragging of an extremity)	Yes	No
		Uncoordinated movements	No	Yes
		Psychomotor Developmental Index ≥90	Yes	No
IV.		Processing		
		Appreciation of object permanency	Yes	No
		Imitative abilities	Yes	No
		Simple problem-solving skills	Yes	No
V.		Mental Activity		
		Goal-directed behaviors	Yes	No
		Attentive procedures	Yes	No
		Average level of activity for age	Yes	No
		Persistent crying/irritability	No	Yes
		Mental Developmental Index ≥90	Yes	No
		Total Optimal _____		
		Total Nonoptimal _____		

Neuropsychological Optimality Score = $\dfrac{\text{Total Optimal ( )}}{\text{Optimal ( ) + Nonoptimal ( )}}$

Source: Aylward 1988.

directed reaching and grasping, secondary circular reactions, object permanence, gross motor skills, fine motor skills, social responsiveness, vocalizations, and language.

Prescriptive Assessment

Prescriptive assessment provides a more comprehensive understanding of the infant's abilities for treatment planning. This is usually obtained through the use of **criterion-referenced assessment** (such as the age at which the infant achieves developmental milestones) that provides information on how the infant performs on a series of activities without comparison to a normative group. The tests are based on a unifying theory of development and provide a framework for intervention programs. Two major criterion-referenced tests for infants are the Albert Einstein Scales of Sensorimotor Development (Escalona and Corman 1969, recently validated in high-risk neonates by Gardner et al. 1990) and the Infant Psychological Development Scale (IPDS, Uzgiris and Hunt 1975). The IPDS is based on Piaget's concept of sensorimotor intelligence and the sequence in which sensorimotor abilities develop. Factor analysis of the IPDS identified three clusters of behavior: causality, object permanence, and imitation. The scales are organized in a developmental sequence and are useful in planning interventions or stimulation in a "logical schematic manner" as a supplement to norm-referenced scales (Ulrey 1982b).

Dissatisfaction with the validity of infants tests has led investigators to develop more direct measures of cognitive ability in infancy. One such measure is the ability to process visual and auditory information (Fagan 1979, Gottlieb and Krasnegor 1985, Zelazo 1981). A method of measuring a child's responses to familiar and unfamiliar visual and auditory stimuli without the reliance on motor movements was introduced by Lewis and Goldberg (1969). These authors argued that the child's ability to habituate and dishabituate to a specific set of visual and auditory events is a function of the capacity for memory of events and perception of change. These functions are related to infant intelligence and may be more predictive of later intellectual outcome.

7.3   Issues in Infant Assessment

Transdisciplinary Assessment

Given the relatively undifferentiated state of the young infant, the value of discrete assessments by discipline can be aided by attempts to integrate findings across disciplines (Foley 1990). Additionally, since development is viewed in a social-environmental context, a comprehensive assessment of infant and family requires a transdisciplinary approach. Originally described by Hutchinson (1978), this approach provides a more holistic view of the child by pooling and exchanging information and skills.

Family Involvement

Also critical to infant assessment is how an infant's development affects and is affected by family functioning. The ability of a family to cope with the often complex and chronic demands of an infant with a developmental disorder may influence the long-term outcome for the infant (Ostfeld and Gibbs 1990). A realization of the importance of family involvement has led to an expanding body of information on the interactional effects of family functioning and infant development (Belsky and Isabela 1988).

Reliability

Obtaining a reliable estimate of a child's ability is difficult in infant testing because of the variability in the infant's behavior and the need to obtain the child's optimal performance. Test results can be compromised because of the infant's limited behavioral and verbal repertoire; the variable states of arousal (Prechtl and O'Brien 1982); the rapid emotional, cognitive and physical development; and inadequate training and experience of the examiner. The behavioral state (e.g., sleep, drowsiness, alertness) is especially critical in neonatal assessment because the quality of the reflexes that are elicited vary as a function of state. Infant state also influences habituation to external stimuli, muscle tone, and deep tendon reflexes (Prechtl 1977). With age, the influence of behavioral state on assessment results lessens, but physical and emotional discomfort, such as hunger, thirst, sleepiness, and motivation remain important variables in testing the young child (Ulrey 1982a). For example, significant differences in preschoolers' fluency in speaking was noted depending on whether the children were seen in the home, at school, or in a clinical setting (Silverman 1971). Temperamental predisposition can also influence test findings. Hertzig (1983) described how different temperamental characteristics, such as the difficult temperament, the slow-to-warm-up temperament, and the easy temperament, can influence test scores. Reliability of infant testing is also a function of the expertise of the examiner whose conclusions must be grounded in a knowledge of infant development and experience and familiarity with a wide range of infant behaviors. Trained and knowledgeable examiners for example, using the Bayley Scales, can reach reliability at the .80 and .90 level (Bayley 1969, Hatcher 1976).

Test Limitations

Some infant assessment instruments are qualitatively and psychometrically limited (Aylward 1988). Additionally, many of the norm-referenced tests of infancy are derived from normal infant population samples, but are often used to assess handicapped infants. The high level of dependence on motor behaviors in many infant tests up to 2 years of age tends to increase the risk of invalid assessment of children with physical handicaps and of underestimation of the cognitive ability of some handicapped children. The reliability of parental report has also been questioned, although recent findings by Creighton and Sauve (1988) indicate a strong correlation between results on the Bayley Scales of Development and parent report using the Minnesota Infant Developmental Inventory (MIDI). The results of their study indicate a potential use for the MIDI as a screening tool for follow-up programs of high-risk infants. Other limitations include the lack of explicit guidelines for administering and scoring certain test items (Aylward 1988, Yang 1979).

Stability and Continuity in Development

A major issue involves the concepts of stability and continuity in infant functions. Some theories of cognitive development (e.g., Bornstein and Krasnegor 1989, Bruner 1966, Piaget 1960) assume that there is a common substrate to cognitive development and that development is linear or continuous. The "continuous" theory holds that if behavioral processes are stable over time, an infant should maintain his or her relative position with respect to other infants. In support of this theory, Lu and co-workers (1989) found a linear increase in the development of mental abilities from birth to 1 year on the Bayley scales; Majnemer et al. (1992) also supported this view of an intrinsically programmed time- and environment-independent progression in an examination of low-risk preterm and normal infants with the Einstein scales. If behavioral and psychological processes are continuous, they should even persist without major change over the life-span. If development is stable and continuous, prediction of outcome, based on early assessment, should be fairly straightforward, and such dimensions as intelligence should be predictable through infancy, childhood, and adolescence into adulthood.

The issues of stability and continuity in infant tests are of great importance to those studying and working with high-risk infants. Although diagnosis in severely compromised infants is fairly clear, prediction of outcome is more complex. In infants in whom organic dysfunction is identified in infancy (e.g., Down syndrome), stability and continuity of impairment from infancy are more reliable, but can be influenced by environmental quality (Shonkoff and Hauser-Cram 1987). In infants with significant impairment (i.e., developmental quotients below 80), prediction rates for later successful intellectual outcome can account for as much as 45 per cent of the variance between early and later measures (Aylward and Kenny 1979). Predictive accuracy is similar in newborns with obvious neurological syndromes, i.e., apathy or hyperexcitability. These, however, are group predictions and do not allow for individual variability in infant development (Aylward et al. 1987).

In children whose test findings and performances are suspect, diagnosis and prediction of outcome are more difficult. Two studies of high-risk infants highlight this point. The first (Coolman et al. 1985) identified 50 per cent of the infants in their study as having mild neuromotor problems and 7 per cent with moderate neuromotor problems. At age 2 years, 75 per cent of the mild group and 50 per cent of the moderate group fell within normal limits. A second study (Aylward et al. 1987) followed 275 infants to age 3 years. Of the infants who were identified as cognitively suspect at the age of 40 weeks, 71 per cent were normal by the age of 3 years. Of those with questionable motor defects, 88 per cent had improved by age 3 years. Of those identified as neurologically suspect at 40 weeks, 93 per cent had improved at 3 years. These studies and others (Touwen 1978) suggest that CNS dysfunction at birth may not be permanent since the majority of infants recover (Aylward 1988). They lend support to the theory that since structural and functional relationships change over time, development is discontinuous. In contrast, Korner et al. (1989) found in two longitudinal studies of preterm infants considerable individual stability of performance across ages with highly significant developmental gains.

In children without organic impairment, continuity of functioning may depend on the behavior under study and the degree to which environmental circumstances endure over time. For example, children who are insecurely attached to parents during infancy have a higher likelihood of manifesting socioemotional difficulties later in life if the unfavorable environment that fostered this insecurity persists over time (Lamb et al. 1985).

The predictability of infant intelligence in non-organically impaired children depends on the method by which it is assessed. The correlations between traditional infant tests in the first 18 months of life and tests of intellectual ability in later childhood are low, although predictibility increases for the seriously delayed child (Bornstein and Sigman 1986, Honzik 1976). McCall (1979) analyzed the results of studies that had attempted to predict intellectual outcome in childhood from infant test scores. Table 7-3 shows the correlations between infant scores at various ages during the first 12 months. The closer together in time the assessments, the higher the correlation. Table 7-4 illustrates the weaker correlation across studies between infant test results and later childhood IQ. "The first and strongest effect is that the correlations increase linearly with the age at which the infant test is administered. . . . The second and weaker trend is the shorter the developmental period spanned, the higher the correlation" (McCall 1979, p. 712).

Table 7-3.   Median Correlations Across Studies Among Infant Test Scores at Various Stages During the First Two Years of Life

	First test period			
Second test period	1–3 mo	4–6 mo	7–12 mo	13–18 mo
1–6 mo	.52	—	—	—
7–12 mo	.29	.40	—	—
13–18 mo	.08	.39	.46	—
19–24 mo	−.04	.32	.31	.47

Source: Adapted from McCall 1979.

Table 7-4. Median Correlations Across Studies Between Infant Test Scores and Childhood IQ

Age of childhood tests (yr)	Age of Infant Tests (mo)			
	1–6	7–12	13–18	19–30
8–18	.06	.25	.32	.49
5–7	.09	.20	.34	.39
3–4	.21	.32	.5	.59

Source: Adapted from McCall 1979.

McCall concluded from his analysis that before 18 months of life parental education and socioeconomic status seem to be the best predictors of intellectual development in later childhood. The poor predictability of infant tests to later childhood is influenced by the qualitative differences between infant tests, which are mostly sensorimotor based, and the verbal-representational tests of later childhood (Gibbs 1990, McCall 1979).

McCall's observations support the view of development as discontinuous. Other authors also support this view. Amiel-Tison (1982) and Prechtl (1977) for example, referred to a silent period in which dysfunction observed during the first few days of life disappears only to resurface later in life. Amiel-Tison (1982) suggested that major changes in sensorineural functions occur during the first 6 months of life, whereas Prechtl (1984) recognized the second month of life as a time of important transitions. For a general discussion of growth spurts see Chapter 4.

In contrast, Siegel (1989) argued that traditional tests of intelligence in infancy and early childhood are predictive of later measures of intelligence. Siegel suggested that discrepancies in the literature regarding the failure of infant tests to predict later development are not a result of the tests per se, but are related to an analytic strategy that uses correlation coefficients. Furthermore, a measurement approach that focuses on the prediction of range rather than an exact score should be used. In assessing stability, Siegel argued that specific rather than global tests should be used (for a more comprehensive review, see Bornstein and Krasnegor 1989).

Information Processing Abilities as Indicators and Predictors of Intellectual Capacity

Several lines of investigation lend support to the hypothesis that information processing procedures, such as visual preference and recognition memory, habituation-recovery, and standard-transformation-return (STR), measure mental ability more accurately than conventional infant tests and predict intellectual functioning in later childhood more precisely (Sontheimer 1989, Zelazo and Weiss 1990).

RECOGNITION MEMORY AND INFANT INTELLIGENCE

Research conducted by early investigators (Fantz and Nevis 1967) established infant recognition as a measure of intellectual ability using a visual-novelty preference paradigm. In their studies, recognition memory was inferred by length of visual fixation, when an infant showed a preference for a novel over a familiar visual stimulus presented simultaneously. Fantz and Nevis (1967) were able to show that recognition memory developed at an earlier age in children of highly intelligent parents compared to children of parents of average intellectual ability. Using a similar technique, Miranda and Fantz (1974) found that the recognition memory of normal children was superior to children with Down syndrome at 13, 24, and 36 weeks of age. Preterm infants matched for conceptual age have shown less advanced recognition memory ability than term infants (Caron and Caron 1981). Moderate predictive validity coefficients of .35 and .57 were obtained between 5- to 7-month infant recognition scores and verbal IQ scores at 5 and 7 years by Fagan and McGrath (1981). Recognition memory and Bayley Mental Development scores in 19 infants with failure-to-thrive were correlated with Stanford Binet-Intelligence scores at 3 years of age (Fagan et al. 1986). Recognition memory (RM) predicted later intelligence with a moderate coefficient of .51, whereas the Bayley scores produced a lower coefficient of .23. Butterbaugh (1988) compared the mean predictive validity coefficients of sensorimotor tests (SM) for normal and high-risk samples from Fagan and Singer's study (1983) with the recognition memory tests from a study by Bornstein and Sigman (1986). Table 7-5 illustrates that the RM tests have stronger correlations with childhood intelligence tests and are more predictive than SM tests.

HABITUATION, RECOVERY AND INFANT INTELLIGENCE

The habituation-recovery paradigm (see Chapter 5) has also been used to measure infant attention and recognition, and studies have attempted to correlate these attributes with later intellectual outcome. In this paradigm a visual stimulus is presented over repeated trials. The decrease in looking time is called

Table 7-5. Mean Predictive Validity Coefficients for Infant Tests Across Normal and High-Risk Samples

Age (yr)	Sensorimotor tests		Recognition memory tests	
	Infant test age			
	0–11 mo		0–7 mo	
	Normal	High risk	Normal	High risk
2–3	.16	.23	.44	N.A.
4–5	.16	.18	.48	.50
6+	.11	.21	.56	.44

Source: Butterbaugh 1988.
N.A. = not available.

habituation. After habituation, a new stimulus is presented. Renewed responding to the new stimulus is called recovery, a measure of recognition memory. Lewis and Brooks-Gunn (1981) found that recovery to novel stimuli after habituation predicted later functioning on the Bayley scales at 24 months better than 3-month Bayley Scores. Bornstein (1990) compiled data from several longitudinal studies correlating measures of habituation (attention) in the first 6 months of life with cognitive outcome measures between 1 to 4 years of age and found a significant association between early habituation and later cognitive development (Table 7-6).

> This relation obtains across different laboratories, across different populations of both normal and at-risk infants, across different measures in infancy, across different modalities including visual and auditory, and for (at least) a small variety of different outcomes in childhood. . . . Although not large in absolute terms, in a climate of belief in instability, these correlations suggest a meaningful degree of stability in individual mental development (Bornstein 1990, p. 159).

Although RM tests show greater predictive validity, their practical application is limited, and currently there is only one commercially available RM test, the Fagan Test of Infant Intelligence (Fagan et al. 1986).

THE STANDARD-TRANSFORMATION-RETURN PROCEDURE

Zelazo and Weiss (1990) argued that, for an information processing measure of infant capabilities to be clinically useful, the time period of measurement should span a larger age range than the 3- to 7-month period used in the visual recognition and habituation literature. The Standard-Transformation-Return (STR)

Table 7-6. Representative Predictive Correlations From Habituation in Infancy

Test	Age (mo)	r
1. Bayley Scale Scores	12	.46
2. Productive Vocabulary	12	.52
3. Bates Language Comprehension	13	.35
4. Belsky Play Competence	13	.36
5. Representational Competence	13	.57
6. Reynell Language Score	24	.55
7. Wechsler Test Score (WPPSI)	48	.54

Source: Bornstein and Krasnegor 1990.
1. Bayley Scales of Infant Development (Bayley 1969); 2. Maternal estimate (Bornstein and Ruddy 1984); 3. Maternal Language Review (Bates et al. 1988); 4. Manual for the Assessment of Performance, Competence, & Executive Capacity in Infancy (Belsky and Most 1981; Belsky et al. 1983); 5. Latent variable of language comprehension and play sophistication (Tamis-LeMonda and Bornstein 1989); 6. Reynell Developmental Language Scales (Reynell 1981); 7. Wechsler Preschool & Primary Scale of Intelligence (Wechsler 1963).

Procedure "assesses the child's ability to create mental representations for events and measures the rate at which these representations are formed and announced" (Zelazo and Weiss 1990, p. 140). In the standard phase the child is provided with an opportunity to create an expectancy for a sequential event referred to as the standard, e.g., a toy car is released at the top of a ramp and is allowed to roll down and tap over a brightly colored object. In the transformation phase the infant's ability to form a mental representation of a discrepancy is assessed, e.g., the car taps the object, but the object does not fall. In the return phase, the infant's ability to recognize and assimilate the reappearance of the familiar standard is assessed, e.g., the car rolls and hits the object, which falls over. Measures of the child's heart rate, visual fixation, smiling, vocalizations, and pointing are recorded. Empirical support for the validity of the STR procedure as a measure of information processing comes from a series of studies (Zelazo and Kearsley 1989, Zelazo and Weiss 1990). Children with developmental delay were followed prospectively to 26 months of age. Seventy-five per cent of children who were categorized as delayed on conventional tests demonstrated intact information processing abilities, despite significant expressive language delays.

7.4   Assessment Tools in the First Two Years of Life

The functions assessed during the period of birth to 2 years and the techniques to measure them are age specific. Techniques that are not age related include morphological methods such as angiography, ultrasound scan, and CT scan; bioelectric measures, such as EEG and evoked potentials. More direct age-related evaluation of neurological status can be obtained through measurement of neuromotor functions.

Newborn and Neonatal Assessment

Assessment in the neonatal period provides an opportunity to determine the extent of any damage that may have been incurred during gestation or birth. The aim of the neonatal neurological examination is to assess the functional integrity and maturity of the CNS and to provide (1) an immediate diagnosis of an evident neurological problem (such as convulsion or coma) that will determine what therapy to begin; (2) an evaluation of day-to-day changes of a known neurological problem, such as an hypoxic episode; and (3) the long-term prognosis of a newborn (Parmelee and Michaelis 1971).

Traditionally, the neurological examination of the neonate has provided an appreciation of the neonate's response to negative stimuli at the midbrain level. The examination has undergone several modifications to increase its sensitivity. Peiper (1963) believed that the newborn functioned at the brainstem level and based his evaluation on observed reflexes also found in anencephalic infants. However, the reflexes were qualitatively different in the anencephalic infant, and those qualitative aspects of the reflexes thought to represent control by the pyramidal tract and motor cortical areas became an important part of the comprehensive neurological examination of Prechtl and Beintema (1965) and of Parmelee and Michaelis (1971).

Traditional neurological methods of assessment of full-term neonates include (1) the Graham Behavior Test for Neonates (Graham et al. 1956), which was revised by Rosenblith in 1961 and renamed the Graham-Rosenblith Test; (2) the neurological examination devised by Andre-Thomas et al. (1960), which was later elaborated by Saint-Anne Dargassies (1977); and (3) the Neurological Examination of the Full-term Newborn Infant by Prechtl and Beintema (1964), revised in 1977 (Prechtl 1977). Other techniques, such as those by Parmelee (1974) and Amiel-Tison (1976), are quicker to administer, but include a more limited range of test items and run the risk of misclassification of infants who do not appear sick but who may suffer from brain damage (Prechtl 1982).

A complete neurological examination includes evaluation of the infant's reflexes and responsiveness to stimulation, as well as muscle tone, physical condition, and general state. The **Dubowitz Scale** (Dubowitz et al. 1970, Table 7-7, Figures 7-1 to 7-4) is a widely used neurological assessment for the estimation of gestational age. This scoring system is based on 10 neurological signs related

Table 7-7. The Dubowitz Scale

	Score
Neurological signs	
Posture	0–4
Square window	0–4
Ankle dorsiflexion	0–4
Arm recoil	0–2
Leg recoil	0–2
Popliteal angle	0–5
Heel to ear	0–4
Scarf sign	0–3
Head lag	0–3
Ventral suspension	0–4
External criteria	
Amount of edema	0–2
Skin texture	0–4
Skin color	0–3
Skin opacity of the trunk	0–4
Amount of lanugo (fluffy hair) over the back	0–4
Plantar creases (on sole of foot)	0–4
Nipple formation	0–3
Breast size	0–3
Ear form	0–3
Ear firmness	0–3
Genitals	0–2

Source: Dubowitz et al. 1970.

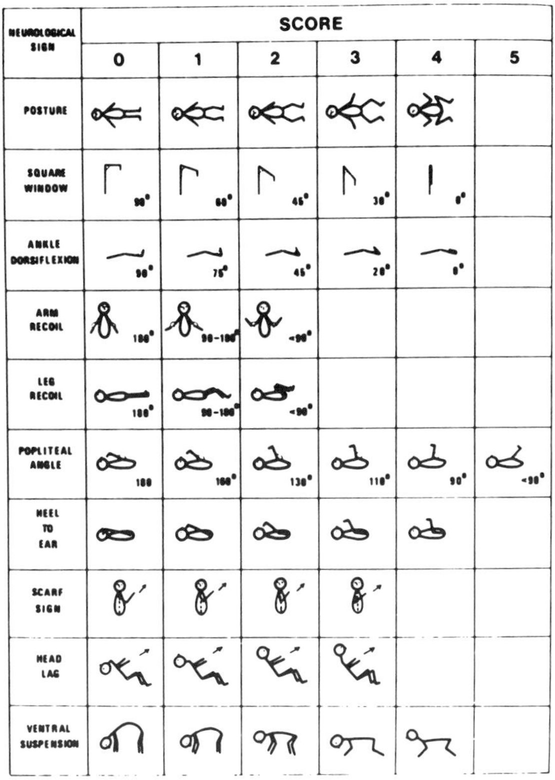

Figure 7-1. Scoring system for neurological criteria (Dubowitz et al. 1970). A total score greater than 70 corresponds to a gestational age of more than 43 weeks, of 50 to 39 weeks, and of 20 to 30 weeks gestational age.

mainly to postures and primitive reflexes suggested by the work of Prechtl and Beintema (1964) and Robinson (1966), as well as 11 external criteria (Farr et al. 1966). Recent research findings note that, when this scale is applied to preterm infants with birth weights of less than 1500 g, it tends to overestimate gestational age under 34 weeks (Sanders et al. 1991). Eyler et al. (1991) reduced the Dubowitz scales into four clinically meaningful clusters validated by factor analysis based on the assessment of 575 preterm infants.

The lengthier neurological examination of Prechtl and Beintema (1964) is used for a more complete examination of the high-risk full-term infant. The administration is standardized, and test items include observations of the infant's state. Six classifications of state are included.

State 1. Regular sleep: Eyes closed, respiration is regular, no movements except startles.

State 2. Irregular sleep: Eyes closed, respiration is irregular, no gross movements, but sudden jerks, startles, and facial expressions occur.

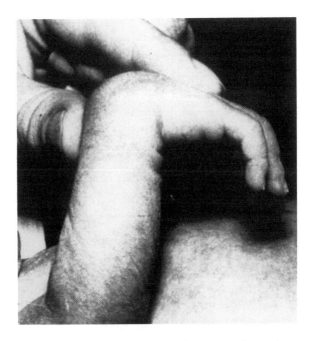

Figure 7-2. Technique for square window (Dubowitz et al. 1970).

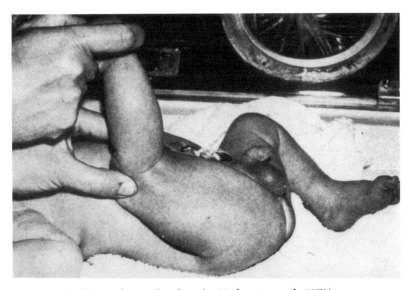

Figure 7-3. Technique for popliteal angle (Dubowitz et al. 1970).

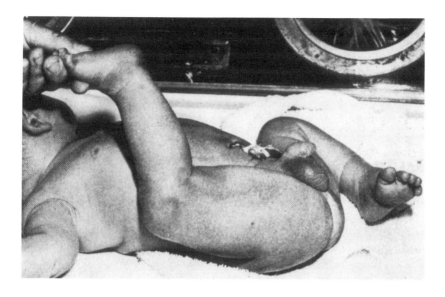

Figure 7-4.   Technique for heel to ear maneuver (Dubowitz et al. 1970).

State 3. Drowsiness: Bursts of writhing activity, the eyes open and close, and have a dull appearance.
State 4. Alert inactivity: The infant is relaxed, has a bright, shiny appearance, but is inactive. Visual search and regular breathing occur.
State 5. Waking activity: Eyes open, spurts of activity involving the whole body, respiration is irregular.
State 6. Crying with significant motor activity.

It is estimated that infants spend 67 per cent of their time in a sleep state, 7 per cent in drowsiness, 10 per cent in alert inactivity, 11 per cent in waking activity, and 5 per cent in crying (Berg et al. 1973).

Spontaneous movement, color and respiration, reflexes, and resistance to passive movement are also included in the standard neurological examination. The final summary incorporates a diagnosis based on the appraisal of posture, motility, motor systems, response thresholds, tendon reflexes, state, crying, pathological movements, hemisyndrome, and reaction type (normal, hyperexcitability, apathetic, and comatose). The assessment by Prechtl and Beintema (1964) was originally conducted on 1500 children with high observer reliability (.80 and .96). Prechtl (1967) reported on the highly significant prognostic value of this examination in a group of 285 high-risk infants followed to 2, 4, and 8 years of age. The correlation between neurological findings and follow-up examinations was highly significant. Using a briefer neurological examination, Amiel-Tison

(1982) was able to identify several clinical indicators of CNS dysfunction in the neonate (Table 7-8).

The classic pediatric neurological assessment of the neonate is based on responses to painful or intrusive stimuli mediated by the midbrain. It directs less attention to the available organized behavior that the infant can demonstrate as reflexive behavior is suppressed in order to attend to more interesting stimuli. To record and evaluate some of the more integrative behaviors of the neonate, Brazelton (1973) developed a neurobehavioral evaluation scale known as the **Brazelton Scale**: the Brazelton Neonatal Behavioral Assessment Scale (BNBAS). The examination consists of 20 elicited reflex items (Table 7-9) and 27 behavioral responses to environmental stimuli during a graded series of procedures, such as talking, holding, and rocking (Table 7-10). Test items on the BNBAS may be grouped into four clusters: (1) attention and social responsiveness, (2) motor and tone capacity, (3) state regulation, and (4) physiological response to stress. Data were collected from a homogeneous group of 54 healthy full-term, white newborns with repeated assessment on days 1, 2, 3, 4, 5, 7, and 10 and provide a picture of the behavioral recovery of a group of newborns who experience minimal trauma during or following delivery (Als et al. 1977). The BNBAS has been used in studies of such issues as the effects of maternal obstetric medication (Tronick et al. 1976), the effects of phototherapy and hyperbilirubinemia (Edgell 1986, Telzrow et al. 1976), seizures (Emory et al. 1989), cross-cultural differences (Brazelton et al. 1976), prenatal care and dietary practices (Lester et al. 1986). Predictive validity of the BNBAS and the neurological examination developed by the Collaborative Study of the National Institute for Nervous Disease and Stroke (NINDS) was measured against the 7-year outcome of a group of 54 infants (Tronick et al. 1976). In this study, the BNBAS was

Table 7-8.   Clinical Features of Neurological Dysfunction in the Neonate

Coma	Areactivity, absence of corneal and sucking reflexes
Lethargy	Hyporeactivity, no crying
Status epilepticus	Repeated seizures and coma
Isolated seizure	With rapid recovery of consciousness after seizure
Hyperexcitability	Jitteriness, tremor, clonic movements bursts of agitation, poor sleep, high-pitched cry, sustained clonus
Hypertonia	Generalized, limited to neck extensors, opisthotonos
Hypotonia	Generalized, upper part of the body, one side of the body (hemisyndrome)
Primary reflexes	No primary reflexes, in particular, Moro reflex is abolished and sucking
Primary reflexes	Poor responses, not reproducible
Ocular signs	Conjugated deviation, setting-sun sign, sustained nystagmus
Intracranial hypertension	Tense fontanelle, distended sutures, particularly the squamous, neck extensors, hypertonia
Abnormal respiration	Irregular, apnea

Source: Amiel-Tison 1982.

Table 7-9. Brazelton Neonatal Behavioral Assessment
Scale—Reflex Behaviors

	Xa	O	L	M	H	A
Plantar grasp						
Hand grasp						
Ankle clonus						
Babinski						
Standing						
Automatic walking						
Placing						
Incurvation						
Crawling						
Glabella						
Tonic deviation of head and eyes						
Nystagmus						
Tonic deviation of head						
Moro						
Rooting (intensity)						
Sucking (intensity)						
Passive movement						
Arms R						
L						
Legs R						
L						

Source: Als et al. 1977.
Xa = response omitted, O = response not elicited, L = low, M =
medium, H = high, A = asymmetry of response.

able to predict 12 out of 15 children classified as abnormal at age 7 years. The
lower false-alarm rate, argued Brazelton, is probably because the BNBAS elicits
higher-order functioning to predict a recovery process (such as alertness, state
organization, and quality of movement) than does the NINDs exam. The assessment of preterm infants can be carried out using the scales developed by
Als et al. (1982) and Korner and Thom (1990).

A more recent assessment tool was derived from a correlation matrix using
factor analysis of items from several neurological examinations. It includes a
neonatal examination, referred to as the Neoneuro (or Neonatal Neurological
Examination, Sheridan-Pereira et al. 1991), and an infant neurological scale, the
Infanib (or Infant International Battery). Results of examinations of 1237
neonates were analyzed. Thirty-two items were grouped into seven dimensions:
hypertonus, primitive reflexes, limb tone, neck support, reflexes, alertness, and
fussy. From the total scores, cut-off points were recommended for four levels
of normality-abnormality. The scoring system is reported to be well based both
theoretically and psychometrically. The quantified scoring system permits evaluation of individual neonates, as well as comparison of samples of neonates on

Table 7-10.   Brazelton Neonatal Behavioral Assessment Scale—Global Descr
and Interaction Repertoire of the Newborn

	Descriptive paragraph			
Attractiveness	0	1	2	3
Interfering variables	0	1	2	3
Need for stimulation	0	1	2	3

What activity did the baby use to self-quiet?

Behavioral items

1. Response decrement to light (2, 3)
2. Response decrement to rattle (2, 3)
3. Response decrement to bell (2, 3)
4. Response decrement to pinprick (1, 2, 3)
5. Orientation inanimate visual (4)
6. Orientation inanimate auditory (4, 5)
7. Orientation animate visual (4)
8. Orientation animate auditory (4, 5)
9. Orientation animate visual and auditory (4)
10. Alertness (4)
11. General tonus (4, 5)
12. Motor maturity (5, 6)
13. Pull-to-sit (3, 5)
14. Cuddliness (4, 5)
15. Defensive movements (4)
16. Consolability (6 to 5, 4, 3, 2)
17. Peak of excitement (6)
18. Rapidity of buildup (from 1, 2 to 6)
19. Irritability (3, 4, 5)
20. Activity (alert states)
21. Tremulousness (all states)
22. Startle (3, 4, 5, 6)
23. Lability of skin color (from 1 to 6)
24. Lability of states (all states)
25. Self-quieting activity (6, 5, to 4, 3, 2, 1)
26. Hand-mouth facility (all states)

Source: Als et al. 1977.
Numbers in parentheses refer to optimal state for assessment.

item scores, subscores, and total scores (Sheridan-Periera et al. 1991). Both subscale and total scores can be used for data analysis and are computer compatible.

In summary, there have been encouraging advances in the neurological and behavioral assessment of neonates over the last 20 years. Prechtl (1982), however, struck a cautionary note:

> The repeated attempts to shorten or modify comprehensive and standard-
> ized methods have hampered rather than promoted progress, as they seem

to have been made without careful reflection on the strategies of the approach, and without necessary expertise in examining the developing brain. One cannot escape the impression, that item collections, which form a scale and produce a score, have a strong appeal despite the fact that what is to be quantified is often expressed only in vague terms (p. 46).

Assessment Beyond the Neonatal Period

The healthy development of infants sets the stage for their entry into the world of preschool, kindergarten, and school. Health care professionals have become involved in the assessment of infants and preschoolers to identify various problems that may affect later functioning. The rationale is "that early identification of problems can lead to early intervention, to correcting or minimizing these problems, or at least to providing supportive resources to the child and family" (Ireton 1990, p. 78).

The areas typically included in assessment of the infant up to the age of 2 years are cognition, memory and learning, language and speech, motor skills, self-help or independence skills, and social-emotional development. Assessment is based on direct testing of the child, combined with parent-rating scales of infant behavior and the home or day-care environment, and draws on tests from neurology and developmental psychology. Table 7-11 (Butterbaugh 1988) provides a selective list of test instruments for infants. A more comprehensive description of infant tests can be found in Frankenburg (1983), Teti and Gibbs (1990), Tramontana and Hooper (1988, 1992) and Ulrey and Rogers (1982).

Traditional infant tests emphasize sensorimotor and visual-perceptual abilities, including fine motor construction, visual motor integration, and gross motor abilities. The Milani-Comparetti (1967) examination provides an opportunity to evaluate reflexes at this age. Signs of possible dysfunction include the persistence of primitive reflexes, irritability, chronic dystonia, a strong hand preference, stereotyped and repetitive movements, and developmental quotients greater than two standard deviations below the mean (Aylward 1988). Tests of infant mental development are among the oldest infant tests and have been used extensively to identify infants at risk for mental retardation. Some of the most commonly used standardized instruments for infants up to age of 2 years have already been mentioned and include the Gesell Developmental Schedules (Knobloch et al. 1980, 1987), the Bayley Scales of Infant Development (Bayley 1969), the Griffiths Mental Developmental Scale (Griffiths 1970), the Cattell Infant Intelligence Scale (1940), the Milani-Comparetti Neuro-Developmental Screening examination (Milani-Comparetti and Gidoni 1967) and the Battelle Developmental Inventory (Newborg et al. 1984). "The best approach seems to be a selection of combinations of items, drawn from existing tests but based on a conceptual framework of functions" (Aylward 1988, p. 243). A developmental neuropyschological approach should incorporate a combination of existing developmental and neurological techniques with age. Development, environment, and neurological impairment form a complex interactive matrix. Psychologists

Table 7-11. Assessment Instruments Used in Early Neuropsychological Testing

Assessment instrument	Description	Information	Comment
Age: Newborn Brazelton Neonatal Behavioral Assessment Scale (Brazelton, 1973)	27 behavioral items (9-point scale), 20 elicited responses (3-point scale)	How infant responds to caretakers and environment; states, habituation, orientation (visual, auditory), muscle tone, activity; "best performance"	(+) Clinical instrument, provides good research information, recovery from stress; (−) some problems with data interpretation and scaling, poor long-range prediction
Prechtl Neurological Examination (Prechtl), 1977; Prechtl & Beintema, 1964)	Approximately 52 items + states, postures, spontaneous activity	Gross state of CNS reactivity (motor activity, states) + specific lesional approach; syndromes identified	(+) Extensively studied, good standardization, provides immediate diagnosis, prognosis, those needing follow-up, behavioral response descriptions; (−) lengthy, perhaps too detailed
Brief Infant Neurobehavioral Optimality Scale (Aylward, et al. 1985)	Reduced version of Revised Prechtl Neurological Examination, 15 items scored in optimal/nonoptimal manner	Screen of CNS intactness (tonus, tendon reflexes, spontaneous activity, some primitive reflexes)	(+) Easily administered, less time-consuming, similar sensitivity and specificity values as Prechtl, summary score; (−) not as much data on states, not as extensive as Prechtl
Parmelee's Neurological Examination (Parmelee et al. 1974)	Divided into two sections—Section I: state observations, 20 items; Section II: crying, activity, tremor, etc.	Active and reflexive muscle tone, primary reflexes, arousal, and spontaneous behavior	(+) Brief—takes 10 minutes to administer, summary score; (−) not as extensive as Prechtl

Table 7-11. Continued

Assessment instrument	Description	Information	Comment
Graham Behavior Test for Neonates (Graham et al. 1956; Rosenblith 1974)	Five scales: pain threshold, maturational level, visual responsiveness, irritability, and muscle tension ratings; pain threshold deleted in revision	Originally designed to differentiate normal and brain-injured newborns; motor function (head control, crawl) tactile-adaptive (cotton over nose), visual tracking, auditory responsiveness, irritability rating	(+) Correlations between neonatal data and early infant data, revision had large sample; (−) long-range predictability fair, used infrequently
Neonatal Neurological Examination (Sheridan-Pereira et al. 1991	32 items, 7 dimensions: hypotonus, primitive reflexes, limb tone, neck support, reflexes, alertness, fussiness.	Normality/abnormality cut-off, combined with Infant International Battery	Quantified scoring system, item scores, subscores, and total scores can be compared to large normative sample
Age: Infancy Gesell Developmental Schedules (Knobloch & Pasmanick, 1974; Knobloch et al. 1987)	Items provided at each of key ages, under five groups; can be scored by observation or history	Key ages: 4, 16, 28, and 40 weeks; 12, 18, 36, and 48 months; gross motor, fine motor, adaptive, language, personal-social	(+) Basis for most examinations of infancy; good screening inventory; (−) not as well standardized as other infant examinations, ratio developmental quotient
Bayley Scales of Infant Development (Bayley 1969)	Mental Developmental Index (163 items), Psychomotor Developmental Index (81 items), Infant Behavior Record	Sensorimotor skills, problem solving, verbal skills, and areas outlined previously in Gesell	(+) Well standardized, good overall assessment of child's strengths and weaknesses, most widely used; (−) questionable predictability, very dependent on motor function

Table continued

135

Table 7-11. Continued

Assessment instrument	Description	Information	Comment
Griffiths Mental Developmental Scale (Griffiths 1954, 1970)	Derived from Gesell, 498 items, most detailed in first 2 years; five areas with several items for each month of age	Locomotor, personal-social, hearing and speech, eye and hand coordination, performance; designed to enable examiner to distinguish normal and abnormal children	Used predominantly in Great Britain, (+) rigorous training; (−) many unreliable items
Cattell Infant Intelligence Scale (1940)	Items arranged on an age scale, drawing from Gesell at early ages and Stanford-Binet from 22 months upwards; 2–36 months	Many motor items at early ages; later ages include more cognitive and language items; provides an IQ score	(+) Smooth transition from infant to early childhood examination, good for testing older children who function at lower levels; (−) small standardized sample (294), IQ concept questionable, not used frequently
Milani-Comparetti Neuro-Developmental Screening Examination (Milani-Comparetti and Gidoni 1967)	Assesses spontaneous behavior, postural control, evoked responses; chart provided with age norms in terms of onset and disappearance of responses 0–24 months	Neuromotor abnormalities—head and body control, movement, evoked primitive reflexes, righting, parachute, and tilting reactions; enables detection of cerebral palsy, developmental delay	(+) Administered in 5–10 minutes, good screening device that can be used with other examinations; (−) tilting reactions need tilt board, which is often not readily available
Age: Toddler/early childhood Merrill-Palmer Scale of Mental Tests (Stutsman 1948); Extended Merrill-Palmer Scales (1969)	Verbal, perceptual-motor, and nonverbal items grouped into 6-month age ranges; extended version has 16 tasks—11/2–6 years, 3–5 years	Perceptual-motor function; extended version—semantic production and evaluation, figural production and evaluation (verbal expression, comprehension, perceptual-motor, and nonverbal skills)	(+) Can be used in language-delayed children, high interest level for children; (−) norms outdated, heavily loaded with perceptual performance items, should be used as a supplemental test, poor predictive validity

136

Table 7-11. Continued

Assessment instrument	Description	Information	Comment
Stanford-Binet (1960; Terman & Merrill 1972)	Age 2–adult, provides IQ score; grouped at half-year intervals from 2 to 5, yearly thereafter	General intellectual abilities; general comprehension, visual-motor ability, arithmetic reasoning, memory and concentration, vocabulary, judgment and reasoning	(+) Used frequently, good predictive utility; (−) unequal distribution of verbal and nonverbal items at different ages, heavy loading of perceptual/performance items at early ages
Stanford-Binet–Revised (Thorndike, et al. 1986)	Items of same type grouped into 15 tests—2–adult	Four areas assessed: verbal, abstract/visual, quantitative reasoning, short-term memory	(+) Differentiates between MR and LD, better reliability, better underlying test theory; (−) new instrument, needs more application
McCarthy Scales of Children's Abilities (McCarthy 1972)	Eighteen component tests divided into five scales: verbal, perceptual-performance, quantitative, memory, and motor; provides a General Cognitive Index, 21/2–81/2 years	Five scales + general cognitive (summary of verbal, perceptual-performance, and quantitative); provides good overview of child's general function (verbal and nonverbal) as well as specific strengths and weaknesses; early detection of LD	(+) Age equivalents available for subtests, includes a gross motor component, best in the 3- to 5-year age range, can prorate; (−) LD children score lower on this test, may give underestimate of child's true abilities, of limited utility for older children

administering and interpreting the assessment results require training affiliated with pediatrics, pediatric neurology, neonatology, genetics, or interdisciplinary clinics.

Summary

Infant assessment provides information which is important in the early identification and diagnosis of central nervous system dysfunction and aids in the formulation of treatment plans. Modern day assessment techniques originated in the early work of Binet and Gesell, who established procedures for standardized assessments and norm-based comparisons of mental ability and general development. Infant assessment today is more holistic and integrative, and provides information, for example, about neuro-motor integrity, language development, social behavior, play and family interactions. Experimental research techniques have provided important procedures for measuring attention and memory in infants. The functions assessed, and the techniques used to measure these functions, vary with the child's age. In the newborn and neonatal period, an important aim of assessment is to provide information about the functional integrity and maturity of the CNS. This is accomplished by the traditional neurological examination and the more recently developed neurobehavioral examinations. Assessment beyond the neonatal period is based on direct testing of the child, parent-rating scales and draws on neurology and developmental psychology and takes into account the social milieu of the child. Some of the test instruments rely heavily on motor behaviors and tend to increase the risk of an invalid assessment of children with physical handicaps. The reliability of the results obtained from infant assessments may be influenced by the infant's temperament and by the inadequate training and experience of the examiner. The predictive validity of traditional infant tests is stronger in infants with significant CNS dysfunction. In non-organically impaired infants, the prediction rate for later intellectual outcome is low, although some authors have demonstrated that this depends on how specific the tests are and how the results are analyzed. There appears to be a growing body of research findings to support the notion of a significant association between infant attention and memory and later cognitive development. A recent trend in infant assessment incorporates a developmental neuropsychological approach that uses a combination of test instruments from developmental psychology and neurology and requires specific training in an interdisciplinary setting.

8

Critical Periods, Plasticity, and Recovery of Function

At first glance the concepts of critical periods and plasticity seem to be opposites, one suggesting rigidity, the other flexibility. On closer scrutiny, however, the ideas are not incompatible. At some developmental stages the organism is more receptive or vulnerable to environmental influences than at other stages, and it is at these times that the labels "critical" or "sensitive" are applied. The ability of the CNS to change in response to these environmental influences is referred to as "plasticity." Both concepts have a direct bearing on the recovery of function after brain lesions.

8.1 Critical Periods

Definitions and Criteria

Essentially, the **critical period** is the time between the emergence anatomically or functionally of a given biobehavioral system and its maturation. The system may be affected in this emergent but immature state (for better or worse) by exogenous stimuli and this effect can be permanent should the system "harden" to maturity (Colombo 1982, p. 263).

The concept of critical periods has its origins in experimental embryology. Working on the effects of inorganic compounds on the development of Fundulus eggs, Stockard (1921) first thought that the development of one-eyed fishes was caused specifically by magnesium ion. Further experiments showed that similar malformations could be produced by other inorganic chemicals administered at appropriate times during development. Although the concept has been attributed to Stockard, he himself gives credit to Dareste for originating the basic idea 30 years earlier. Stockard, and later Child (1941), went on to

139

specify that the more rapidly growing tissues are most sensitive to interference (Dennenberg 1968). In line with this early work, the concept of critical periods in development refers to stages of maximum sensitivity to exogenous stimuli.

The criteria for a critical period include (1) an identifiable onset and terminus; (2) an intrinsic component (i.e., the organism's sensitivity must be triggered by some maturational event); and (3) an extrinsic component, i.e., an external stimulus to which the organism is sensitive (Nash 1978).

The main areas of critical-period research have been visual development in the cat, imprinting in precocial birds, and socialization in dogs (for a comprehensive bibliography in these areas, see Colombo 1982). This research indicates that the period begins not with a sudden change but rather with a gradual rise in sensitivity to the critical stimulus. This increase in sensitivity reaches a plateau that can last from hours to days or years, depending on the behavior under investigation. The increase is in part a reflection of biological maturation, but it may also be triggered or extended by external stimuli. For example, Garey and Pettigraw (1974) noted that synaptic vesicles in the feline visual cortex could be reduced by limiting visual input.

The termination of a critical period may also be gradual, but is generally less so than the onset. It remains controversial whether the critical period ends as a result of intrinsic or extrinsic factors, but current data suggest that biological factors probably set an outer limit on the period.

The intrinsic component consists of the neurobiological changes that underlie the sensitivity to stimuli. Most critical periods are paralleled by periods of rapid development. In mammalian visual development the critical periods for binocular vision correspond to the postnatal development of the visual cortex (age 4 to 12 weeks in the cat, the first 9 weeks in the rhesus monkey, and the first 3 years in humans) when cells compete for cortical synapses (Colombo 1982).

The extrinsic component consists of the critical stimuli or events that can influence an organism's development. In some cases the nature of the extrinsic factor remains nonspecific. Lenneberg (1967) argued that a child must be exposed to language before age 14 if language is to be acquired and used. In contrast, such specific stimuli as exposure to light and ocular movement of the eyes are critical in the development of cortical binocularity (Freeman and Bonds 1979).

Critical Periods During Prenatal Development

At the cellular level there is some support for the critical period hypothesis. For example, in his study of the nerve fibers that connect the retina and the optic tectum in the frog, Jacobson (1978) was able to specify the exact point in development at which a disruption of the prespecified connections is irreversible. During the early stages of development the optic nerve can be severed and the eye inverted, but the nerve will regenerate and the eye will develop normally. At larval stage 31 and beyond, inversion of the eye causes the frog to have permanently inverted vision. Sperry (1963) attributed this developmental process to the biochemical specificity, or chemospecificity, acquired by each retinal ganglion cell.

There is also a great deal of gross embryological support for the hypothesis. **Teratogens**—agents capable of producing a deformed fetus—if introduced at particular times, produce a range of congenital anomalies. The organ systems most affected are those that show maximum cellular growth at the time of teratogenic introduction. Those systems that have either passed or not yet reached the rapid-growth stage are spared (Hamburger 1954). During the fertilization and implantation period in humans, which lasts from conception to 17 days gestation, toxic agents can interfere with all cells and result in death. The embryonic period from 18 to 55 days is the time of organ differentiation and characteristically shows extreme sensitivity to teratogenic agents. Exposure to toxic agents during this period produces both functional and morphological deficits.

Several principles of teratology require emphasis:

1. The critical period for teratogenesis is the phase of organ differentiation; this period corresponds approximately to the first trimester in humans.
2. Susceptibility to teratogens, however, depends on the genotype of the conceptus, thereby resulting in different effects in different species.
3. A variety of different teratogens may produce the same malformation.
4. A variety of malformations may result from a single teratogen.
5. Manifestations of deviant development vary with exposure.

The developmental defects arising from teratogenic influences include developmental arrest, agenesis (absence of an organ), hyperplasia (abnormal increase in cell numbers), and aberrant development. Teratogenic agents that cause abnormalities during the embryonic stage include infections, drugs, environmental pollutants, and metabolic deficiencies, which are discussed in detail in Chapters 14 and 15. Best known among the infections are syphilis, toxoplasmosis, rubella, cytomegalovirus, and herpesvirus—the STORCH agents. Among drugs, thalidomide is infamous for producing **phocomelia**, a shortening of the limbs. Studies have shown that the critical period for phocomelic defects is between 20 to 40 days after conception. Tetracycline has been implicated as causing eighth (auditory) nerve damage and multiple skeletal anomalies. Alcohol abuse during pregnancy has been correlated with microcephaly, cardiac defects, growth retardation, and developmental delay (Howard and Hill 1979, Schroeder 1987).

Among the various environmental pollutants associated with gross abnormalities, mercury, DDT, carbon monoxide, and lead have been studied most extensively. In addition, radiation injury in the embryo or fetus has been recognized for some time and depends largely on age at time of exposure. If the exposure takes place in the first 1 or 2 weeks, resorption of the embryo is probable (Wald 1979). Between the second and sixth weeks, the effect is on the particular organs undergoing development at that time. With increasing gestational age, more subtle generalized effects may occur, leading to deficits in growth and development. Human anomalies reported to have been induced by irradiation include microcephaly, hydrocephaly, mental deficiency, blindness, and spina bifida. Dobbing (1968) noted a relationship among maternal proximity to the center of the Hiroshima atomic bomb explosion, gestational age of less than 15 weeks, and the incidence of microcephaly and mental retardation.

The relationship between the severity and number of malformations and size of the teratogenic dosage occurring in the embryological period is fairly well established. During the period of fetal development, lasting from the 56th day to birth, the fetus becomes less susceptible to gross malformations, and the primary effect of exposure to noxious environmental influences is reduction in cell size and number (Howard and Hill 1979). The relationship between subteratogenic or marginally teratogenic doses and development has also been studied. A dose-response relationship has been hypothesized (Butcher et al. 1975) and is illustrated in Figure 8-1. The curve describes the increase in the number of gross malformations associated with large teratogenic doses during a period of rapid growth in the CNS. The right-hand curve describes a similar relationship for embryo lethal effects. The left-hand curve suggests that, in addition to embryo lethal and teratogenic effects, a given dose of a CNS teratogen may also produce functional impairments, including possible learning impairment or abnormal activity patterns.

The idea that behavioral deficits may result from low doses of teratogens during fetal development finds support in the animal research of Dobbing

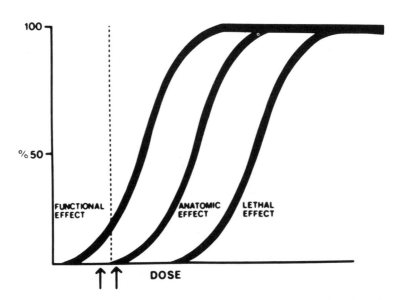

Figure 8-1. Dose-response relationships for agents teratogenic to the CNS (Butcher et al. 1975).

(1968), Hicks and D'Amoto (1966), and Hutchings et al. (1975). For instance, excessive levels of vitamin A in fetal rats can produce motor disturbances and behavioral patterns resembling those of children with so-called minimal brain dysfunction. In neonates, injection of a protein synthesis blocker, cycloheximide, in 15- to 30-day-old rats resulted in increased intraspecies aggressiveness, whereas injections in 35- to 50-day-old rats did not exert a substantial influence (Rylov and Anokhin 1992). Motor activity response to amphetamine given in adulthood is related to the timing of administration of cocaine during a critical period between 1 and 10 days, but not during days 11 to 20 (Hughes et al. 1991). In young children, the timing and duration of thyroid hormone deficiency have been related to specific critical periods with different outcomes (e.g., poorer visuospatial and verbal skills) at age 5 (Rovet et al. 1992). Rovet et al. (1990) also established critical periods of sensitivity of different brain regions to the effects of diabetes. Children with onset before age 5 were poorer in visuospatial abilities, whereas those with later onset were poorer in verbal skills.

Dobbing (1968) asserted that there is a **vulnerable period**, rather than a critical one, at the time of rapid brain growth in humans, beginning at approximately 25 weeks gestational age. During this period, maturation of axonal and dendritic growth, glial multiplication, myelination, and growth in size take place (Figure 8-2). Nutritional stunting in rats has been used as an animal model to test the hypothesis (Dobbing 1968). Restriction on growth during this period

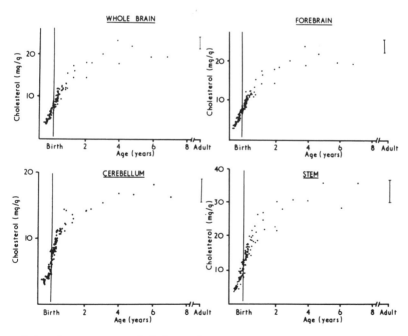

Figure 8-2. Concentration of cholesterol per unit fresh weight in whole brain, forebrain, cerebellum, and stem during growth (Dobbing and Sands 1973).

retards development and reduces the ultimate size of the brain. In behavioral terms, deficits of function rather than physical anomalies appear. The testing of Dobbing's hypothesis is far from complete and has involved experimental work with animals and observational studies with human populations at risk. Results indicate that deprivation during the time of rapid brain growth produces subtle behavioral deficits in learning ability. Although such species as the rat show distinct fetal development periods similar to humans and can be used for animal model studies (Winick 1976), generalizations across species and inferences about consequences in the human fetus remain speculative at best.

Critical Periods in Postnatal Development

Although the concept of critical periods is well established in embryological terms and in many cases can be defined precisely, the issue of whether the concept has equal validity in behavioral and psychological terms after birth has raised considerable debate.

Traces of the critical period hypothesis can be found in Freud's notion of the origin of human neuroses in early infancy and in his belief that early infancy is an especially sensitive period of development. The early work of Lorenz in 1937 (Lorenz 1970) also emphasized the importance of critical periods in the formation of primary social bonds in birds (imprinting). Later, McGraw (1946) suggested a critical period for the learning of motor skills in infancy. The idea of critical periods was also promulgated by Scott (1958) to explain socialization in dogs. The concept of educational readiness and stage-dependent theories of development, such as those of Piaget, imply a critical period hypothesis (Connolly 1973). The hypothesis has been expanded to include three major aspects of postnatal development: (1) the effects of early experience; (2) the establishment of basic social relationships, in particular the formation of attachment; and (3) learning.

CRITICAL PERIODS AND EARLY EXPERIENCE

Over the last 40 years, an extensive literature on the effects of early experience has accumulated. Not only can genetically based characteristics be extensively modified by early experience but early experiences are also one of the principal sources of individual differences in behavior. In humans, studies ranging from the effects of environmental deprivation (Fujinaga et al. 1990) to the effects of early musical training on the acquisition of absolute pitch (Cohen and Baird 1990) have been reported. The main evidence, however, comes from animal experimentation.

Sensory deprivation studies in animals indicate that there is a genuine critical period during which suitable experiences must occur if the visual system is to develop and function normally. Rearing laboratory animals in the dark results in neuroanatomical and neurochemical changes that lead to later defects in visuomotor coordination and degenerative changes in several regions: the retina, the lateral geniculate body of the thalamus, and the granular and supragranular layers of the visual cortex (Riesen 1975, Toyama et al. 1991). There is a relationship between the time of onset and length of light deprivation and the severity of effects (Rosinski 1977). A few hours of light exposure after the first opening of the eyes will reduce the neuroanatomical effects of subsequent visual deprivation (McVicker-Hunt 1979).

A relationship between specific environmental stimuli and physiological change has been demonstrated in experimental work with cats. Exposure to horizontal, vertical, or slanted lines or to stroboscopic light alters cell response in the lateral geniculate nuclei and changes the shape of the cortical response (Cremieux et al. 1992, Rosinski 1977). If this procedure is carried out for only one eye, a shrinkage of cells in the corresponding lateral geniculate nucleus occurs, but at the same time more cells are driven by the normal eye than would be found if binocular vision had not been interfered with (Cynader 1982, Hubel and Wiesel 1965). The critical period for such interference in kittens lasts from 2 to 5 weeks (Van Sluyters and Freeman 1977).

Clinical reports and psychophysical studies suggest that there is a similar sensitive period for the development of the human visual system that occurs sometime during the first 2 years; that susceptibility may continue up to 4 to 5 years. Hickey (1977) described a period of susceptibility for the parvocellular layer (X cells) of the lateral geniculate nucleus that might extend through the first 12 months; the period of rapid growth occurs in the first 6 months. Hickey also suggested a period of susceptibility for the magnocellular layer (Y cells) of the lateral geniculate nucleus that might continue until the end of the second year; the period of most rapid growth occurs in the first 12 months. During development the X and Y cells may compete for synaptic space relaying to cortical cells. By maturing faster, the X cells may gain an advantage that would show up when the system is visually deprived. These mechanisms may play a role in the effects of deprivation on monocular and binocular vision.

Comparisons of how early experiential enrichment and/or deprivation affects brain development in experimental animals support the idea of a sensitive period in early development. The basic model has been to compare the effects of pet-reared or enriched conditions (EC) with cage-reared or isolated conditions (IC) on both biochemical and morphological characteristics of the brain. In general, EC produce a brain that is heavier and thicker, especially in the occipital lobes (Bennett et al. 1964). Weight and thickness have proved to be a function of corresponding differences in dendritic volume, glial density, and size of nerve cell bodies (Greenough 1976).

Similar research paradigms on contrasting conditions for laboratory-reared animals have also highlighted the importance of EC for improved performance (Dennenberg 1968, Hebb 1949). EC also clearly improve recovery of function in lesioned rats (Rose et al. 1992). Conversely, the debilitating consequences of IC seem to be long lasting. Harlow and Harlow's (1965) famous studies demonstrated that monkeys reared from birth in social isolation are unable to mother successfully in adulthood. The results of most experimental animal studies that include measures of both CNS and behavioral variables support the view that the developing brain is sensitive to the effects of environmental deprivation.

CRITICAL PERIODS FOR BASIC SOCIAL RELATIONSHIPS

The notion of the effects of early environmental deprivation on animal brain structure and early learning has its counterpart in the study of basic social relations.

In human development the view that maternal deprivation in the first few years of life, through institutionalization or hospitalization, leads to later maladaptive behavior was clearly expressed in the work of Spitz (1945), verEecke (1989), and Bowlby (1951). They hypothesized a critical period for the development of social bonds that lasted from birth into the preschool years. The estimated length of the critical period varies from author to author. Goldfarb (1943) assumed that the critical period for social bonding terminates at age 3. Bowlby's so-called affectionless psychopaths were found to have been maternally deprived after the first 6 months, whereas Spitz's studies suggest that the first 3 months are critical. J.P. Scott (1958) set the critical period for the establishment of social relations even earlier: between 4 and 6 weeks. Dennenberg (1968) has suggested that the human equivalent for successful use of an enriched environment begins roughly at 6 months. Reviews of these studies by Orlansky (1949), Pinneau (1955), and Kagan et al. (1978) indicate that the early infancy period may be sensitive rather than critical to the development of social relationships.

The concept of the development of attachment, or filiative, behavior also includes a sensitive period during which infant and mother establish social relations (Ainsworth 1973). Klaus and Kennel (1976) suggested that the sensitive period for the establishment of social relations occurs during the immediate perinatal period. They attempted to show that children of mothers who were allowed to interact with their infants immediately after birth showed more attachment later. Bowlby and Ainsworth asserted that a lack of constant mother-infant contact during the first 2 years would render the children incapable of forming permanent, affectionate bonds. Others have argued that early experience may serve to "tune" the neuroendocrine system, altering the threshold and duration of emotional stress reactions (Levine and Mullins 1968). Strong social networks have also been reported to have a positive effect on recovery from closed head injury in childhood and later (Bach-y-Rita and Bach-y-Rita 1990, Wagner et al. 1990).

Ethological studies of imprinting (Lorenz 1970, Moltz 1968) made it clear that, at least in some animals, there is a short critical period for the establishment of social ties. In birds this period occurs 20 to 28 hours after hatching, and in dogs it occurs between 3 and 9 weeks (Scott 1958). The human equivalent of imprinting according to Caldwell (1962) begins soon after birth and can be described as visual pursuit. Visual pursuit is initially based on discrimination and occurs in response to isolated stimuli characterizing the mother. Toward the end of the infant's learning period, responses to far more subtle cues and groups of cues occur in such a way that individuals not possessing the total group of cues will be rejected, i.e., anxiety toward strangers arises. The critical period, in this case, is regarded as the length of the learning period required for the establishment of the discriminative filiative response. Such attachment to the mother is usually established between 6 and 9 months of age in human infants.

CRITICAL PERIODS FOR LEARNING

The existence of critical periods for learning was first noticed in children, rather than in animals. McGraw (1946) described varying periods for learning different motor activities that depended on the degree of opportunity and stimulation.

Of special interest to neuropsychologists is the concept of critical periods for language acquisition and its relation to cerebral lateralization, as discussed in Chapter 5. According to Lenneberg (1967), natural language acquisition can occur only during the critical period that begins at age 2 years and ends around age 14. After puberty, the basic acquisition of language is unlikely to occur because of a loss of cerebral plasticity upon completion of the cerebral lateralization of language function.

Other researchers have questioned Lenneberg's theory. Some argue that the development of lateralization is complete by the age of 5 years. Although a critical period for language acquisition may exist, its neurological substrates are not necessarily tied to the development of lateralization (Krashen 1973, Milner 1975). Still others have placed the critical age for transfer of language functions to one hemisphere at the age of 1 year (Woods and Carey 1979), as discussed in Chapter 5. Kinsbourne (1976) asserted that lateralized functions exist from birth, i.e., lateralization is invariant.

The case of Genie, an adolescent girl who was isolated for 11 years before she acquired a language, provides evidence to support a sensitive period hypothesis for language. Genie emerged from isolation at the age 13 years 9 months with no verbal abilities, and was faced with the problem of acquiring a first language (Curtiss 1977). Despite this handicap, Genie has shown steady progress in language learning. Her speech is similar to that of normal younger children with an equivalent mental age. (At 16 years, her mental age was 5 years 8 months). Her vocabulary is large, but she has difficulty in learning formal rules of language. It seems that Lenneberg's critical period for language learning should rather be regarded as a sensitive period. That such sensitive periods extend over a longer period of time is also suggested by studies of second-language learning. In adult immigrants, performance on a test of grammar declined continuously over age of arrival in an English-speaking country until adulthood (Johnson and Newport 1991).

Conceptual Issues

The critical period concept has been subject to considerable confusion. One reason for this has been its application both to periods during which a specific type of stimulation or experience was beneficial for normal development and to periods during which the organism was susceptible to the harmful effects of noxious stimuli. Colombo (1982) has characterized the differences as "need periods" versus "vulnerable periods." Fox (1970) recommended the use of the term "critical period" for times during which normal development needed to be triggered by stimuli and the term "sensitive period" for times during which the organism is especially vulnerable to harmful influences. Moltz (1973) used the term "contingent" instead of "critical" need and "noncontingent" instead of "sensitive." Unfortunately, none of these divisions serves a heuristically useful purpose since it has not been shown that the two types of periods have different biological bases.

Another conceptual issue relates to what is described as "continuation versus noncontinuation of plasticity" (Colombo 1982). In behavioral development, most examples of deprivation during critical periods show that the effects are followed by some behavioral recovery. Moltz (1973) suggested that critical periods after which the organism has the ability to recover be distinguished from periods after which no recovery is observed. Krashen (1973) proposed "strong" and "weak" forms of the critical period hypothesis, depending on the amount of plasticity remaining in the developing system after the end of the period. Thus, Moltz and Krashen base their distinctions of critical period phenomena on recovery from deprivation or adverse experience. Reports of recovery, however, have been behavioral, rather than anatomical or physiological.

A third issue relates to the levels of assessment used to measure effects during critical periods. Effects are more clear cut and time bound when they are assessed biologically, rather than behaviorally.

8.2   The Concept of Plasticity

The term **plasticity** refers to the capacity of the CNS to adapt or change after environmental stimulation. Two major research issues dominate current discussions of plasticity. The first relates to the concept of developmental plasticity and is supported by studies involving the surgical alteration of neural connections in animals. The second issue focuses on neural plasticity and the recovery of function in children and adults.

Developmental Plasticity

Surgical alteration of neural connections in laboratory-reared animals indicates that there is a neonatal period of plasticity. In contrast to the classical notion that afferent cells either degenerate or survive without afferentation after surgical lesions, recent research suggests that afferent cells may form new connections by a process called **synaptic reorganization**. This process forms the basis of the concept of neural plasticity (Brauth et al. 1991, Cotman and Nieto-Sampedro 1982, Gazzaniga et al. 1979, Lynch 1974).

Three forms of synaptic reorganization have been observed: sprouting, spreading, and extension. Gazzaniga and his colleagues have described these three forms in lesion studies of the afferent system of the dentate gyrus in the hippocampus (Figure 8-3). **Sprouting** of new axons increases the number of terminals in the normal dendritic area. **Spreading** is the development of terminals in new target areas. **Extension** refers to the termination of afferents on cells that are not the normal targets.

Other evidence to support the concept of developmental plasticity comes from animal brain surgery. By artificially manipulating environmental conditions, researchers have been able to show parallel anatomical, biochemical, and physiological changes in the nervous system. Studying bullfrog tadpoles with mid-thoracic transection of the spinal cord, Brenner and Stehouwer (1991) showed that behavioral recovery depended, at least in part, on the axonal growth of fibers across the transection site. Reference has already been made to the effects

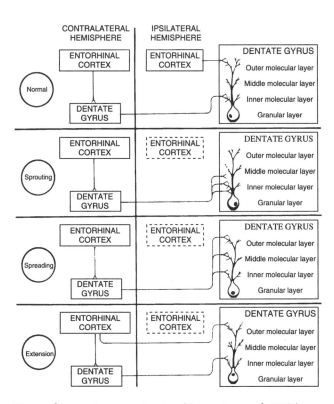

Figure 8-3. Types of synaptic reorganization (Gazzaniga et al. 1979).

of enriched and isolated conditions on brain weight and size. Hirsch and Jacobson (1975) noted other anatomical changes in the visual cortex of animals reared totally in the dark: decreases in the size of the neurons, the length of the dendrites of certain types of cells, and the number of synapses on the dendrites to other types of cells.

The experimental literature indicates that neural plasticity can be seen in three ways

1. *Spared function*: For example, the removal of the optic tectum in neonatal hamsters resulted in spared visual functioning in adulthood (Schneider 1974). Rats with cingulate lesions in infancy showed normal spatial navigation and normal hippocampal EEGs; brains were smaller and had a thinner cortex, but showed normal dendritic arborization similar to controls (Kolb and Wishaw 1991). Kolb (1989) also demonstrated a strong correlation between dendritic arborization and behavioral recovery.

2. *Maladaptive behavior.* Schneider (1974) also showed that, when the superior colliculus is lesioned on one side in neonatal hamsters, retinal projections spread to the remaining side and also to the contralateral tectum. As adults, these hamsters made inappropriate turning responses when presented with food in certain parts of the visual field.

3. *Restoration of function.* In the same series of experiments, Schneider (1974) showed that, when severed, the anomalous connections to the lesioned superior colliculus result in the restoration of normal turning behavior.

8.3 Behavioral Plasticity and Recovery of Function

A central theme in the study of critical periods in brain development is that the effects of disturbances are likely to be more profound and longer lasting for a growing brain than for a mature brain. Chemicals, drugs, infections, and other factors may cause gross malformations in the developing brain, whereas the same insults to the mature brain may produce no demonstrable harm or only a transient effect. There are two exceptions to this concept. The first is the greater resilience of the immature brain to hypoxia, which is explained by its lower metabolic rate (Robinson 1981). The second relates to the effects of mechanical disrupting events, such as trauma, infarction, local inflammation, and necrosis (death of tissue). Experimental studies with animals and clinical reports on humans show that there is greater functional recovery from these disrupting events if they occur in infancy. One explanation is that the younger brain recovers better because of its greater neuronal plasticity (Brunner and Altman 1974, Huttenlocher 1990), but this view has been a focus of debate for the last few years.

Models of Recovery

The mechanisms of recovery can be explained by several models (Figure 8-4), reviewed by Almli and Finger (1992), Bach-y-Rita (1990), Chelune and Edwards (1981), and Finger and Stein (1982).

The **equipotentiality model** of Lashley (1938) was derived from studies with rats and attempted to account for recovery through mass action of the remaining parts of the system, which maintain function because of an inherent redundancy in brain systems.

Another common explanation of the recovery process is **vicarious functioning**. Munk (1881) suggested that functions lost after injury are taken over by other areas of the brain, areas whose functions may be sacrificed to fulfill the role of the damaged area or areas that had been functionally dormant. This idea is also used to explain the hypothesis of preferential immature plasticity. In young brains, cells are assumed to be less committed to specific functions so that they can take over the functions of damaged parts of the brain more easily (St. James-Roberts 1979). Recovery has also been explained on the basis of "**behavioral substitution**," i.e., the use of similar neurophysiological processes to achieve the original end by different behavioral means (Goldberger 1974).

Denervation supersensitivity is another possible explanation for the synaptic reorganization that may underlie recovery (Stavraky 1961). After dener-

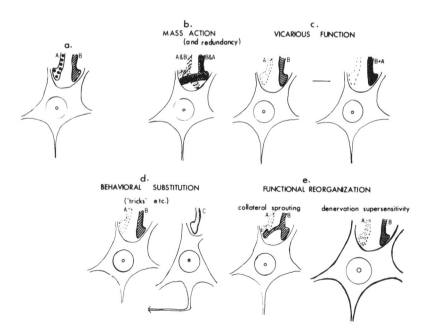

Figure 8-4. Models of recovery of function: (a) large neuron; (b) mass action; (c) vicarious function; (d) behavioral substitution; (e) functional reorganization (Goldberger 1974).

vation in a damaged area, the remaining fibers or postsynaptic processes may become overly sensitive to residual neurotransmitters. It is possible that small amounts of neurotransmitters leaking from prelesion neurons could activate new postlesion pathways. As a result, new synaptic connections and functional restoration might be achieved (Tsukahara 1981). The synapse renewal can be viewed as an extension of "natural synapse turnover," which has been demonstrated both for the peripheral and various parts of the CNS in animals, especially in periods of hibernation or pregnancy and in response to environmental changes to increase or decrease specific activity (Rutledge et al. 1974, Thorbert et al. 1978).

Von Monakov (1911) formulated the concept of **diaschisis** to help explain recovery. He suggested that damage to one part of the nervous system deprives other areas of normal stimulation and leads to a state of shock. Even undamaged areas may be malfunctional. With recovery, the undamaged portions of the brain resume normal functioning. Some support for this theory from cerebral blood flow and metabolic studies has been reviewed by Hecaen and Albert (1978).

Animal Studies

It is commonly assumed that age is a crucial factor in neuronal plasticity, although some investigators have recently challenged this view. Those who consider age an important variable argue that functional localization is poorly defined in the young infant. If there is enough unallocated reserve in the cortex, cognitive functions can be assumed by areas not traditionally serving this role, i.e., by vicarious functioning. The early experimental work of Kennard (1938) supported the notion of greater neural plasticity in infants. Her findings showed that unilateral lesions in the precentral (motor) cortex of newborn monkeys have minimal effects compared with the same lesions in adults. The contralateral and ipsilateral motor areas seem to take over for the damaged tissue. At the age of 2 months, the animals appeared undamaged, in contrast to the adult monkeys who were permanently hemiplegic. Later studies (Kennard 1942), however, showed that those lesioned infant monkeys when tested in adulthood had learning deficits, thus refuting the idea of full neural plasticity in infants. Recent work by Yamasaki and Wurtz (1991) showed that recovery of function after middle temporal lesions in monkeys has a rapid phase that depends on the surviving portions of the lesion area, and then a slower phase that depends on areas outside the superior temporal sulcus.

A new line of research examines the effect of grafts of fetal basal forebrain tissue on the recovery of function (Iversen and Dunnett 1990, Sprick and Sprick 1991). Such transplants have been described as "living mini-pumps" that release or diffuse trophic substances, such as GABAergic basal ganglia outflow from the transplant and from the damaged host brain, which may partially restore neuronal and behavioral functions after lesions (Lescaudron and Stein 1990). Olton and Shapiro (1990) found that rats with fimbria-fornix lesions showed better behavioral recovery after tissue grafts by the restoration of normal hippocampal unit activity, rather than by reorganization of new neural networks.

The question whether the immature brain is less vulnerable to injury was also taken up by Goldman (1974) and others (see Rakic and Goldman-Rakic 1982). Goldman showed that removal of the dorsolateral prefrontal cortex in prenatal, infant and adult monkeys had different effects. Learning of a delayed-response task in monkeys with prenatal and infant lesions seemed to be unaffected, whereas the adults failed to learn. Follow-up examination of the infant monkeys, however, demonstrated that learning deficits could emerge later. If dorsolateral damage occurred prenatally, however, little or no deficit was found when the monkey reached adulthood. Goldman offered an alternative to the idea of neuronal plasticity of the immature brain by suggesting that parts of the cortex are pre-programmed for tasks that are taken up at different ages. She hypothesized that the dorsolateral prefrontal cortex is not used to solve delayed-response tasks in the infant monkey but develops that function later (Robinson 1981). A similar view of developmentally determined constraints on long-term recovery in rats emerges from a study by Brennan et al. (1990).

Human Studies

The concept of plasticity in the immature brain has been extensively applied to studies of language acquisition and hemispheric lateralization, particularly to studies of infantile hemiplegia, hemispherectomy, callosotomy, and childhood aphasia. Careful scrutiny of these studies suggests that the degree of plasticity may be related to the site, nature, and severity of the injury.

Basser's (1962) work with hemiplegic subjects has been put forward in support of the hypothesis of greater neural plasticity in infants. In this study of 102 children and adults with onset of hemiplegia in infancy, verbal performance was unaffected by the side of hemispheric damage and age at onset of hemiplegia. Equally optimistic results were reported by Obrador (1964), who described intact sensorimotor functions, praxis, and language, no matter which hemisphere was preserved. In a comparison of residual function after hemispherectomy for tumors in adults and for intractable epilepsy in children, Gardner et al. (1955) noted greater deficits for adults. Similar reports of a lessened impact on young children after hemispherectomy were presented by Krynauw (1950), Cairns and Davidson (1951), and Hillier (1954); persisting deficits have been ascribed to the "crowding" of functions of both hemispheres into one (Levin et al. 1984). Studies of agenesis of the corpus callosum and callosotomy before the age of 8 years suggested that "interhemispheric communication during ontogeny can be assumed by other pathways that may be competing with callosal connections during cortical maturation" (Lassonde et al. 1991, see Chapters 9 and 21).

In spite of good recovery, children with unilateral lesions typically show an overall decrement in intellectual functions when compared to controls, although the form of such a deficit may depend on the site of lesion and Performance IQ seems to be affected more (Aram et al. 1985, Rutter 1982). Annett (1973) found that 41 per cent of hemiplegic children with left hemispheric damage had language problems, compared to 15 per cent of children with right hemispheric damage. Language difficulties in complex tasks after left hemispherectomy were also reported by Dennis and Kohn (1975). After head injury, children seem to recover better than adults, but this generalization does not hold when more sensitive psychometric instruments are used (Miner et al. 1986). Classical aphasias seem to be an infrequent longterm symptom (Fletcher et al. 1987), although Woods and Carey (1979), Ewing-Cobbs et al. (1985), and others demonstrated continuing subtle language deficiencies in these children with more detailed testing. In particular, written language skills were more affected in young children.

Fletcher et al. (1987) stressed that the effects of head injury in children are related to the sequence of development of cognitive growth. The injury disrupts the developmental sequence, i.e., it slows the rate of subsequent development, but may also lead to deviant patterns of development. Skills affected in the younger child may be basic to the later development of more complex, apparently unrelated deficits, e.g., learning disabilities. Therefore, recovery studies, instead of focusing on simple age effects, should shift to a "fuller appreciation of the complexities of development" (p. 288). Kolb (1989) pointed out that frontal lobe injury in the first year of life almost invariably leads to lowered IQ and poor performance on tests sensitive to frontal lobe function in adulthood, whereas frontal lobe injury in later childhood has a somewhat better outcome, although severe social difficulties are common sequelae. He concluded that, at least for this part of the brain, the earliest lesions produce the worst behavioral outcome.

In sum, recent studies have produced limited evidence for greater neuronal plasticity after early lesions in children (Goodman 1989a). Finger (1989) argued that, although an injury may trigger neuronal growth, the ensuing changes may not always be beneficial for the individual (e.g., inappropriate, fast-growing connections, exaggerated growth, misconnections) and that recovery, if it does occur, may be an epiphenomenon.

Summary

The term "critical period" encompasses many phenomena within one abstract concept. In embryonic development the concept is well established and can be defined precisely. The issue of whether critical periods exist for fetal development is still debatable. Dobbing speculated that a critical period exists during which the organism is sensitive to subteratogenic influences, particularly malnutrition. His hypothesis has been supported by animal research. When applied to behavioral development, the term "critical periods" can be useful only if accompanied by (1) an approximate onset and terminus of the period, (2) exact specifications of the critical stimulus to which the organism is most sensitive, and (3) exact specification of the critical system that will be affected later on (Colombo, 1982).

Others have argued that the term is an oversimplification and a misnomer because such relationships should probably be better described as time-relationships, a term that does not imply a critical relation. Nevertheless, the importance of light experience in the normal development of the visual system of laboratory-reared animals and the possibility of the need for similar experiences in the development of the human visual system seems to reflect a critical period, as does the period for imprinting in birds. Time intervals in human development are much larger, the variability of the response much greater, and the ability of the organism to adjust much more complex so that the application of the critical period concept is difficult.

Two types of plasticity of the CNS have been proposed. The first relates to the ability to modify adaptive behavior and depends on experience and the anatomical and physiological characteristics of the CNS. The second relates to recovery after damage. The recovery is facilitated by two mechanisms. Diaschisis accounts for some recovery and seems to be unrelated to age, although the concept is insufficient by itself to explain all recovery phenomena; recovery may occur where functional overlap between systems is possible or where systems can be duplicated.

9

Disconnection Syndromes

Just as damage to a cortical region can lead to behavioral disturbances, so can lesions of connections between cortical regions. A **disconnection syndrome** is defined anatomically as "the effects of lesions of association pathways, either those which lie exclusively within a cerebral hemisphere or those which join the two halves of the brain" (Geschwind 1965, p. 242). Thus, a disconnection syndrome is the result of a lesion of either cortical association fibers, which connect cortical regions within a hemisphere, or of commissural-interhemispheric fibers, which connect similar regions across the two hemispheres. The behavioral effects of such disconnections are relatively predictable when they occur after brain damage in adults.

9.1 Disconnection Syndromes in Adults

The early history of the concept of disconnection syndromes has been reviewed by Dimond (1972), Gazzaniga (1970), Geschwind (1965, 1970, 1975), and Joynt (1974). Carl Wernicke (1874) introduced this concept when he predicted that an aphasic syndrome (conduction aphasia) could result from the disconnection of the sensory speech zone from the motor speech area by a single lesion in the left hemisphere. Dejerine (1892) first described definite symptoms resulting from a lesion of a commissural system, the corpus callosum, when he presented a case of alexia (loss of the ability to read) without agraphia (loss of the ability to write). The patient had a lesion in the left occipital lobe, blocking sight in the right visual field (hemianopia), and in the splenium of the corpus callosum. Dejerine interpreted this case as a disconnection of the speech area in the left hemisphere from the remaining right visual cortex. As a result, the patient could read correctly using the right visual cortex, but not the left. However, the information from the right visual cortex could not be transmitted to the speech area because the corpus callosum was damaged.

156

A few years later, Liepmann (1900–08) demonstrated disconnections in several patients that led to disorders of voluntary movement (apraxias). In 1937, Trescher and Ford described a patient in whom the posterior half of the corpus callosum was sectioned during the surgical removal of a colloid cyst of the third cerebral ventricle. The resulting behavioral deficits, including loss of the ability to name letters placed in the left hand or read in the left visual field (hemialexia), were attributed to a disconnection syndrome. Ferro et al. (1983) described a patient with transcortical motor aphasia, left arm apraxia, and optic ataxia; a study of the lesion confirmed that crossed-visual reaching passes through the posterior two-fifths of the corpus callosum and that these fibers are arranged in ventrodorsal fashion. In contrast, interhemispheric tactile transfer seems to be located in the anterior part of the trunk of the corpus callosum (Bentin et al. 1984).

"Split-Brain" Studies

In 1940, Van Wagenen and Herren sectioned the corpus callosum, either partially or fully, in ten patients for the relief of epileptic seizures. Their reasoning was that doing so would stop the spread of the seizure across the hemispheres through the corpus callosum. The surgery limited the seizures successfully, and resulting disturbances in behavioral functioning were minimal and temporary. Akelaitis and his colleagues (1940–44) reported an extensive series of such "**split-brain patients**" who showed little evidence of deficits in psychological test performance or everyday behavior. The work of Akelaitis and Van Wagenen, therefore, seemed to argue against lasting behavioral disconnection symptoms resulting from the commissurotomy.

The impetus for further study of disconnection effects came from animal experiments conducted by Sperry and Myers in the 1950s (reviewed by Sperry et al. 1969). They split both the optic chiasm and the cerebral commissures in cats and found that functions in each of the two hemispheres could be trained independently. However, they had to go to great lengths to obtain these results. After splitting the chiasm and corpus callosum, they covered one of the cat's eyes, thereby restricting visual input to only one hemisphere since it could not be relayed either by the commissures or by the visual system. They then presented certain discriminations to the cats, which were learned almost normally. However, when subsequently the opposite eye was covered to test for residual memory of the discriminations, no learning could be demonstrated. In this way Sperry and Myers showed that the hemispheres could apparently function independently of each other and suggested that the normal role of the cerebral commissures is to transfer information between hemispheres. Their vivid animal demonstration of disconnection symptoms resulting from a split corpus callosum forced a re-examination of corpus callosum sections in humans.

Two neurosurgeons, Bogen and Vogel, reported in 1962 the case of a patient who underwent commissurotomy in a successful attempt to control epileptic seizures (reviewed by Bogen 1979). Encouraged by the results, they performed

split-brain operations in other severely epileptic patients. Sperry and his associates then began extensive psychological studies of these patients. They developed new techniques, appropriate to humans, that allowed strict lateralization
of visual and somesthetic stimuli to one hemisphere and demonstrated many of
the disconnection effects predicted by the original theory, such as an inability
to transfer certain types of information between the hemispheres (Sperry et al.
1969). Geschwind and Kaplan (1962) identified similar human disconnection
symptoms in a patient with a tumor in the corpus callosum.

In 1965 Geschwind reviewed much of the early evidence for disconnection
effects and presented the case for the use of anatomical knowledge in the prediction of symptoms resulting from fiber tract disruptions. His monograph has
been influential in contemporary neuropsychology because it argues for a strict
localizationist (or "connectionist") view of brain structure and function, a view
not fully accepted by many neuropsychologists at that time and one that is still
debated.

More recent studies have confirmed that callosotomy interferes with the interhemispheric transfer of information as tested with sophisticated examinations.
Generally, the procedure is effective in reducing specific types of seizures and
does not affect general intellectual functioning (Sass et al. 1988). In a series of
18 patients with partial and total corpus callosotomy, however, Sass and co-
workers found defects of speech and language function in patients in whom the
language-dominant hemisphere did not control the dominant hand; some patients with pre-existing mild to moderate unilateral motor dysfunction also
showed further unilateral deterioration. Joseph (1986) described a callosotomy
case with complete reversal of cerebral dominance for language and emotion in
addition to the typical disconnection syndromes.

Types of Disconnection Syndromes

Disconnection syndromes in adults can be divided into two major groups
(Geschwind 1970): (1) those resulting from lesions of interhemispheric commissures (i.e., the corpus callosum and/or the anterior commissure) and (2)
those resulting either from lesions of association pathways within one hemisphere or from a combination of lesions of association pathways with other
lesions.

Commissural disconnection syndromes in adults usually result from surgical
intervention, tumor, or interruption of the blood supply to the corpus callosum
or immediately adjacent structures. The full syndrome includes (1) the inability
to match a stimulus object held in one hand to an object held in the other hand;
(2) the inability to match an object seen in one visual field to one seen in the
other field; and (3) several disabilities restricted to the left side of the body
related to the presence of speech in only one hemisphere, such as the inability
to carry out verbal commands with the left hand, to name objects placed in the
left hand, and to write legibly with the left hand. These deficits have been

consistently demonstrated in a number of patients and are interpreted as evidence that information is not transferred from one hemisphere to the other (Bogen 1979, Gazzaniga 1970). However, specialized tests are needed to demonstrate these deficits, and they are not seen in every patient (Trevarthen 1975). Quantitative differences in the ability to name by touch or on sight have been reported by Spreen et al. (1966), suggesting that the results of disconnection are not necessarily an all-or-none phenomenon.

Disconnection syndromes resulting from lesions in other association pathways have not been studied as extensively as the callosal syndromes. Two examples of the latter type are alexia without agraphia (pure word blindness) and conduction aphasia. Writing to dictation—spontaneously and by copying—is preserved in **alexia without agraphia**, but patients cannot read what they have written. A combination of lesions in the left occipital (visual) cortex and the splenium of the corpus callosum is usually found. Hence, the transfer of visual information (only available in the right hemisphere because of the left occipital lesion) to the reading (posterior language) area of the left hemisphere is disrupted.

In **conduction aphasia** the patient generally has normal or only mildly defective comprehension of written or spoken language and fluent though paraphasic speech (substituting or reversing phonemes, syllables, or whole words), but shows a striking difficulty in repeating phrases spoken by the examiner (Damasio 1991). The lesion spares Wernicke's area of the superior temporal region, as well as Broca's area in the inferior frontal gyrus, but typically involves the arcuate fasciculus (a fiber tract in the supramarginal gyrus) connecting these two areas (see Damasio and Damasio 1980 for other lesions). Since Wernicke's and Broca's areas are intact, language comprehension and speech output are both preserved. However, the pathway for speech running from Wernicke's area through the arcuate fasciculus to Broca's area is damaged, likely accounting for the aphasic aspects of speech, as well as the peculiar defect in repetition. Tanabe et al. (1989) reported conduction aphasia in a 10-year-old boy without buccofacial or ideomotor apraxia after removal of an arteriovenous malformation. Damage was confined to the left supramarginal gyrus invading the arcuate fasciculus. The aphasia cleared up rapidly after surgical recovery.

9.2   Commissural Disconnections in Children

For several reasons—in particular, compensatory mechanisms and the effects of development—complete disconnection syndromes have not been found in children. In reviewing the behavioral effects of lesions of the connections between cortical areas in children, however, we follow the division into two types of disconnection syndromes, as we did for adults, to permit a comparison of the adult and childhood syndromes.

Surgical Disconnection

Commissurotomies for epilepsy have been performed in children. One report (Luessenhop et al. 1970) indicated that for three older children (two aged 3 years, one aged 7 years) the procedure was very effective in controlling seizures. A fourth child (aged 4 months) continued to have seizures, possibly because they were bilateral in origin. A tendency to neglect and even deny the presence of the left arm for several months after surgery was noted in the 7-year-old child. The authors suggested that there were no obvious behavioral disconnection symptoms in these children, although detailed testing was not carried out.

Benes (1982) reported preliminary results on the neurological and neuropsychological sequelae of transcallosal disconnection surgery in 15 children with a mean age of 10 years. The surgery was performed in most cases to remove a tumor located in the midline of the brain below the corpus callosum. The surgical approach therefore disconnected most of the commissural fibers. Benes did not use standardized psychometric tests to evaluate these cases postoperatively, but did report several disconnection symptoms similar to those observed in the adult disconnection cases (Campbell et al. 1981). After the operation, the patients were described as showing signs of tactile anomia and apraxia in the left hand, as well as such other symptoms as hypokinesia (low levels of motor activity) and deficit in recent memory. However, this brief report did not quantify the findings nor state the number of children in whom these signs appeared. Research on the effects of neonatal sectioning of the corpus callosum in young animals suggests that subtle disconnection signs are evident (Jeeves 1972), similar to those observed in the Benes (1982) study.

A study by Geoffroy et al. (1983) reported that sectioning of the corpus callosum (rather than complete commissurotomy) was successful in controlling seizures in 14 children. Surgical morbidity was reduced, and electrophysiological and psychological function, especially memory, improved more than in reported adult cases of commissurotomy. Lassonde et al. (1988) found that older callosotomized children showed disconnection deficits similar to those found in adults, but that the youngest patient with complete callosal transection, as well as six patients with callosal agenesis, demonstrated a high level of accuracy in interhemispheric tasks. A finding common to all patients was that they required more time to accomplish cross-integration of relatively complex visual and tactile information. M.J. Cohen et al. (1991) reported similar results.

Agenesis of the Corpus Callosum

Callosal agenesis is a condition in which the corpus callosum fails to develop properly. Although rare, callosal agenesis has been studied extensively by neurologists and neuropsychologists interested in disconnection effects in children (Bigler et al. 1988; Grogono 1968). Agenesis can occur together with mental handicap, epilepsy, characteristic eye lesions, vertebral anomalies, and abnormal

EEG patterns, in a syndrome called **Aicardi's syndrome** (Diani and Jancar 1984).

NEUROLOGICAL DATA

Callosal agenesis is thought to result from an arrest in the development of the primitive commissural plate, which forms in the second week of human fetal life (Dignan and Warkany 1977, Loeser and Alvord 1968a and b) and can be detected by both neonatal ultrasound (Deeg et al. 1986, Skeffington 1982) and MRI (Byrd 1989) scanning. Two main forms have been described: **total callosal agenesis**, in which all the fibers of the corpus callosum are absent, and **partial callosal agenesis**, in which some callosal fibers remain and develop anteriorly (Ettlinger 1977). The difference between the two forms is attributed to different timing in the arrest of development. The cause of the arrest in development is thought to be mechanical, infectious, or possibly hereditary in nature (Lynn et al. 1980). Toriello and Carey (1988) described callosal agenesis occurring with facial and other physical anomalies as a possible autosomal recessive syndrome.

Other defects often associated with callosal agenesis include those of midline CNS development, such as **holoprosencephaly** (failure to develop the cleavage of the prosencephalon), cysts of the septum pellucidum, and of non-midline CNS defects, such as microcephaly, a radial patterning of sulci in the hemispheres, and defective cortical lamination. These associated defects may sometimes be sufficient to explain the behavioral deficits of patients with callosal agenesis. The condition seems to produce a unique pattern of cerebral organization. Bossy (1970) and Stefanko and Shenk (1979) have demonstrated the occurrence of an extra bundle of longitudinal fibers (Probst's bundle) running in the medial wall of either or both hemispheres. Loeser and Alvord (1968a) suggested that these fibers represent the decussating axons that normally would have crossed the midline as commissures but that under this condition terminate ipsilaterally. In this case, callosal agenesis represents a failure to develop the major interhemispheric connections, rather than just an absence of the corpus callosum.

BEHAVIORAL STUDIES

Callosal agenesis in children allows tentative behavioral comparisons between disconnection syndromes in adults and children. Many behavioral studies of these children, often similar in form to adult split-brain studies, have been conducted. One obvious limitation of direct comparisons and of application to normal brain functioning lies in the pathological conditions of the patients: split-brain data are based upon a neurologically abnormal population (epileptics), and callosal agenesis patients often show accompanying neurological or behavioral deficits, such as enlarged ventricles and low IQ. Another limitation of any comparison is that children born with incomplete commissures acquire behavioral patterns without these connections, whereas adults with commissurotomy have a long history of development with intact connections. Hence, split-brain surgery and callosal agenesis are two very different situations.

Several psychological studies of acallosal children by Jeeves (1965, Jeeves et al. 1988a and b) demonstrated deficits in bimanual coordination similar to patients with partial callosotomy. This series of patients had below-average intelligence and impaired visuomotor coordination, and were generally considered clumsy. They showed (1) problems with bimanual coordination of movement of a pen across a screen if visual feedback was withdrawn, (2) slowing of "crossed" (those involving interhemispheric transfer) compared with "uncrossed" reaction times, and (3) an inability to transfer movement aftereffects (Milner et al. 1985). Jeeves and co-workers concluded that the anterior part of the corpus callosum is crucial for interhemispheric integration of the lower motor system in each hemisphere.

Solursh and colleagues (1965) reported the case of a 14-year-old acallosal boy with an IQ of 107 whom they compared with ten control subjects on several psychological tasks. His initial learning of transfer from the contralateral to the ipsilateral hand on a tactual formboard was impaired, but his "over-learning" performance was not affected. He did show some other problems with integration of information across the midline: he could not tap correctly with one hand the same number of times he had tapped with the other hand, although he could identify objects by name and pointed equally well with either hand. No deficits on tasks of lateralized visual field presentations or dichotic listening were found.

Lehman and Lampe (1970) studied nine cases of callosal agenesis, mainly with tactile tasks. They found that the patients were unimpaired on visual tasks, but failed to show transfer of tactile maze learning, whereas controls had no difficulty on any of the three transfer tasks. Interhemispheric transfer of tactile information develops gradually in children up to age 11 (Quinn and Geffen 1986, Roeltgen and Roeltgen 1989).

In marked contrast to their findings with split-brain patients, Saul and Sperry (1968) reported normal test scores on a variety of measures for a 20-year-old college student with callosal agenesis. All of the cross-integration tasks were essentially normal. Dimond (1972a) noted that in this patient the anterior commissure was enlarged to 1.5 times its normal size, which may have aided cross-integration.

No auditory deficit was found in dichotic listening tasks given to acallosal patients by Bryden and Zurif (1970) and by Ettlinger et al. (1972). However, Lassonde et al. (1990) did find acallosal subjects to be more strongly lateralized on dichotic listening, whereas patients with callosotomy showed a more variable pattern of lateralization. In a comprehensive series of studies, Ettlinger and colleagues (1972, 1974) could show no difference between agenesis and control groups on visual and tactile, crossed and uncrossed tasks. Their results are somewhat clouded, however, by the inclusion of both complete and partial callosal agenesis patients in their experimental group; these types of patients may differ in the extent of their remaining abilities.

Several acallosal patients ranging in age from 19 to 30 years were tested by Ferris and Dorsen (1975). They found low intelligence and deficits in the following areas: bimanual coordination, transfer of kinesthetic learning, and complex visuomotor performance. The usual laterality differences for language were absent. Ferris and Dorsen suggested that in acallosal patients each hemisphere duplicates the functions of the other hemisphere in order to compensate for the loss of the corpus callosum.

Dennis (1976) gave two acallosal children a series of tactile discrimination tasks both for same- and opposite-hand comparisons and contrasted them with two hydrocephalic and two normal control subjects. The children were asked whether one or two fingers had been touched with the eraser end of a pencil and, if it was two, how many fingers were between the fingers that had been touched. The tasks require both discrimination and accurate localization. In a second experiment, the children were asked to identify common objects, letters, and simple shapes as being the same or different, with the same or the opposite hand. They were then touched with a fairly thick nylon filament and asked which part (distal or proximal) of four fingers had been touched. Dennis found that acallosal patients were deficient in transfer of information from one hand to the other. However, they also had difficulty identifying the locus of stimulation on the same hand, even though they could discriminate one- and two-finger stimulation accurately with either hand. She suggested that subjects with callosal agenesis lack inhibitory activity normally mediated by the corpus callosum, which is necessary to acquire differentiated sensation and movement for each hand. Apparently, acallosal patients can compensate during interhemispheric transfer with their presumed alternate brain organization, i.e., a possibly bilateral functional development. However, they could not adequately differentiate sensation in the same hand. Using results of more sophisticated language tests, Dennis (1981) concluded that one behavioral function of the corpus callosum during development is to suppress ipsilateral information. This theory, based only on case studies, should be interpreted with some caution.

In a neuropsychological examination of two acallosal preschool-aged children, Field et al. (1978) found low intelligence and impaired visuomotor and bimanual coordination. One of the patients showed more disconnection symptoms than the other. Gott and Saul (1978) examined two 19-year-old acallosal patients with sensitive neuropsychological tests. The two patients did not demonstrate the major defects of cross-integration reported after commissurotomy. Pirozzolo et al. (1979) described a 60-year-old acallosal man with normal intelligence who showed no evidence of a disconnection syndrome. Bruyer (1985) and Temple and Villarroya (1990) also found acallosal patients who were basically asymptomatic except for slight motor disturbances, whereas Sanders (1989) reported poor syntactic sentence comprehension in a 6-year-old acallosal girl compared to three controls matched for age and verbal IQ. Poor rhyming retrieval skills have also been observed (Temple et al. 1989).

Other case reports include those of Martin (1981), Teeter and Hynd (1981), Sauerwein and Lassonde (1983), and Lassonde et al. (1991). Sauerwein and his colleagues studied two siblings, an 18-year-old woman and a 10-year-old boy, who both showed total agenesis of the corpus callosum. They administered an extensive series of kinesthetic, somesthetic, and motor bimanual integration tasks and compared the results with those of matched controls. There were no differences between the acallosal and the control subjects on any of the transfer tasks; both acallosal subjects, however, were slow in bimanual operations. The authors suggested that, rather than assuming a bilateral organization of functions in these patients, the increased use of ipsilateral and/or subcortical pathways should be considered as a more plausible explanation for the absence of disconnection symptoms.

Martin (1981) analyzed the visual processing skills of a 22-year-old male with callosal agenesis. This subject could name letters presented to the sides of the visual field better than he could localize them. Martin suggested that the anterior commissure could be capable of transferring information on the characteristics of such stimuli but that spatial information might be carried only by the posterior regions of the corpus callosum, which were absent in this patient.

In an extensive review of the cognitive functioning of 29 reported cases of agenesis of the corpus callosum, Chiarello (1980) addressed two basic questions: do acallosal subjects manifest split-brain symptoms, and is the corpus callosum necessary for the establishment of lateralization? In answer to the first question, many behavioral studies indicate that, unlike commissurotomy cases, acallosal patients show very few symptoms of disconnection, but lasting impairment in visuo- or spatial motor functioning often accompanies callosal agenesis. With regard to the second question, Chiarello concluded that there is no definite evidence that the corpus callosum is needed for the lateralized development of functions, although it may play a role in the satisfactory performance of some lateralized functions once they are established.

9.3 Implications

Disconnection syndromes are still to some extent a theoretical concept in developmental neuropsychology. Their presence in children cannot be demonstrated with certainty, even though cases of agenesis of the corpus callosum lend some support to the concept. Explanations for the failure to find disconnection syndromes in children generally invoke the concept of plasticity or reorganization of function (Chapter 8). In addition, several compensatory mechanisms have been suggested, particularly in regard to commissural disconnections (Chiarello 1980, Gott and Saul 1978, Jeeves 1979).

Among the proposed behavioral strategies is cross-cueing. This involves the subtle communication of information from one hemisphere to the other by a learned maneuver, such as tapping the object on the table, thereby sending auditory information to the other hemisphere. Gazzaniga (1970) described several elegant examples of cross-cueing in his split-brain patients. Generally, such behavioral strategies do not satisfactorily account for the paucity of disconnection effects in children since one would expect improved performances (due to practice) over time. In a long-term follow-up of two acallosal patients, Jeeves (1979) showed that essentially the same pattern of disconnection deficits was present after 15 years.

Among the possibilities for reorganization of brain function that have been suggested are (1) the bilateral representation of function in each hemisphere (i.e., "equipotentiality," Ferris and Dorsen 1975, Sperry 1970); (2) the increased use and elaboration of ipsilateral pathways (Dennis 1976, Jeeves 1979, Reynolds and Jeeves 1978); and (c) the increased use of noncallosal commissures, such as the anterior commissure (Ettlinger et al. 1972, 1974, Gott and Saul 1978). Although each of these neurological mechanisms could account, at least in part, for the lack of disconnection symptoms in children, none can explain all the varied findings satisfactorily. However, they are not mutually exclusive, and there could be individual differences in the cases that would make an explanation by one or the other mechanisms more satisfactory (Chiarello 1980). Lassonde et al. (1991) noted that "the remarkable plasticity seen in acallosal and young callosotomized patients may be related to a critical period in development co-inciding with a phase of synaptic overproduction and redundancy that would favor reinforcement of alternative neural pathways" (p. 481). The length of this period is estimated to reach up to early adolescence and possibly beyond, as demonstrated in cross-sectional studies of normal children (Hatta and Moriya 1988). This length is consistent with developmental MRI studies of the corpus callosum in normal children (Holland et al. 1986).

Summary

This chapter presented similarities and differences between disconnection syndromes seen in adults and hypothetical disconnections in children. Although many of the differences can be explained by the assumption of compensatory mechanisms referring to the plasticity of the young brain or equipotentiality of behavioral functioning in the two hemispheres, the proposed similarities among the syndromes (across ages) may indicate some continuities and shared basic principles of brain function between the child's and the adult's brain. The child's brain, however, is not a direct replica of the adult brain. A "disconnection syndrome" therefore still remains a theoretical concept in children.

10

Classification, Epidemiology, and Research Designs

10.1 Classification

Classification systems for disorders and diseases are of necessity designed for the convenience of the major disciplines involved. Psychiatry uses a system based on the psychiatric disorders, DSM-III-R (American Psychiatric Association 1987, replaced by DSM-IV in 1994). Psychologists and educators prefer to focus on intellectual functioning and impairment, adaptive abilities, or personality characteristics. For neurologists, the neurological disorders are the primary focus. A panel on developmental neurological disorders (National Institute of Neurological and Communicative Disorders and Stroke 1979) recommended a mixed system. Neuropsychological diagnostics can and does make use of all of these classification systems.

Generally, classification systems have coped with the priorities of different disciplines by developing a multiaxial system (Rutter et al. 1988) that allows users to choose their own primary system while considering another system on a different axis in space. DSM-III-R lists the clinical psychiatric syndrome on axis 1, personality and developmental disorders on axis 2, physical disorders on axis 3, psychosocial stressors on axis 4, and adaptive functioning on axis 5. Intensive research has shown only moderate reliability and validity for all axes (Achenbach 1988). In addition, Tanguay (1984) suggested that DSM-III pays insufficient attention to developmental issues. Others have even argued that "elementary principles of philosophical enquiry do not support the assumption that reality comes packaged in well-bound categories waiting to be discovered" (Dumont 1984, p. 326) and that any classification scheme of neuropsychological interest draws arbitrary lines through a spectrum of behavioral, intellectual, emotional, and social disabilities. Although the point of these objections to classification systems is recognized, such boundary lines are necessary in clinical practice and for a systematic presentation of the disorders described in this book. They also have considerable socioeconomic implications because they pro-

166

vide cut-off points for those who receive state-supported care and special training and those who do not (e.g., for the Developmental Disabilities Bill of Rights Act 1978).

One simple way to visualize overlapping classification systems is to consider psychological impairment as the horizontal dimension and etiology as the vertical dimension. A given patient or group of patients could then be described in terms of both the horizontal and vertical axis. For example, the newly released ICD-10 (World Health Organization 1993) provides a major code, 31X, for intellectual status in mental retardation (310 borderline, 311 mild, 312 moderate, 313 severe, 314 profound) and then amplifies the major code by specifying the associated physical condition in an additional code after the period, e.g., .311.411 represents mild mental retardation with anencephaly. Similarly DSM-III-R uses 317.00 for mild mental retardation, 318.00 for moderate, 318.10 for severe, 318.20 for profound retardation, and 319.00 for unspecified mental retardation. It provides special codes for developmental reading (315.00) and language and speech disorders (315.39). There is no limit to the number of additional axes that can be used. Such a multiaxial system was incorporated in DSM-III-R, ICD-10, and the Manual on Terminology and Classification in Mental Retardation (American Association on Mental Retardation 1992). The three major classification systems are designed to be compatible. ICD-10 is by far the most detailed and comprehensive medical classification system available; it uses 17 major disease coding areas, as well as supplementary codes for health hazards and external causes of injury and poisoning.

Table 10-1 presents an abbreviated overview of the AAMR system. It is the only one of the three classification systems specifically designed to deal with developmental disorders of gestation, infancy, childhood, and adolescence relevant for the psychological status of the person, whereas the other two deal with all psychiatric (DSM) or all diseases in adults and children generally. DSM and ICD are rather cumbersome to use, and the numbering systems would be discontinuous if used in the context of childhood disorders. For these reasons, we present the AAMR system as an example; it is designed along the lines of etiology similar to that used in Part III of this book and is relatively brief.

The AAMR system divides causes into prenatal, perinatal, and postnatal. Within each of these major categories, specific groups of disorders (e.g., C. inborn errors of metabolism) are listed, followed by an additional subclassification by major subgroups (e.g., C.1 amino acid metabolism disorders); the specific disorders are then listed as a third code (e.g., C.1.a. phenylketonuria). This system is more detailed and does not match the decimal system used by its predecessor (Grossman 1983).

10.2   Epidemiology

Although data on the frequency of occurrence of the disorders included in the AAMR systems are available, they come mainly from hospitals and institutions,

Table 10-1. Simplified AAMR Etiological Classification

I. Prenatal causes
   A. Chromosomal disorders
      1. Autosomes
         Example: q. trisomy 21 (Down)
                  r. translocation 21 (Down)
      2. X-linked mental retardation
         Example: e. Fragile X syndrome
                  f. Fragile X phenotype (no fragile site)
      3. Other X chromosome disorders
         Example: a. XO syndrome (Turner)
                  c. XXY syndrome (Klinefelter)
   B. Syndrome disorders
      1. Neurocutaneous disorders
         Example: q. Sturge-Weber syndrome
                  f. tuberous sclerosis
      2. Muscular disorders
         Example: d. Duchenne muscular dystrophy
      3. Ocular disorders
         Example: Leber amaurosis syndrome
      4. Craniofacial disorders
         Example: f. Craniofacial dysostosis (Crouzon)
      5. Skeletal disorders
         Example: g. Hereditary osteodystrophy (Albright)
      6. Other syndromes
         Example: a. Prader-Willi syndrome
   C. Inborn errors of metabolism
      1. Amino acid disorders
         Example: a. Phenylketonuria
      2. Carbohydrate disorders
         Example: b. Galactosemia
      3. Mucopolysaccharide disorders
         Example: a.1. Hurler type alpha-L-iduronidase deficiency
      4. Mucolipid disorders
         Example: c. Mucolipidosis type 4
      5. Urea cycle disorders
         Example: e. Arginase deficiency (arginemia)
      6. Nucleic acid disorders
         Example: a. Lesch-Nyhan syndrome
      7. Copper metabolism disorders
         Example: a. Wilson disease
      8. Mitochondrial disorders
      9. Peroxisomal disorders
         Example: b. Adrenoleucodystrophy
   D. Developmental disorders of brain formation
      1. Neural tube closure defects
         Example: b. Spina bifida
                  c. Encephalocele
      2. Brain formation defects
         Example: c. Hydrocephalus
                  d. Lissencephaly
      3. Cellular migration defects
         Example: c. Heteropia of gray matter

Table continued

Table 10-1. Continued

       4. Intraneuronal defects
          Example: a. Dendritic spine abnormalities
       5. Acquired brain defects
          Example: b. Porencephaly
       6. Primary (idiopathic) microcephaly
   E. Environmental influences
       1. Intrauterine malnutrition
       2. Drugs, toxins, and teratogens
          Example: f. Alcohol (fetal alcohol syndrome)
       3. Maternal diseases
          Example: f. Maternal phenylketonuria
       4. Irradiation during pregnancy
II. Perinatal causes
   A. Intrauterine disorders
       1. Acute placental insufficiency
       2. Chronic placental insufficiency
       3. Abnormal labor and delivery
       4. Multiple gestation
   B. Neonatal disorders
       1. Hypoxic-ischemic encephalopathy
       2. Intracranial hemorrhage
          Example: a. Subdural
       3. Posthemorrhagic hydrocephalus
       4. Periventricular leucomalacia
       5. Neonatal seizures
       6. Respiratory disorders
          Example: a. Hyaline membrane disease
       7. Infections:
          Example: b. Meningitis
               c.1. Encephalitis, cytomegalovirus
       8. Head trauma at birth
       9. Metabolic disorders
          Example: a. Hyperbilirubinemia
     10. Nutritional disorders
          Example: b. Protein-caloric malnutrition
III. Postnatal causes
   A. Head injuries
       1. Cerebral concussion
       2. Cerebral contusion or laceration
       3. Intracranial hemorrhage
       4. Subarachnoid hemorrhage (with diffuse injury)
       5. Parenchymal hemorrhage
   B. Infections
       1. Encephalitis
          Example: a. Herpes simplex
       2. Meningitis
          Example: c. Hemophilus influenzae, Type B
       3. Fungal infections
       4. Parasitic infestations
          Example: b. Malaria
       5. Slow or persistent virus infections
          Example: b. Rubella (progressive rubella panencephalitis)

169

Table 10-1. Continued

C. Demyelinating disorders
    1. Postinfection disorders
    2. Postimmunization disorders
    3. Schilder disease
D. Degenerative disorders
    1. Syndrome disorders
       Example: a. Rett syndrome
    2. Poliodystrophies
       Example: c. Friedreich ataxia
    3. Basal ganglia disorders
       Example: b. Huntington disease (juvenile type)
    4. Leucodystrophies
    5. Sphingolipid disorders
    6. Other lipid disorders
E. Seizure disorders
    1. Infantile spasms
    2. Myoclonic epilepsy
    3. Lennox-Gastaut syndrome
    4. Progressive focal epilepsy (Rasmussen)
    5. Status epilepticus-induced brain injury
F. Toxic-metabolic disorders
    1. Acute toxic encephalopathy
    2. Reye syndrome
    3. Intoxications
       Example: a. Lead
    4. Metabolic disorders
       Example: c. Cerebral anoxia
G. Malnutrition
    1. Protein-caloric (PCM)
    2. Prolonged intravenous alimentation
H. Environmental deprivation
    1. Psychosocial disadvantage
    2. Child abuse and neglect
    3. Chronic social/sensory deprivation
I. Hypoconnection syndrome (Disturbance of Neuronal Connectivity)

Source: American Association on Mental Retardation (AAMR) 1992.

so that only cases severe enough to require hospitalization or institutionalization are counted. Also, many diseases occur most frequently in developing or newly industrialized countries where reliable epidemiological data are difficult to obtain. Moreover, such statistics do not necessarily follow the AAMD or ICD systems, but often use a classification system of their own. Table 10-2 presents some available statistics reorganized to follow the Grossman (1983) classification. The first column is based on a complete survey of severely and profoundly retarded persons over age 10 in Quebec (McDonald 1973), the second relies on referrals to mental retardation clinics in the United States (DHEW 1973), and the third is based on a survey of patients in mental institutions in the United States (DHEW 1966). The figures indicate the importance of each disorder in

Table 10-2. Frequency of Occurence of Childhood Disorders

	Severely retarded at age 10 (%)[a]	Clinics, (%)[b]	Institutions (%)[c] First admission	Residents
.0 Infections and intoxications				
.01 Prenatal infection		2.1	6.6	5.6
.02 Postnatal infection	10	4.0		
.03 Intoxication		1.7	2.2	1.4
Hyperbilirubinemia	1.5	.8		
.1 Trauma or physical agent				
.11 Prenatal injury		1.4		
.12 Mechanical injury at birth	7	2.1		
.13 Perinatal hypoxia		5.3	10.8	8.4
.14 Postnatal hypoxia				
.15 Postnatal injury	1	2.5		
.2 Metabolism or nutrition				
.21 Neuronal lipid storage		.6		
.22 Carbohydrate disorders	21	.5		
.23 Amino acid disorders		.9		
.24 Nucleotide disorders			2.0	1.7
.25 Mineral disorders				
.26 Endocrine disorders		.4		
.27 Nutritional disorders		1.2		
.28 Other				
.3 Gross brain disease (postnatal)				
.31 Neurocutaneous dysplasia		1.1		
.32 Tumors		.2	.6	.4
.33 Cerebral white matter				
.34 Specific fiber tracts				
.35 Cerebrovascular system				
.36 Unknown cause with structural reaction		10.1	15.6	5.9
.4 Unknown prenatal influence				
.41 Cerebral malformation		2.5		
.42 Craniofacial anomaly				
.43 Status dysraphicus		8.4	27.4	23.4
.44 Hydrocephalus				
.45 Hydranencephaly				
.49 Other prenatal causes		8.2		
.5 Chromosomal abnormalities				
.50 A group chromosomes (1, 2, 3)				
.51 B group (4, 5)				
.52 C group (6-12)				
.53 D group (13-15)				
.54 E group (16-18)				
.55 F group (19-20)	23	7.8		
.56 G group (21-22)				
.57 X chromosome				
.58 Y chromosome				

Table continued

171

Table 10-2. Continued

	Severely retarded at age 10 (%)[a]	Clinics, (%)[b]	Institutions (%)[c]	
			First admission	Residents
.6 Gestational disorders				
.61 Prematurity		5.3		
.62 Small for date	3			
.63 Postmaturity				
.7 Following psychiatric disorders				
.8 Environmental influences			29.1	35.7
.81 Psychosocial disadvantages				
.82 Sensory deprivation				
.88 Unknown cause for functional reaction		33.3		
.9 Other conditions				
.91 Defects of special senses				
.98 Other (unspecified)			5.6	17.6

[a]McDonald 1973. Frequencies based on severely and profoundly retarded in province of Quebec (IQ less than 50). 5.4/1000 of all live births.
[b]Department of Health, Education, and Welfare (DHEW) 1973. Covers children served in mental retardation clinics.
[c]Department of Health, Education, and Welfare (DHEW) 1966. Covers all patients in institutions for the mentally handicapped in the United States.

terms of need for public care and intervention, not of actual incidence. It is noticeable, for example, that the widely researched inherited metabolic disorders (such as phenylketonuria), for which medical science has developed reliable screening, diagnosis, and treatment methods, account for only a small fraction of the total. The unknown-cause categories (unknown prenatal and environmental influences) without effective treatment account for more than 50 per cent of the total number of disorders, even in recent surveys of epidemiological studies (McLaren and Bryson 1987). It is likely that the percentage of cases falling into the unknown-cause categories would be even higher if the general population incidence were known. Table 10-3 presents prevalence rates based on a larger-scale British survey.

Incidence rates are based on live births only, i.e., on the surviving population affected by a disorder. The effect of spontaneous and induced abortions and of perinatal death is difficult to estimate. The Medical Research Council of Canada has published partial figures that suggest that the survivors are only a small portion of those affected by many disorders. Down syndrome, for example, is reported to have a frequency of 1.4 live births per thousand, but a perinatal death rate of 3.3 and a spontaneous (within 28 weeks of gestation) abortion rate of 15 per thousand. For sex chromosome disorders, the rates are 0.22 per thousand live births, 1.2 for perinatal death, and 7.2 for spontaneous abortion. For children with structural abnormalities, the live-birth rate is 0.25, the perinatal

Table 10-3.   Prevalence of Handicapping Conditions in Children under 16 (1981 census)

Twelve most frequent conditions	N	Estimated prevalence[a]
Mental handicap	16,347	8.03
Cerebral palsy, all types	10,151	5.10
Down syndrome	6,978	3.61
Deafness	3,616	2.02
Spina bifida and hydrocephalus	3,307	1.76
Spina bifida only	3,440	1.68
Epilepsy	2,368	1.20
Heart disease	1,687	1.06
Blind, vision deficit	1,754	0.93
Hydrocephalus	1,692	0.91
Autism-maladjusted behavior disorders	2,005	0.86
Other central nervous system disease	1,414	0.79

Source: Bradshaw and Lawton 1985.
[a]Per 10,000 UK population. Based on survey of 75,000 severely disabled children.

death rate 1.2, and the spontaneous abortion rate 1.1 per thousand (Kessner et al. 1973).

Neonatal mortality has dropped gradually from 35.7 per 1000 live births in 1930 to 18.7 per 1000 in 1960, and to 8.4 per 1000 in 1980 (Wegman 1981). However, this improvement is almost entirely due to better survival of low-birth-weight infants as a result of improved perinatal medical care. The major causes of death in newborns are listed in Table 10-4. These figures not only reflect the magnitude of problems related to pre-, peri-, and postnatal development but also highlight the need to study the early phases of development in normal and affected children and to make a detailed analysis of their neuropsychological deficits.

The discussion in the following chapters of specific factors in abnormal development is restricted to a few examples. This reflects in part the spotty knowledge available about these conditions. It would be pointless to describe conditions that have been insufficiently studied and do not have a well-established link with psychological sequelae or to describe multiple examples with similar outcomes. Even within this selection, it is obvious that clear-cut cause-effect relationships are the exception, rather than the rule. Prediction of the exact consequences of exposure of these factors remains hazardous at best.

10.3   Research Designs

In the subsequent chapters of this book, we draw from a variety of research designs that permit the investigator to examine the relationships among variables over time. These designs differ with respect to the control exerted over threats

Table 10-4. Causes of Neonatal Death in 1094 Autopsies[a]

	Weight at birth			
	Whites		Blacks	
	<2500 g	>2500 g	<2500 g	>2500 g
Birth injuries	5.1	5.4	6.0	8.1
Sepsis	1.6	1.3	3.1	3.8
Pneumonia	8.0	18.1	15.9	23.7
Hyaline Membrane disease	14.7	10.1	17.0	6.5
Erythroblastosis	9.0	8.7	1.3	.5
Pulmonary hemorrhage	5.4	10.1	5.6	11.8
Subarachnoid hemorrhage	4.5	4.7	6.7	4.8
Congenital malformation	24.4	41.6	15.0	<8.0
Aspiration of amniotic fluid	35.9	43.6	34.9	42.5

Source: Niswanger and Gordon 1972.
[a]Total in excess of 100 per cent because more than one condition may be present in the same case.

to internal and external validity and in their cost efficiency (Figure 10-1). The more elaborate designs are most appropriate for the study of normal development and have been rarely used with abnormal or clinical populations.

Cross-Sectional Designs

A **cross-sectional design** focuses on the relation among variables or attributes when measurement is taken only once. The three types relevant in neuropsychology are prevalence, retrospective, and prospective study designs.

Prevalence studies investigate the presence, absence, and/or level of an existing attribute in different population subgroups, e.g., age groups, brain-damaged versus non-brain-damaged groups. For example, a group of children with cerebral palsy and a suitable control group may be studied to determine the prevalence of visual anomalies, or a group of language-impaired children may be compared to a suitable control group with respect to the occurrence of middle-ear disease. Comparing the performance of children of different ages on a task is a common use of this design in developmental psychology.

In **retrospective studies**, a group is defined by a particular attribute (e.g., congenital malformations), and a suitable control group without this attribute is established. Histories are then investigated to determine the frequency of occurrence of a preceding attribute variable in each group. For example, a group

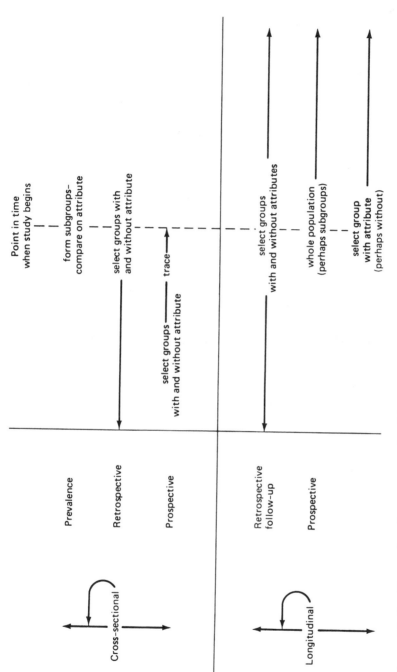

Figure 10–1. Time-ordered cross-sectional and longitudinal research designs.

of children with malformations and a suitable control group without malformations can be established. The investigator can then determine whether the mothers of these children took a particular drug during pregnancy.

In **prospective** (also called retro-follow-up) **studies**, data from the subject's history are used to identify a group for which a certain attribute occurred previously and a suitable control group without the attribute. The selected subjects are then traced, located, and assessed to determine the frequency of occurrence of an attribute or variable. For example, an investigator may go through hospital records and establish a group of children born to mothers taking a particular drug during pregnancy and a control group of children born at the same time whose mothers did not take that drug. These children will then be located and assessed for a specific psychological or physical deficit.

Longitudinal Designs

Longitudinal designs involve the measurement of the relationship among variables or attributes at two or more points in time. Two types of longitudinal designs are retrospective follow-up (also called nonconcurrent) and prospective follow-up (also called concurrent, forward looking, follow-up).

In **retrospective follow-up studies**, a group with an attribute and a suitable control group without the attribute are established. The design is similar to the cross-sectional retrospective design except that here both groups are reassessed at periodic intervals, rather than only once. For example, a group of learning-disabled schoolchildren and a suitable control group may be identified and historical information concerning pre-, peri-, and postnatal events obtained. These children may then be assessed at regular intervals throughout their academic careers.

Prospective studies may use a general population sample or select specific groups from the population. If a general population sample is used, an entire population is measured on a particular variable or set of variables and then followed over time. For example, the Collaborative Perinatal Study (Broman et al. 1975) used this design to investigate the relations between adverse conditions surrounding birth and subsequent neurological and cognitive deficits in infancy and childhood. Data were collected on mothers admitted for prenatal care in 12 university-affiliated hospitals (1) during prenatal visits, (2) at admission for delivery, and (3) during labor and delivery. The children born to these mothers were examined as neonates and at specific intervals through age 8 years.

Alternatively, specific groups who are at risk or have been exposed to a particular factor and a suitable control group may be selected and followed over time. Identifying children who showed different degrees of jaundice at birth and assessing their cognitive abilities at specific intervals throughout childhood represents an application of this design.

The major advantage of the retrospective design is its economy. Information is obtained quickly from available data. The retrospective design may be the only feasible approach when studying rare diseases. Examining the five clinic-referred persons out of one million with a rare disorder would be much more practical than collecting prospective data on a million persons in an effort to identify these five. One major disadvantage of retrospective designs is the problem of **backward contingency probabilities** (Gottfried 1973): the selected sample of subjects is an unknown proportion of the affected population and therefore does not represent the true frequency of such individuals in the population. In the example of malformed children and the relationship to drugs taken by the mothers during pregnancy, there may actually be a number of mothers who took the drug and whose children were not malformed. In a retrospective sampling design, they would not be detected, and only an indirect estimate of risk could be provided.

Other potential sources of bias include incomplete or inaccurate historical information and attrition before testing due to the attribute. Knowledge of the present attribute (i.e., congenital malformation) may affect the recollection of facts concerning the events surrounding birth, a selection bias first noted in hospital studies by Berkson at the Mayo Clinic (**Berksonian bias**). In a neuropsychology clinic, such bias may arise if only learning-disabled children known to have sustained early brain injury are referred for assessment. Generalization of findings to the general population of learning-disabled students would not then be possible.

Prospective designs provide more direct evidence of risk and are most valuable when specific hypotheses have already been developed from previous retrospective studies. Subjective bias involved in identifying the initial attributes is decreased with the use of a prospective design. However, prospective designs are time-consuming and difficult to execute and are inefficient for studying rare attributes. They are also not suitable for exploratory research where the examiner may wish to look at a large number of factors of doubtful significance.

Studies using a cross-sectional design are easier, quicker, and less expensive to conduct. However, these designs lack necessary controls for internal and external validity. For example, when age has been used to divide a population into groups, the assumption must be made that, if the behavior of younger and older children from the same population is measured, the behavior of the older child will indicate how the younger will eventually behave. This assumption is faulty since it is not possible to determine whether other influences, such as year of birth, may affect the results. The year or decade in which a person was born may affect performance, which suggests that the developmental course of the particular cohort may differ from cohort groups born earlier or later (**cohort effects**). For example, the cohort effect has been implicated in discrepancies between cross-sectional and longitudinal studies of IQ over time. The influence of cohort effects increases as the time span of the investigation lengthens.

Longitudinal designs give a direct estimate of intraindividual change and interindividual differences. However, these designs lack controls for the effect of repeat testing (**practice effects**) and other threats to internal validity. They are restricted in external validity since only one cohort is studied. Longitudinal designs are also vulnerable to the effects of attrition, which may be related to the subject characteristics and thus bias the remaining subjects further.

The **time-lag design** was developed specifically to identify cultural-historical effects and compare subjects from different cohorts when they reach a certain age. For example, an investigator may wish to compare children born in four different years (1976, 1979, 1982, 1985) when they reach 11 years of age— 1987, 1990, 1993, 1996 (Table 10-5). One disadvantage of this design is that it confounds possible differences in cohort with differences in year of measurement (Achenbach 1978).

To avoid the confounding of age, cohort, and time-of-study effects, sophisticated designs have been developed to control these variables explicitly by the use of sequential extensions of the three traditional designs—cross-sectional sequential, longitudinal sequential, and time-lag sequential.

Cross-sectional sequential designs involve samples from several birth cohorts assessed at successive times. That is, new samples are drawn from each cohort for each set of observations. The major advantage of this approach is that it does not require that the same subjects be retained from one observation period to the next; therefore, the effects of attrition and initial selection for stability do not threaten its validity. The major disadvantage of this design is that changes in individuals cannot be identified over time; only the average

Table 10-5. Design of a Combined Longitudinal and Cross-Sectional Study

1973		1974		Grade in school each year of measurement 1975		1976	N in 1976	Control group designation
K	→	1	→	2	→	3	62	Longitudinal Block A
				1	→	2	23–26	Cohort Control 1
						1	33	Cohort Control 2
				2			34–40	Retest Control 1
						3	32–40	Retest Control 2
3	→	4	→	5	→	6	77	Longitudinal Block B
				4	→	5	36–37	Cohort Control 1
						4	34–36	Cohort Control 2
				5			34–40	Retest Control 1
						6	37–40	Retest Control 2
6	→	7	→	8	→	9	80	Longitudinal Block C
				7	→	8	32	Cohort Control 1
						7	35	Cohort Control 2
				8			33–40	Retest Control 1
						9	37–40	Retest Control 2
9	→	10	→	11	→	12	73	Longitudinal Block D
				10	→	11	32–33	Cohort Control 1
						10	38	Cohort Control 2
				11			33–40	Retest Control 1
						12	34–40	Retest Control 2

Source: Klausmeier and Allen 1978.

change in functions can be determined. Baltes et al. (1977) noted that "cross-sectional sequences require fairly strict assumptions about linearity and additivity if inferences about average change functions are to be useful and valid" (p. 135). Another disadvantage of this type of design lies in uncontrollable random fluctuations in sampling.

Longitudinal sequential designs compare samples from several birth cohorts over the same longitudinal period. The major advantage of this type of design is the amount of information collected, which allows cross-sectional comparisons of cohorts at any point in the study, comparisons of the longitudinal course of development in each cohort over the course of the study, and time-lag comparisons as subjects reach a particular age in successive years. This design also makes it possible to obtain longitudinal data on relatively long periods of development in less time than it takes the development to occur (Achenbach 1978) and allows the investigator to determine whether changes in behavior are attributable to cultural-historical changes, age changes, or an interaction of the two. As with all longitudinal designs, attrition may affect the results.

Time-lag sequential designs entail taking observations on two or more samples from each cohort as they reach two or more ages in different years. This design yields information specifically related to the effects of cultural-historical changes with fewer observations than other designs. However, the design is vulnerable to uncontrollable random fluctuations in sampling from the same cohort.

Baltes et al. (1977) noted that a greater degree of internal validity could be accomplished when cross-sectional and longitudinal sequences are used simultaneously. The authors recommended (1) that sequential data are best used for descriptions of intraindividual changes in various cohorts and (2) that explanatory interpretations of the observed changes and interindividual differences in change be left to subsequent or parallel research.

Klausmeier and Allen (1978) used a time-lag sequential design to study the cognitive development of children. Children at four grade levels were tested each year for 4 years. Control groups were incorporated into the design to evaluate possible cohort and retest effects for the groups studied longitudinally. Two cohort control groups of the same age as the groups under study, one born a year later and one born 2 years later, were established, as well as two retest control groups of the same age. Each of the retest control groups was tested only once. One group served as a control for the cohort control that had been assessed twice, and one group served as a control for the groups studied longitudinally over 4 years. Table 10-5 illustrates this sophisticated research design.

As pointed out above, studies with sophisticated time-ordered research design are difficult to conduct with clinical populations. They require carefully selected population samples of considerable size and carefully developed research assessment methods. For this reason, a majority of clinical studies still rely on limited samples and assessment methods followed over an essentially unplanned period of time or on retrospective information with or without good documentation. In the following chapters, studies with less-than-ideal research qualities are quoted and contradictory results from such studies reported. Caveats for studies of limited scope and reliability are pointed out. However, it should be remembered that even a single-case report can make a substantial contribution if it opens up a new avenue of research. For example, Drake's (1968) first findings of anomalous brain development at autopsy of a learning-disabled child have since been replicated in several studies and form the basis for a host of theories about the causation of learning disabilities. **Single-case studies** can also be conducted with considerable sophistication when used as a specific research design for the testing of specific treatment or educational approaches.

Summary

The merits of several classification systems for the discussion of disorders of neuropsychological significance in the remaining chapters of the book was discussed in the first part of this chapter. The second part reviewed some basic aspects of epidemiology and presented some tables for the incidence and prevalence of childhood disorders. In a final part, we reviewed several research designs frequently used in the study of neuropsychologically relevant populations. Such designs, developed with great sophistication for the study of larger normal populations, unfortunately are only infrequently used in neuropsychological studies, although they set a standard which eventually should be attained even for clinical research.

III

Disorders of Development and Their Consequences

This part of the book deals with the link between neural development in early life and factors that interfere with it. Some of these factors, such as gross malnutrition of the mother, lack of breathing at birth (asphyxia), severe illness of the mother during pregnancy, or serious brain damage during birth, are obvious causes of developmental abnormalities; they often result in spontaneous abortion or a stillborn child. Other factors, such as a mild infection of the mother during pregnancy or premature birth, are more subtle. Whether gross or subtle, however, these influences do not always result in predictable consequences of impaired function in the child.

This section provides an overview of such factors and examines in detail a few of the important ones, the effects of which on child development have been fairly well established. The description of even short-term sequelae is often difficult; the results of studies may be quite variable and at times contradictory. To take but one example, early descriptions of the **XYY male**, a clearly defined chromosomal disorder resulting from nondysjunction of the sex chromosomes, suggested a definite association with an increased incidence of aggressive and violent criminality since the first studies found such males with greater frequency in prison populations (Jacobs et al. 1965, Sandberg 1963). This apparent demonstration of a well-defined relationship between chromosomal error and relatively complex behavioral consequences (as well as greater physical height) but without other disabling results was greeted with enthusiasm by a variety of researchers, especially in psychology and behavioral genetics. After more than a decade of research, a sobering review by Owen (1972) concluded that no consistent personality or behavioral characteristics can be predicted on the basis of the XYY complement if the effect of using highly selective prison populations is taken into account. Similar negative results were reported by Witkin et al. (1976) and Theilgaard (1984) after a comprehensive study of 4139 tall young men in Denmark.

If relations between influences in early life and later psychological problems or behavioral abnormalities are to be demonstrated, we must rely on the methods of longitudinal research described in Chapter 10 and critically evaluate existing long-term follow-up studies. Often this is not a yes-or-no matter, but rather a question of exploring the interaction of numerous factors accompanying the growth of the individual. For instance, malnutrition during pregnancy usually exists alongside neglect, poor educational opportunities, an unsanitary environment, and poor health care. To focus single-mindedly on one factor and its effect on prenatal or neonatal neural development under such circumstances would be a mistake; yet it is necessary to carefully analyze each factor individually if we want to move beyond generalities.

A general comment on the findings reported in these chapters and the examination of the individual may be in order: even for such obvious chromosomal defects as Turner syndrome or such genetic defects as phenylketonuria, the search for specific cognitive neuropsychological characteristics is often fraught with contradictory or weak evidence. The lack of uniform psychological findings is due to variations in expressivity of a gene, predisposing factors in the individual, treatment, environmental factors, age at onset, and selective locations in the brain for causative factors, especially infections and intoxications. For example, only 50 per cent of women with Turner syndrome show the full syndrome. As a result of the interaction of these numerous factors, group results may be weak when comparisons with other handicapped groups are made. Studies of nonhuman primates have successfully attempted to delineate both maternal and paternal risk factors in greater detail (Sackett 1984). It follows then that each individual should be examined and treated as an individual case, rather than as a member of a group.

This reasoning applies particularly to the person with mental handicap. Just because a person's IQ is below 70 does not mean that no special abilities or disabilities can be found. Although many of our general-purpose tests, especially intelligence tests, "bottom out" at low levels of intelligence, a careful screening with specifically designed tests with low bottom items may reveal specific strengths and weaknesses of the individual.

11

Chromosomal and Genetic Disorders

This chapter deals with two major forms of disorders that are often loosely described as genetic but that differ greatly in origin: (1) **inherited disorders**, i.e., disorders involving genetic transmission, and (2) **chromosomal disorders**, i.e., defective formation of the genetic material itself. Inherited disorders are presumed to be carried by certain genes or combinations of genes and are primarily disorders of metabolism (C in the AAMD system). Chromosomal disorders (AAMD category A) form a distinct group of defects of the chromosomal configuration (**karyotype**), which are clearly recognizable in the laboratory and result from unknown or suspected environmental influences. The two groups overlap since some chromosomal defects may be inherited.

Both inherited and chromosomal disorders are part of the "**genetic load**" (Frazer 1962), which has several components: (1) the spontaneous mutation of genes and/or chromosomes (i.e., the extent to which a population is impaired because of recurrent mutations); (2) genetic incompatibility between the parents, which results in reduced fitness or disorder in the child; and (3) genes predisposing to a certain disorder already present in the population that are combined in sexual reproduction. Hence, the genetic load for defects is present in the population—as part of its genetic variability—and cannot be eliminated entirely. "We can only strive to keep it to a minimum; the ideal homozygote will never be found" (Frazer 1962).

11.1 Genetically Transmitted Disorders

A full listing of genetically transmitted disorders would exceed the scope of this chapter by far. McKusick (1992) provides a regularly updated catalogue of human genetic disorders (as well as physical and mental characteristics) that follow Mendelian rules of inheritance.

In Mendelian inheritance, autosomal dominant, autosomal recessive, and X-linked transmission are distinguished. The term "**autosomal dominant transmission**" refers to any transmission via chromosomes other than the sex chromosomes that requires only the gene from one parent for the occurrence of the disorder or trait in the offspring. **Autosomal recessive transmission** requires the combination of two genes, one from each parent, for the trait or disorder to occur in the offspring. **X-linked transmission** refers to any disorder affecting one sex selectively and hence presumably transmitted by a gene located on the sex chromosomes. In addition to these basic forms of single-gene transmission, inheritance through the interaction of several genes (polygenic), inheritance of genetic predisposition (which may or may not lead to the disorder later in life), and inheritance based on single or multiple genes whose expression depends on environmental influences (interactive) have been described.

One group of genetically transmitted disorders is neurocutaneous dysplasia (.31), exemplified by neurofibromatosis (von Recklinghausen disease), which has an autosomal dominant pattern of transmission. Numerous neurofibromas of the skin and the peripheral nerves cause a "café-au-lait" appearance in parts of the body. Neurofibromatosis is reported to be as common as Down syndrome (1 per 3000 live births) and frequently involves the eyes and the optic pathways (Rosner 1990). MRI scans show a spectrum of abnormalities that are not necessarily correlated with cognitive difficulties, school problems, or findings during the clinical neurological examination (Duffner et al. 1989).

The most important of the genetic disorders of early development affect metabolism. More than 100 different forms have been described. As Table 11-1 indicates, groupings are usually made on the basis of the specific substance that cannot be metabolized properly (e.g., C5. mucolipid disorders; C2. carbohydrate disorders) or which endocrine function is affected (C9. endocrine disorders). In most cases, the genetic transmission is autosomal recessive. In fact, studies have found unusual neuropsychological profiles in otherwise normal and healthy heterozygotes, e.g., deficits on spatial and constructional tests for parents of children with metachromatic leukodystrophy, a deficiency of arylsulfatase (Kohn et al. 1988). Galactosemia, the condition in which enzymes for the metabolism of milk sugar are lacking, is a recessive autosomal disorder; it not only produces generalized, severe neonatal manifestations but also can be responsible for the later onset of a distinct neurological syndrome (Takano et al., 1989). Late onset at age 30 in twins with generalized seizures, progressive ataxia, and apraxia has also been reported (Friedman et al. 1989).

Most of these disorders have been discovered fairly recently. Once the substance that cannot be metabolized is known, treatment by proper diet or hormones becomes possible. For example, early screening and treatment of newborns with congenital hypothyroidism results in mostly normal intellectual and behavioral characteristics at age 7 (Rovet et al. 1986).

Table 11-1.   Inborn Errors of Metabolism Detected by Screening of Infants Born in Massachusetts Between 1967 and 1973

Disorder	Number screened	Number found	Presumed incidence
Phenylketonuria	1 012 017	66	1:15 000
Hyperphenylalaninemia	1 012 017	60	1:17 000
MSUD	872 660	5	1:175 000
Galactosemia (classical)	588 827	5	1:120 000
Homocystinuria (with hypermethioninemia)	480 271	3	1:160 000
Tyrosinemia (permanent)	438 907	0	—
Iminoglycinuria	350 176	37(?)	1:9000(?)
Cystinuria	350 176	23	1:15 000
Hartnup disease	350 176	22	1:16 000
Histidinemia	350 176	20	1:18 000
Argininosuccinic aciduria	350 176	5	1:70 000
Cystathioninuria	350 176	3	1:120 000
Hyperglycinemia (nonketotic)	350 176	2	1:175 000
Propionic acidemia	350 176	1	<1:300 000
Hyperlysinemia	350 176	1	<1:300 000
Hyperornithinemia	350 176	1	<1:300 000
Fanconi syndrome	350 176	1	<1:300 000
Rickets, vitamin D-dependent (with hyperaminoaciduria)	350 176	1	<1:300 000

Source: Wortis 1980.

Phenylketonuria

Phenylketonuria (PKU) is a well-known disorder of amino acid metabolism. Discovered by Folling in 1934, it has an autosomal recessive mode of transmission. An enzyme, phenylalanine hydroxylase, that normally oxidizes the protein phenylalanine to tyrosine in the liver is altered in PKU and does not function properly. As a result, phenylalanine accumulates in many parts of the body and acts as a toxin to impede development, especially of nerve tissue. Autopsy reports on persons with PKU showed defective myelination with an excessive number of oligodendrocytes and astrocytes (Knox 1960). The early observation of an overflow of phenylalanine through the kidneys—with an excessive green coloring by phenylpyruvic acid in the urine and a distinctive odor—led to the detection of the disorder in newborns.

The estimated frequency of PKU at birth is 1 per 18,000 births (Tischler and Lowry 1978). Since carriers of a recessive disorder would have to be 300 times more numerous than those actually affected by the disease, approximately 1.3 per cent of the population would be expected to be carriers of one gene for PKU (heterozygotes). The clinical effects described below are by no means uniform in children with detected PKU; further biochemical analyses have shown that what seems to be a single entity may have to be divided into several enzyme mutations and levels of severity, some of which may not require dietary treatment at all.

The clinical picture of the untreated child includes severe mental retardation, decreased attention span, and lack of responsiveness to the environment. Neurologically, these children suffer from seizures, spasticity, hyperactive reflexes, and tremors (Jervis 1963), as well as abnormal EEG patterns. Affected persons are somewhat shorter than average and have a small head; have light hair, eyes, and skin; and show a tendency to develop dermatitis (because the lacking amino acid is involved in pigmentation). All of these findings are rarely present in a single individual, however.

Relatively simple and effective screening methods for newborns have essentially eliminated cases of untreated PKU in most developed countries. The question of whether rigorous treatment with a low-alanine (low-phe) diet for children with low phenylalanine blood levels may be harmful (because important proteins are removed from the diet) has led to modifications in the treatment approach (Hanley et al. 1970).

The length of time for which dietary restrictions are necessary is still a topic of debate. In an earlier study, Smith et al. (1978) followed 52 PKU children between the ages of 5 and 15 who were returned to a normal diet. Twenty-six of these children had been on the restrictive diet since before the age of 4 months, and 26 had begun treatment later. After the return to a normal diet, a significant decline in mean IQ of five to nine points was observed. In contrast, Schmid-Rüter (1978) in Germany followed 22 early-treated and 17 late-treated PKU patients after a relaxed diet was instituted, but did not find a decline in overall IQ. However, the early-treated groups showed no further decline after discontinuation of the restricted diet. More recent studies showed some deterioration in intelligence generally and on choice reaction times specifically after discontinuation of the diet treatment (Clarke et al. 1987). These authors used a triple-blind design study in which PKU adolescents with unrestricted diets since the age of 8 to 10 years were assigned randomly to periods of high-phe and low-phe diets. This study supported similar findings by Chang et al. (1983) in which treated girls and boys achieved growth parameters, including weight, height, and head circumference, similar to those of normals, although weight-height ratios still correlated positively with IQ scores.

As a result of these studies, the recommendation that the special diet be discontinued at age 8 was altered to call for a moderate diet after age 8 to avoid the effects of rising phenylalanine levels, which may occur even then.

Early clinical studies concentrated on the intelligence deficit. Berman et al. (1961) found that treated PKU children were more intelligent than their untreated siblings, but were inferior to matched control subjects with similar neurological findings. In untreated cases, IQs were usually reported to be well below 50. This discrepancy in IQ tended to decelerate with age after treatment was started, suggesting that treatment should be started as early in life as possible.

Later studies followed up different variants of PKU. Berman and Ford (1970) separated 33 classical PKU cases with blood phenylalanine levels higher than 20 mg/dl from 24 children with 6 to 9.99 mg/dl (variant form) and 7 with less than 4 mg/dl (transient variant form). All had been treated promptly. Although the mean IQ of the total group was 97, that of the variant-form children was 111, and that of the transient variant form was 102. Compared with other family members, the variant and the transient variant forms showed no IQ loss, but the classical group showed an 11.5-point IQ drop. This study suggests some decrement in intelligence in classical PKU, despite treatment. Speech and language skills also were found to be poorer (Ozanne et al. 1990).

Anderson (1975) also reported three different levels of response to increased levels of phenylalanine, suggesting differences in enzyme systems, in the nervous system response to metabolic alterations, and probably in mutations at the major genetic locus as well. In the Collaborative Perinatal Study, similar results were found in 167 PKU cases: with treatment carried out between birth and 6 years of age, neither of the two low phenylalanine blood levels were found to be damaging (Williamson et al. 1981). The neurological status of these children was essentially normal. Average IQ at age 4 was 93, which represented a small but statistically significant difference relative to sex- and age-matched siblings (mean IQ 99). At age 6, the average IQ was 98 for 132 children remaining in the study compared with an average IQ of 103 for matched siblings. Treatment was designed so that half the group (randomly assigned) was intended to maintain a phenylalanine level below 5.4 mg/dl and the other half between 5.5 and 9.9 mg/dl. No IQ differences between the two treatment groups were found. In an attempt to determine the variables most important for outcome IQ, a stepwise regression analysis was done on both treatment variables (phenylalanine measurements and days of exposure to high levels of phenylalanine before treatment was started) and nontreatment variables—mother's IQ, father's years of schooling, family coping pattern, and father's age. Three important factors emerged: (1) mother's IQ ($r = .499$), (2) how well parents adhered to the dietary regimen ($r = .400$) and (3) age when first treated ($r = .327$). The importance of these factors has been confirmed in several studies. In addition, studies by Holtzman et al. (1986) and Barclay and Walton (1988) found that the age when control in dietary treatment is lost (i.e., phenylalanine concentration persistently exceeds 15 mg/dl) is the best single predictor of IQ at the age of 8 to 10 years (Table 11-2). The study also suggested that treatment should be continued after the age of 8 years.

Table 11-2.   IQ Scores of Children with PKU, Unaffected Siblings, and Parents According to Age when Dietary Control in Patients was Lost (SD in brackets)

	PKU Children				Siblings			Parents
Age at Loss[a]	N	8 years	N	10 years	N	8 years	N	
<71 mo.	29	94.4 (11.8)	29	93.9 (12.5)	17	109.3 (9.9)	31	105.5 (10.3)
72–95 mo.	46	99.7 (12.7)	43	98.4 (12.2)	27	108.9 (8.9)	46	108.6 (9.0)
>96 mo.	38	103.6 (10.9)	30	104.6 (11.9)	18	100.7 (12.5)	39	109.1 (12.4)

Source: Holtzman et al. 1986.
[a]Age at beginning of the first of three consecutive 6-month periods in which the indices of dietary control exceeded 15 mg/dl.

Studies of the specific nature of the PKU-related mental deficiency are rare since larger groups of children with PKU are not readily available to be contrasted with other retarded children. Chamove et al. (1973) simulated the condition in rhesus monkeys by feeding them a diet high in amino acids. They found permanent mental retardation if the diet was fed either prenatally or for 3, 6, or 12 months postnatally, suggesting that the damage occurs quite early in life. A second study, by Chamove and Molinaro (1978), explored the PKU-related behavior in more detail. Using a food-motivated operant situation, the authors described a "primary frustration reaction to reward that is an energizing emotional response." This excessive and disruptive emotional response to non-reinforcement was similar to the behavior of monkeys with frontal brain lesions. The authors called this "an emotionality interpretation of the PKU learning deficit" and speculated that the PKU damage is most pronounced in the frontal lobes since that area tends to be the last part of the brain to myelinate fully. Hence, extended to humans, one could call this a frontal lobe damage hypothesis to explain the behavior of PKU children. Welsh and Pennington (1988, Welsh et al. 1990) found support for this theory. Comparing early-treated PKU children with unaffected, IQ-matched peers at preschool age, they found average or above-average IQ and memory performance, but a selective impairment of "executive functions" in the PKU group, i.e., poor planning and perseveration. The executive function composite score correlated negatively with concurrent phenylalanine levels.

Other authors tried to describe a specific neuropsychological deficit in PKU subjects. In addition to poor choice-reaction time mentioned above, visual-perceptual and perceptual-conceptual difficulties have been reported (Brunner et al. 1987, Faust et al. 1986–87, Fishler et al. 1987, Mims et al. 1983). Craft et al. (1992) found lateralized deficits in visual attention and right visual field impairment in male, but not in female, PKU children; the authors attributed this finding to the PKU-related dopamine depletion that disrupts left hemisphere function. However, at least one study (Pennington et al. 1985) ascribed this pattern to right hemisphere and prefrontal area damage. Even in treated schoolchildren with PKU, educational problems, especially in arithmetic and spelling, are often reported.

Another effect of PKU described in the earlier literature is "unpleasant" behavior. Untreated children were not friendly, placid, or happy; rather, they were described as being restless, anxious, jerky, tearful, hyperactive, irritable, sometimes destructive, with uncontrollable temper tantrums, night terrors, and occasionally noisy psychotic episodes (Wright and Tarjan 1957). Dietary-treated children have been characterized as being less persistent and more intense (Schor 1983, 1986), field-dependent (Davis et al. 1986), and hyperactive (Realmuto 1986). The SQ (social quotient) was found to decrease significantly after dietary treatment was discontinued (Matthews et al. 1986).

Stevenson et al. (1979) used Rutter's rating scales for teachers and parents to measure deviance of a neurotic and antisocial type in 99 early-treated PKU children and 197 IQ- and age-matched controls. Twenty-four per cent of the

PKU children were identified by their parents and 40 per cent by their teachers (as compared with 20 per cent of the control group) as having either type of behavior problem. Neurotic deviance ratings were found in 31 per cent of the PKU boys and 15 per cent of the PKU girls, in contrast to 24 per cent of the boys and 10 per cent of the girls in the control group. Twenty-four per cent of the PKU boys and 13 per cent of the PKU girls were classified as antisocial, in contrast to 12 per cent of the boys and 13 per cent of girls in the control group.

The subjects were treated PKU children with a mean IQ of 89.7 in males and 83.2 in females. Among girls, the neurotic behavior was more often found in those with IQs below 70. In the higher IQ ranges, no significant differences between PKU and control groups were noted. Stevenson and collaborators commented that the PKU children had the highest behavioral deviance rate among the groups studied, with the exception of children with multiple lesions above the brainstem, who had similar rates. They speculated that several factors may be responsible for this high rate:

> a direct effect of the raised blood phenylalanine levels on brain cell metabolism,
> an effect of raised phenylalanine blood levels on brain growth and development in early life,
> psychological effects of the prolonged abnormal diet on both the child and family,
> a genetic mechanism linking PKU vulnerability to psychiatric disturbances.

11.2   Chromosomal Disorders

A great many chromosomal abnormalities have been described and Table 11-3 presents a partial list of the most frequently occurring syndromes. Basically, they represent an unexplained failure of chromosomes to develop properly (**chromosomal dysgenesis**) during the formation of the oocyte or spermatocyte or during conception and germination, resulting in an irreversibly abnormal chromosome makeup in the embryo. Major forms include the presence of extra chromosomes—for example, in (1) **trisomy** three chromosomes of a particular type are present instead of two; (2) **translocation**, mismatched chromosome pairs or portions of a chromosome in the fertilized ovum; and (3) structural abnormalities involving partial or complete **deletion** of a part of the chromosome, e.g., short-arm deletion. Even within each of these syndromes, molecular geneticists have been able to describe many specific variants (Latt et al. 1984).

Many fetuses with chromosomal disorders abort spontaneously. Among live newborns, 1 out of 200 has a significant chromosomal abnormality; about one-third of these abnormalities affect the autosomes and two-thirds the sex chromosomes (Hook 1981). As shown in Figure 11-1, many chromosomal abnormalities have a relationship to the age of the mother. Chromosomal errors are usually the result of **nondysjunction**; that is, chromosome pairs may remain

Table 11-3. Incidence of Chromosomal Errors in Consecutive Infants

Jacobs et al. (pooled data)		
Both sexes	Frequency
Trisomy	
13	1/10 000
18	1/10 000
21	1/1000
	1/830
Males	
XYY	1/1100
XXY	1/1100
Other	1/1700
	1/400
Females	
XO	1/10 000
XXX	1/1100
Other	1/3300
	1/770
Euploid autosomal rearrangement	
Both sexes	1/520
Anuploid autosomal rearrangement	
Both sexes	1/2000
Sex chromosome male and female	1/500
Autosomal trisomies	1/830
Autosomal rearrangement	1/420
	1/179

Berger (pooled data)	
Autosomal trisomies	Frequency
13	1/7100
18	1/3700
21	1/670

Lubs and Ruddle: Number of chromosome abnormalities in 4500 consecutive newborns	
Type of abnormality	Chromosomal abnormalities (No./1000)
Translocations	1.37
XXY	0.92
Trisomy G	0.69
XYY	0.69
XXX	0.69
Trisomy D	0.23
Trisomy E	0.23
XO	0.23

Source: De Myer 1975.

attached as two chromosomes in one of the oval cells during the final cell division while the other cell has no portion of the particular chromosome. A similar process may occur immediately after fertilization during the first few cell divisions; this results in some parts of the embryo having a normal complement of chromosomes, whereas other parts have a trisomic complement, a condition described as **mosaicism**.

Chromosomal abnormalities almost invariably result in physical abnormalities. Most of these are easily detected in the newborn, although a strikingly high proportion (25 per cent) of children with Down syndrome (trisomy 21, also translocation 15/21 and mosaic form of trisomy) are unrecognized at birth. Partial trisomy of chromosome 15 with mild to moderate stigmatization has been found in a subgroup of autistic children (Gillberg et al. 1991).

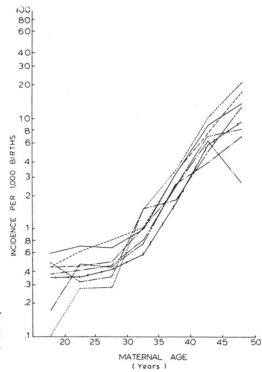

Figure 11-1. Incidence rates of Down syndrome by maternal age at birth from selected studies, 1923–1964 (Lilienfield 1969).

Mental retardation is a common consequence of autosomal, but not necessarily of sex chromosome, disorders. The intelligence of Down syndrome children can range from extremely low to IQs up to 70, but on average falls below an IQ of 50. The intellectual development and specific neuropsychological characteristics of children with Down syndrome are described in detail in Chapter 28.

Nondysjunction of the sex chromosomes produces various **sex chromosomal anomalies** (more or less than two sex chromosomes, both aneuploid and mosaicism), such as 45 XO (Turner syndrome), 47 XXX, 47 XYY, and 47 XXY (Klinefelter syndrome). A 10-year follow-up study from birth of 51 such children, compared to their normal siblings (Robinson et al. 1983), revealed that the physical manifestations are relatively minor: XXY boys and XXX girls are significantly taller and show some problems in muscular and motor development, male adolescents have small testicular volume, and XO girls are relatively small. Intelligence is generally within normal limits although a majority of scores are at the lower range of the scale. XXY boys and XXX girls are at greater risk for speech and language disorders, although such disorders are more frequent in the total group as well. A Danish study of language-impaired children found that 8 out of 92 children showed chromosomal abnormalities, but only two were XYY sex chromosomal trisomies (Friedrich et al. 1982). Learning disorders and neuromaturational lag were reported to be more frequent in XXY males and XXX females than in other children (Mandoki et al. 1991). Other authors have also noted a risk for language-based dyslexia in XXY boys (Bender et al. 1986b, Graham et al. 1981). Bender et al. (1986a) produced neuropsychological profiles for various sex chromosome disorder groups indicating that verbal IQ is often lower, that language and auditory memory impairments are common, and that spatial abilities and neuromotor skills are frequently impaired as well. Many of the subjects with sex chromosome anomalies were classified as learning disabled. Emotional disorder was more frequent in the group as a whole, particularly when family stress was high. All findings were less pronounced in children with mosaic anomalies.

A series of studies of XXY males has focused on the hormonal pattern as a potential cause of "minor irreversible impairment" (Theilgard 1984). Netley and Rovet (1987, 1988) concluded from their studies that these males had a stronger right-to-left inhibition during maturation, leading to a right hemisphere dominance for verbal and nonverbal cognitive processing, as well as to lower-than-average activity levels and tendencies toward social withdrawal during puberty. They also proposed that the total finger ridge count, a dermatoglyphic index relating to variations in mitotic cell division rate, was also related to hemispheric specialization. The authors generalized their model to stages of both normal and abnormal sex chromosome maturation in terms of ability pattern and hemispheric specialization (Figure 11-2), somewhat like Geschwind and Galaburda (1987, see Chapter 5).

Turner Syndrome

First described by Turner in 1938, this example of a chromosomal disorder drew attention not only because of its physical characteristics but also because of highly specific psychological abnormalities. The basic form of **Turner syndrome** results from a missing sex chromosome (usually written as 45, XO) due to nondysjunction in the meiotic division of either parent or in the first mitotic division after fertilization. Hence, no relationship with maternal age has been found. Since the second sex chromosome determines the sex of the individual, Turner syndrome infants are female. Mosaic forms have also been reported.

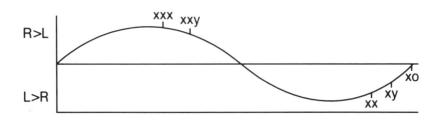

Figure 11-2. Stage of hemispheric maturation in X aneuploid and normal males and females during early cognitive development (Netley and Rovet 1988, Rovet and Netley 1983).

The physical appearance is characteristic: short in stature (less than 5 feet tall), undeveloped or poorly developed primary sex characteristics, sexual dysfunction in puberty and adulthood, webbed neck, low posterior hairline, broad chest with widely spaced nipples, and a deformed bend of the forearm (deviating to the midline of the body in an extended position and called cubitus valgus). Generally, individuals with mosaic forms have fewer abnormalities. The structure of the brain has not been studied systematically, but there are usually no neurological abnormalities. Spontaneous abortions are quite frequent; in fact, it has been reported that 95 to 98 per cent of XO fetuses fail to survive (Hecht and MacFarlane 1969). Treatment with female hormones has had limited success in furthering sexual development during puberty, although sterility is irreversible.

Turner syndrome has attracted considerable interest in neuropsychology because of a cognitive impairment that was thought to be highly specific. Although mental retardation is rare and only mild if it occurs, striking defects in the perception of form and space have been described (Figure 11-3). Alexander et al. (1966) found a mean IQ of 101 in a sample of 18 cases, but the verbal IQ was 112 on average, in contrast to a performance IQ of only 81. Factor scores revealed specific disabilities on such Wechsler subtests as Digit Span and Arithmetic (factor: freedom from distractibility) and Block Design and Object Assembly (factor: perceptual organization, Shaffer 1962). The ability to draw a human figure or reproduce geometric designs, map-reading skills, and word fluency usually are clearly defective; girls with Turner syndrome tend to have problems finding their way into and out of buildings or city districts. In a study of 67 Turner syndrome females, ranging in age from 6 to 31 years and compared with matched controls, Garron (1977) found no increase in the incidence of mental deficiency (mean IQs 96 and 98, respectively) nor was intelligence re-

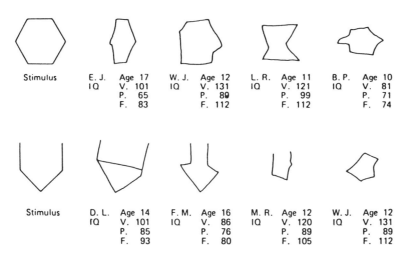

Figure 11–3. Drawings of two stimulus figures from the Benton Visual Retention test by girls with Turner syndrome (Alexander et al. 1966).

lated to the karyotype (XO or mosaic) or to the number or specific types of physical stigmata. Garron did confirm, however, that these subjects had specific difficulties in tasks requiring spatial and numerical abilities. On average, the performance IQ was 17 points lower than the verbal IQ.

Nyborg and Nielsen (1977) also reported poor scores on tests for the recognition of embedded figures, maze tasks, and the rod-and-frame test, which requires the subject to adjust a luminescent rod within a luminescent frame to the exact vertical position in a dark room; the frame may be tilted to varying degrees. The average normal error is about 6 degrees from true vertical, but Turner syndrome females showed an average of 12 degrees of error. The authors also reported that estrogen treatment tended to improve rod-and-frame test results.

These findings led to the speculation that the cognitive defect is based on a right hemisphere deficiency (Kolb and Heaton 1975), specifically the right parietal area (Money 1973). This interpretation is based on the view that spatial perception is more closely related to right hemisphere function. However, it does not explain the deficits in word fluency and the memory-for-rhythm test of Seashore (Silbert et al. 1977). Shucard et al. (1992) also found poor performance on measures specific to spatial skills, as well as visual ERP amplitude asymmetry consistent with the spatial deficit. Waber (1979b) conducted a comprehensive examination of 11 teenage to young adult women with Turner syndrome and 11 controls matched for background, age, and overall IQ. She found that the patient group performed significantly more poorly on tests of word fluency, perception of left and right, visuomotor coordination, visual memory, and motor learning. They also showed a higher incidence of left-ear advantage on the dichotic listening test, but their performance on other tests (including the perceptual organization factor on the Wechsler test, face recognition, a roadmap directional sense test, the spatial part of the California Test of Mental Maturity, and finger tapping) did not differ significantly from that of the control group. Waber concluded that it is questionable whether a specific defect in spatial ability exists. Rather than using a hemisphere-specific model, she preferred the interpretation that both cerebral hemispheres in the frontal and parietal areas may be involved in Turner syndrome. Waber has taken Luria's theoretical position that "early alterations in brain development have a generalized rather than localized effect on brain function in later life." She also noted that the performance of women with Turner syndrome resembles that of prepubertal children; hence, the syndrome may reflect lack of pubertal changes or a maturational lag, since all the functions found impaired in patients improve markedly in normal children between the age of 6 and 10 years. Similarly, McGlone (1985) rejected a focal CNS dysfunction interpretation, based on her detailed study of speech lateralization and somatosensory right-left differences in 11 13- to 18-year-old Turner syndrome subjects. Additional supporting evidence comes from Lewandowski et al. (1984), Pennington et al. (1985), and Tsuboi and Nielsen (1976), who found in Turner syndrome patients an EEG immaturity similar to the EEG patterns of girls 6 to 9 years of age, but no lateralized abnormalities.

Nor did Reske-Nielsen et al. (1982) find consistent localized lesions in the autopsied brains of two Turner syndrome patients.

One specific finding of interest in Waber's (1979b) study is the lack of ear lateralization in dichotic listening. Netley (1976) and Netley and Rovet (1982) had reported similar findings. Both authors suggested that sex hormones may be necessary for the lateralization of language to the left hemisphere.

Several reports (Nielsen and Sillesen 1981, Trunca 1980) indicated that Turner syndrome women are socially immature and unassertive, show poor peer relationships, and have significant behavior problems. To rule out the possibility that this impression simply reflects the fact that they are short and sexually immature, McCauley et al. (1987) compared a group of 17 Turner syndrome girls between 9 and 17 years of age with 16 controls matched for height, age, verbal IQ, and family socioeconomic status. They confirmed that Turner syndrome subjects performed more poorly on spatial, attentional, and short-term memory tasks, but in addition these girls were also inferior in the ability to discriminate affect in characters from television clips. The authors concluded that this latter deficit may underlie psychosocial problems found in Turner syndrome samples.

Further speculation centers around the possibility that Turner syndrome may reflect an exaggerated "female" pattern of behavior, since visuospatial skills have been reported to be more poorly developed in females generally (Wittig and Peterson 1979; see Chapter 6). Waber (1977) rejected this interpretation since many other nonspatial deficits are present. However, the findings in Turner syndrome do raise the question of the role of the second X chromosome, since this defect is obviously not related to survival. Turner syndrome females tend to show poor development of physical sex characteristics, consistent with their genetic status. Gartler et al. (1973) suggested that the second X chromosome is important in many tissues for the first few cell divisions and that the lack of this chromosome may lead to irregular somatic growth patterns, which are reflected both in the physical abnormalities of Turner syndrome women and in abnormal patterns of their CNS development (Rovet and Netley 1982). The second X chromosome becomes inactive during later development in most parts of the body except for the ovaries.

Fragile-X Syndrome

The occurrence of a fragile site on the long arm of the X-chromosome (at Xq27 [Figure 11-4]) was first described by Lubs (1969), but the clinical manifestations and importance of the **fragile-X syndrome** for mental development were not studied in detail until the 1980s. Rogers and Simensen (1987) estimated its prevalence as 1 in 1350 males and 1 in 2033 females, suggesting that it accounts for up to 10 per cent of all persons with developmental handicap and is second only to Down syndrome among the etiologies of mental retardation associated with cytogenetic abnormalities. In females, the second X chromosome may mask

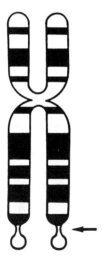

Figure 11-4. Fragile-X chromosome. Arrow points at fragile site.

the effects of the faulty one. However, some 20 per cent of males who inherit the defect are unaffected carriers, and only one-third of females who are carriers are affected (Hagerman and McBogg 1983). The inheritance pattern is not understood fully. Defects associated with fragile-X syndrome in males include enlarged testicles (hyperorchidism) (which are always present), and, less frequently, long thin faces, midface hypoplasia, simple oversized ears, an elongated forehead, and double-jointedness. Low synaptic density and poor development of synapses in the brain have been described. Reiss et al. (1991) found abnormalities of the posterior fossa in MRI scans of 14 fragile-X males: the size of the cerebellar vermis was decreased and the fourth ventricle increased in comparison to a normal control group. In addition to mental retardation, psychological defects range from learning disabilities, hyperactivity, aggressiveness, and unusual hand movements to autism. However, Wright et al. (1986) reported that only 1 of 40 autistic children had a fragile-X syndrome, and Gillberg et al. (1985) who studied ten such cases emphasized that a number of other pathological factors were present and that no direct association between fragile-X and autism should be inferred.

Mean IQs of 26 for males and 49 for females have been reported by Rogers and Simensen (1987). These authors found neuropsychological test patterns that suggested diffuse dysfunction without consistent lateralizing signs. Long-term follow-up shows a decline in IQ, specifically at the time of onset of puberty (Hodapp et al. 1990). Some investigators reported a specific speech and language deficit that could not be explained solely by mental retardation (McLaughlin and Kriegsman 1980), but others did not confirm this finding. Early treatment with folic acid has shown some promise (Hagerman et al. 1986). Dykens et al. (1993) provided a detailed review of fragile-X research.

Summary

A large number of developmental defects are genetically transmitted. Of this group, the disorders of metabolism have been studied intensively. The development of the child with phenylketonuria was chosen as an example. A second group of disorders occurs because of defects in the genetic material, i.e., the chromosomes. The best-known example is Down syndrome, which may result from the nondysjunction of chromosome 21 or translocation, although an inherited form has also been described. Because of the special interest for neuropsychological theory, the development of the XO female (Turner syndrome) and of the male with fragile-X syndrome was described in some detail. A variety of specific cognitive deficits in addition to general mental handicap have been described and their neuropsychological meaningfulness continues to be debated.

12

Structural Abnormalities

This chapter deals with one major group of congenital defects, the structural malformations, or **dysmorphias**, that are present at birth. These contrast with the congenital disorders involving physiological functions, such as metabolism, that were discussed in the preceding chapter. Structural abnormalities are usually of undetermined origin. One structural abnormality, agenesis of the corpus callosum, was discussed in Chapter 9 because of its impact on neuropsychological theory.

A group of structural abnormalities in which hands and feet are formed adjacent to the shoulders and hips (phocomelias) became notorious in the 1960s when about 15,000 babies were born with this malformation before thalidomide, a widely prescribed sleeping medication, was recognized to be the teratogenic agent.

Not all malformations are evident upon physical examination at birth. It has been reported that two-thirds of the malformations recognized at the age of 12 months were not detected at birth (Aase 1990). Unrecognized malformations include some forms of hydrocephalus and microcephaly, as well as minor neuroanatomical defects. Depending on their effect on an individual's life, some defects may be discovered only accidentally at autopsy, e.g., heteropia, misplaced groups of nerve cells. **Dandy-Walker syndrome**, which involves abnormal development of the posterior fossa and cerebellum and obstruction of the fourth ventricle, is often recognized during the first 2 years of life because of increased intracranial pressure, although it is usually not apparent prenatally or immediately after birth. Symptoms may, in fact, not appear until later in childhood, and in some instances the condition may remain asymptomatic into adulthood (Lipton et al. 1978). Ultrasonographic prenatal diagnosis has been reported to be successful in uncovering many cases (Newman et al. 1982).

Defects that are of neither medical nor cosmetic consequence (e.g., single palmar crease) have been termed **minor physical anomalies** (MPA). They are usually present at birth and remain relatively stable in childhood (Quinn and Rapoport 1974). Multiple minor malformations, however, tend to be associated

198

with major malformations (Smith 1971). Waldrop et al. (1968, Table 12-1) have suggested a weighted scoring system for MPAs.

12.1 Structural Abnormalities of the Central Nervous System

Malformations of the CNS, particularly the brain itself, are naturally of primary importance for neuropsychological development (Sarnat 1991). The incidence of these abnormalities ranges from 2.5 to 3.0 per 1000 children under the age of 12 months (Table 12-2). Since spontaneous abortions occur frequently with these disorders, the recorded incidence represents only a very small portion of the actual incidence. Table 12-2 includes only anencephaly and hydrocephaly,

Table 12-1. Minor Physical Anomalies and Their Significance in Scoring Weights

Head	
Fine electric hair (very fine, does not comb down)	1–2
Two or more hair whorls near crown of head	0
Head circumference 1 to 11/2 standard deviations above norm	1–2
Eye	
Epicanthus (vertical skin fold covering or partially covering the lacrimal caruncle)	1–2
Hypertelorism (unusually wide-set eyes, e.g., more than 32 mm according to 7-year-old Caucasian norms)	1–2
Ears	
Low-seated ears (below the line set by nose bridge and outer corner of the eye)	1–2
Adherent ear lobes	1–2
Malformed ears (asymmetrical, shape or protrusion)	1
Soft and pliable ears (jellylike feel)	0
Mouth	
High-steeped palate (roof of mouth forming an angle, rather than an arch)	1–2
Furrowed tongue (one or more deep grooves)	1
Tongue with smooth-rough spots (localized thickening of the epithelium)	1
Hand	
Curved fifth finger (inward curve)	1–2
Single transverse palmar crease (simian crease)	1
Feet	
Third toe longer than second	1–2
Partial syndactylia of two middle toes (webbing extending to the nearer toe joint)	1–2
Big gap between first and second toe (with flat base across gap at least the size of half the width of the second toe)	1

Source: Waldrop and Halverson 1971.

Table 12-2. Incidence of Anencephaly, Spina Bifida, and Hydrocephalus in Newborns (per 1,000 Births)

Disorder	WHO[a] Worldwide	NIHCS[b] Whites	NIHCS[b] Blacks	Male/female Ratio[c]
Anencephaly	1.05[d]	0.99	0.24	0.5
Hydrocephalus	0.87	1.4	1.3	NA
Spina bifida without hydrocephalus	0.55	0.66	0.68	0.7
Spina bifida with hydrocephalus	0.26			
Total	2.47	3.05	2.22	NA

[a]Stevenson et al. 1966.
[b]Myrianthopoulos and Chung 1974.
[c]Slater 1963.
[d]Values in the first three columns are per 1000 births.

omitting many other brain malformations, such as microcephaly, which occurs relatively frequently (Figure 12-1), and the many faults in development of the bones of the skull, face, and mouth (cranio-facial-oro syndromes), often including malformations of the fingers (digital syndromes).

The many syndromes combining structural abnormalities of the body and head are described in detail by Duckett (1981) and Jones (1988). Distinctions

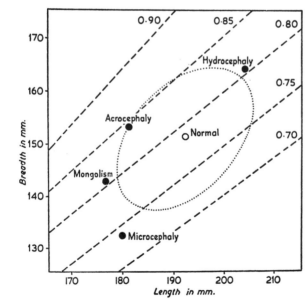

Figure 12-1. Mean head length and breadth in adult males (Penrose 1963).

are made between complete and partial lack of brain development (anencephaly), disproportionately small brain development (D6. microcephaly, micropolygyria), and enlarged head development, often with hydrocephalus (D2. macrocephaly).

Primary microcephaly is usually distinguished from secondary microcephaly. The rare, primary form is hereditary with autosomal recessive transmission (Figures 12-2 and 12-3), while other forms of microcephaly occur secondary to disorders of pregnancy or birth (Figures 12-4 and 12-5) or are associated with chromosomal disorders, e.g., cri-du-chat syndrome, short-arm deletion of a group 5 chromosome.

Another group of conditions results from premature closure of some of the bones of the skull (craniostenosis). Premature closure of the coronary bones results in a flat, short head (brachycephaly); early closure of the lateral bones results in asymmetric head shapes; upward and forward extension of the head, face, and eyes (oxycephaly) results from early closure of all bony connections. Another malformation of importance is **status dysraphicus**, the incomplete closure of the membranes surrounding the brain and the spinal cord (the caudal neuropore; Figure 2-1). Among the forms of this condition are **meningoencephalocele** (D1), a protrusion of the meningeal membranes and brain through a cranial defect, and **meningomyelocele**, a protrusion of the spinal cord and

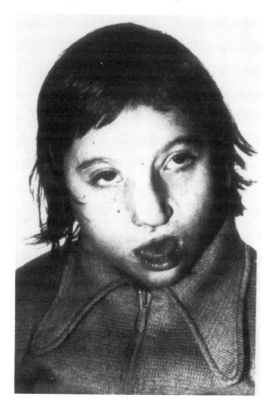

Figure 12-2. Microcephaly with damage to chromosome 13. Age 4.5; height 96 cm, head circumference 41 cm; cleft lip, jaw, and palate (Neuhaeuser et al. 1981).

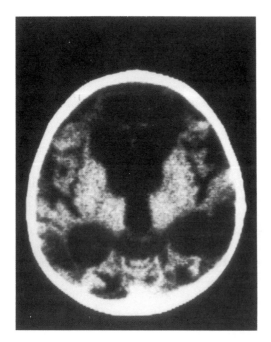

Figure 12-3. Tomography in micro-hydrocephaly of a 1-year-old child with postpartum hypoxia; enlargement of ventricular system and subarachnoid space (Neuhaeuser et al. 1981).

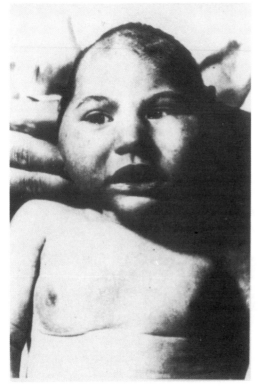

Figure 12-4. Microcephaly of exogenous prenatal origin. Hydrocephalus externus, cerebellar hypoplasia. Age 3 months, head circumference 29 cm; generalized seizures, muscle hypertonus, normal karyogram (Neuhaeuser et al. 1981).

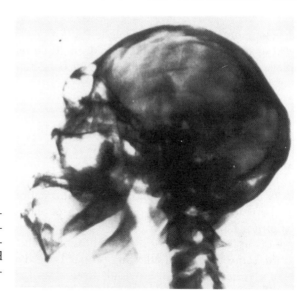

Figure 12-5. X-rays (lateral) of a 33-year-old individual with endogenous microcephaly. Height 162 cm, head circumference 45.3 cm (Neuhaeuser et al. 1981).

its covering membranes through a defect in the vertebral column. Another major form of status dysraphicus that affects psychological development is hydrocephalus internus and externus—the abnormal enlargement of the skull and the brain ventricles or subarachnoid space. The extent of the hydrocephalic condition is often described by Evans' ratio, defined as anterior horn width divided by internal skull breadth as determined in a CT scan (Figure 12-6). Schizencephaly presents with abnormal clefts in the gray matter of the cortex, an abnormal ventricular system, and other associated cerebral abnormalities. In hydranencephaly, a special case of anencephaly, there is a failure of cortical

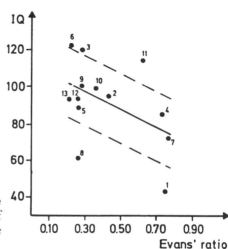

Figure 12-6. Intellectual performance (expressed as Evans' ratio) at the time of investigation in 13 shunted hydrocephalic children (Bottcher et al. 1978).

development that does not include the lower temporal and occipital lobes, as well as increased cerebrospinal fluid, multiple malformations, and a congenital single umbilical artery. For a review of congenital neurological malformations, see Icenogle and Kaplan (1981).

12.2   Etiology

Although structural defects have been associated with some well-defined disorders (e.g., chromosomal abnormalities), the exact causes for most defects remain unknown. Basically, most CNS malformations are defects of the formation of the neural tube during the induction period (third and fourth week of gestation). A fault in the separation of the mesenchymal and neuroectodermal tissue disrupts the normal growth and fusion of the neuroectoderm (neural tube), at the same time often affecting proper bone development from mesenchymal tissue. Other abnormalities result from disorders of nerve cell migration and proliferation during the second through the sixth month of gestation.

What leads to these disorders is still open to speculation. Genetic factors are suggested by the fact that neural tube defects occur less frequently in males and in African-Americans and that the incidence rate tends to be higher in the relatives of affected persons (Carter 1974). Fishman (1976) believed that a multifactorial genetic transmission can be assumed. Wide differences in frequency depending on geographical distribution (e.g., 4.5/1000 in Belfast versus 0.1/1000 in Bogota and Ljubljana) suggest both racial and nutritional factors. Among environmental factors, drugs, irradiation, excessive intake of vitamins and even of tea, and withholding zinc from the mother's diet are related to increased incidence (National Institute of Neurological and Communicative Disorders and Stroke 1979, Table 12-3). A recent large-scale study (Milunski et al. 1989) claimed that neural tube defects occur less frequently in women who use multivitamins including folic acid during the first 6 weeks of pregnancy. A higher incidence among infants born during winter months, first-borns of very young mothers, and the youngest children of older mothers has been reported. The relationship to maternal infections, especially the cytomegalovirus, is discussed in Chapter 14.

Finally, retarded brain development in the fetus affects the neuroendocrine balance. In particular, absence of the hypothalamus results in the lack of growth stimulation and, in addition, to the failure to accelerate labor; hence, the anencephalic or microcephalic fetus is likely to be exposed to additional perinatal stress (Swaab et al. 1978). Except for major damaging infections, none of the genetic or environmental factors has been shown to have a direct causal relationship; they probably should be regarded as contributing interactively to the etiology of structural defects.

Table 12-3. Known Causes of Developmental Defects in
Humans

Cause	Incidence (%)
Known genetic transmission	20
Chromosomal aberration	3–5
Environmental causes	
Radiation	<1
Therapeutic	
Nuclear	
Infections	2–3
Rubella virus	
Cytomegalovirus	
Herpesvirus hominis	
Toxoplasma	
Syphilis	
Maternal metabolic imbalance	1–2
Endemic cretinism	
Diabetes	
Phenylketonuria	
Virilizing tumors	
Drugs and environmental chemicals	2–3
Androgenic hormone	
Folic antagonists	
Thalidomide	
Organic mercury	
Some hypoglycemics (?)	
Some anticonvulsants	
Potentiative interactions	?
Unknown	65–70

Source: Wilson 1973.

12.3   Development of the Child with Meningomyelocele

The development of the newborn with a CNS anomaly depends upon the size
and location of the defect, especially as it affects brain development. With anencephaly, early death is likely. Microcephaly, porencephaly, and hydrocephalus
tend to be associated with developmental retardation, although the degree of
retardation is highly variable. Fusco et al. (1992) even reported a case of normal
intellectual development in a child with hemimegalencephaly (congenital overgrowth of one hemisphere), although most children with this abnormality suffer
from hemiparesis, mental retardation, and seizures. No specific psychiatric or
personality profile for hydrocephalic children has been identified (Donders et
al. 1992). Meningomyelocele is chosen as an example here because of its special
neuropsychological interest.

Meningocele usually is evident as a sack-shaped bulge in the dorsal region,
although in some instances it may be so small as to be undetectable by visual

inspection and may be asymptomatic (spina bifida occulta). The defect is a herniation of the spinal cord and its membranes. It is often referred to as spina bifida because of the associated lack of closure of the vertebral laminae that normally cover the spinal canal. Spina bifida without meningocele occurs fairly frequently (5 to 10 per cent of all newborns, according to Scarff and Fronczak 1981), but meningomyelocele, or spina bifida cystica, is relatively rare (approximately 5 per 1000, Ferguson-Smith 1983). If the spinal cord tissue is bulging into the sack (meningomyelocele), paralysis may occur depending on the location along the spinal cord. If the bulge is located in the sacral region, only bladder and bowel functions may be affected; if lumbar and lower dorsal regions are involved, paraplegia and sensory loss usually follow. In rare instances, the defect occurs in the upper dorsal or cervical region, producing paralysis and sensory loss in all functions below that level (Reigel 1982). Meningomyelocele is frequently accompanied by other CNS malformations. In all cases, the risk of infection is high, although the hernia may be closed surgically. Mental development depends, of course, on the magnitude of the cerebral defect.

Several other abnormalities are frequently associated with meningomyelocele (Gilbert et al. 1986): hydrocephalus occurs as a result of the partial closure of the cerebrospinal fluid ducts (aqueduct of Sylvius) connecting the fourth ventricle and the subarachnoid space; midline white matter structures (corpus callosum and internal capsule) are measurably reduced in size (Fletcher et al. 1992); the cerebellum and the medulla protrude into the upper spinal canal at the cervical level (Arnold-Chiari syndrome); the medulla shows an S-shaped kinking; parts of the visual and auditory system, as well as some of the cortical gyri, remain underdeveloped; the thalami may be fused, and complete or partial agenesis of the corpus callosum and of the olfactory tract and bulb may be present; and aberrant migration of cells during embryogenesis results in clusters of nonfunctional neurons in many parts of the brain (possibly producing epileptogenic foci). Seizures have been reported in 17 per cent of children with myelomeningocele (Noetzel and Blake 1991).

Pregnancy is usually normal, but early detection by amniocentesis is possible. Severely affected embryos are frequently aborted spontaneously. After birth, the defect is usually closed to prevent infection and damage to the herniated tissue; the hydrocephalus is shunted by insertion of a drainage tube to relieve the pressure. Bottcher and colleagues (1978) reported significant reduction in ventricular size of 13 successfully shunted hydrocephalic children.

The subsequent development of children with meningomyelocele and hydrocephalus has been studied widely. Intellectual functions usually remain at a mildly retarded to low-average level; IQ scores are commonly between 70 and 90, but range widely (Dennis et al. 1987, Erickson 1990, Friedrich et al. 1991, Wills et al. 1990) depending on the degree of hydrocephalus present. A study of four dizygotic and six monozygotic pairs of twins discordant for hydrocephalus (Berker et al. 1992) even reported reciprocity in the degree and nature of above-average intellectual development, despite drastically reduced cerebral mantle size in the hydrocephalic twin.

As a group, however, such children tend to show impaired concentration and visuo-perceptual difficulties (Miller and Sethi 1971). Difficulties in manual sensory functions, including sensitivity for touch, joint, and position awareness, and stereognosis are present, a primary cause of clumsiness in hand use (Hamilton 1991) and possibly of the drawing and handwriting problems reported by Reid and Sheffield (1990) and Ziviani et al. (1990). Brunt (1984) described an apraxic tendency in children with meningomyelocele. A survey of 527 children with meningomyelocele found an associated increase of urinary tract infections and bowel problems in more than 90 per cent of these children (Lie et al. 1991). Relatively good predictions about later achievement have been made as early as the second year of life (Fishman and Palkes 1974).

Nielsen (1980) examined a series of 30 unselected meningomyelocele cases in Denmark younger than the age of 18 months and attempted to follow them over a 5-year period. There were 19 girls and 11 boys in the sample. Only four did not require a shunt operation. At the age of 6 to 18 months, Cattell IQs ranged from 25 to 110 with a mean of 81; at age 3 years, the Minnesota Preschool Scale IQs ranged from 50 to 128 with a mean of 91; and at age 6 the WISC IQs ranged from 94 to 117 with a mean of 98 for the 8 children remaining in the study. Although these group differences may be influenced by sample attrition, those children who were retested on all occasions showed a definite gain in IQ level; correlations among measures ranged from .56 (between 6-month Cattell and 3-year Minnesota) to .84 (between 18-month Cattell and 3-year Minnesota). The authors interpreted the increase as the result of overcoming the early period of surgery with its frequent, lengthy hospitalizations. Most studies found no significant sex differences in IQ scores, although Lawrence and Tew (1971) found girls to be more retarded than boys. Shunt insertion tended to be associated with slower psychomotor development.

McLone et al. (1982) reported lower IQ scores (mean of 72) in 128 shunted children with meningomyelocele than in 39 nonshunted children (mean IQ of 102). However, this difference was almost entirely attributable to the occurrence of CNS ventriculitis. Fruehauf (1976) followed 36 hydrocephalic children who were shunted during the first year of life. Retesting in the first grade (up to age 9) showed an increase in developmental quotients for 60 per cent of the children from those obtained during the first 3 years of life; 10 per cent showed a decrease. Children in a subgroup with significant gains had less severe brain damage and early shunting. The developmental quotient was computed from a variety of measures, but rose mainly because of improved motor development (Ozeretzki Scale). The IQ remained stable over the years with a mean of 77 for the total group. Recent longitudinal studies of 56 (Jensen 1987) and 26 (Borjeson and Lagergren 1990) shunted children with meningomyelocele even recorded a mean IQ of 90. More than 75 per cent attended normal school and only 33 per cent received remedial instruction; no sex differences were found. These reports are confirmed in a study by Lord et al. (1990).

Surprisingly, many children with meningomyelocele acquire good verbal skills, although this has been characterized as an ability to learn words and speech at a superficial level. Several studies reported higher Verbal than Performance IQ results. The verbal-performance discrepancy obtained regardless of whether a shunt is inserted in the left or the right hemisphere (Grant et al. 1986). Hadenius and colleagues (1962) were the first to describe the verbal skills of meningomyelocele children as "**cocktail party syndrome**": a facility for chattering without knowing what they are talking about. Hurley et al. (1990) described such speech as "hyperverbal behavior with shallow intellect" with a glib, chatty, superficial quality. Irrelevant verbal production is noted (Foltz and Shurtleff 1972). Cutlatta and Young (1992) described the linguistic ability of children with spina bifida as being equal to normal children at the concrete level; however, they give more "no-responses" or irrelevant answers at more abstract levels of communication. This latter finding was not confirmed in the study of Byrne et al. (1990). Considering the results of the Nielsen follow-up study discussed above, it is possible that the cocktail party syndrome may result from frequent hospitalizations and illness, as well as by frequent physical handling because of paralysis; these circumstances may provide many more superficial child-adult interactions than other pediatric patients with or without hydrocephalus would normally receive. However, increased verbal imitation is found as early as the first 2 years of life (Morrow and Wachs 1992).

Children with hydrocephalus are also reported to show an "uneven growth of intelligence during childhood, with non-verbal intelligence developing less well than verbal intelligence" (Dennis et al. 1981, Fletcher et al. 1992). Dennis and colleagues proposed a somewhat different explanation for the relatively good verbal intelligence of hydrocephalic children: although increased verbal stimulation and contact through handling may play a role, their proposed factor is impaired development of the vertex and the occipital cortex, which block the cerebral aqueduct and result in visual abnormalities, motor deficits, and seizures. The child gains limited visuospatial experience and thus develops poor nonverbal intelligence. Grant's (1985) study emphasized that the deficit does not represent a general right hemisphere dysfunction; rather it is based on an asymmetrical cortical thinning or stretching in an antero-posterior direction and for this reason is more likely to disrupt visual rather than somatosensory processes as proposed by Dennis et al. (1981). Hurley et al. (1983) confirmed that sensorimotor tasks, such as the Tactual Performance Test, are not affected in most hydrocephalic children.

Another proposed explanation for this finding is the resilience of language (also described as "primacy of language") in the developmental period as compared to other cognitive functions (Dennis et al. 1987). In a sample of 75 hydrocephalic children ranging in age from 6 to 14 years, Dennis and colleagues found a steady progression of word-finding, fluency and automaticity, immediate sentence memory, understanding of grammar, and metalinguistic awareness (detecting syntactic anomalies) across age, although at a gradually slowing rate compared to normal children. Hydrocephalics with pre- or perinatal disturbances showed better language development, and those with intraventricular hydrocephalus did more poorly, especially on word-finding tasks. Children with spinal dysraphia did more poorly on verbal fluency tasks, but not on other language functions. The limits of the resilience of language were especially evident in later acquired or higher levels of academic skills. For example, Grant et al. (1986) found lower reading accuracy. A study by Barnes and Dennis (1992) of 50 6- to 15-year-old children with early hydrocephalus reported that primarily the understanding or comprehension of words and paragraphs was impaired in this group, whereas word recognition and reading of "pretend" words were not different from that of age- and education-matched controls. Murdoch et al. (1991) summarized the communicative impairments in children with neural tube disorders.

Few reports on later development have been published. As expected, academic difficulties, especially in arithmetic, are common in this population (Andrews and Elkins 1981, Shaffer et al. 1985). A report by Rinck et al. (1989) indicated that, in spite of extensive histories of surgery, most of the 38 adolescent survivors were mainstreamed into regular classroom settings. The continuing impairment of visual-cognitive skills was documented by Simms (1986) in a relatively unimpaired group of learner drivers with meningomyelocele and hydrocephalus; all subjects showed poor performance on relevant tests.

In a preliminary study of 119 young people (89 with cerebral palsy and 30 with meningomyelocele with hydrocephalus), Anderson (1979) found that only 48 per cent were without marked or borderline personality disorders compared to 85 per cent of a nonhandicapped control group. The incidence of psychological disorder was highest for meningomyelocele girls. The nature of the disorder was most frequently described as being neurotic, rather than conduct or mixed disorder (72, 15, and 5 per cent, respectively). Misery and depression, lack of self-confidence, self-consciousness, and fearfulness were most frequently mentioned. Ratings of the overall quality of life suggested that 41 per cent led an isolated and lonely life, 38 per cent had a very restricted social life, and only 21 per cent had satisfactory social lives (as compared to 93 per cent of the controls). Dependency on the family was high. Quality of life was closely related to severity of handicap.

Laurence and Tew (1971, Tew and Laurence 1975) noted the high incidence of maladjustment and emotional problems, even in nonhydrocephalic children with spina bifida. In children with hydrocephalus, Laatsch et al. (1984) noted that caretakers more frequently listed higher levels of aggression, increased moodiness, and somatic complaints. Breslau (1985) and Wallander and Varni (1989) confirmed the frequent occurrence of behavior problems, social incompetence, and poor social adjustment in larger samples. These problems were less severe in the absence of mental retardation and when good social support from both family and peers was provided (Fernell et al. 1991, Wallender et al. 1989).

12.4 Psychological Development in Children with Other Anomalies

Numerous studies of children with other CNS malformations, especially hydrocephalus, have been published. Some of these studies have already been described in the preceding section. A general finding is the strong association between malformations, on the one hand, and impaired development of brain and intellect, on the other. The finding of a higher verbal than performance IQ in hydrocephalic children has been confirmed in recent studies (Fletcher et al. 1991, Westerveld et al. 1991). These studies also found more left-handedness in these children and concluded that a reorganization of hemispheric specialization takes place. However, such a reorganization is "brittle" and tends to lead to a cognitive decline, particularly if the number of shunt revisions in left-handers is taken into account. Bigler (1988), in a review of studies of hydrocephalus, stressed that, although a variety of cognitive and perceptual-motor deficits are frequently found, there is "no common neuropsychological pattern" (p. 81) and little systematic relationship between ventricular size and type and degree of psychological impairment can be shown. Donders et al. (1990) reviewed the methodological issues and emphasized that the most significant predictor variables for intellectual status at age 5 to 8 years for hydrocephalus that was shunted during the first year of life are medical problems in infancy and ocular defects.

Some debate has arisen about the association between minor physical anomalies (MPAs) and the development of intelligence and occurrence of behavior problems. MPAs have no influence on attractiveness ratings (Rapoport and Quinn 1975), so that a direct influence on social interaction with peers is unlikely. Riese (1984) studied 120 full-term and 140 preterm neonates and found that full-term, but not preterm, male infants had higher MPA scores than females. However, the relationship between MPA scores and a variety of newborn behavioral measures was tenuous at best. In school-aged boys, hyperactive, disruptive, impulsive behavior has been reported to be associated with the number of minor anomalies. In girls, an association with passivity, low activity level, withdrawal, and chronic anxiety has been noted. Anomaly scores (based on the number and significance of physical anomalies) were also negatively correlated with IQ, although this was independent of the association with the inhibited behavior in girls (Waldrop and Goering 1971, Waldrop et al. 1976).

In a normal Danish birth cohort between 10 and 13 years of age, Fogel et al. (1985) did not find sex differences in MPA scores, but confirmed a strong association with hyperactive behavior in boys and with inhibited behavior in girls. The authors view MPAs as markers of nervous system anomalies because they originate in the same embryonic layer that produces the CNS. Deutsch et al. (1990) confirmed the frequent occurrence of MPAs in 6- to 14-year-old boys with attention deficit disorder (ADD) and speculate that they are transmitted by an autosomal dominant mode with partial penetrance because ADD probands who are not dysmorphic (have MPAs) have non-ADD relatives who are, a finding first reported by Firestone et al. (1978). For college-aged youth, Paulhus and Martin (1986) reported a significant correlation between MPA scores and lifestyle factors (physically active, aggression/misbehavior, clumsiness), and with emotionality, masculinity, sociability, and extraversion (based on factors from a multiple-choice questionnaire and interviews) in males, but not in females. Other studies have claimed a relationship between MPAs and a predisposition for violent (Mednick and Kandel 1988) and recidivistic violent behavior (Kandel et al. 1989) during late adolescence, but Crowner et al. (1987) found no such link in violent adult psychiatric inpatients.

MPAs have also been described as "markers" for behavioral or learning disabilities (Marino et al. 1987; Matthews and Barabas 1985) and as part of the "latent genetic structure" of attention deficit disorder (Deutsch et al. 1990). Shprintzen and Goldberg (1986) reviewed several physical anomaly syndromes and found that learning disabilities are a common feature in children, particularly if the syndrome occurs only in a mild form. Finally, a possible link between MPAs and autism (Mariner et al. 1986, Rosenberger-Debiesse and Coleman 1986) and with a predisposition for schizophrenia (Green et al. 1987, Guy et al. 1983) has been claimed.

Summary

Numerous structural malformations have been described in the literature. They arise from maldevelopment during the induction period or during the periods of rapid growth pre- and postnatally. Although some causes have been isolated, the etiology of most disorders remains unknown. The psychological development of children with structural malformations is usually affected to some degree requiring careful examination.

Long-term follow-up shows high infant mortality and severe impairment in most disorders, whereas a few produce little evidence of overt impairment. Although some improvement of mental functions during childhood, especially in shunt-operated hydrocephalics, has been noted, long-term mental development is frequently limited. Behavioral problems and specific patterns of speech arise probably as the result of the need for intensive handling and hospitalization during infancy and the continued need for assistance, especially in children with severe motor impairment (meningomyelocele and hydrocephalus).

13

Prematurity and Low Birth Weight

The questions of prematurity and low birth weight and the implications for later development are consistent with the theme of risk and vulnerability discussed throughout the book. This chapter deals with the assessment of preterm and low-birth-weight infants, major risk factors associated with these conditions, and the long-term outcome of prematurity and low birth weight.

One of the earliest definitions of **prematurity** was provided by the World Health Organization in 1949: a birth weight of 2500 g or less became the single criterion for prematurity. Two considerations seemed to influence this decision. First, birth weight is easily measured and universally noted in records, whereas gestational age, the other main index of prematurity, is more difficult to determine (Kopp and Parmelee 1979). Second, mortality and morbidity rates are highest for infants of low birth weight. Premature infants defined according to birth weight, however, constitute a heterogeneous group that includes those with congenital abnormalities, those born of mothers with small stature, those born early with weight appropriate for age, and infants born early who are clearly undernourished for age (Drillien 1964). When it became accepted that not all neonates of 2500 g or less at birth are premature, the designation **low birth weight** (LBW) was applied to them instead. Improvements in perinatal and neonatal care reduced the mortality rate and increased the need for differential diagnosis. In response to this need, the World Health Organization (1961) redefined prematurity to include infants with a birth weight of 2500 g or less who were born before 37 weeks of gestation. Thus, we now have two criteria for prematurity: low birth weight and immaturity. Within this still broad definition, premature infants can be divided into three major subgroups. The first includes infants born before 37 weeks whose weight is appropriate for gestational age, designated **preterm AGA**. Infants born before 37 weeks whose weight is small for gestational age, designated **preterm SGA**, form the second group; they are also called small-for-date (Eichorn 1979, Kopp and Parmelee 1979). Cutting across these two groups is a third group, identified by **very low birth weight**

(**VLBW**) (below 1500 g) or **extremely low birth weight (ELBW)** (below 1000 g). This group includes infants born very early but at a weight appropriate for gestational age and a distinct subgroup of infants who may be born either early or close to term who suffer from **intrauterine growth retardation** (IUGR), which is defined as birth weight falling below the tenth percentile for gestational age (Harel et al. 1989, Figure 13-1). The distinction between preterm AGA, preterm SGA, and VLBW is of more than academic interest because of the differences in etiology and outcome.

The estimation of gestational age can be based on the onset of last menses, amniocentesis, ultrasound, ophthalmological assessment, or neurobehavioral indicators. A widely used neurological assessment for the estimation of gestational age is the Dubowitz scale (see Chapter 7).

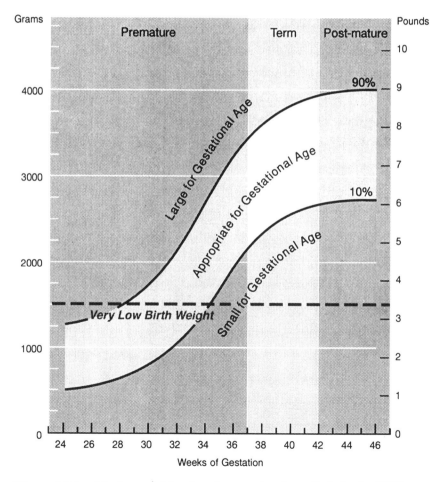

Figure 13-1.   Newborn weight chart by gestational age (Lubchenko 1976).

Despite the refinement of other measures to assess maturity, birth weight remains a useful indicator, and many earlier studies focused on the sequelae of low birth weight alone, rather than using a combination of criteria (Caputo and Mandell 1970, Harper and Weiner 1965). Although earlier research focused on birth weight below 2500 g, more recent studies have focused on infants weighing less than 1500 g (Goldson 1992, Hack et al. 1991, Robertson et al. 1992). Other studies have included birth weight and gestational age (Kurtzberg et al. 1979), gestational age alone (Amiel-Tison 1980), or a combination of age, weight, and body measurements (Caputo et al. 1981).

13.1 Major Risk Factors Associated with Prematurity

Approximately 5 to 8 percent of all infants in North America and Europe are born before 37 weeks and have birth weights of less than 2500 g. About 1 per cent are born with very low birth weight. In affluent societies, at least two-thirds of LBW infants are born preterm, whereas in developing countries most LBW births are due to IUGR (Barros et al. 1992). The exact causes of prematurity in many cases are not clear, although numerous factors are implicated.

Individual risk factors contributing to prematurity include the mother's age, previous pregnancy history, cigarette smoking, weight gain during pregnancy, and prepregnancy weight, as well as birth order (parity) and family income and education. There is an increased rate of premature births among women younger than 20 and older than 35 years (Placek 1977). The tendency to repeat preterm delivery accounts for 25 per cent of LBW infants among second births in Norway (Bakketeig 1977). In Canada, a previous preterm birth doubles the risk of having a LBW infant (Meyer et al. 1976). Income and education are inversely associated with the likelihood of prematurity (Garn et al. 1977), and smoking during the second half of pregnancy has been associated with a decrease of 200 g in the average birth weight (Davies et al. 1976). The difference in birth weight is most pronounced in babies born to mothers in the lower socioeconomic strata (Rush 1981). In Brazil, significant risk factors for IUGR include low socioeconomic status, low maternal height, low prepregnancy weight, short birth interval, and smoking during pregnancy (Barros et al. 1992).

To examine the individual contribution of risk factors to birth weight, Keller (1981) conducted a multiple regression analysis of data collected in a perinatal project. Table 13-1 illustrates the relative contribution of each variable. The most important factors are weight gain, prepregnancy weight, last prior birth weight, smoking, and previous pregnancy outcome.

Several medical complications pose risks for the premature infant. Some center around the infant's ability to receive sufficient oxygen. Respiratory problems are among the most common complications experienced by the preterm infant. The failure to breathe normally may be the result of immaturity of the lungs. In addition, hypoxia or drug-induced respiratory distress can pose risk (Rigatto and Brady 1972). The significance of these respiratory problems is discussed in

Table 13-1.   Percentage of Variance in Birth Weight "Explained" by Various Factors Among Multiparous Women[a]

	Variance explained	
Factor	White (n = 8326)	Black (n = 10 723)
Weight gain	6.6	8.2
Prepregnancy weight	6.0	4.6
Last prior birth weight	6.0	4.6
Cigarettes/day	3.2	1.4
Previous pregnancy outcome	1.0	1.7
Parity (order of pregnancy)	0.3	0.4
Mother's age	0	0
Annual income	0.1	0.1
Height	0	0
Maternal diseases	0.2	0.4
Fetal attributes[b]	2.6	1.6
Complications of pregnancy and labor	7.3	6.5
Total explained variance (multiple R squared)	33.3	29.5

Source: Keller 1981.
[a]Based on linear regression analysis (Weiss and Jackson 1969).
[b]Includes sex, congenital malformations, and Coombs test for blood antibodies to detect erythroblastosis.

Chapter 17 in the section on Anoxia. In most cases, 8 minutes is the upper limit of anoxia (lack of oxygen) that the premature infant can tolerate. Infants surviving longer periods of asphyxia show varying degrees of brain injury (Werthmann 1981). Partial deprivation of oxygen (hypoxia) presents a more subtle but equally threatening hazard. If asphyxia is followed by abnormal behavior, such as apneic spells (disturbances of breathing), apathy, and altered muscle tone, a syndrome of hypoxic-ischemic encephalopathy may result (Robertson et al. 1992). When hypoxic distress is not treated, small areas of brain circulation are closed down with a permanent loss of function. The outcome can range from severe disabilities, including early seizures, spasticity, or hypotonia, to more subtle effects that are not evident until childhood (Werthmann 1981).

The premature infant is vulnerable to a series of conditions that, if left untreated, can seriously influence later development. Risk is conceptualized as a physical-environmental factor that could adversely affect development. For example, prenatal exposure to toxic substances is a potential risk factor. Vulnerability refers to the characteristics of the infant that increase the probability of adverse effects on development (Greenbaum and Auerbach 1992). Some researchers have attempted to deal with risk and vulnerability through the development of screening assessments and cumulative risk scores (Apgar 1953, Field et al. 1979, Hines et al. 1980, Littman and Parmelee 1978, Prechtl 1968, Siegel 1992). A meta-analysis of six major perinatal risk scales was conducted by Molfese (1989), who reduced 303 individual items from five scales to 108 items that were shown to be the best predictors of infant outcome. These items, in turn, formed the basis of a new composite risk scale that predicted a greater number of outcome measures than three of the five original scales. The amount of variance accounted for by the new composite score was increased by adding measures of maternal personality characteristics, such as anxiety and depression, and life stress events.

The vulnerability of the VLBW and the ELBW infant to complications of birth deserves special consideration. This group includes infants born preterm (some as young as 24 weeks) whose weight is appropriate for gestational age, as well as those born preterm who are small for gestational age as a result of intrauterine growth retardation. Most IUGR infants fall below the third percentile for growth standards and weigh between 500 and 1500 g. Failure to grow may be due to impaired fetal oxygen or nutrient transport or the exchange of metabolic waste and is influenced by such maternal conditions as toxemia, smoking, drug and alcohol use, viral infections, structural features of the uterus, or placental or fetal abnormalities (Kopp and Parmelee 1979). Preterm infants with weight appropriate for gestational age usually catch up in growth, whereas IUGR infants remain smaller (Barros et al. 1992, Villar and Belizan 1982).

After delivery, the VLBW infant is extremely susceptible to complications. Neonatal morbidity may include respiratory distress, necrotizing colitis, septicemia, meningitis, hypoglycemia, hypothermia, intraventricular hemorrhage, periventricular leukomalacia, and a recirculation of arterial blood to the lungs (Hack et al. 1992).

VLBW alone may influence developmental outcome. Parkinson et al. (1981) followed 60 SGA infants, each of whom had undergone serial ultrasound measures of head growth before birth. They found that children whose head growth had slowed before 34 weeks gestation were more likely to be of shorter stature at 4 years. Those who had slow head growth starting before 26 weeks gestation had lower developmental quotients at a 4-year follow-up and were found to have difficulties with concentration, balance, and coordination at the 6-year follow-up. Small head circumference in VLBW infants persisting beyond the first year of life has also been shown to affect intellectual, language, and visuomotor outcome at the age of 8 (Hack et al. 1991, Lucas et al. 1992). VLBW in combination with medical complications and specifically with intracranial hemorrhage leads to a greater compromise of developmental outcome (Ford et al. 1989).

13.2 Comparisons Between Low-Risk Premature and Full-Term Infants

The neurobehavioral development of premature infants has been extensively examined for some time. As early as 1945, Gesell and Amatruda reported that prematurity alone neither retarded nor accelerated the inherent development sequences. Similarly, Saint-Dargassies (1966) examined the neurological matu-

ration of infants from 28 to 41 weeks conceptual age and concluded that neurological development unfolds at a predetermined rate, regardless of the time
of birth. These studies, which compared full-term newborns at 40 weeks with
preterm infants tested at 40 weeks corrected conceptual age (i.e., gestational
age plus age from birth), agree that the two groups show many similarities.

Most studies on the developmental outcome of the preterm infant use a
correction for gestational age to allow for the disadvantage of biological maturity
and to separate delay associated with prematurity from that caused by CNS
damage. Some studies reported that, when correction is applied to infants born
more than 8 to 12 weeks preterm, a skewed distribution occurs so that overtly
abnormal infants fell within the normal range (Miller et al. 1984, Parmelee and
Schultz 1970).

More recent studies suggest that preterm infants at 40 weeks corrected age
show differences in neurobehavioral performance relative to full-term infants
(Ferrari et al. 1983, Piper et al. 1985). EEG maturation is often delayed (Cioni
et al. 1990). Differences in activity states and development, including inferior
performances on visual and auditory orienting, inferior motor performance, and
weak state regulation, have been noted. Using the Assessment of Preterm Infant
Behavior Scale, a scale designed to measure the behavioral repertoire of preterm
infants, Als and her colleagues (1982, 1988) found significant behavioral differences between full-term and preterm infants. Overall, the preterm infants as a
group at 42 weeks corrected age had moderate difficulties with autonomic, motor, and state organization and great difficulties in coming to a steady, focused
alert state; they also displayed more autonomic lability and motoric stress.

Studies of sensory functioning in the preterm infant have demonstrated an
unevenness of development. Fetal tactile, auditory, and visual modalities are not
equally developed at the time of preterm birth (Gottlieb 1971, Table 13-2). The
fetal tactile system develops first and is functional at 4 months of gestation
(Hooker 1952). The fetal auditory system is not functional before 8 months of
gestation (Parmelee 1981). The visual system continues to develop throughout
pregnancy, and structural changes occur as late as 9 months of gestation (Mann
1969). Some researchers argue that, because the normal environment for the
developing sensory system is intrauterine, extrauterine conditions do not provide
optimal support for development. One would therefore expect the visual system,
which is not mature at preterm birth, to be most seriously affected by premature
exposure to the extrauterine environment. Following this line of reasoning, the
tactile system would not be affected and the auditory system less affected than
the visual. Results from several studies support this hypothesis (Caron and Caron 1981, Parmelee 1981, Rose 1981, Siqueland 1981, White and Brackbill
1981).

Comparative studies on tactile processing in full-term and preterm infants
with a mean conceptual age of 38 weeks show that the preterm infant's performance, as measured by cardiac responsiveness, is only slightly deficient (Field
et al. 1979, Rose et al. 1976). Studies on auditory processing also describe preterm infants of less than 36 weeks conceptual age as less responsive (Als et al.

Table 13-2. Ontogenetic Sequence of Sensory Function in Neonates Whose Condition at Birth Is Normal After 265-Day Gestation

Function	Approximate day of onset	Type of evidence	Source
Tactile	Prenatal day 49	Behavior	Hooker 1952
		Histology	Humphrey 1964
Vestibular	Prenatal day 90–120	Behavior	Minkowski 1928
		Histology	Humphrey 1955, Langworthy 1933
Auditory	Prenatal day 210 or earlier	Behavior	Fleischer 1955
	Prenatal day 180 or earlier	Physiology and histology	Bredberg 1968
	Prenatal day 147 or earlier	Physiology	Weitzman and Graziani 1968
Visual	Prenatal day 180 or earlier	Physiology	Ellingson 1960
	Prenatal day 154 or earlier	Physiology	Engel 1964

Source: Gottlieb 1971.

1979, Katona and Berenyi 1974). Cortical auditory evoked potentials (AEP) to consonant-vowel syllables were recorded at 40 weeks in full-term infants and 40 weeks conceptual age in VLBW infants and later at 1, 2, and 3 months (Kurtzburg et al. 1984). The VLBW infants exhibited significantly less mature AEPs than the full-term infants. By 3 months all infants exhibited mature AEP morphology and topography. These findings led the authors to conclude that the relative immaturity of the cortical mechanisms of speech processing in some VLBW infants might contribute to a later speech and language disorder, a finding confirmed in a study by Vohr et al. (1989).

The most marked differences between preterm and full-term infants have been found in visual processing. Fantz and Fagan (1975) described a shorter attention span for preterm infants 10 weeks after delivery than for full-term infants 5 weeks after delivery. Sigman and Parmelee (1976) identified a preference for familiar rather than novel stimuli in preterm infants at 4 months corrected conceptual age. Using a visual recognition task, Rose (1981) found that preterm infants could not discriminate between familiar and novel stimuli until 12 months corrected age, whereas full-term infants demonstrated such discriminations at 6 months. In a study of the ability to process categorical information, preterm infants at 33 weeks conceptual age responded only to changes in detail of stimuli, whereas full-term infants at 33 weeks could respond to both changes in detail and configuration (Caron and Caron 1981). These studies suggest that the premature infant shows a less mature response pattern to visual processing.

The temperament of preterm infants between 4 and 8 months conceptual age was studied to investigate whether prematurity poses a risk for subsequent social interaction (Oberklaid et al. 1986). Infants born preterm did not differ significantly on any temperament dimensions.

In summary, the differences between sensory processing abilities in preterm and full-term infants overall are minimal, and many of them disappear if adjustments are made for conceptual age. These differences are not evenly distributed across modalities: more significant differences are found in visual than in auditory and tactile processing. The lag or deficit in some areas of sensory processing can be explained as the result of exposure to the extrauterine environment before the sensory system has completed maturation. There seems to be an inverse relationship between the degree of maturation of the sensory system at preterm birth and the impact on the system of exposure to the extrauterine environment. The evidence for uneven development in the premature infant and the hypothesis of maturational readiness fit well with Gottlieb's (1971) theoretical framework on the development and maturation of sensory functions.

There have been several studies of supplemental extrauterine stimulation, including auditory (Katz 1971), tactile and kinesthetic (Korner 1985, 1986, Scardafi et al. 1986), rhythmic rocking (Thoman et al. 1991), and multimodal stimulation (Scarr-Salapatek and Williams 1973). Among the dependent variables have been growth measures, activity levels, performance on development assessments, visual orientation, and recognition memory. Most studies cite some benefits of supplemental stimulation, including weight gain, increased activity level, improved visual and auditory responsivity, and better performance on development assessment scales, especially for motor development (Field 1980). Continued stimulation programs beyond the hospital stay have also demonstrated sustained effects. Follow-up studies describe better performance in exploratory behavior, parent-infant interaction (Garber 1988), and on the Bayley Scales of Infant Development (Siqueland 1973, Sostek et al. 1979).

The evidence suggests that at 40 weeks conceptual age the neurological and behavioral status of the premature infant without complications is generally similar, but less mature, than that of the full-term infant. Infants born prematurely have temperament profiles similar to infants born at term. Differences reflect an uneven development across sensory modalities for the premature infant, particularly in visual and auditory orienting and perception, motor performance, and state regulation. During the first year of life differences have been noted in visual recognition and memory. However, the overall differences between term and preterm infants without complications are small and may fall within the variability of performance for the full-term range (Touwen 1980). Infant stimulation has been shown to be beneficial.

13.3   Outcome of Prematurity

A synthesis of current research findings on outcome is difficult because of the heterogeneity of the samples in published studies. Study groups of premature infants differ in gestational age, birth weight, adequacy of intrauterine growth for gestational age, and number of complications, and each of these variables has a number of possible causes and different outcomes. In addition, variations in experimental parameters, including different assessments and observation techniques, hinder the comparison within and between groups. Neurobehavioral findings are difficult to relate to underlying brain function in the newborn infant. Perinatal cerebral damage produces few characteristics that would allow the localization of areas of dysfunction (Kurtzberg et al. 1979). Equally important, the immature brain has the capacity for functional restoration in later development; this restoration, described in Chapter 8, limits the degree to which neural damage occurring in early life remains apparent.

Neonatal neurological abnormalities are not necessarily predictive of later development, although prediction improves when neonatal behavioral data are included (Cohen et al. 1992, Hunt 1981, Tronick and Brazelton 1975). However, low developmental test scores, which suggest behavioral delays, may not necessarily predict performance later in life. Some authors have reasoned that qualitative changes in the infant's behavior and skills are responsible for the lack of predictive ability (McCall 1976b). The association between early infant status and later intellectual outcome is further complicated by the mediating effects of the environment on growth (Drillien 1964, Knobloch and Pasamanick 1966, Sameroff and Chandler 1975). Except in cases of gross damage to brain structures in infancy, these mediating effects can be potent in altering outcome. Knobloch and Pasamanick (1966) referred to a **continuum of reproductive casualty** triggered by prematurity, in which perinatal complications, depending on their severity, can result in brain damage with sequelae ranging from death, cerebral palsy, and mental retardation at the severe end of the continuum to less severe disorders of behavior and adjustment at the other end. Sameroff and Chandler (1975) argued equally cogently for a continuum of caretaker causality; that is, of the strong effects of the social and economic environment on infant development.

Outcome of Preterm Births above 1500 Grams

Many of the earlier studies that helped record the effects of prematurity and low birth weight have become less relevant because of changes in neonatal care. Also, studies carried out before 1970 generally did not differentiate preterm low birth weight from intrauterine growth retardation and thus cannot be directly compared to recent studies. The pattern of development in terms of growth and morbidity between preterm LBW and IUGR is different (Barros et al. 1992). Current research focuses not only on major handicaps but also on subtle learning disabilities and social dysfunction, which may not be apparent until later childhood (Mitchell 1980).

Early longitudinal studies indicated that low-birth-weight infants were at increased risk for neurological sequelae such as cerebral palsy and seizures (Lilienfield and Parkhurst 1951, Lilienfield and Pasamanick 1954). The risk for

LBW and VLBW infants was three and ten times more than for full-term infants. This increased risk, and the etiological factors that contributed to that risk, was established in a study of a large cohort of infants born in the United States and followed prospectively in the Collaborative Perinatal Study (Hardy et al. 1979, Niswander and Gordon 1972). Reports from other countries were consistent with the U.S. experience (Abramowicz and Kass 1966). These findings were instrumental in the emergence of modern perinatal care.

In many of the earlier studies of outcome of prematurity and low birth weight, the incidence of serious handicap ranged from 10 to 40 per cent. A major handicap in these studies would preclude attendance at a regular school class and is associated with an IQ below 70, definite cerebral palsy, and/or severe deafness or vision loss (Lancet 1980). A minor handicap was associated with an IQ below 84, slight hearing or visual defects, and early childhood convulsive disorders that no longer required medication (Commey and Fitzhardinge 1979). Although older studies set the incidence of serious mental handicap as high as 40 per cent, the rate in present-day industrialized nations ranges from 5 to 15 per cent (Davies and Stewart 1975, Hagberg 1975). In the last 15 years the morbidity rate for major handicap has remained constant, although there have been significant reductions in the neonatal mortality rate (Hack et al. 1991).

Korner and her colleagues (Korner et al. 1993) have demonstrated the predictive validity of a new Neonatal Medical Index (NMI) for mental and motor development of LBW preterm infants up to 3 years. The NMI is a summary score of a select number of clinically salient items that are available on a medical chart during the neonatal period. It reflects how ill low-birth-weight and preterm infants were during their hospital stay. The NMI classifications range from I to V, with I describing those preterm infants who are free of significant past medical problems and V describing infants with serious complications. The NMI classification is based on two major criteria. The first considers birth weight with and without complications. For example, infants with a birth weight of more than 1000 g who experienced no major medical complications would fall into classifications I and II. Infants born at less than 1000 g or heavier infants who had experienced major medical complications would fall into categories III, IV, or V. The second considers the need for and duration of mechanically assisted ventilation (ventilatory care or intubation on continuous positive airway pressure [CPAP] or mask or nasal CPAP).

Details for computing the NMI are found in Table 13-3 and Table 13-4. Korner and her colleagues found that the NMI during the neonatal period is predictive of later cognitive and motor development to age 3 years primarily for infants born at or less than 1500 g. In infants weighing 1500 g or less, the effects of neonatal complications continued to affect development adversely to at least 3 years. Infants who had the most difficult course during their hospital stay and who received NMI scores of V obtained the lowest developmental quotients at 12, 24, and 36 months. In heavier infants, the developmental effects of sociodemographic factors predominated to 2 years and beyond. Despite these group findings, there were some exceptional infants born at less than 1000 g who

Table 13-3. Instructions for Computing the Neonatal
Medical Index (NMI)

Steps	NMI classification
Step 1	
Birth weight <1000 g	III
Birth weight ≥1000 g	
Assisted ventilation ≤ 48 hours	II
or a day or more on oxygen	
No assisted ventilation *and*	I
no days on oxygen *and*	
no RDS *and*	
no patent ductus *and*	
no apnea (for bradycardia)	
Step 2. Recode to the highest applicable NMI	
Assisted ventilation for 3-14 days *or*	III
Theophylline used for apnea or (bracycardia) *or*	
PVH-IVH grade 1 or 11 *or*	
Patent ductus requiring indomethacin *or*	
Exchange transfusion for hyperbilirubinemia	
Assisted ventilation for 15-28 days *or*	IV
Major surgery *or* (resuscitation for apnea	
of bradycardia while on theophylline)	
29 or more days on assisted ventilation *or*	V
Meningitis (confirmed or suspected) *or*	
Seizures *or*	
PVH-IVH grade III or IV *or*	
Periventricular leukomalacia	

Source: Korner et al. 1993.

obtained developmental quotients that were almost indistinguishable from infants who had minimal or no medical complications.

Studies of the relationship between prematurity and school performance (Caputo and Mandell 1970, Caputo et al. 1979, Rubin et al. 1973) reported that reading, writing, arithmetic, and language difficulties are seen more frequently in school-aged children who were born prematurely, regardless of the degree of prematurity, because of lower levels of intelligence and behavioral difficulties. One study (Rubin et al. 1973) reported that 17 per cent of preterm children aged 7 years repeat a grade and 6.8 per cent are in special classes, compared with 11.5 per cent and 2.5 per cent of normal children, respectively. A follow-up study of 874 children with low and high birth weight (Lagerstrom et al. 1989) indicated that at age 13 low-birth-weight boys had no significantly inferior school performance compared to high-birth-weight boys; however, low-birth-weight girls suffered significantly in their school performance. Other authors

Table 13-4. Criteria for Classifying the Neonatal Medical Index

I.	Birth weight greater than 1000 g; free of respiratory distress and other medical complications; no oxygen required; absence of apnea or bradycardia; no patent ductus; allowable complications are benign heart murmur and need for phototherapy.
II.	Birth weight greater than 1000 g; assisted ventilation for 48 hours or less and/or oxygen required 1 or more days; no periventricular hemorrhage-intraventricular hemorrhage (PVH-IVH); allowable complications are occasional apnea and/or bradycardia not requiring theophylline or related drugs; patent ductus arteriosus (PDA) not requiring medication, such as indomethacin.
III.	Assisted ventilation for 3–14 days and/or any conditions listed under III below.
IV.	Assisted ventilation 15–28 days or more and/or any condition listed under IV.
V.	Assisted ventilation 29 days or more and/or any condition listed under V.

Conditions requiring a classification of III, IV, or V, regardless of length of time on assisted ventilation:

III.	Birth weight less than 1000 g; PVH-IVH grade I or II; apnea and/or bradycardia requiring theophylline; patent ductus requiring indomethacin; hyperbilirubinemia requiring exchange transfusion. Exclude conditions listed under IV or V.
IV.	Resuscitation needed for apnea or bradycardia while on theophylline; major surgery including PDA (exclude hernias, testicular torsion, and all conditions listed under V).
V.	Meningitis confirmed or suspected; seizures; PVH-IVH grade III or IV; periventricular leukomalacia.

Source: Korner et al. 1993.

also found that differences in academic abilities between preterm and full-term children are not significant if socioeconomic status is taken into account (Bayley 1970, Douglas 1976).

In a 10-year follow-up study of 64 premature infants, Caputo and colleagues (1981) recorded a mean WISC-R IQ of 100.3 for preterm infants compared to 108 for full-term infants. The lower preterm mean was clearly in the normal range. The Performance Scales of the WISC-R and the results on the Bender Gestalt test were, however, significantly lower. The authors concluded that the premature infant in later life demonstrates a slight deficit in cognitive functioning that involves visually mediated, particularly visuomotor, functioning. Since very few of their subjects were visually impaired and there was no obvious neurological impairment, it was suggested that the visual system deficit originates in the CNS and is based on subtle brain dysfunction or limited brain cell growth.

Another 7-year follow-up study assigned preterm infants to three groups according to degree of prematurity, with group 1 being the least premature (Grigoroiu-Serbanescu 1984). Continuous progress in emotional and intellectual development in children to ages 6 and 7 was seen in preterm group 1 of boys and girls, and among girls in group 2; "stagnant" development was found in boys in group 2 and in both boys and girls in group 3. This analysis of the "developmental rhythm" in preterm children over a 7-year period suggests that very small premature children have an "oscillating evolution," with periods in which they do not differ from full-term children and with periods of regression. Hence, studies covering only preschool years may lead to different conclusions than do longer-term studies. These conclusions would support a discontinuous theory of development.

Als and her colleagues (1989), however, argued very strongly for continuity of development. In their comprehensive follow-up of preterm infants, status during the neonatal period predicted the results of a neurophysiological measure (BEAM), a neuropsychological assessment, and a play observation at age 5. The low-threshold reactive newborns showed much greater difficulty in spatial organization, attentional capacity, and sequential processing at follow-up.

In the context of modern perinatal care, low birth weight and preterm delivery (excluding VLBW) are not risk factors for severe impairment if the maternal, fetal, and placental systems have been functioning optimally and if no complications occur. Unfortunately, a preterm delivery is often symptomatic of dysfunction in one of these systems, and there seems to be an increasing risk of medical complications with decreasing birth weight and younger gestational age. Low-birth-weight infants (excluding VLBW) remain three times more likely than full-term infants to have adverse neurological sequelae (Papile et al. 1983). However, research findings suggest that premature infants in the upper range of low birth weight are only minimally intellectually impaired, if at all. Although full-term infants seem to score slightly higher on IQ tests, the mean score for premature groups is within the average range (Grioroiu-Serbanescu 1984, Silva et al. 1984). A mild lag in cognitive and language function for AGA preterm infants was also reported by Vohr et al. (1989) and Casiro et al. (1990, 1991).

Outcome of VLBW Infants Below 1500 Grams

The long-term outcome of preterm birth of VLBW babies presents a different picture. VLBW infants are a relatively new group who have been able to survive because of increased understanding and improvement in neonatal intensive care. This group of infants is not homogeneous and includes newborns who weigh between 500 to 1500 g, as well as those who are appropriate for gestational age and those who are small for gestational age.

Reports of VLBW babies during the early 1960s indicated a high mortality rate (75 per cent) and a high incidence of serious mental and physical handicap.

In a study of 69 subjects with birth weight below 1500 g, Drillien (1958) reported that 10 per cent were ineducable, 18 per cent were physically handicapped, and 18 per cent required remedial instruction. Altogether, 49 per cent of surviving infants below 1360 g birth weight had visual handicaps. Drillien predicted that the survival of VLBW infants would be paralleled by an increase in the incidence of handicap. This hypothesis was supported by a study by Lubchenco et al. (1963), who noted an incidence of visual handicaps, cerebral palsy, or mental retardation in 63 per cent of the sample. In contrast, the outcome of infants born in New York between 1942 and 1952 who weighed 1000 g or less and who received nonintrusive supportive care was described more positively in a study by Dann et al. (1958). After the age of 4 years, 73 of the 116 survivors had caught up in height, few had neurological handicaps, and 16 per cent had IQs below 80. The infants with the highest IQs were in families with higher socioeconomic status. These early studies are important because, even without neonatal intensive care, some VLBW infants did survive and did well (Goldson 1992, Koops and Harmon 1980, Stewart 1986).

Many of the noted impairments in VLBW infants have proven to be amenable to improved methods of delivery and neonatal care. The prevention and treatment of birth trauma, birth asphyxia, hypoxia, hypothermia, hypoglycemia, and hyperbilirubinemia, for example, have certainly improved the prognosis of the VLBW infant. Table 13-5 (Commey and Fitzhardinge 1979) shows the incidence

Table 13-5. Incidence and Mortality of Major Neonatal Complications and Proportion Showing Handicap at 24-Month Follow-up

	Total	Mortality, %	Months followed	Handicapped, %
Total population[a]	109	26	71	49
Asphyxia	68	29	43	48
CNS depression on admission	48	48	25	76
Mechanical ventilation	46	39	28	46
Respiratory distress syndrome	26	46	14	57
Primary or late apnea	45	31	28	46
Seizures	20	65	7	57
Intracranical hemorrhage (clinical or autopsy diagnosis)	19	89	2	100
Meningitis	4	25	3	67
Hyperbilirubinemia needing exchange transfusion	19	26	14	71
Hypoglycemia	14	21	11	73
Necrotizing enterocholitis	6	33	4	0
None	25	0	22	36

Source: Commey and Fitzhardinge 1979.

[a]More than one complication may have occurred in the same infant.

and mortality of major complications and the proportion with a handicap among VLBW infants at a 24-month follow-up.

Studies between 1970 and 1980 optimistically reported a better survival rate and outcome for VLBW infants. Yu and Hollingsworth (1979) noted a 60 per cent survival rate among infants with birth weights of 1000 g and less, with a 44 per cent survival rate among infants weighing less than 751 g. At a 1-year follow-up, they reported no abnormalities. At University College Hospital in London, as few as 10 per cent of surviving VLBW infants had a severe handicap. The 5-year follow-up of 85 children found approximately 90 per cent without handicap, 4 per cent with physical handicap including spastic diplegia or partial vision, and 4 per cent as mentally handicapped with a mean IQ of less than 72 (Lancet 1980, Rawlings et al. 1971, Reynolds et al. 1974).

Less optimistic findings were reported by other authors. Kitchen et al. (1984), for example, found that the survival rate for VLBW infants increased from 37.1 to 68.3 per cent between 1966–1970 to 1980–1982, but that neurodevelopmental outcome was poor and impairments were similar in frequency to the 1966–1970 cohort. The incidence of strabismus, myopia, and small head circumference decreased, but that of cerebral palsy increased, and mental development scores remained the same. Molteno et al. (1990) found that poor postural control (head and trunk righting at 4 months) was also related to locomotor development at 12 and 14 months. Casiro et al. (1990, 1991) found significant language delay at the age of 3 years, especially in infants with neurological abnormalities. A study by Kitchen et al. (1984) followed 351 ELBW infants (500 to 999 g) and found a survival rate of 24.4 per cent. The incidence of severe functional handicap was 22.5 per cent, 29.2 per cent had mild-to-moderate handicap, and 48.3 per cent had no handicap. There was a 13.5 per cent incidence of cerebral palsy and a 3.4 per cent prevalence of sensorineural hearing loss. At the age of 2 years, the mental development index on the Bayley Mental Scales was 91.1 and the mean psychomotor index 87.7. At follow-up at the age of 5.5 years, 60 per cent had no impairment, 10 per cent had severe sensorineural hearing loss, 10 per cent had mild-to-moderate impairment, and 20 per cent had minor neurological abnormalities. Three of the children had spastic diplegia. The mean full-scale IQ on the Wechsler Preschool and Primary Scales of Intelligence (WPPSI) was 101.8, although 40 per cent of the survivors had some learning difficulty. A 5-year follow-up study of 79 VLBW infants by Roussounis et al. (1993) showed significant intellectual impairment on the WPPSI scales mostly for boys, although they were not emotionally and socially different from normal-birth-weight peers. VLBW subjects with motor coordination difficulties did poorly on arithmetic and visuospatial tasks. Saigal et al. (1992) also found 31 per cent of 114 8-year-olds born with ELBW to be non-right-handed as compared to 19 per cent for controls, a finding confirmed by Ross et al. (1992). Similar outcomes have been reported by other authors (Hoy et al. 1991, Klein et al. 1989, Orgill et al. 1982, Ruiz et al. 1981). Weisglas et al. (1992) found that ventriculomegaly and intraparenchymal damage detected by neonatal cerebral ultrasound were the best predictors of poor neurodevelopmental outcome at 3.5 years of age.

A summary of ten studies between 1970 and 1978 shows that survival rates averaged about 58 per cent (Levene and Dubowitz, 1982). The incidence of major neurological handicap ranged from none in Coventry, England, to 44 per cent in Toronto, Canada. The high incidence in Toronto is due to the number of at-risk infants who arrive in poor condition from other centers. In addition, infants who are both SGA and preterm are at greater risk for adverse neurological handicap. Tables 13-6 and 13-7 show the survival and outcome of infants with weight below 1500 g and below 1000 g. Although the average survival is lower than for infants with birth weights above 1500 g, the average incidence of major handicap is similar (about 22 per cent).

The financial impact of medical and nonmedical expenditures on the parents of VLBW infants can be significant. Recent data from the United States suggests that costs for a VLBW delivery average at least five to six times that for a full-term delivery ($29,000 versus $4600) and may increase to as much as $150,000 for the smallest infants. The monthly costs of care for VLBW infants during the first 3 years of life can be as much as 60 times those of the average child (McCormick et al. 1991).

The long-term outcome of VLBW infants in their school years is marked by reports of increased behavioral problems; problems in motor, visuomotor, and perceptual skills; and language and reading difficulties (Astbury et al. 1985, Eilers et al. 1986, Hack et al. 1991, Hirata et al. 1983, Klein et al. 1985, Saigal et al. 1991, Vohr and Garcia-Coll 1985). Between 20 to 37 per cent of children born after 1965 with VLBW were learning disabled (Hunt et al. 1982). Some had difficulties with visual perception (Klein et al. 1985), although the majority of such learning problems occur in VLBW children who also have major neurological abnormalities (Aram et al. 1991). Drillien et al. (1980) reported that 60 per cent of VLBW infants who attended normal school had shown transient signs in the first year of life and at age 7 years had poor scores on all measures used, including the WISC-R, Bender Gestalt, and school achievement tests. Those children who were able to attend normal school showed no evidence of intrauterine insult or perinatal complications and were neurologically normal.

Longitudinal studies assessing the outcome of SGA infants compared to preterm infants have yielded varying results (Fitzhardinge and Stevens 1972, Parmelee and Schulte 1970, Vohr et al. 1979). Neligan et al. (1976) in a comprehensive study reported that both the preterm and very SGA children (fourth percentile for weight and age) performed significantly less well on a wide range of measures at ages 5, 6, and 7 years. The major conclusion of the Neligan study was that, in terms of intelligence and behavior problems as reported by parents, it is better to be born too early (preterm) than too small (small for gestational age). Silva et al. (1984) reported similar findings in a large sample of children from Dunedin, New Zealand, with the SGA children significantly disadvantaged at each age at 3, 5, 7, and 9 years in intelligence and parent-reported behavior problems.

Table 13-6 Summary of Survival and Outcome from Nine Follow-Up Studies of Infants with Birth Weight $\leq$ 1500 g Conducted in the 1970s

Group	Time period of births	Survival rate (%)	SGA (%)	Born in hospital	Major CNS handicap	Significant cerebral palsy	Neonatal retardation (developmental quotient <80)	Age of assessment
Toronto (Fitzhardinge et al. 1976)	1970–1973	48	47	Nil	33/75 (44%)	14/75 (18.7%)	35/75 (46.7%)	>2 years
Sydney (Mercer et al. 1978)	1971–1975	55	35[a]	All	11/88 (12.5%)	2/88 (2.3%)	8/88 (9.1%)	Mean 4 years
Hammersmith, London (Jones et al. 1979)	1971–1975	48	32	All	7/104 (6.7%)	3/104 (2.9%)	3/104 (2.9%)	>23 months
Coventry (Hommers and Kendall, 1976)	1973–1974	54	21	?		0/42	2/42 (4.8%)	9–31 months
McMaster, Hamilton (Horwood et al. 1982)	1973–1977	77[b]	?	All	21/134 (15.7%)	—	—	1½–6 years
Hamilton (Saigal et al. 1982)	1973–1978	63	18	76%	11/104[c] (10%)	24/104 (23.1%)	9/104 (8.7%)	2 years
Toronto (Fitzhardinge et al. 1978)	1974	66	19[a]	Nil	44/149[d] (29.5%)	13/149 (8.7%)	40/149 (26.8%)	>2 years
New York State (Knoblock et al. 1982)	1975–1979	53	?	All	22/96 (22.9%)	—	—	>1 year
Cleveland (Hack et al. 1979)	1975–1976	65	26[a]	?	27/160 (16.9%)	—	—	Mean 2 years
Melbourne (Kitchen et al. 1982)	1977–1978	68	?	87%	53/297 (17.8%)	35/297 (11.8%)	28/297[e] (19.4%)	>2 years

Source: Levene and Dubowitz 1982.

[a]Refers only to those infants followed up.

[b]Only infants of 1000–1499 g.

[c]30% major CNS handicap in the ventilated subgroup.

[d]53% major handicap rate among infants born with weight below the third centile for gestation.

[e]Number of infants with mental development index $\leq$ 68.

Table 13-7. Summary of Survival and Outcome of Infants with Birth Weight ≤1000 g from 11 Centers

Group	Time period of births	Survival rate (%)	SGA (%)	Born in hospital	Major CNS handicap	Significant cerebral palsy	Neonatal retardation (developmental quotient <80)	Age of assessment
University College Hospital, London (Stewart et al. 1977)	1966–1974	32	?	47%	2/27	1/27	2/27	>15 months
Sydney (Mercer et al. 1978)	1971–1975	19	?	All	3/9	0/9	3/9	Mean 4 years
Los Angeles (Pomerance et al. 1978)	1973–1975	40	?	45%	9/27	?	8/27	1–3 years
Hamilton (Saigal et al. 1982)	1973–1978	32	?	76%	9/37	—	—	2 years
Toronto (Pape et al. 1978)	1974	47	33	None	13/43	2/43	9/43	>18 months
Illinois (Bhat et al. 1978)	1974–1976	31	40	48%	3/16	—	3/23	10–36 months
Pennsylvania (Kumar et al. 1980)	1974–1977	26	5	All	2/50	—	2/50	?
Cleveland (Hack et al. 1979)	1975–1976	40	?	?	7/32	—	—	Mean 2 years
New York State (Knoblock et al. 1982)	1975–1979	20	?	All	5/9	—	—	>1 year
Syracuse, New York (Ruiz et al. 1981)	1976–1978	34	18	45%	10/38	4/33	6/28†	8–15 months
Columbia (Driscoll et al. 1982)	1977–1978	48	38	56%	7/23 (30%)	2/23	3/23	18–36 months

Source: Levene and Dubowitz 1982.

In conclusion, long-term follow-up of VLBW and ELBW infants tells us that significant advances in perinatal care have resulted in improved survival and developmental outcome for these infants. ELBW and VLBW infants who were delivered in centers with appropriate perinatal and/or tertiary care nurseries using aggressive therapy did better. Although more infants are surviving, a large percentage have some handicap. Of the ELBW and VLBW infants who survive, 20 to 60 per cent have minor difficulties, and 10 to 20 per cent have significant sequelae. There is a high proportion of children with visuomotor disturbance and learning difficulties and who require special education. Outcome varies and is guarded if the VLBW infant has postnatal complications, such as broncho-pulmonary dysplasia, hyaline membrane disease, or intracranial hemorrhage (Landry et al. 1984, Meisels et al. 1986, Palmer et al. 1982, Sostek et al. 1987). SGA infants have a poorer outcome than preterm infants. Stjernquist and Sven-ningsen (1990), however, reported that even ELBW (500–900 g) infants with very poor Brazelton scores, often with intracranial hemorrhage after birth, showed a highly variable behavioral repertoire, with repeated short periods of alertness and high performance when they reached term.

Prematurity and Low Birth Weight in Relation to Psychopathology

In several studies prematurity has been found to be associated with an increase in emotional and behavioral disorders in later childhood. However, this rela-tionship is confounded with low socioeconomic status (SES), illegitimacy, and poor maternal health (Chamberlain et al. 1976). In a prospective study by Rob-inson and Robinson (1965), the premature group seemed to have more behavior problems than would be expected in the general population, but when controls who were carefully matched for SES were chosen, the differences disappeared. The authors concluded that the social pathology associated with prematurity accounts for most of the children's psychopathology. Davie et al. (1972) studied all low-birth-weight children born during 1 week in 1958 in the United Kingdom and compared their social adjustment at the age of 7 years with normal-birth-weight children. No significant differences in emotional and behavior disorders were found.

However, Drillien (1961, 1964) reported that in a prospective study infants with very low birth weight (below 1360 g) showed a greatly increased incidence of behavior and emotional problems when they reached school age. Seventy per cent of the children were described as hyperactive, restless, insecure, and having poor concentration. To a lesser extent, immaturity, anxiety, passivity, and ag-gressiveness were found. The majority of the children were neurologically im-paired and showed sensory disability, epilepsy, or language retardation. Szatmari et al. (1990a) also found an increased rate of attention deficit with hyperactivity, but not of conduct and emotional disorder, in 82 5-year-old children born with ELBW. It seems that the ELBW and VLBW child is especially vulnerable to emotional and behavioral disorder. This is consistent with the finding that these children are also at risk for generally retarded development and perceptual disorders.

In a prospective study, 60 children were examined in utero by serial ultrasound measurement of head growth (serial ultrasonic encephalometry, Parkinson et al. 1981). Forty-five small-for-date children born at a gestational age of at least 37 weeks were selected for follow-up. Birth weight was below the tenth percentile for gestational age and was adjusted for sex, birth order, mother's height, and mother's mid-pregnancy weight. Normal-weight babies were matched for age, sex, birth order, socioeconomic class, and race. No infant in either group had a history of intrauterine infection or of chromosomal or congenital anomaly at birth. The children were re-examined between 5 and 9 years of age, and teacher ratings of emotional and behavioral factors were obtained. The results showed that balance and coordination problems in childhood were more frequent if head growth slowed before the 26th week of pregnancy. Children whose head growth slowed before 34 weeks of gestation were found to be shorter at age 4, independent of social class. The children most likely to have scholastic and behavior problems were boys whose head growth slowed before 34 weeks and after 26 weeks of gestation, particularly if they came from lower social classes. These boys were found to be clumsy, worried, fidgety, unadaptable, and unable to concentrate, whereas girls with the same slowness of head growth cried, bullied, and were irritable. Children of both sexes with slowed head growth had more problems with reading, writing, drawing, and concentration. This carefully controlled study confirmed the findings of Drillien's study.

Pasamanick and Knobloch's (1960) retrospective study of psychiatrically disturbed children found a significant increase in birth complications; 40 per cent of the disturbed children also showed a hyperkinetic syndrome. However, most prospective studies have found no relationship between perinatal complications and emotional disorder. Werner and Smith (1977) found a relationship between perinatal complications and later behavioral and emotional status, but noted that poor psychosocial status greatly increased the incidence and severity of psychopathology. No particular type of psychopathology could be specified. Wolff (1970) examined retrospectively the perinatal history of 100 children with psychiatric disorders and found no differences in the number or severity of perinatal complications compared with a control group matched for age, sex, and social class.

Summary

Preterm birth and LBW do not necessarily place the child at risk for normal development. The complications associated with prematurity either during pregnancy, delivery, or postnatally increase the likelihood of an abnormal outcome. The probability of poor outcome is higher with birth weights of less than 1500 g and SGA; VLBW also increases susceptibility to complications of medical procedures because of immaturity. During the early years, hazardous complications can be associated with developmental problems. Longer follow-up studies show a higher incidence of developmental and learning problems among the lighter and younger infants. However, environmental factors assume increasing importance over time (McGauhey et al. 1992, Schrader 1986). There seems to be a significant interaction among the degree and type of complications associated with prematurity, the age and weight at preterm birth, the caregiving environment, and intellectual outcome. Furthermore, biological risk status may potentiate the effect of the environmental factors, in that adverse social/caregiving environments have a greater deleterious effect on infants born at risk, thereby creating a "double hazard" for some infants (Escalona 1982).

14

Infections

Infectious organisms and intoxicants (to be discussed in Chapter 15) are two groups of more than 800 teratogenic agents that can cause structural or functional deviations in development. An annotated catalog of the complete list of agents is provided by Shepard (1975). For a detailed discussion the reader is referred to Johnson and Kochlar (1983). This chapter provides an introduction to the topic and a more detailed description of the effects of HIV, rubella, and cytomegalovirus infections, and of meningitis as examples of pre- and postnatal infections that have been studied more extensively.

14.1   Prenatal Infection

Infections affecting the CNS may be caused by bacteria, viruses, rickettsiae, fungi, protozoa, and helminths (Johnson 1982). During the prenatal period, only those infectious agents that cross the placenta are of importance to the developing fetus. The clinical effects of severe prenatal infection have been known for a long time: severe retardation, convulsions, **chorioretinitis** (inflammation of the layer of eye tissue carrying blood vessels and the retina), and micro- or hydrocephaly. More recently, the production of IgM, one of the immunoglobulins, has been used as an indicator of whether an infection occurred during the prenatal period. IgM does not cross the placenta, but is produced by the fetus in response to infection and therefore can be used to survey the frequency of prenatal infection. By this measurement, 6 per cent of all living newborns are presumed to have had an intrauterine infection (DeMyer 1975). However, this figure does not include infections acquired from the mother's birth canal during birth or those acquired before the fifth to sixth month of pregnancy since IgM levels do not respond to infections during these periods.

Only a small proportion of maternal infections produce clear-cut psychological consequences in the child. The best-known infections during pregnancy are the

STORCH agents: Syphilis (treponema pallidum), Toxoplasma gondii (toxoplasmosis), Rubella (German measles), Cytomegalovirus (cytomegalic inclusion body disease, one of the many forms of the herpesvirus) and Herpes simplex. Together these STORCH agents account for about 20 per cent of all prenatal infections. The remaining 80 per cent of infections are caused by a variety of infectious agents, including mumps, hepatitis, chicken pox, and coxsackie-virus group B (Nahmias et al. 1976). The relationship between the time of infection and the severity and type of damage has already been discussed in Chapter 8.

The mechanism of damage to the fetus often remains unexplained and the effects on the future development of the child obscure. One reason for the lack of information is that many infections of the mother show only mild or no clinical signs and hence remain undetected. Alternatively, the infection may invade the cerebrospinal fluid and cause a narrowing (stenosis) of the cerebral aqueduct. This may lead to the development of hydrocephalus in the infant, although at that time serological evidence of a viral infection can no longer be obtained. Johnson (1974) found, for example, that newborn hamsters inoculated with mumps and influenza viruses later developed malformations of the brain without evidence of a destructive inflammatory lesion.

HIV Infection

Much recent research has focused on infants infected with the **human immunodeficiency virus** (**HIV**) who then develop a pediatric **acquired immunodeficiency syndrome** (**AIDS**), now the ninth leading cause of death in children (Fletcher et al. 1991a, Pizzo and Wilfert 1992). The infection originates from a parent with HIV infection (intrapartum transmission) or from transfusions of infected blood. A description of the neuropathology is provided by Scaravilli (1993). Fetal progressive encephalopathy with calcification of the basal ganglia after an incubation period between 2 months and 5 years has been reported (Belman et al. 1986, Berger and Levy 1993, Ragni et al. 1987). A follow-up study by Belman and co-workers (1988, Ultmann et al. 1985) of 61 children showed acquired microcephaly or poor brain growth, cognitive deficits, and bilateral pyramidal tract signs in virtually all subjects. Ten children developed classical CNS lymphoma or Kaposi's sarcoma and CNS infections, and 11 showed subacute, but steady deterioration. In 30 children the course was more indolent, starting with a plateau, but with further neurological deterioration in 13, whereas 17 remained static with cognitive and/or neurological deficits. A second study (Diamond 1990) compared carefully matched groups of 28 HIV-seropositive with 22 seronegative children over the age of 15 months born to seropositive mothers and raised in foster care; 48 children were immunologically and neurologically stable, and 2 showed signs of progressive encephalopathy. The seropositive group showed significantly more neurological involvement and different cognitive patterns, including deficits on the Bayley scales, the Stanford-Binet, and other intelligence scales, although weight, height, and head circumference measures did not differ significantly. A study of 18 HIV-positive children by Condini et al. (1991) came to similar conclusions; infected children produced shorter sentences in communication and were less advanced on speech production tasks than noninfected children. Figure 14-1 shows a schematic representation of different encephalopathic courses, assessed with the individual growth approach recommended by Fletcher et al. (1991a). Bennett (1987) stressed the psychosocial consequences. In older children, there is likely to be some similarity to three clusters of HIV infection described for adults: normal cognitive performance; psychomotor slowing, forgetfulness, and affective disturbance; and global cognitive deficit with euthymic mood (Van Gorp et al. 1992).

Congenital Rubella

Since the first description by Gregg in 1941, **rubella** infection has perhaps become the best-known and most feared complication of pregnancy. Rubella epidemics were recorded in some years, as in 1964, with fetal infections ranging from 4 to 30 per 1000 births. However, with the advent of rubella vaccine in 1969, the incidence rate in North America has rapidly decreased to 0.1 in 10,000

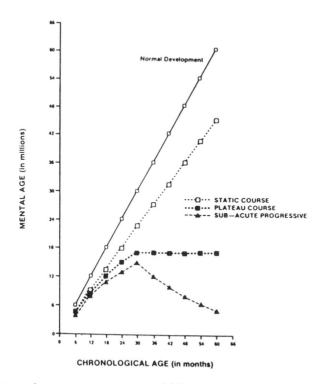

Figure 14-1.   Schematic representation of different encephalopathic courses (Browers et al. 1990).

live births. In 1988, only 221 cases were reported in the United States (Massachusetts Medical Society 1989).

If acquired before the thirteenth week, maternal rubella results in abnormalities in 50 per cent of the infants (Hardy 1973). Infections during the first trimester of pregnancy result in morphological abnormalities in almost all pregnancies. More recent studies have shown that the risk extends well into the second trimester, though with diminishing severity (Hardy 1973, Ueda et al. 1979). A risk is even present if the maternal infection occurs after the last menstrual period but before conception, although in such cases the incidence of spontaneous abortion is very high (Ueda et al. 1979). Subclinical rubella occurs at least as often as the clinically apparent infection and poses the same amount of risk to the fetus (Knox et al. 1980). Maternal rubella infections may produce rubella syndrome in the child, the effects of which extend to many areas of function and include mild disease or an inapparent infection at birth. Even an inapparent infection, however, can cause significant problems later in life (Tables 14-1 to 14-3).

The clinical picture of the rubella syndrome often includes low birth weight, meningoencephalitis, microcephaly, psychomotor and mental retardation, cataracts and pigmented retinopathy of the eye, and abnormalities of the ear, heart, and major blood vessels. A 9- to 12-year follow-up study of 29 nonretarded

Table 14-1. Neurological Abnormalities Noted in 32 of 64 Survivors of Maternal Rubella Followed to 18 Months[a]

Motor deficits			Other neurological abnormalities	
Tetraparesis		20	Hyperactivity and restlessness	16
With general spasticity	4		Hypotonic shoulder girdle	16
With hypotonia	9		Lateral rotation of feet	14
With spasticity of lower			Incoordination of swallowing	
extremities	4		mechanism	8
With athetosis	1		Strabismus (in infants without	
			cataracts)	7
With asymmetrical involvement	1		Head retraction and back	9
of upper extremities			arching	
Paraparesis		2	Hypertonicity on stimulation	8
With spasticity	1		Stereotyped movements	12
With hypotonia	1		Abnormal associated movements	
Hemiparesis		2	movements	3
			Tremors	2
Monoparesis		2	Cutis marmorata	4
Severe motor delay		6	Apparent unawareness of	
With hypotonia	5		environment	8
With intermittent hypertonus	1		Mental retardation (no	
			progress in adaptive	
			behavior)	11

Source: Desmond et al. 1970.
[a]Findings confined to 18-month examination.

Table 14-2. The Johns Hopkins Rubella Study: Fetal Outcome by Gestational Age at Time of Maternal Rubella

| Completed weeks of gestation | No. | Died[a] | | Survived | | | | |
		Fetal	Later	Severe	Moderate	Mild	? Normal	Normal
Preconception	5	2	2	1	—	—	—	—
0–4	23	2	4	11	6	—	—	—
5–8	28	2	1	7	9	7	1	1
9–12	14	—	—	3	3	7	1	—
13–16	10	1	1	2	3	1	2	—
17–20	7	1	—	1	—	2	1	3
21–30	11	—	—	1	2	2	2	4
31–45	4	—	—	—	—	1	2	1
	102	8	8	26	23	20	9	9

Source: Hardy 1973.
[a]Two additional deaths occurred between 4 and 5 years of age.

children who had congenital rubella suggested that an increasing number of manifestations not detected during infancy occur during childhood (Desmond et al. 1978). Among the 29 children, manifestations during the first 2 years of life included abnormal muscle tone and reflexes (69 per cent), delays in motor development (66 per cent), feeding difficulties (48 per cent), and severe to profound hearing loss (79 per cent). Between 3 and 7 years, poor balance and motor incoordination (69 per cent) and such disturbances as short attention span, distractibility, perseveration, and emotional instability (66 per cent) were noted, and hearing losses increased to 86 per cent. At age 9 to 12 years, 25 of the 29 children showed residual deficits, including learning problems (52 per cent) and deficits in tactile perception (41 per cent). The number of children with overt driven hyperkinesis was recorded at 66 per cent at age 3, but decreased to 17 per cent by age 9 to 12. Learning problems predominated in later years, despite normal-range measured intelligence (WISC-R IQ of 85 and higher). Feelings of isolation and low self-esteem were common. Fourteen of the children required a total communication program, including sign language, at school. The authors concluded that the primary problems of rubella children differ in each phase of childhood.

In a second follow-up study (Desmond et al. 1985), 53 adolescents between 16 and 18 years of age were found to have multiple handicaps, including neurosensory impairment, hearing loss, cerebral dysfunction, and organic behavior syndromes. Those with severe to profound hearing loss diagnosed before the age of 18 months used total or manual communication as adolescents. Van Dijk (1982) presented similar results about the behavior and learning problems of 81 Australian children with congenital rubella who had cataracts and/or hearing impairment. Late-onset progressive panencephalitis related to the original rubella infection—an infectious process affecting both the gray and white matter

Table 14-3. The Johns Hopkins Rubella Study: Status of Surviving Children with Congenital Rubella at 4 to 5 Years of Age

Intelligence[a] (IQ Score)	No.	Percent	H/O maternal rubella	Birth weight <2501 g	Cardiac	Auditory	Other abnormalities				
							Visual	CNS	Other minor	Small head	None
Above average ≥110	20	11.7	13	3	7	15	1	3	6	11	4
Average 90–109	49	28.6	20	7	15	21	—	7	12	22	11
Low normal 75–89	31	18.1	14	12	14	17	4	10	9	20	1
Borderline 70–74	22	12.0	6	10	8	12	7	9	6	21	—
Defective <70	49	28.6	24	25	23	28	21	30	2	38	(1)
Total Number	171	—	77	57	67	93	33	59	35	112	16 + (1)
%		100.0	45	33	39	54	19	34	20	65	9

Source: Hardy 1973.

[a]Distribution of defects in 171 children with congenital rubella by IQ score at 4 to 5 yr of age. The Stanford-Binet was used where possible. Other tests, such as the Merril Palmer, Leiter, and Cattell, were given where the child was deaf or otherwise unable to take the Binet.

of the brain—may occur as late as the second decade of life (Townsend et al. 1975, Weil et al. 1975).

Similar findings were reported by Chess et al. (1978) in a larger study group; they examined 243 children with congenital rubella at age 2.6 to 5 years and again at age 8 to 9 years. At the first examination, they found mental retardation in 37 per cent, reactive behavior disorders in 15 per cent, behavior disorder in conjunction with neurological damage in 3.3 per cent, and autism in 7.4 per cent. They stressed that autism is frequently associated with mental retardation and that all the autistic children were infected during the first trimester of pregnancy. Of the 210 children returning for re-examination at age 8 to 9, 25.7 per cent were mentally retarded; 18.1 per cent showed reactive behavior disorders, such as moodiness and rebelliousness; 12.4 per cent showed behavior disorder in conjunction with neurological damage, 6.2 per cent were autistic; and 2.4 per cent had neurotic behavior disorders. Thus, with increasing age, behavior problems increased in frequency as these children are exposed to the increased demands of school and society (Ziring 1977). Reviewing the 25-year outcome of 50 individuals who had congenital rubella, Menser et al. (1967) found that some degree of mental deficiency was present only in 5 and severe mental deficiency only in 1 case. Forty-seven had severe hearing loss, 26 had cataracts or chorioretinopathy, 11 had congenital cardiovascular defects, and 40 had speech defects. Despite evidence of chromosomal abnormalities in many infants with congenital rubella, 6 of the 11 married females had normal off-spring. The authors pointed out that the socioeconomic adjustment of the group as a whole had been underestimated in previous assessments; only four of their subjects were unemployed. "The developmental potential of many patients had been assessed erroneously during the preschool period" (Menser et al. 1967, p. 1347).

The great variability in the type and degree of psychological deficit has been ascribed to differences in the age of the fetus at the time when the mother acquired the rubella infection. Yet, very few systematic correlations between gestational age and symptoms or their severity have been clearly established. One study of outcome in relation to gestational age is illustrated in Tables 14-2 and 14-3 (Hardy 1973). In addition to gestational age, the physical condition of the mother, the amount of virus to which the fetus has been exposed, the virulence of the strain, and the immune response of both mother and fetus have been described as factors determining the effects of rubella infection during pregnancy.

Congenital Cytomegalovirus Infection

Among the many varieties of the herpesvirus (including herpes simplex, herpes zoster, and Epstein-Barr virus), **cytomegalovirus (CMV)** has been identified as one of the most common causes of intrauterine infection. In a worldwide study, Krech (1973) found CMV antibodies in 40 per cent of healthy blood donors in industrialized countries and in 100 per cent of donors in developing countries. Discovered in 1956, this virus is estimated to infect between 0.5 and 2.4 per cent of all newborns, although fewer than 5 to 10 per cent of those infected show clinical manifestations of the disease during infancy (Starr 1979). Since the infection remains subclinical in most adults as well, maternal infection often remains undetected, unless a serological examination is carried out.

The effects of invasion by the virus can be widespread and include enlargement of the spleen and liver, intrauterine growth retardation, various congenital deformities, and damage to the developing visual and auditory system (Johnson 1977). After long-term follow-up, Pass et al. (1980) reported that, of 34 newborns with clinical evidence of infection and with the virus isolated from urine, 10 had died and all but 2 of the 23 patients remaining in the study showed evidence of CNS or auditory handicaps. Microcephaly was present in 70 per cent, mental retardation in 61 per cent, hearing loss in 30 per cent, neuromuscular disorder in 35 per cent, and chorioretinitis or optic atrophy in 22 per cent of the children when seen at an average age of 4 years (ranging from 9 months to 14 years). These results are essentially in agreement with studies by Berenberg and Nankervis (1970) and Niedt and Schinella (1985). In a review, Eichhorn (1982) linked CMV infection to IQ scores and also reported that the incidence of school failure in CMV-infected children is 2.7 times greater than in matched controls and 8 times greater than in random controls.

There has been growing interest in exposed children who do not have clinical symptoms during the neonatal period and in whom the infection is not recognized. CMV has the capacity to survive and to replicate in the tissue for months or years after perinatal or intrauterine infection. Studies by Kumar et al. (1973) and by Melish and Hanshaw (1973) suggested that, in 5 to 10 per cent of these asymptomatic cases, neurological symptoms may develop later. Reynolds et al. (1974) reported that, of 18 children followed up to 5 or 6 years of age, more than half developed sensorineural hearing loss, and there was a trend toward subnormal intelligence. Asymptomatic CMV infection has also been associated with school failure (Hanshaw et al. 1976) and schizophrenia (Albrecht et al. 1980).

The similarity between the long-term sequelae of CMV and of those of another prenatal infection, Toxoplasma gondii virus, should be pointed out (Holliman 1988, Stagno 1980). Wilson and colleagues (1980) reported that 92 per cent of the children in a long-term follow-up study of toxoplasmosis during pregnancy showed late-developing effects, including a gradual decrease in IQ from an average of 97 to 74, over a 5-year period.

14.2 Postnatal Infections

Most children are subjected to numerous infections, only a few of which have more than a temporary effect on their well-being. Of concern here are those postnatal infections that have been shown to affect the development of the nervous system, especially if the infection involves brain tissue (**encephalitis**) or the membranes of the brain (meningitis). Well-known examples are measles, rubella, and mumps. Some cases may be related to inoculation with serum or vaccines, others to autoimmune reactions. However, even infections not involving the brain may affect cognitive development. For example, persistent otitis media has been shown to affect the language development of the child (Teele et al. 1990, see Chapter 27).

Meningitis

Meningitis is an inflammation resulting from infection by one of the numerous bacteria (e.g., meningococcus, pneumococcus, staphylococcus), viri, and fungi that can invade the meninges via the middle ear, the paranasal sinuses, the bone of the skull, or the bloodstream. In the newborn, meningitis may be a complication of birth: premature rupture of the membranes may allow bacteria into the fetal environment. The clinical picture often emerges slowly, but at its peak often includes neck rigidity, clouding of consciousness, increased reflex activity, and seizures. A persisting defect is usually the result of damage to the blood supply (end arteries) serving the meninges and to brain tissue because of swelling. The latter complication leaves nonfunctional necrotic tissue after the infection, usually more thickly at the base of the brain. Some blood vessels may become thrombosed and produce small infarctions, frequently affecting the brain as well (meningoencephalitis). The brain is swollen and shows ventricular dilation; cerebrospinal fluid ducts become obstructed. Abscesses of the infection into the brain can occur (Bigler 1989).

The rapidly progressive and often fatal **neonatal bacterial meningitis** (still fairly frequent, 1500 cases per year in the United States) is usually distinguished from the bacterial or viral meningitis occurring in older children and adults. Later in life, the clinical picture is often less obvious, although the destructive effects on brain tissue can be more pronounced.

Before the advent of antibiotics, approximately 60 per cent of patients infected with bacterial meningitis suffered severe, permanent neurological damage; this figure has since dropped to 30 per cent. In addition, about 20 per cent have significant difficulty with school work (Lawson et al. 1965, Smith 1954). Sell and co-workers (1972a, 1972b) reported that over 18 per cent of the children who had suffered from bacterial meningitis had lasting neurological sequelae, 7 per cent were mentally retarded, and others had impaired intelligence relative to their siblings (Figure 14-2). Only half of the children recovered without sequelae (Sell 1983). Following 88 children for at least 1 year after infection, Feigin and Dodge (1976) found that one died and nine were affected by hemiparesis or quadriparesis, although this condition cleared up in six of them within a year. Thirteen of the children had IQs between 80 and 90, and ten were below 80. Several authors noted clinically significant hearing defects and poor brainstem evoked potentials in children after meningococcal meningitis (Jiang et al. 1990).

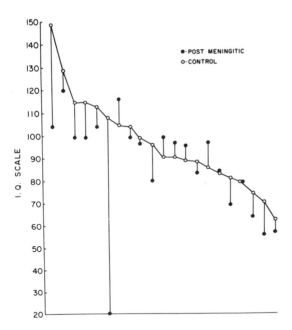

Figure 14-2. IQ results of postmeningitis subjects compared with control sibling pairs (Sell et al. 1972b).

Kresky et al. (1962) found high average intelligence, but a marked discrepancy between verbal and performance parts of the WISC, favoring the verbal part, in many postmeningitis subjects. In addition, 20 per cent of their sample had school difficulties that could not be explained solely on the basis of IQ. Using a matched control group, Wright and Jimmerson (1971) examined 11 children approximately 8 years after they had been hospitalized because of hemophilus influenzae meningitis at an age ranging from 4 months to 5.5 years. They found significant differences in Full-Scale IQ, Verbal and Performance IQs, and on ten Wechsler subscales, but not on the Bender-Gestalt test or six Frostig test variables. Thus, their results indicated not a specific visuomotor impairment, but rather a more general cognitive deficit.

Summary

This chapter dealt with the effects of infections. As examples, congenital HIV and rubella infections were described, which have been studied for their effects on psychological, behavioral, and clinical development well into adolescence. Less is known about cytomegalovirus infections, which are present in a sizeable proportion of newborns, but which show obvious effects only in a small number of these children. Recent research has concentrated on cytomegalovirus' long-term effects, since the virus infection may persist subclinically for many years and show clinical manifestations only at a much later age. In addition to the late occurrence of neurological symptoms, the possible link between subclinical infections and development of intellect, learning problems, and even schizophrenia has opened intriguing hypotheses for future follow-up research. As an example of postnatal infection, the sometimes devastating effects of meningitis were described.

15

Toxic Damage

Exposure of the mother during pregnancy or of the child after birth to any type of toxin may result in acute or chronic intoxication of the fetus and various forms of short- and long-term impairment during childhood. One example of an intoxication during pregnancy is toxemia of pregnancy (**gestosis**), which is presumed to result from a variety of pathological conditions. These are essentially metabolic disturbances in the mother that may cause nausea, vomiting, gastric pains, headache, hypertension and edema (pre-eclampsia), and sudden convulsions and even coma (eclampsia).

Another maternal intoxication, **neonatal jaundice** (hyperbilirubinemia, kernicterus), occurs because of blood type incompatibility between the mother and fetus. Other intoxications by environmental pollutants, such as carbon monoxide, DDT, mercury, lead, arsenic, quinine and so on, were described in Chapter 8 as they relate to critical periods of gestation. The thalidomide tragedy focused attention on intoxication with prescribed and nonprescribed drugs (Stimmel 1982), including the use of multiple antiepileptics (Dodson 1989), barbiturates, and psychotropic drugs (Boer and Swaab 1985). The fetal alcohol syndrome and the teratogenic effects of smoking during pregnancy also have been studied in detail. Although many of these effects have been known for a long time, it was usually assumed that the placenta functioned as a protective barrier and that all potentially toxic material would be filtered out. However, the protective function of the placenta is poorly understood; in fact, it is likely that the placenta may actually maintain an unusually high concentration of certain toxic elements, such as mercury. Deficiencies of certain trace elements, such as zinc and copper, may also have a damaging effect on the neurological development of the fetus.

Postnatally, various toxins tend to affect the developing organism adversely (Isaacson 1992). Best known are the effects of lead (Smith et al. 1989) and carbon monoxide poisoning. Marlowe et al. (1984) found a significant association between hair-metal concentrations of lead and problem behavior in the classroom, and Rimland and Larson (1983) concluded from an analysis of 51 studies that high levels of minerals, especially lead and cadmium, are associated with undesirable behavior. Petit et al. (1983) related postnatal lead exposure to hippocampal morphological development, as well as to behavioral changes. Hawk et al. (1986), in an independent replication of an earlier single-blind study, demonstrated that IQ in African-American children of a low socioeconomic status drops from 94 (with a lead level of 5 PbB) to 75 (with a blood lead level of 45 PbB), resulting in a correlation of −.456 after the elimination of confounding variables. Exposure to mercury vapors during early adolescence has been shown to have lasting effects on visuoperceptual, constructive, and nonverbal memory skills and conceptual abstraction far in excess of the effects found in adults with similar exposure (Yeates and Mortensen 1994). Anesthetics, hypnotics, and even mild exposure to various chemical neurotoxins, such as arsenic, strychnine, and DDT, can have toxic effects (Allen 1975). Hartman (1988) provides an up-to-date reference on the subject of neurotoxicology.

15.1 Hyperbilirubinemia

The excessive formation and retention of **bilirubin**, the yellow-brown-reddish bile pigment formed in the liver, spleen, and bone marrow, may be the result of failure in one or more steps of the normal process of metabolism and excretion and may be related to the destruction of red blood cells. The accumulation of bilirubin results in the clinical picture of neonatal jaundice. Bilirubin is found in increased amounts in all newborns due to accelerated production from degraded fetal hemoglobin, decreased hepatic uptake of bilirubin, and increased enterohepatic circulation. High bilirubin levels are present in about 50 per cent of all newborns between the second and fourth day of life; levels vary, depending on gestational age, birth weight, and many other factors, such as the degree of hypoxia, drug ingestion, delayed cord clamping, and infection. Blood type incompatibility has for some time been recognized as one cause of seriously toxic hyperbilirubinemia, although improved treatment has greatly reduced its incidence. A distinction between water-soluble (conjugated) and fat-soluble (nonconjugated) bilirubin levels is made since only the latter tends to be associated with increased risk to the newborn.

At high levels of accumulation, **kernicterus** (nuclear jaundice) occurs, and the result is death or severe nervous system damage for the survivors. Damage is primarily the result of (1) depression of cell respiration and (2) impaired protein synthesis primarily affecting neural tissue in areas of high susceptibility (basal ganglia, thalamus, hippocampus, and brainstem nuclei) and in other areas of the CNS with a higher level of blood flow. On autopsy of low-birth-weight infants who died from other causes, the typical yellow staining of the basal ganglia has been observed even if the bilirubin level was as low as 15 mg/dl.

The best-known cause of kernicterus is autoimmunization of the mother against one of the Rh+ blood group factors. In this case antibodies (agglutamins) against red blood cells containing the Rh+ factor are formed in the mother's blood system and may ultimately cross the placenta and destroy fetal red blood cells (**erythroblastosis fetalis**). In the past, death during the first months of life occurred in 75 per cent of all infants, but it can usually be prevented now by blood exchange in the infant before birth. Infant mortality is now less than 5 per cent (Dekaban 1970). The danger of kernicterus in a first-born child is quite low since sensitization of the mother builds up slowly, but it rises in subsequent pregnancies because of increased antibody formation. Injection with immune globulin during pregnancy markedly decreases the incidence of erythroblastosis fetalis.

This mechanism of the disorder is a good example of the complex interaction of many factors in intoxications. In this case, the brain defect results from an intoxication that is ultimately determined by genetic factors.

Sequelae in survivors with bilirubin encephalopathy have been studied for some time. Snyder et al. (1945) found that, among an undifferentiated mentally retarded population, the incidence of Rh-incompatibility between parents was twice as high as that in the normal population. This finding suggested that, at that time, kernicterus remained unrecognized and untreated and resulted in mental retardation without specified causes and without gross physical abnormalities.

More recent studies indicate that the incidence of mental retardation, cerebral palsy, and other major handicaps after transfusion is very low (Bowman 1975, Greg and Hutchinson 1969, Phibbs et al. 1971). For example, in Bowman's study, 74 of 87 intrauterine transfusion survivors were completely normal on extended follow-up. If kernicterus does occur, gross physical disorders are common, including choreoathetosis, torsion spasms, localized hypertonicity with serious impairment of voluntary movements, grimacing, hearing and speech defects, difficulty in chewing and swallowing, and maintaining eye fixation. Little improvement during the long-term development of these infants has been reported.

Further studies of hyperbilirubinemia have concentrated on the long-term effects of moderate elevations of bilirubin levels (physiological hyperbilirubinemia) in the newborn. The earliest effects are hypotonia and stupor, which may not be recognized. Severe hyperbilirubinemia of the newborn shows classical signs after the first year of life, including athetosis, deafness, paralysis of eye gaze, and mental handicap. Boggs et al. (1967) found in an 8-month follow-up significantly lower motor scores on the Bayley Developmental Scales if bilirubin levels at birth exceeded 15 mg/dl.

At low levels of concentration (between 12 and 17 mg/dl), Edgell (1986) found effects at the age of 3 days as indicated by a lowered alertness-activity-control dimension of the Brazelton Scale, although socioeconomic status, length of delivery, and gestational age also contributed to this effect. At the age of 8 months only a weak relationship with cognitive tasks and temperament was found; this effect was overshadowed by socioeconomic status, length of delivery, and consumption of alcohol in a multivariate predictor set of variables. Phototherapy tended to accentuate the effects produced by bilirubin level, especially in male infants.

Since damage to the hippocampal areas may affect learning and retention, long-term studies with 4- to 8-year-old children have focused on potential cognitive defects. Johnston et al. (1967) and Upadhyay (1971) found poor attention span, motor hyperactivity, and poor motor coordination, but no IQ deficit, in children whose neonatal bilirubin level was greater than 20 mg/dl; a study by Rubin et al. (1979) failed to confirm this result. A study of 6-year-old children who had neonatal jaundice found impairment of auditory-verbal memory on the Token Test, and that children who had received phototherapy did more poorly than children who had not (Lenhardt 1983). In another 6-year follow-up of infants with lower concentrations of bilirubin (12–17 mg/dl), Heppenstrijdt (1988) found no correlation between total concentration and overall neuropsychological performance, but noticed a subtle reduction in fine motor coordination and speed, tactile perception, auditory verbal memory, and speed and accuracy on a complex task involving planning and mental flexibility; this study also found a significantly higher incidence of mild peripheral sensorineural hearing loss.

The breakdown into conjugated and nonconjugated bilirubin counts began to be used in follow-up studies in the 1970s. Johnson and Boggs (1974) found that cognitive impairment cannot be demonstrated with increases in the total bilirubin but that children with nonconjugated bilirubin levels of more than 15 mg/dl had deficits not only in fine motor integration but also in visual perception and expressive language.

15.2   Other Intoxications Before and After Birth

Prenatal Intoxications

Many drugs administered to the mother can cross the placenta and affect the fetus. Those studied include sedatives and hypnotics, local anesthetics (Dodson 1976), and anticonvulsants. Even exposure of the mother to PCB through cooking oil and its thermal degradation products may cause persistent developmental delay in newborns (Yu et al. 1991).

A study of babies born to cocaine-using mothers compared to a matched control group showed that cocaine-exposed infants had smaller head circumference, more obstetrical complications, lower performance on the habituation cluster of the Brazelton scale, and poorer scores on a newly developed stress scale measuring abnormal reflex behavior and autonomic instability (Eisen et al. 1991). They did not differ on sex distribution, chronological age, birth length, or postnatal complications. However, high cigarette and alcohol use in the same mothers was also present. In a stepwise regression analysis, alcohol use contributed to the stress scale, but not to the Brazelton and other scores. Cocaine use by mothers was thought to have a negative impact on birth weight and head circumference. Link et al. (1991), however, found no abnormalities in MRI studies of infants exposed to cocaine prenatally; the authors suggested that adverse outcome may be due to changes at the neurotransmitter or cellular, rather than the gross morphological level. An unusually high incidence of language delay (94 per cent) and of autism (11.4 per cent) has also been observed in children with perinatal cocaine exposure (Davis et al. 1992). One study of infants born to mothers who used marijuana indicated that the normal rate of CNS development may be subtly depressed up to the age of 30 days, but no effects on mental, motor, and language outcome up to the age of 24 months were found (Fried 1989). The effects of maternal substance abuse were reviewed by Zagon and Slotkin (1992).

The **fetal alcohol syndrome** (FAS) in children of alcoholic mothers and in experimental animal studies has attracted particular attention during the past 20 years (Abel 1981, Overholser 1990, Rosett and Sander 1979). The first description by Jones (1973) of "a characteristic pattern of malformation," including facial malformations, intrauterine growth retardation, and neonatal neurobehavioral dysfunction, stimulated a large number of studies. These three characteristics still form the minimal criteria for diagnosis of the FAS syndrome. Among the neonatal neurobehavioral dysfunctions, increases in time periods with eyes open, in body tremors, in head orientation to the left, and in hand-to-mouth behavior, as well as decreased vigorous body activity, have been described (Jones 1977). Animal experiments have yielded similar findings, as well as evidence of decreased protein synthesis; delayed myelination of the fetal brain; digital impairment; eye, cardiac, and neural abnormalities; and cardiovascular, genital, and head malformations (Streissguth et al. 1980). Although the mechanism of damage has been described as being mediated by hypoxia, direct toxicity of ethanol or acetaldehyde may also be involved. In an analysis of the world literature on 492 cases of FAS and based on seasonal alcohol sales and alcohol-related office statistics in eight countries, Renwick and Asker (1983) suggested that the timing of the ethanol damage may be early, as expected, but that the sensitive period may extend to as late as the 18th to 20th week of pregnancy.

The relatively low reported incidence (0.4 to 3.1/1000 births, Abel 1984) of FAS suggests that alcohol intake during pregnancy alone does not necessarily cause the full FAS syndrome. Factors related to socioeconomic level, such as poor nutrition or excessive smoking, are likely to contribute to it. Abel (1984) also considered the weight, age, and parity of mother and genetic susceptibility as additional risk factors. The facial dysmorphology is similar to that found in children of mothers with PKU, of epileptic mothers who took Dilantin during pregnancy, and of mothers who were exposed to other teratogens. In a 10-year follow-up of 11 children with FAS, 2 had died, 1 could not be located, and the remaining 8 children were growth-deficient and dysmorphic (Streissguth et al. 1985).

Hanson et al. (1978) proposed a syndrome compatible with FAS (CFAS, also described as "**partial FAS**") including four features: (1) small for gestational age, (2) microcephaly, (3) short palpebral fissures, and (4) multiple dysmorphic features. Zuckerman and Hingson (1986) stressed, however, that the risk for CFAS in their study of 1384 infants born to mothers who had two or more drinks daily during pregnancy was not significantly different from that of non-drinkers. In contrast, the risk was 5 times higher for marijuana users, 2.6 times higher for women who gained less than 5 pounds during pregnancy, and 2.8 times higher for women who were exposed to x-rays. Other studies have shown a marginal reduction in birth weight, length, and head circumference for infants born to alcohol-using mothers (Day et al. 1991, Ernhart et al. 1985), although confounding variables, such as smoking, dietary restrictions, drug use, and malnutrition, often were not sufficiently controlled. Korkman et al. (1989) reported that IQ scores in 2-year-old children of drinking mothers were negatively related to the length of alcohol use during pregnancy, whereas the risk of attention problems and hyperactivity persisted even if the mothers gave up drinking during the later stages of pregnancy.

In a major follow-up study, Streissguth et al. (1992) selected 250 pregnant women who were heavy or moderate drinkers and 250 light or infrequent drinkers and abstainers in the Seattle area. Measures included delivery data, Brazelton examinations on day 1, operant head turning and sucking on day 2, Bayley scale and other examinations at 8 and 16 months, WPPSI and WISC scores, and achievement and other testing at age 4 and 7 years. In contrast to Zuckerman and Hingson (1986), the authors concluded that there were deficits at all ages, which were directly related to the level of alcohol exposure, "suggesting no non-effect level of exposure" (p. 196). In the 4-year-olds, poor attention span, longer reaction times, and deficits in fine and gross motor function, memory, attention, and achievement were observed; at age 7, characteristic behaviors included "distractibility, impulsivity, poor cooperation, poor organization, poor recall of information, and a rigid approach to problem solving" (p. 197). This study used multiple regression analysis to control for birth order, maternal education, nutrition, and caffeine and tobacco use. Maternal cigarette use was related to poor attention and poor orientation to the board on a computer-controlled vigilance task. A more indirect effect of alcoholism by either father or mother was reported by Steinhausen et al. (1984) who found heightened psychiatric risk, although some improvement in psychiatric status and psychological functioning was noted in a follow-up at the age of 3 years.

Postnatal Intoxications

Among the postnatal intoxications, chemical neurotoxins in industry and the environment, such as lead, mercury, manganese, solvents, alkyl halides, organophosphates, and gases, have received considerable attention (Hartman 1988, Wilson 1977). Lead intoxication has been the subject of considerable research. Lead intoxication occurs when infants are exposed to lead-based paints and to dust, soil, and air with high lead content, which are usually found in the vicinity of ore smelters, foundries, brass works, battery factories, printing operations, and other plants. Epidemic levels of lead absorption in approximately 2700 children near an ore smelter in El Paso, Texas, were reported by Landrigan et al. (1975). Low-level lead intoxication from exhaust fumes in heavy traffic areas and other sources has been investigated (Hankin et al. 1973, Needleman 1980, Needleman et al. 1974). Exposure is much more likely in relatively poor urban districts and hence is associated with low socioeconomic levels.

Lead intoxication affects virtually all tissues of the body by causing degeneration of nerve cells, neuronal loss, decreased myelination, and reactive gliosis. Necrosis of neural tissue probably occurs because of the occlusion of small blood vessels. Neural tissue involvement in acute intoxications is indicated by pallor, irritability, vomiting, deterioration of consciousness, seizures, and focal neurological signs. Survivors of this acute lead encephalopathy usually show significant mental handicap. Whether long-term subclinical intoxication causes a lead neuropathy with decreased reflexes, motor weakness, hypesthesia, and reduced nerve conduction velocity is still under investigation. Children with sickle-cell anemia, a hereditary disorder of hemoglobin, are especially vulnerable to lead neuropathy. In animal studies, raising the lead content of maternal milk has been shown to increase lead levels in the blood and brain tissue of the newborn. The rodents showed increased motor activity, aggressiveness, tremor, and self-grooming (Golter and Michaelson 1975, Overmann 1977).

Lead poisoning during pregnancy has mainly been studied in more severe cases (Angle and McIntire 1964, Palmisano et al. 1969). Hyperactivity in children is associated with increased blood levels of lead (David et al. 1972). Intelligence test scores are inversely related to lead blood levels (Beattie et al. 1975, Klein et al. 1974). Marlowe et al. (1983) found elevated lead and cadmium concentrations in a significantly higher proportion of hair samples from mild and borderline retarded children than in a control group of children in grades 7 to 12. Unfortuantely, many studies are confounded with socioeconomic factors related to living in areas where lead exposure is likely. These same factors render inconclusive many of the earlier studies of low-level lead exposures (Lansdown et al. 1974, Rutter 1980).

Solvent abuse in childhood and adolescence was reviewed by Thomasius (1986), who noted that resulting neuropsychological impairments, encephalopathies, and atrophy of the cerebellum and the corpus callosum often remain permanent. Lower overall intelligence, especially on tests involving visual processing, has been reported (Zur and Yule 1990).

Summary

This chapter dealt with the effects of various toxins on the developing embryo, fetus, or child. As an example of neonatal toxic damage, the mechanism of neonatal jaundice (which in one of its forms, Rh-incompatibility, is ultimately related to genetic factors) was described. Again, we are only at the beginning of fully detailed behavioral follow-up studies, since it is mainly the more seriously elevated bilirubin levels with and without kernicterus that have been studied and low levels of unconjugated bilirubin may also be related to cognitive and motor development in infancy and later childhood. New research into the fetal alcohol syndrome was also described. Our example for postnatal toxic damage to the nervous system, lead neuropathy, has been the subject of intensive study. The consequences of acute lead encephalopathy are well established. Whether continuous low-level exposure to such environmental hazards as gasoline fumes may have significant adverse effects on the child's development is not fully established and has yet to reach a consensus among researchers.

16

Nutritional Disorders

The World Health Organization estimated in 1983 that 300 million children, mostly living in the developing world, sustained growth retardation secondary to malnutrition (WHO 1983). Protein-calorie malnutrition (PCM) and protein-energy malnutrition (PEM) are generic terms for a wide spectrum of nutritional deficiencies in early life that vary in type, timing, and severity. These deficiencies are distinct from the malnutrition secondary to medical conditions, such as cystic fibrosis, or from genetically determined metabolic disorders, such as phenylketonuria. Protein-calorie deficiencies are also distinct from highly selective deficiencies of specific vitamins, such as vitamin A deficiency, a primary cause of preventable blindness in infancy and childhood, or of minerals, e.g., iron deficiency anemia or iodine deficiency disorder. These selective deficiencies usually occur in the context of a diet that is otherwise adequate.

Two clinically notable syndromes are present in the PCM spectrum of disorders: kwashiorkor and marasmus. If severe enough, a predominantly protein-deficient diet in the young child may present clinically as a syndrome known as **kwashiorkor,** whereas a predominantly energy-deficient diet may result in a syndrome termed **marasmus** (Table 16-1). These syndromes are accompanied on the spectrum of nutritional deficiencies by severe combined deficiencies sometimes called **marasmic-kwashiorkor** and by common and chronic **subclinical nutritional deficiencies** characterized by notable protein, caloric, or combined shortages.

Both marasmus and kwashiorkor are postnatal syndromes. However, in Third world settings, the infant at risk for a nutritional deficiency has typically been subjected to direct prenatal stunting because of poor maternal nutrition and also because of the influence of nutritional deficiencies spanning generations that have weakened the mother's ability to carry the fetus to term without obstetrical difficulty. A poorly developed placenta and a very small maternal pelvis interfering with fetal development are two examples of the influence of generational malnutrition on the pregnant mother.

Table 16-1 Salient Features of Kwashiorkor and Marasmus

	Marasmus	Kwashiorkor
Age of maximum incidence	6–18 months	12–48 months
Emaciation	3+	1–2+
Edema	None	1–3+
Fatty infiltration of liver	None to 1+	3+
Skin changes	Infrequent	Frequent
Serum albumin	Almost normal	Markedly decreased
Serum enzymes		
Lipase	Normal	Markedly decreased
Amylase	Normal	Decreased
Esterase	Slightly decreased	Decreased
Serum lipids		
Triglycerides	Normal	Normal
Cholesterol	Normal	Lowered
Nonesterified fatty acids	Increased	Increased

Source: Suskind 1977.

Nutritional deficiency rarely occurs as an isolated phenomenon. Usually, it is associated with several concurrent environmental and health-related features. The entire set of deprivations has been termed the "**malnutritional milieu.**" These features include increased risks of infection, secondary dehydration, infected water supplies, inadequate medical facilities and care, insufficiencies in the quality and quantity of maternal care and environmental stimulation, inadequate sanitation, poor education, and inadequate income. The association between malnutrition and infection is particularly important. Although malnutrition may make an individual more susceptible to infection, the presence of an infection can prolong the acute consequences of the malnutrition. Any statements about the later mental consequences of malnutrition need to be placed in the context of an early life of deprivation. This is particularly true in evaluating research if explicit control over other deprivational factors is lacking.

The development of the CNS depends upon the availability of proper nutrients in adequate amounts to supply both the raw energy to fuel growth and the essential building blocks of growth at a biochemical level. Proteins, carbohydrates, fats, water, minerals, and vitamins must be part of a balanced diet (Table 16-2). For example, the human body cannot readily use fat-soluble vitamins, such as A and D, if adequate supplies of fats are not also available from the diet.

When adequate amounts of nutrients are not available from the diet, they are drawn initially from biochemical stores accumulated within the body. If need persists, nutrients are catabolized from the cells and organs of the body themselves. If the deprivation is severe and prolonged, continued somatic wasting, coma, and death may occur. However, if an adult is moderately or even severely malnourished on an acute basis and then nutritionally rehabilitated and supplemented, weight gain again ensues, and little, if any, permanent anatomical or

Table 16-2 Essential Human Nutrients

Carbohydrate		
Fat		
Protein		
Water		
Minerals		
Calcium	Iron	Cobalt
Phosphorus	Zinc	Chromium
Potassium	Selenium	Fluorine
Sulfur	Manganese	Silicon
Sodium	Copper	Vanadium
Chlorine	Iodine	Nickel
Magnesium	Molybdenum	Tin
Vitamins		
A	Riboflavin	
D	Niacin	
E	Pyroxidine	
K	Pantothenic acid	
C (ascorbic acid)	Folacin	
B6 (Thiamin)	B12	
Biotin		

chemical changes are observed. Permanent neurological deficits are not usually observed when the duration of the protein-calorie deprivation episode occurs during adulthood. However, specific vitamin deficiencies can cause temporary or permanent neurological damage and neuropsychological deficits. The loss of thiamine from the diet—a finding often associated with severe alcoholism—may result, for example, in the permanent amnestic syndrome that is part of the Wernicke-Korsakoff syndrome (Adams and Victor 1993). Sklar (1986) reported a case of B_{12} deficiency in a 7-month-old son of a mother who was a strict vegetarian; the child presented with lethargy and failure to thrive, and laboratory data revealed macrocytic anemia and methylmalonic acid in the urine. This child responded well to vitamin B_{12} supplements and was developmentally normal by 11 months of age.

The developing organism does not always have this recuperative ability. Once subjected to PCM or PEM deficiencies and their attendant milieu of deprivation, the infant or child may suffer permanent changes in both somatic and CNS status (Lozoff 1989). Tissues that undergo the most rapid development during the period of the deficiency may be most vulnerable, which corresponds to the Dobbing hypothesis (Dobbing 1968) of critical growth periods (Chapter 8).

The primary concern of this chapter is the extent to which early life nutritional deprivation influences functional abilities in later life. Whether structural changes in the CNS actually mediate subsequent losses of function has been the subject of experimental work with animals, but few human studies have been reported.

16.1 Physical and Biochemical Brain Alterations

Prenatal Deficiency

The developing fetus has two buffers to protect it from inadequate nutrition: (1) direct nutrition from the consumption of food by the mother and (2) the placental transfer of nutrients stored by the mother. It has been said that the fetus has a "parasitic" relationship with the mother, thriving fairly successfully to the detriment of the mother when she is moderately malnourished. However, this bit of science folklore has been contradicted by research indicating that the fetus is, in fact, affected by insufficient maternal food intake.

It is difficult to determine the optimal level of nutrients needed for the normal development of the fetus because nutrients are ingested by the mother, not the fetus. The amounts that actually cross the placenta remain unclear (Zamenhof and van Marthens 1978). Furthermore, the actual quantities and qualities required by the fetal organism are not known. Previously, it had been assumed that fetal and maternal nutritional needs were identical, but fetal needs for amino acids unique to early life place this assumption into serious doubt. The fetus does require **glucose,** the main source of biochemical energy, which is stored as glycogen in the placenta and the fetal liver. These stores form important short-term reserves in the organism's response to perinatal stress. The fetus also requires amino acids for protein synthesis; these are absorbed in the maternal small intestine from food proteins and cross the placenta to the fetus. Vitamins and essential fatty acids are required, but only in such small amounts that maternal stores can usually provide them regardless of the nutritional status of the mother. Since the fetus can extract minerals, such as iron, from its mother even when her daily iron intake is inadequate, it is not very vulnerable to a prenatal mineral deficiency.

The importance of maternal biochemical stores as a defense against the consequences of prenatal malnutrition was apparent in the **Hongerwinter** of 1944 to 1945 in the larger cities of Western Holland. During this time of deprivation, the result of a transportation embargo imposed by the Nazi occupation forces in reprisal for a strike by Dutch rail workers, maternal stores of pregnant women were sufficient to offset, partially or fully, severe deficiencies of available nutrients (Stein et al. 1975). Below a threshold value of food intake, however, fetuses were vulnerable to some extent in the third trimester in terms of intrauterine growth and early postnatal mortality. Birth weight was affected to a greater degree than either body length or head circumference. Follow-up with males at the time of their military induction at age 19 showed, however, that no variation in performance on the Raven Progressive Matrices test was associated with prenatal exposure to famine, either early or late in gestation (Stein and Susser 1976). Similarly, variance in the prevalence of mental retardation was related neither to conception nor to birth during the famine.

Severe malnutrition very early in pregnancy—during the period of rapid neuronal proliferation when the fetus is extremely vulnerable—usually results in a failure to maintain embryonic implantation and ends with a spontaneous abortion. Moderate malnutrition throughout the period of pregnancy or more severe deficiencies later in gestation usually allow the fetus to survive, but result in changes in the growth of both the placenta and the fetus. Winick (1976) reported that changes in the placenta accompany and usually precede changes in the fetus. For this reason, the placenta has proven to be useful for experimental investigation to evaluate indirectly the types of changes presumed to occur in fetal tissue (Beaconsfield et al. 1980).

At birth, the most visible clinical manifestation of prenatal malnutrition is small size for gestational age, indicating intrauterine growth failure due to maternal malnutrition. This growth failure is of the Type I form, in Brasel's (1974) classification of prenatal growth failures. The size and weight of all body organs, including the brain, are decreased below normal ranges. In contrast, intrauterine growth failure due to placental insufficiency (Brasel's Type II) provides a good deal of brain "sparing" compared to other organs. Interventional studies in several cross-cultural settings have shown that birth weight is heavier when deprived mothers are provided with nutritional supplements during pregnancy (Lechtig 1985).

Reduction in gross brain weights of offspring as a result of maternal deprivation has been demonstrated both experimentally in animals and clinically at autopsy. The weight reduction is attributable to the reduction of cellular proliferation during pregnancy, which mostly involves neurons (**hypoplasia**), whereas malnutrition during the first year affects mostly glial cells and myelination. The number of microneurons, the proliferation of which continues beyond the early peak period, may also be reduced. Winick and Rosso (1969) and Zamenhof and van Marthens (1978) independently determined that the decrease in brain weight corresponds to about a 15 per cent reduction in brain cell number.

Postnatal Deficiency

Experimental evidence concerning the influence of nutritional deficiencies on postnatal brain development has generally been consistent with Dobbing's hypothesis: ongoing development is impaired in those cell types, tissues, and regions that show a maximal velocity of growth at the time of the nutritional deficiency. Once rapid growth of the CNS has ended and development has stabilized, malnutrition has little permanent influence on the status of the brain if the child is returned to a full diet.

Significant decreases in nerve cell number are not observed when the organism has had adequate prenatal but inadequate postnatal nutrition. However, the number of glial cells may be permanently reduced as a consequence of early postnatal deprivation. The primary effect of postnatal nutritional deficiency is an overall reduction in the size of both neurons and glial cells. This effect is generally reversible when subsequent food intake provides adequate nutrition. The elaboration of neuronal processes may also be stunted: given the reduction in both glial cell number and size, the extent of myelination in the brain is reduced, although the composition of the myelin is not grossly abnormal. In animal studies, the cerebellum shows greater reduction in cell number because the critical period for cell proliferation occurs later there than in the cerebrum or the brainstem.

Marasmus and kwashiorkor are clinical manifestations of life-threatening malnutrition after birth. However, in most cases of chronic malnutrition some degree of prenatal maternal malnutrition has also occurred. Postmortem examinations of the brains of marasmic infants, as well as experimental animal studies, indicate that there is a quantitative reduction in cell number and cell size, rather than the presence of a particular pattern of neuropathology. The quantity of myelin is reduced, but aberrations in myelin composition do not occur to any significant degree. Persistent alterations in auditory evoked potentials as a consequence of marasmus, despite rehabilitation, have been reported (Barnet et al. 1978). In kwashiorkor, cell size is reduced, but the number of cells may be unaffected. In one study, the EEGs of recovered kwashiorkor children differed from those of their siblings and peers who did not suffer severe clinical malnutrition, as well as from those of a high-SES group of the same age who had no nutritional deficiencies of any kind. The abnormal EEGs revealed less alpha activity and more slow-wave activity, indicating neuronal alterations (Bartel et al. 1979). A CT head scan study reported from a center in South Africa noted severe cerebral atrophy or shrinkage in the absence of neurological abnormalities in a small number of children with severe kwashiorkor (Househam and deVilliers 1987). At the time the CT scans were taken, the children had been hospitalized for at least a week and were medically stable and normally hydrated. This center reported a follow-up study with essentially the same findings, but noted that the severe cerebral shrinkage resolved after nutritional rehabilitation was complete (Househam 1991).

Basic research has suggested that the brains of animals that were inadequately nourished during both prenatal and postnatal periods of rapid brain development show a greater cumulative stunting than those affected during either period alone. Winick (1976) reported a reduction of 60 per cent in brain weight in that situation compared to a reduction of approximately 15 per cent with either prenatal or postnatal deprivation alone (Figure 16-1).

16.2   Behavioral Alterations

The consequences of nutritional deficiencies are examined by follow-up investigation of retrospectively or prospectively identified individuals who have suffered some degree of early-life nutritional deprivation. Causes cannot be directly investigated in the study population, but must be inferred from human case studies and animal experiments. No study has combined both behavioral and later autopsy data from human patients with nutritional deficiencies. To provide the most relevant cognitive information, follow-up studies of children exposed to nutritional deficiencies should cover the breadth of neuropsychological func-

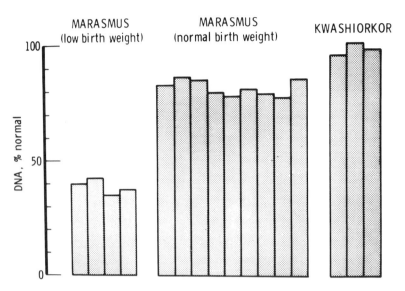

Figure 16-1. Comparison of brain cell numbers in marasmus, marasmus plus low birth weight, and kwashiorkor (Winick 1970).

tioning, as well as provide information on adaptive, motivational, and social maturity. Unfortunately, no available study meets this ideal. Most examine the long-term consequences of malnutrition by using a global measure of intellectual function, such as the Wechsler or Stanford-Binet IQ scales. Others have sought to examine specific abilities, such as the development of cross-modal integrative capacities (i.e., identifying similarities and differences across sensory modalities) or language development.

Groups that differ in nutritional history are also likely to differ in the malnutritional milieu described above (e.g., show a differential risk for infectious disease), clouding any inferences of direct causality (Figure 16-2). As one solution to this perplexing difficulty, Cravioto and his associates (Cravioto and DiLicardie 1975) performed prospective research, collecting premorbid information from a large group of infants who subsequently may or may not become malnourished. A second approach has been to use animal (usually rat) models to study behavioral consequences just as they were used to study brain development (Fleischer and Turkewitz 1984). This approach has been of limited success because even in laboratory rats maternal care (Crnic 1976) and environmental stimulation (Levitsky and Barnes 1972) have been shown to exert potent early-life influences on cognitive abilities in adulthood.

The quality of the control groups employed in malnutrition studies is important. These groups usually are made up of peers matched for age and sex and include individual groups of siblings, neighbors, or members of the community with the same socioeconomic status (SES), as well as members of the com-

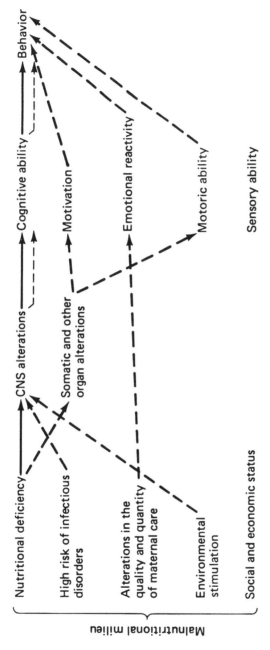

Figure 16-2. Structural challenges in examining the consequences of inadequate early life nutritional disorders.

munity or of neighboring communities with a higher SES and a smaller probability of suffering from nutritional deprivation. Although the use of siblings is helpful in controlling family-child interactions and familial idiosyncracies, it is likely that siblings in these families also have suffered some degree of subclinical malnutrition. Comparisons limited to index versus sibling groups may therefore underestimate the deficits (Hertzig et al. 1972), whereas use of different communities may overestimate these deficits. The specific locales from which both malnourished and control groups are drawn may add their own unique social and environmental factors that also make cross-cultural comparisons difficult.

Although easier to execute, retrospective designs do curtail the value of information gathered on the long-term consequences of early-life nutritional deficiencies. A retrospective design cannot provide information about premorbid nutritional status, standard medical diagnosis of the nutritional deficiency, and the percentage of the population of interest that died as a result of the deficiency. Retrospective studies of subclinical malnutrition are even less powerful because the presence of an early-life deficiency is generally inferred only from anthropometric measurements such as head circumference.

Marasmus Follow-Up Studies

Marasmus typically is manifested during the first 6 months of life. Before marasmic presentation, the infant's low-calorie diet often is also low in protein. The marasmic child shows a failure to grow, usually weighing less than 60 per cent of the age-expected norm. In many cases, the marasmic infant has been stunted from conception because of the mother's insufficient nutrition and biochemical stores, as well as the effects of nutritional deficiency endemic to her population for generations. The generational factor may have influenced, for example, the anatomy of her pelvic region and the efficiency of her digestive and metabolic systems.

Starvation of the infant is usually exacerbated by any abrupt and premature weaning; breast milk is frequently replaced by diluted and dirty infant formulas. Muscle and organ wasting, the loss of subcutaneous fat, and minimal hair growth are common. Edema is absent in marasmus (but is a cardinal feature of kwashiorkor). Without medical intervention, death from starvation compounded by infection is a common outcome. Successful nutritional rehabilitation can avert death, but the infant usually returns to an environment that will continue to supply insufficient nutrition. Head circumference and, by inference, brain size are diminished. Stunting of physical stature may be observed compared to same-aged peers, even after successful nutritional rehabilitation.

Results have shown fairly consistently that marasmic infants perform significantly more poorly than controls on global scales of mental ability, such as the Wechsler, Binet, and Bayley scales. Early studies were retrospective. Brockman and Ricciuti (1971) examined the categorization behavior of marasmic infants after successful hospitalization and rehabilitation. A control group of children, matched for age and sex, was drawn from a day-care center in an urban slum community. The previously malnourished infants performed less well on the task than the more adequately fed control group. McLaren and colleagues (1973) examined performance on the Stanford-Binet test for groups of nutritionally stunted and control Lebanese children who were between 3 and 5 years of age at follow-up. Rehabilitated marasmic children, subclinically malnourished children, the siblings of both groups, and a control group matched for age and SES were tested. Global mean IQ values were lower by one standard deviation or more for the marasmic and subclinical groups compared to the two control groups.

A series of reports by Galler and her collaborators (1984, Galler et al. 1983a and b, 1984a and b, 1990) describe a detailed and carefully controlled examination of the outcome of marasmus in a sample of schoolchildren in Barbados. The sample was composed of all children admitted to a hospital from 1967 through 1972 who met a clinical diagnosis of moderate-to-severe marasmus. For inclusion in the malnourished sample, children had to have had a birth weight of at least 5 pounds (to exclude any children exposed to significant fetal growth retardation); normal Apgar scores at birth; and no history of any other neurological disorder. A sample of 129 boys and girls between the ages of 5 and 11 years was evaluated on a spectrum of measures, including physical status, soft neurological signs, intellectual performance (on a modified and shortened version of the WISC), grades in school, and classroom behaviors. A comparison group of 129 peers was also evaluated on these measures. The authors considered Barbados to be a suitable location for this type of research because of its well-documented health care and nutritional support delivery system, its population that was at least 95 per cent literate and its relatively stable and industrializing economy.

Compared to the control group, the malnourished children showed statistically significant lower IQ scores (Figure 16-3). Group means differed by 12 IQ points. Socioeconomic differences between the two groups were not significantly associated with the IQ differences. Teachers who rated classroom performance without knowledge of the children's nutritional history indicated that the malnourished children showed significantly more attentional problems, reduced social skills, poorer physical appearance, and greater emotional instability than did control children. These behavioral characteristics were independent of IQ scores and were observed more frequently in boys. In elementary school, previously malnourished children were noted to perform less well than control peers in eight of nine academic subject areas. The researchers attributed the difference to classroom behaviors, rather than to reduced IQ performances, because of a relatively stronger statistical association (Figure 16-4).

The performance of the previously malnourished children on the standard high school entrance examination was significantly lower than the performance of the comparison group. Lower scores were associated with teacher ratings of attentional problems in the classroom, lower IQ scores, and poorer academic performance. The group differences remained significant even when conditions in the home environment were statistically controlled. Galler and Ramsey (1989)

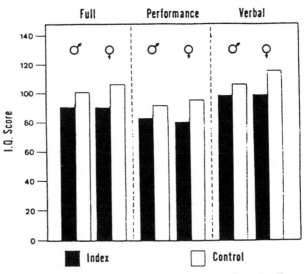

Figure 16-3. IQ scores of malnourished and normal children (Galler et al. 1984).

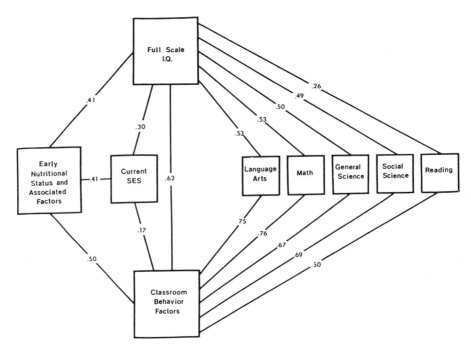

Figure 16-4. Multifactorial model of the relationship between malnutrition and school performance (Galler 1984).

reported the presence of residual attentional deficits and increased distractibility in these children relative to controls through the age of 15 years, both in school and at home.

In sum, infants who have had clinically diagnosed marasmus during the first year of life and have then been rehabilitated show lasting mental deficits on global measures of intelligence. The work of Galler and her colleagues has indicated that a specific cognitive deficit in attention may be observed even after successfully treated children develop into adolescence.

Kwashiorkor Follow-Up Studies

Kwashiorkor usually appears clinically between the first and third years of life. It is not observed in the early months of life because breast milk provides the infant with adequate protein and with some protection from infection. Kwashiorkor may develop when the baby is weaned to a protein-deficient diet. The consequences of a lack of adequate protein are compounded by the severe diarrhea that is present in over 90 per cent of kwashiorkor cases (Gomez et al. 1955). Edema is a common feature of kwashiorkor, resulting in the typical image of the starving infant with a greatly bloated stomach and sparse, depigmented hair. The child is often apathetic, somnolent, and indifferent to his or her surroundings. These children have intermittent periods of monotonous crying and/ or echolalia. Low serum levels of **albumin** (the main blood protein) are characteristic of kwashiorkor.

Studies of children who have sustained kwashiorkor in infancy present more varied neurobehavioral findings than those of the marasmic infant. An earlier notion that later-childhood deficits are generally less severe in kwashiorkor than in marasmus (Pollit and Thompson 1978) has been questioned by more recent findings (Galler et al. 1987a).

Birch and his colleagues (1971) examined the performance of Mexican children who had been hospitalized between 6 and 30 months with a diagnosis of kwashiorkor. Their performance was compared to that of their nearest-aged sibling who did not show signs of a clinical nutritional deficiency. At follow-up, the children were between 6 and 13 years of age and had been out of a hospital for at least 3 years. Full-scale, Verbal, and Performance IQ scores all were significantly lower in the patient group than in the group of siblings. For example, the malnourished group's mean Full-scale IQ was 68.5 compared to the mean of 81.5 for siblings. An analysis of the subtest scatter (i.e., variability in performance within the intelligence test) showed no indication of potential specific deficiencies.

In contrast, studies by Bartel and colleagues (1977a and b) and Evans and colleagues (1971) failed to find significant differences between groups of children who had a history of kwashiorkor and controls without evidence of clinical levels of malnutrition. Bartel and co-workers examined 31 children aged 5 to 14 years who had been diagnosed and treated for kwashiorkor by age 3. The performance of these children was contrasted with that of two control groups:

their nearest-aged siblings and an age-matched group of peers from the same community. The three groups showed similar performance on all tasks—the Tactual Performance test, Tactual Form Recognition, the Category test, and the WISC mazes subtest—but they differed on levels of alpha- and slow-wave activity observed on the EEG (Bartel et al. 1979). Evans and colleagues compared children who had a documented history of kwashiorkor with their adequately nourished siblings on the New South African Individual Scale of Intelligence and the Goodenough-Harris drawing task. The groups performed similarly on these tests.

The Barbadian studies of Galler and her colleagues described above were extended to include a sample of children who had kwashiorkor during the first year of their lives and were then remediated (Galler et al. 1983a, 1989, and 1990). When these children were between the ages of 11 and 18 years, they were examined with a Barbadian version of the WISC. Their performances were significantly below those of the control group, which had been selected using the same criteria that were discussed in the prior subsection. WISC performance showed no significant subtest scatter. The previously malnourished children also performed more poorly on a set of Piagetian conservation tasks. Motor performance, as measured by the Purdue Pegboard, was also examined in these children. Those with histories of either clinical syndrome performed more poorly than controls on aspects of the motor task. Their right (dominant) hand performance was not significantly slower. However, slowed performances on other subtests, including the Assembly task, were statistically significant. Lower high-school entrance examination test scores were noted in the group with a history of kwashiorkor relative to the control group. As with the Barbadian marasmus group, these entrance examination differences were not attributable to home conditions.

In sum, kwashiorkor and its related milieu, even when the malnutrition is treated successfully, are associated with cognitive and motor impairments in later childhood.

Follow-Up Studies of Subclinical Nutritional Deficiency

Whereas studies of marasmus and kwashiorkor rely upon a medically diagnosed and documented early-life condition, the follow-up study of children with less severe nutritional deficiencies has to rely on more indirect, anthropometric measures, such as size and weight for age. Despite this difficulty in classifying nutritional status, an early and carefully designed study by Cravioto, DiLicardie, and Birch in 1966 remains useful in providing information about the cognitive consequences of subclinical deficiencies.

Children in the upper and lower quartiles for height in cross-sectional samples of 6- to 11-year-olds from both a poor rural community and a high-SES urban community in Chile were chosen for evaluation. The purpose of the evaluation was to determine relationships between presumed nutritional history and cognitive cross-modal integrative capacities in the visual, kinesthetic, and haptic sensory modalities. In general, the high-SES urban group performed better on the tasks than did the rural group. In the rural group, the lower-height quartile (i.e., those who were presumed likely to have suffered from early-life deficits) performed less well than the upper quartile, whereas quartile status (which is presumed to be unrelated to nutritional status in high-SES) was not related to cross-modal performances in the urban group.

Other studies of subclinical malnutrition, some discussed by Pollit and Thompson (1978), have explored the effect of nutritional and psychoeducational intervention programs on mental development. An investigation by McKay and colleagues (1978) found a narrowing of the differences between deprived and control children after a treatment program that combined nutrition, education, and health care. Zeskind and Ramey (1981) reported a similar amelioration of the effects of fetal malnourishment in a 3-year follow-up study. Ricciti (1981) suggested that under optimal rehabilitation conditions the long-term effects of subclinical malnutrition may be completely eliminated, a suggestion contradicted by Lozoff (1989).

In an important prospective study, Cravioto and DiLicardie (1975) analyzed the relation between the conditions of a child's upbringing—especially the nutritional history—and the course of the child's physical growth, mental development, and learning. The setting of the study was a stable population in an agricultural community in southwest Mexico. A census 1 year before the study cohort was born determined the similarity between the cohort's families and the community as a whole (population 5637). Eighty per cent of the villagers were under 35 years of age, reflecting the reduced life expectancy in the region. Most of the adults were seasonal agricultural laborers. Illiteracy was common. Many households had substandard sanitary facilities. Malnutrition affected a large proportion of the village population and ranged from mild to clinically severe.

The entire cohort of infants born during a 12-month period in 1966 and 1967 was then followed for 7 years at dozens of data-gathering times. Demographic, nutritional, and social background data indicated that the families of the children in the study were representative of the community as a whole.

Of the 300 infants born during the 12-month period, equal numbers were boys and girls. The mean birth weight was 2898 g; 12.3 per cent of the cohort had a birth weight below 2500 g. The total first year mortality was 6.4 per cent. During the first 5 years of life, 22 children (14 girls and 8 boys) were clinically diagnosed as suffering from severe malnutrition: 15 had kwashiorkor and 7 had marasmus. By the end of the first 38 months of life, 72 (26 per cent) of the 276 children surviving in the cohort, including 14 of 19 clinically malnourished children, showed growth failure relative to normative expectations. The first indication of growth failure in clinically malnourished children appeared an average of 7.7 months before the diagnosis of clinically severe malnutrition was made.

The 19 surviving children with severe malnutrition before the age of 39 months were matched for gestational age, weight, and length at birth with children from the cohort who were not clinically malnourished, but who probably suffered from some degree of nutritional deficit. A language age was determined for each child by the Gesell method; the malnourished children showed poorer language development than their matched cohort mates. Early language development (e.g., babbling) was very similar for the two groups during the first year of life, when only one severe case of malnutrition had been diagnosed. As time passed and more children were recognized as suffering from malnutrition, differences in language development favorable to the control children became evident. The differences became more marked at each successive testing period.

In addition to the global measure of language development, a specific test of bipolar concept formation was administered on several occasions. The ability to recognize the difference between such concepts as big-little, in-out, and long-short was evaluated by this test. Serial testing at nine points between 26 and 58 months of age indicated that the malnourished children had a poorer grasp of bipolar concepts than control subjects. The difference continued beyond the time of clinical recovery.

Family variables were examined in relation to test performance. Very little in the **family "macro-environment"** (a term employed by the authors to refer to such variables as literacy, family size, and sanitation) correlated with test performance; neither did age, height, weight, educational level, personal cleanliness, or sources of income account for a significant portion of the variability in test performance. The **family "micro-environment,"** however, was strongly associated with nutritional status. It basically represented the stimulation the child received at home, including the stability of adult contact, vocal stimulation, need gratification, emotional climate, avoidance of restrictions, breadth of experience, aspects of the physical environment, and available play materials. The strong association between nutritional status and the micro-environment was present even at the age of 6 months when only one infant was diagnosed as being severely malnourished. Cravioto and DiLicardie concluded that a deficit in the child's "micro-environment" was important in determining which children suffering from chronic, subclinical deficiencies would eventually develop clinically diagnosable severe malnutrition. A follow-up study by Cravioto and Arrieta (1979) showed that intensive infant stimulation at home was effective in the rehabilitation process. In a study in Kenya, Espinosa et al. (1992) also reported that better nourished children were more active and happy and showed more attention and leadership behavior in playground behavior; this finding pertained even when the effects of family education, SES, and school attendance were considered. However, a combination of factors, including family characteristics, education, and nutrition, provided the best prediction of cognitive status of Kenyan children in a 5-year follow-up (Sigman et al. 1989, 1991).

Summary

PCM and PEM, if untreated, have fatal consequences. Once treated, later-life behavioral and cognitive functioning may be disordered relative to the norm.

Radiological and electrophysiological findings may be observed beyond the period of malnutrition, although human autopsy studies examining the brains of previously malnourished individuals await definitive analysis. Cognitive deficits have yet to be examined in malnourished children from a truly neuropsychological perspective, i.e., by examining performance on all significant dimensions of cognition. When subsets of important brain behavior functions are examined, intellectual functioning is often lower to a degree, specific attentional problems may be elicited, slowed motor findings may be observed, and academic achievement may be poorer relative to the norm. The environment of these children has been examined more carefully during the past decades (Levitsky 1979), and relations among aspects of the malnutritional milieu are now routinely entered into research protocols examining outcome. The nutritional deficiency is accepted as one single element in an entire milieu of deprivation that includes inadequate medical facilities, maternal care, and environmental stimulation.

Early-life malnutritional milieu does influence later-life cognitive abilities. Follow-up studies of marasmic infants indicate a consistent and severe cognitive deficit, whereas studies evaluating kwashiokor are less consistent. Recent studies even suggest that severe malnutrition may be attenuated or, under optimal rehabilitation conditions, avoided completely. Deficiencies also seem to produce long-lasting consequences. Animal studies of behavioral consequences of early-life nutritional stunting, in which better control over both deficiency and rehabilitation is possible, suggest that nutrition per se is not the only aspect of the milieu but that maternal care and environmental stimulation must be considered as important additional factors.

17

Anoxic Episodes

The maturing fetus and neonate are subject to alterations in the availability of oxygen and oxygenated blood during gestation, delivery, and the period immediately after birth. Maternal disease and cardiovascular difficulties, contractions of the uterus during delivery, the cutting of the umbilical cord, and numerous other conditions may interfere with normal oxygen supply. In most of these situations the reduction in oxygen is relatively minor, transient, and amenable to natural physiological and metabolic compensation without the risk of serious complications. However, a serious reduction in available oxygen (**hypoxia**) and a termination of oxygen supply (**anoxia**) are not uncommon perinatal complications. A systemic reduction in oxygen level decreases blood flow to local tissue and results in ischemia; therefore, the entire clinical picture is variably called anoxic ischemia, hypoxic ischemia, or **hypoxic-ischemic encephalopathy** (**HIE**). These terms are sometimes used interchangeably; we use "anoxic episode" as a general term. Anoxic episodes and their immediate consequences account for the greatest percentage of neurological difficulties encountered during the perinatal period. They are responsible, for example, for many of the convulsive disorders that occur in the neonatal period (Rose 1977), particularly when the episode falls into the moderate-to-severe category (Hill and Volpe 1989a).

An anoxic episode involves more than simply a drop in the amount of available oxygen. A decrease in available oxygen leads first to natural defense mechanisms, e.g., increased cerebral blood flow and an increase in the brain's fractional extraction of oxygen. Other adaptive mechanisms include a decrease in energy-consuming processes and a biochemical switch from **aerobic energy generation** (occurring in oxygen) to less efficient **anaerobic energy generation** (in the absence of oxygen) (Richardson 1993), as well as a rapid depletion of the brain's very limited reserve of energy—ATP, **adenosine triphosphate. Asphyxia** (i.e., lack of breathing, the breakdown in respiratory gas exchange) results in the accumulation of biochemical waste products, such as carbon dioxide and lactic acid, which are generated anaerobically from spent energy supplies. These waste products are toxic and can contribute to the neurological problems created by the anoxic episode.

An anoxic episode can also lead to cardiac arrest and stagnation in the neonate's systemic blood circulation. Towbin (1970, 1971) examined the neuropathological consequences of anoxia and anoxia-induced hemorrhage. Based on autopsy studies, he proposed a three-stage process. First is the anoxic episode itself. This event results in systemic circulatory failure (stage two), which in turn causes local venous infarction (stage three). In the brain, systemic venous congestion increases venous pressure relative to the surrounding tissue. This surrounding tissue readily undergoes diffuse infarctional damage as the blood stagnates in the veins. Extravasation (i.e., leaking) of blood into surrounding tissue results in a serious perinatal complication: intracranial hemorrhage. However, the relationship between anoxia-induced venous stagnation and intraventricular hemorrhage has been examined and criticized by de Courten and Rabinowicz (1981a and b) and others, who argue that a more suitable explanation of the intraventricular hemorrhage is not the increased vascular pressure but rather decreased tissue pressure, as seen in dehydration.

The brain is the organ most vulnerable to damage during an anoxic episode because it has a large and constant metabolic demand for oxygen and because neurons do not regenerate after cell death. The brain is also vulnerable to anoxia-induced vascular stagnation because of the proportionally large amount of blood flowing through it at any given time.

The period around birth is the time of greatest risk for an anoxic episode. Yet, it has also proven to be the period during which the organism can best react successfully, within limits, to an anoxic episode. Since oxygen reduction is inherent in birth because of pressure upon the placenta during delivery and the cutting of the cord, this resiliency is protective of the species in an evolutionary sense.

The premature infant is at especially high risk for an anoxic episode because it is essentially unprepared for the birth process. The prematurely born infant is not ready to begin respiration and may require immediate intervention to avert asphyxiation. **Surfactant** is a complex surface-active substance in the lungs that is necessary for normal respiration (Notter and Shapiro 1981). Surfactant, which is predominantly composed of phospholipids, lowers the surface tension of lung tissue to allow respiration to occur. An adequate supply of surfactant has developed in the lungs by the time of a full-term birth, but is not available in sufficient quantities for the premature infant. This condition is known as the **respiratory distress syndrome** (RDS) or hyaline membrane disease. Until the 1980s, when treatments became available, RDS was the leading cause of death in infants born before the 37th gestational week (Dabiri 1979).

Immediate and sustained intervention is necessary for babies with RDS. However, even intervention in such cases is hazardous: **hyperoxia** (i.e., a state of too much oxygen) has toxic consequences and may result in chronic lung disease and blindness due to retrolental fibroplasia (Stern 1973, see also Chapter 25);

hypercarbia, too much carbon dioxide waste product, coexists with the over-abundance of oxygen and may also contribute to the observed toxic damage.

The long-term neurobehavioral sequelae in survivors of prenatal and perinatal anoxia have long been of interest in medical care. Beginning with Little in 1861, an anoxic episode during the time surrounding birth has been regarded as a primary determinant of both mental retardation and cerebral palsy. The development of laboratory techniques in the 1940s to measure blood gases and pH levels provided relatively improved forms of measurement. Clinical and physiological advances thus stimulated empirical research, particularly during and after the 1950s. Gottfried (1973) carefully reviewed the results of major research up to the early 1970s. Since then, several long-term, prospective follow-up investigations have been completed and are discussed later in this chapter.

17.1 Causes

When discussing anoxic episodes, it is useful to delineate three categories of causal factors according to time of occurrence: (1) gestational, (2) parturitional, and (3) neonatal. Hill and Volpe (1989b) reported the temporal occurrence of anoxic episodes resulting in neonatal encephalopathy as follows: gestational, 20 per cent; parturitional, 30 per cent; combined gestational and parturitional, 35 per cent; neonatal, 10 per cent; and other, 5 per cent.

The *gestational* causes can be described as either maternal or placental. Maternal cardiac arrest, for instance, commonly results in total oxygen deprivation in the fetus. Maternal infectious diseases, diabetes mellitus, pre-eclampsia, and toxemias can reduce the amount of oxygen available to the fetus. Severe anemia and bleeding in the mother are also factors for the occurrence of a fetal anoxic episode. Disorders in the structure or function of the placenta, such as an infarction of placental tissue, may not permit adequate levels of oxygen to cross it and reach the fetus (Naeye 1977). If the mother is suffering from malnourishment, the placenta may be underdeveloped and therefore may transport less than optimal amounts of oxygen to the fetus.

During *parturition*, abrupt fetal separation from the placenta, placental compression due to uterine hypertonicity, birth trauma, and placenta previa can reduce the availability of oxygen to the fetus. In **placenta previa,** for example, the fetus cannot be delivered normally because the placenta has shifted from its usual position to partially or completely block the fetus's exit from the uterus. Continuing compression of the fetus against the placenta may hinder the transport of oxygen and nutrients to the fetus. An additional parturitional cause of an anoxic episode is perinatal traumatic brain trauma. Localized brainstem damage is often seen and may cause anoxic damage by interfering with CNS control over respiration and other vital systemic functions.

Gestational- and parturitional-induced anoxic episodes often continue to have a negative influence on perinatal status after delivery and require immediate postnatal respiratory intervention. These newborns show clinical signs of oxygen deprivation (e.g., color change) and consistently low Apgar scores. However, the extent and severity of a prenatal anoxic episode are poorly measured by these signs, even when the condition continues beyond birth. Thus, an anoxic episode before birth is far more difficult to diagnose than a perinatal episode. The advent of new technologies in the 1980s, such as magnetic resonance imaging and ultrasonography, offered some potential as in vivo diagnostic modalities for anoxic episodes and any consequent focal and diffuse brain lesions; the radiological knowledge base continues to expand.

Neonatally, failure to begin respiration (i.e., **asphyxia neonatorum**) or subsequent apneic spells after the onset of breathing prevent environmental oxygen from reaching the neonate. Some of the factors that can interfere with normal respiratory activity are an incompetent or underdeveloped respiratory or circulatory system, perinatal brain trauma, traumatic injury to the lungs, and pneumonia.

17.2   Defining the Anoxic Episode

Several diagnostic difficulties confront any evaluation of the reported neurobehavioral consequences of anoxia because the validity of a single construct "anoxia" is untenable for any group analysis. Direct measures of anoxia, such as oxygen saturation and oxygen content in blood samples, normally vary so widely in early life as to be of little use in any long-term predictive sense (Graham et al. 1962). Even different perinatal measures of anoxia show less correlation among themselves than might be anticipated (Broman 1979). The definition of the anoxic episode ideally includes not only the amount of time that the neonate does not breathe but also measurements of blood pressure, oxygen saturation, red blood cell count, blood sugar levels, and fluid/electrolyte balance. The Apgar score at specific times during the first half-hour after birth is a common clinical measure.

For the full-term infant, careful neurological evaluation can aid in the determination of the severity of the resulting encephalopathy, more so than for the premature baby. Both Hill and Volpe (1989a) and Fenichel (1983) provided their own clinical descriptions of this range of severity. Levels of severity are described in Table 17-1. In a related study, Lipper and colleagues (1986) attempted to quantify as a "post-asphyxial score" results from the neurological examination of full-term infants during the first 24 hours of life, incorporating consciousness level, cranial nerve findings, sensory motor findings, reflexes, and the presence of increased intracranial pressure or seizures. Nevertheless, the neurological examination on the first days of life is of only limited prognostic value (Hill 1993). A review of the relation between asphyxia at birth and subsequent encephalopathy that also provides a useful discussion of definitional problems was published by Nelson and Leviton (1991).

The consequences of an anoxic episode vary widely depending upon cause and the duration of the deprivation. Age and developmental status at the time

Table 17-1 Severity of Encephalopathy in Anoxic Episodes: Presentation and Outcome

MILD

Presentation: Hyperalertness, uninhibited reflexes, and jitteriness, lasting less than 24 hours
Outcome: Not associated with neurological sequelae

MODERATE

Presentation: Lethargic, suppressed primitive reflexes, seizures
Outcome: 20 to 40 per cent develop neurological sequelae, especially if presentation exceeds 1 week

SEVERE

Presentation: Comatose, flaccid tone, suppressed brainstem functions, seizures, increased intracranial pressure
Outcome: "Major" neurological sequelae, e.g., seizure disorder, mental retardation, cerebral palsy

Source: Hill and Volpe 1989a.

of deprivation are important. Velocity of the reduction in oxygenation is another important factor. In addition, secondary complications arising from the episode are important when long-term outcome is examined. The child's prognosis, for example, may be especially poor if there is associated intraventricular hemorrhage or if neonatal seizures occur as a result of the anoxic episode. A good prognosis often is associated with the presence of only a mild encephalopathy (or none at all) during the neonatal period (Hill and Volpe 1989a).

17.3 Neuropathology

Infants who survive an anoxic episode with gross CNS damage show various neuropathological patterns. Common patterns are listed in Table 17-2 and are described below. In addition, focal or multifocal ischemic brain damage may occur.

The typical neurological consequence is **neuronal necrosis,** i.e., regions of cell death. This necrosis is more common in the full-term infant with an anoxic episode than in the prematurely born baby. Necrosis is selectively, but not ex-

Table 17-2 Typical Patterns of Neuropathology in Anoxic Episodes

Neuronal necrosis
Periventricular leukomalacia
Watershed necrotic infarction
Status marmoratus
Intraventricular/periventricular hemorrhage

clusively, located in cortical regions. Neurons in the CA1 region of the hippo-campus and cerebellar Purkinje cells are also especially vulnerable to an anoxic episode. Thalamic and brainstem necrosis has also been reported (Volpe 1981). With increasing severity of the insult, a more diffuse pattern of necrosis is observed. For the premature infant, diencephalic neuronal necrosis and a specific pattern of necrosis that involves the pontine nuclei and the hippocampal subic-ulum have been reported (Hill and Volpe 1989b).

Paradoxically, severely asphyxiated infants who die very soon after the episode do not show neuronal damage because the many cellular changes (e.g., loss of Nissl substance, nuclear pyknosis, hypertrophied astrocyte cells) begin to appear only 24 to 36 hours after the episode (Norman 1978).

In addition to these changes in the cell body, damage to the fibers that form CNS white matter also occurs as a consequence of the anoxic episode. **Periventricular leukomalacia,** for instance, is characterized by necrosis of white matter. It occurs primarily in the premature infant who has suffered an anoxic episode (Volpe 1981). Demyelination occurs principally in the regions adjacent to the anterior and the temporo-occipital horns of the lateral ventricles and in the corona radiata. A propensity to involve the region of opticothalamic radiation has been reported, as has occasional cortical blindness (Dubowitz et al. 1985). This is a coagulation necrosis characterized by a loss of distinctiveness in cellular architecture and a homogenization of cellular components (Hill 1993). The lesions appear as many small areas of coagulated, homogenized tissue surrounded by liquefied areas. Necrosis is usually bilateral but not necessarily symmetrical. If the episode was a severe one, the leukomalacia may be complicated by a hemorrhagic inflow into the necrotic tissue (Hill et al. 1982).

Although this pathological condition was originally described in the mid-nineteenth century (Virchow 1867), Banker and Larroche (1962) provided the first detailed autopsy descriptions of periventricular leukomalacia, which they found in 20 per cent of their sample of severely oxygen-deprived babies. A decade later, Armstrong and Norman (1974) reported only one-third that inci-dence. They attributed the difference to improvements in neonatal intensive care. In the 1980s, neuroradiological refinements allowed Dubowitz and col-leagues (1985) to determine the developmental patterns of periventricular leu-komalacia, which have since been replicated by Keeney and colleagues (1991). This neuropathological pattern of anoxic episodes has been clearly identified by MRI (Keeney et al. 1991). Lesions that are initially hemorrhagic become cystic and then atrophic, all clearly discerned by MRI.

Another common pattern of anoxic neuropathology is the **watershed ne-crotic infarction,** also referred to as parasagittal cerebral injury (Volpe 1981). These infarcts occur in "**watershed areas**" of the cerebral cortex and subcor-tical white matter, i.e., the boundary zones at the periphery of the outlying branches of the major cerebral arteries. Because of their intermediate locations relative to the major arteries, watershed zones are most vulnerable to necrotic damage when there is a drop in arterial blood pressure and a loss of oxygenated blood. The lesions are bilateral and often symmetrical. There is a suggestion in the literature that the posterior watershed regions are more commonly affected than the anterior regions.

Status marmoratus is a relatively rare lesion of the basal ganglia that can be observed in some full-term babies who have suffered an anoxic episode (Volpe 1976). The major neuropathological features are neuronal loss, astrocytic gliosis, and increased myelination of astrocytes in the basal ganglia. Excessive myelination results in the marbled appearance at autopsy that gave rise to the name. Commonly the thalamus is also affected, to the degree that it is now common to group the two sites together when referring to status marmoratus (Hill and Volpe 1989b).

Intraventricular hemorrhage (i.e., bleeding into the ventricles) with **periventricular parenchymal hemorrhage**—bleeding into the brain tissue surrounding the ventricles—is a relatively common consequence of anoxic episodes in premature infants (Volpe 1989).

Towbin's (1969a, 1970) autopsy findings on 600 brains from both premature and full-term infants revealed an important change in the locus of CNS damage depending on the infant's age when the anoxic episode occurred. Premature infants, particularly those between 22 and 35 weeks of gestational age, suffered cerebral infarction damage in periventricular areas, which contain the residue of the germinal matrix. This residual matrix is structurally weak tissue from which, earlier in development, brain cells began the migration to their permanent positions. The leaking of stagnated venous blood from this region into the lateral ventricles typically results in an intraventricular hemorrhage. Full-term infants, on the other hand, suffered diffuse cerebral cortical damage rather than periventricular damage because, by the time of term, the germinal matrix tissue has disintegrated and become insignificant. If hemorrhage occurred in full-term infants, extravasation of blood was observed from the superficial, convex venous drainage system that spans the cerebral cortex.

17.4   Neurobehavioral Consequences

The possible consequences of an anoxic episode range from immediate death or overwhelming neuropathology through various neurological consequences to the absence of any mental and neurological sequelae. The more severe the episode, the greater the probability of death. For example, 22.8 per cent of infants in the Collaborative Perinatal Study who suffered intrauterine anoxia died during the perinatal period (Niswander et al. 1975). The percentage of neonatal deaths was higher (52 per cent) in infants who suffered very severe oxygen deprivation at birth, i.e., a delay of spontaneous respiration for at least 20 minutes and/or apparent stillbirth (Scott 1976).

Three neurological sequelae are accepted as primary consequences in survivors of anoxic episodes: (1) the motor features of cerebral palsy, (2) mental retardation, and (3) seizures (Hill and Volpe 1989b). Mental retardation is of particular concern in children when significant necrosis has occurred in the cerebral hemispheres. Seizures are described in Chapter 20.

Given the diagnostic complexities and clinical variability of anoxic episodes, however, it is difficult to generalize in any clinically useful manner about long-term consequences. This is particularly true when one broadens mental consequences beyond retardation and includes the specific deficits of known neuropsychological syndromes. There also has been speculation in the literature about the presence of "subclinical lesions" causing cognitive deficits as a result of perinatal anoxic episodes (Fuller et al. 1983, Murdoch et al. 1991, Towbin 1971). Freeman and Nelson (1988) provided a critique of these speculations and suggested that this issue has been overstated.

Infants who suffer an anoxic episode in early life are at greater risk for later mental retardation (Gottfried 1973). Yet, risk is not synonymous with occurrence: mental retardation is not an inevitable consequence of an early-life anoxic episode. However, the factors that influence the probability of occurrence are not well understood. Data from the Perinatal Study indicate that mental retardation among children who had consistently low Apgar scores at birth is associated with cerebral palsy (Nelson and Ellenberg 1981, see Chapter 24). Overt CNS damage accompanying an anoxic episode in early life increases the risk of mental retardation in later infancy and childhood (Broman 1979). Fifteen per cent of the follow-up sample examined by Mulligan and colleagues (1980) were intellectually impaired, although the median IQ score of 108 on the Stanford-Binet intelligence test for the entire sample was clearly in the average range. All but one of the intellectually impaired children had associated neurological impairments. An 18-month follow-up of 62 full-term newborns treated for postasphyxial encephalopathy by Fitzhardinge and colleagues (1981) found that major intellectual impairments were present in 47 per cent, as reflected by Bayley DQ scores below 70. An additional 8 per cent had developmental quotients between 70 and 85. Hydrocephalus and spastic hemiplegia, quadriplegia, or diplegia were present in most of these cases with intellectual impairment. The authors noted that the CT scans taken during the first 2 weeks of life and at 6 months were highly predictive of outcome and served to identify the neurological damage in these children.

Despite these high rates of death and frank neuropathology, many infants do survive an anoxic episode with little, if any, major neurological sequelae. These infants have been the subject of many investigations to determine what, if any, selective learning or cognitive deficits they suffered. Gottfried's (1973) conclusions after reviewing the literature were that little specific information could be gleaned from the literature but that, when present, cognitive deficits after an anoxic episode are more prevalent in infants and preschoolers than in older children and adolescents.

There have been three large-scale longitudinal studies on learning and cognitive deficits suffered by survivors of anoxic episodes: the St. Louis prospective study conducted in the 1950s and 1960s by Graham, Corah, and their colleagues (Corah et al. 1965, Graham et al. 1962); the Collaborative Perinatal Study of the 1970s (Broman 1979); and the Canadian prospective study of Robertson and Finer (1985, Robertson et al. 1989). Several smaller prospective studies have also been reported (e.g., Aylward et al. 1989).

In the St. Louis study, children who had suffered prenatal or postnatal anoxic episodes were assessed at 3 and 7 years of age, along with a group of normal children matched for age, sex, race, and SES. The follow-up data included information concerning intellectual, neurological, anthropometric, conceptual, perceptual-motor, and personality status.

At 3 years of age, the anoxic group performed significantly more poorly than the control group on all tests of cognitive functioning. These included the Stanford-Binet intelligence test and tests of concept formation and vocabulary. Conceptual skills were found to be more impaired than was vocabulary. No impairment on perceptual-motor functioning was observed. The anoxic group contained more children with either positive or suggestive neurological findings at follow-up than the non-anoxic group. The cognitive impairment was more severe in children who had a postnatal anoxic episode than in children with a prenatal episode. However, Naeye and Peters (1987) did demonstrate a relationship between prenatal anoxia and poor IQ scores.

At 7 years of age, intelligence test differences between anoxic and control groups had dissipated to such a degree that the two groups were no longer significantly different in their performance. Only one WISC subtest differed significantly between the two groups: Vocabulary. In contrast to the third-year findings, the anoxic group performed more poorly on tests of perceptual-motor functioning and perceptual attention than did the controls.

The Collaborative Perinatal Study findings indicated that an anoxic episode was a very weak predictor of later-life cognitive status. However, the anoxic group did show lower performances on cognitive tasks than did the non-anoxic controls at three ages: 8 months, 4 years, and 7 years. The differences between the groups were not very large and were more pronounced at 8 months than at 7 years.

Children in the Robertson and Finer study were born between 1974 and 1979 and then examined 3.5 years and 8 years later. The study attempted to rate the severity of the initial encephalopathy as mild, moderate, or severe. As one would expect, outcomes were clearly associated with initial severity. Children with severe encephalopathies had either died at the time of follow-up or had suffered severe handicaps. Moderate encephalopathies resulted, at 8 year follow-up, in death in 6 per cent, handicaps in 20 per cent, and reading disabilities in 35 per cent. Children with mild encephalopathies were free of handicapping conditions (e.g., cerebral palsy). These children showed intellectual performances, performances on a test of visuomotor copying (i.e., the Beery test), and mean length of expressive linguistic utterances all within normal ranges.

Aylward et al. (1989) studied a large number of maternal/prenatal medical-biological, perinatal, and asphyxia-related variables in relation to socioeconomic and behavioral-developmental ("optimality" rating) measures in a follow-up of

608 newborns at the age of 36 months. Although all variables contributed mi...ly to the outcome measures at 36 months, the socioeconomic and behavioral-developmental variables showed the highest predictive value. Campbell et al. (1989) also stressed that mother-infant interaction at the time of discharge from the hospital was a strong indicator of developmental outcome at the age of 2 years, suggesting that such interaction may be indicative of the severity of the handicap of the newborn.

Visual and auditory disorders resulting from brainstem damage are common, especially when severe neuro-developmental handicaps are also present (Groenendaal et al. 1989, Zhang and Jiang 1992).

Unfortunately, these studies have generally stopped soon after the children enter school, so that they provide no information on the development of academic and learning problems. The Canadians did examine their sample through the age of 8 years, however.

To summarize the neurobehavioral consequences, a perinatal anoxic episode alone is a very weak predictor of later childhood disability in surviving children. The data of the Perinatal Study suggest that the episode per se accounts for only a small percentage of the observed variability in later intellectual and cognitive test performance. For example, an 8-year-old boy who suffered 5 to 15 minutes of anoxia and a coma of 15 hours after nearly drowning fully recovered and demonstrated very superior intelligence (Johnstone and Bouman 1992). The St. Louis and other studies suggest that, although statistical differences between groups may be observed, inferences about prognosis in individual children are highly tenuous. Clinical neurological beliefs about the relation between outcome and severity of the initial encephalopathy (expressed most notably by Volpe and colleagues) are in accord both with quantitative scores as proposed by Lipper and colleagues (1986) and with objective neurobehavioral data, as reported by Robertson and Finer, for instance.

Summary

An examination of early-life anoxic episodes and their consequences in later life cuts across many of the topics that have been discussed in this part of the book. The occurrence of an anoxic episode is intricately related to prematurity and the risks inherent to being born unprepared for the demands of independent functioning. Advances in hospital care tend to keep smaller and smaller babies alive and have a direct impact on the course of the anoxic episode and its consequences. Anoxic episodes are also associated with perinatal brain damage, convulsive disorders, and secondary hemorrhage. The frailty of nutritional balance in the prematurely born child with respiratory distress presents additional neuronal risks.

Although oxygen deprivation, to some degree, is part of the normal course of perinatal life, a clinically diagnosable anoxic episode places the infant at risk for a wide variety of deficits.

Neuropsychological attention to children with a history of perinatal anoxic episodes is directed initially at determining the presence and severity of mental retardation and then the nature and severity of any features of cerebral palsy if present. If there is an accompanying seizure disorder, deficits specific to it (and its medications) need to be considered. Children with documented mild perinatal episodes or presumed episodes require very careful attention to the medical record (e.g., Apgar scores) and a careful examination of the major cognitive domains, e.g., visual perception, language acquisition.

The imprecision in diagnosing anoxic episodes would suggest that at least some of the population of children who are developmentally disabled in later life may have experienced undiagnosed anoxia in early life. Adopting the concept of a continuum of reproductive casualty, some authors have hypothesized the existence of subclinical anoxic neuropathology that results in later-life neuropsychological difficulties, such as learning or language disabilities and minimal brain damage, a debatable, if not overstated issue.

An anoxic episode is a very weak predictor of later childhood disability. Findings from the Collaborative Perinatal Study indicate that the episode per se accounts for only a very small percentage of the variability of later intellectual and cognitive test performance. Inferences about the prognosis of individual children are highly tenuous. However, this weak predictive value is not unexpected given the wide range in causation, severity, complications, and possible outcomes.

18

Traumatic Brain Injury

Traumatic brain injury (TBI) is the primary cause of death in childhood and adolescence, accounting for half of all deaths during those periods (Fenichel 1988). The emphasis in this chapter is on perinatal trauma and traumatic injuries during the first 2 years of life.

Advances in obstetrical care and technology have resulted in steady reductions in the incidence of perinatal brain trauma at birth. Our understanding of the complexity of the neonatal period has also increased. Because of these advances, severe forms of perinatal mechanical trauma are rarer now. In addition, many neonates who do sustain injuries are now immediately subjected to rigorous intensive care that previously was unavailable. Care for the newborn has also become more sophisticated because of advances in diagnostic sophistication. Diagnostic imaging of the neonatal brain, such as by CT scan, has become invaluable in the early diagnosis of intracranial hemorrhage, permitting immediate intervention for a specific diagnosis that in earlier times might have been made only at autopsy.

After birth, epidemiological studies, such as that done at the Mayo Clinic (Annegers et al. 1980), have delineated three age periods during the life-span when there is a distinctly higher incidence of specific head injuries. Although young adults are at the greatest risk for trauma (usually as a result of motor vehicle accidents), the very young and the elderly have the greatest risk for head injury from falls (Figure 18-1).

Traumatic head injuries during early childhood often occur when exploring toddlers fall. They may fall from furniture, down a flight of stairs, or out of a window. As unrestrained passengers in quickly stopping or colliding automobiles, children may be thrown up against the dashboard or windshield. Older children may fall from bicycles or become involved in sporting mishaps. Head trauma also is a common result of child abuse.

The degree to which the brain itself is damaged by a head injury depends to some extent on certain pathological and secondary complications, to be dis-

279

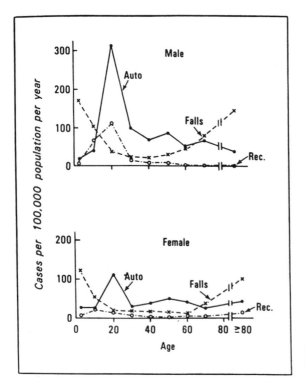

Figure 18-1. Risk of head injury by age (Annegers et al. 1980).

cussed briefly below. The degree of brain trauma in survivors is reflected along a continuum of severity, including no injury, mild head injury, moderate head injury, and severe head injury (Table 18-1). Increasing knowledge in the area has led to an attempt to broaden the mild range of damage to include both modest (trivial) and mild brain injury and to broaden the severe range to include both severe and profound (very severe) brain injury. However, terminology and defining criteria in the field lack uniformity.

By far the most common postnatal head injuries are mild ones, accounting for 89 per cent of all cases among children (i.e., under the age of 19 years) admitted to hospital or dead at the scene in the San Diego County epidemiological study (Kraus et al. 1987). In this study, 76 per cent of the injuries in infants younger than 1 year of age were mild injuries; this percentage increased during the first decade of life. As would be expected, outcome is clearly related to initial severity. In the San Diego County study, the overall in-hospital fatality rate was 3 per cent, but for children with severe head injuries, the rate jumped to 59 per cent, with half dying during the first 24 hours after admission (Kraus et al. 1987). Data from the multicenter Traumatic Coma Data Bank indicated that the mortality rate for severely head-injured children aged 0 to 4 years was 62 per cent with only 12 per cent showing "good recovery" (Levin et al. 1992).

The same data indicated that older children (aged 5 to 10 years) have a 1-year mortality rate of 20 per cent and a "good recovery" rate of roughly 65 per cent.

18.1.   Pathology and Secondary Complications

The characteristics of head injuries vary. Whether the trauma results in a closed or penetrating (or open) head injury is one basic distinction. **Closed head injuries** are the most common form and may result from falls, motor-vehicle accidents, or other physical impacts. Injuries during the birth process form a special group of closed head injuries. Adult **open head injuries** typically result from penetrating projectiles (e.g., bullets), but in children they are more commonly due to self-injury or playmate-caused injury when children play with sharp objects and toys.

Head injury may result in damage to the skull, brain tissue, and cerebrovascular system. Skull fractures, cortical contusions, and diffuse axonal injuries (DAI) may occur. Damage to intracranial blood vessels can result in subdural or epidural hemorrhages (which then can exert secondary mass effects upon brain tissue) or intracerebral hemorrhage. Edema and increased intracranial pressure may be acute complications, although "diffuse cerebral swelling" has been observed more frequently in children than in adults (Shapiro and Smith 1993).

Age differences in the physical dynamics of head trauma have been described. For example, the infant brain is less prone to traumatic cortical contusions and lacerations than is the child's or adult's brain; this difference is attributable to the relative immaturity of the skull and its smoother inward-facing surfaces. The skull is also thinner and, because of unfused suture lines, is more pliable in infants; therefore, it is more easily fractured and deformed (Shapiro and Smith 1993).

Table 18-1   Classification of Head Trauma

MILD HEAD INJURY
Glasgow Coma Scale higher than 12; Abbreviated Injury Scale score of 1 (concussion, but awake on initial observation); no neurosurgical intervention.
MODERATE HEAD INJURY
Glasgow Coma Scale score of 9 to 12, who were hospitalized for at least 48 hours who also had neurosurgical intervention or an abnormal CT head scan; Abbreviated Injury Scale score of 2 (concussion with minimal loss of consciousness).
SEVERE HEAD INJURY
Glasgow Coma Scale score of 8 or lower; Abbreviated Injury Scale score of 3 and above: 3 (cerebral contusion), 4 (subdural hematoma), 5 (diffuse cerebral injury), and 6 (unsurvivable). Levin et al. (1992): Lowest post-resuscitation Glasgow Coma Scale score of 8 or lower.

Source: Kraus et al. 1987.

In addition to the physical characteristics of the skull, other age-related differences may alter the effects of head injury in infants and younger children. Strich (1969) believed that the shearing strains that result in diffuse axonal injury may be less pronounced in small brains; others have raised the issue whether the partially myelinated brain may be less prone to mechanical distortion. The epidemiological differences in the causes of head trauma (Table 18-2) suggest that head-injured infants and young children, as a group, may be less often subjected to the severe rotational forces that more commonly result in DAI-inducing shearing injuries, since these forces are more common and potent in motor vehicle accidents than in the more common pediatric low-velocity falling accidents. There are also age-related differences in the recovery process, as discussed in the first section of this book.

The nature of the neurological damage and the occurrence of secondary complications help determine the need for acute medical and rehabilitative care, as well as the long-term neuropsychological consequences of traumatic brain injury. Table 18-3 lists several important neurological features of acute head injury. The physiological response to and recovery from the injury can be divided into acute, post-acute, and long-term stages, although these stages may be referred to by different names. The nature of these stages may change depending upon an individual's age, and there are no hard-and-fast rules for temporally defining them. Roughly, the **acute stage of recovery** can be thought of as the time period from the injury through the first few months after the injury. The acute period might also be considered to correspond more closely to the period of medical instability only and, if present, to coma (or less severely reduced consciousness) and subsequent post-traumatic amnesia (PTA). Resolution of edema and the physiological mechanisms of recovery are other important factors during the acute stage. The **post-acute stage of recovery** roughly corresponds to the period from 3 to 6 months to about 1 year after the injury. However, the post-acute stage can alternatively be considered to begin once PTA has cleared. Finally, the long-term stage begins about 1 year after the injury. It is during this final stage that the presence of residual (i.e., permanent) deficits can be determined. The **long-term stage of recovery** alternatively may be considered to begin once the patient is felt to be ready to re-enter the community, the home, or the classroom. Staging is not generally relevant for mild injuries.

18.2 Perinatal Traumatic Damage

Birth poses unique traumatic risks. There is increased risk of CNS injury due to purely mechanical causes, such as stretching, compression, shearing, and twisting. These physical forces arise from the passage of the fetus through the birth canal during the stages of labor and the final extraction of the neonate from the mother.

Figure 18-2 depicts the normal traverse and the requisite twists and turns of the fetus's head and body during labor. The complex events that comprise a

Table 18-2 Brain Trauma in the First Year of Life Compared to All Ages (0–19 years) by Cause and Percentage of Moderate-to-Fatal Injuries in the San Diego County Study

Age Group	Cause, % [Moderate-to-Fatal Injury, %]				
	Falls	Motor vehicle	Assault	Sports	Other
<1 year	69	7	17	2	6
	[8]	[50]	[56]	[100]	[67]
1–19 years	24	37	10	21	8
	[7]	[29]	[34]	[6]	[20]

Source: Adapted from Kraus et al. 1987.

normal vaginal delivery are associated with cranial molding and stretching, as well as with rapid changes in the pressure impinging upon the fetus's head. The fetus's progress through the birth canal is difficult enough during a normal, uneventful delivery. However, it can easily become more difficult because of a wide variety of complicating factors, such as, an inelastic birth canal that is physiologically not prepared for delivery of a premature infant, a large baby relative to a small birth canal, or fetal orientations during delivery that are not in the normal vertex position, i.e., head first exiting the birth canal. The use of forceps (Figure 18-3) to extract the neonate during the final stage of delivery may sometimes fracture the skull and damage underlying brain tissue.

A common cause of complications during delivery is the malpositioning of either the placenta (e.g., placenta previa, as described in Chapter 17) or the fetus. The breech presentation (i.e., buttocks first, head last) occurs commonly and has been associated with increased mortality rates relative to non-breech births (National Institutes of Health 1981).

The fetus can assume a variety of presenting positions immediately before labor begins. The normal presentation is the **vertex position,** in which the cranium is the first part of the baby's body out of the birth canal. **Face presentations** twist the head away from the normal body axis. In the **breech presentation** (Figure 18-4), the head is the last part of the baby's body to be removed from the mother, subjecting it to potentially more severe mechanical stresses for a longer period of time. A **cesarean section** may be necessary when

Table 18-3 Acute Neurological Features of Traumatic Brain Injury

Presence of coma
Coma severity (Glasgow Coma Scale)
Coma duration
Presence and location of focal lesions, e.g., contusions
Presence of diffuse lesions
Secondary neurosurgical complications, e.g., hematomas
When coma resolves, length of post-traumatic amnesia (PTA)

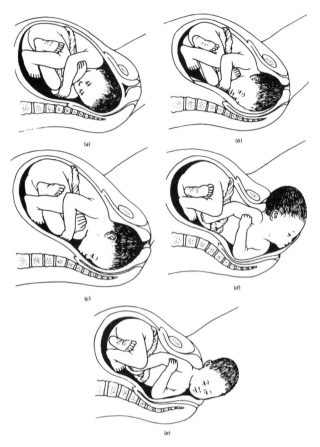

Figure 18-2. Mechanisms of normal labor: (a) engagement, descent flexion, (b) internal rotation, (c) beginning extension, (d) completed extension, (e) external rotation (restitution), (f) external rotation, (g) expulsion (Ross Clinical Education Aid #13, Ross Laboratories, Columbus, Ohio).

fetal or placental malpositioning prevents a normal vaginal delivery: the fetus is surgically removed by incising through the uterus to prevent serious injury to the neonate, as well as to the mother, that might ensue during a complicated vaginal delivery.

Perinatal mechanical brain injury may result in two neurological conditions: intracranial hemorrhage and CNS tissue damage. Intracranial hemorrhage is the most common manifestation of perinatal CNS trauma and may, itself, cause further CNS tissue damage because increased intracranial pressure may displace brain tissue against the skull. Hemorrhage is discussed more fully in Chapter 19. Tissue damage may occur, however, in the absence of any hemorrhagic conditions. Both may coexist in a wider complex of problems, including anoxic episodes and neonatal seizures.

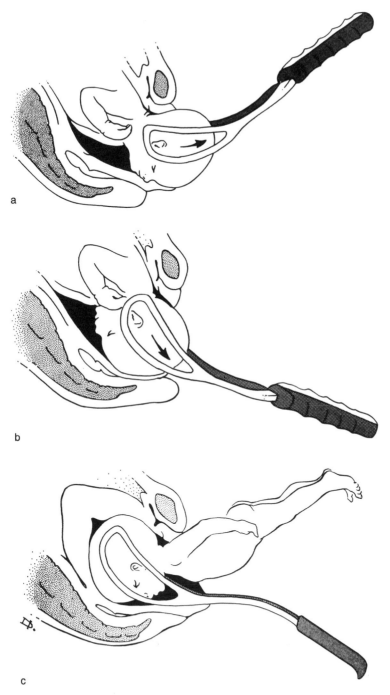

Figure 18-3. Forceps application: (a) in normal position, (b) in normal position showing change in force and direction, (c) with aftercoming head (Oxorn 1980).

285

18.3   Acute Deficits in Postnatal Traumatic Damage

Acutely after the injury, children may lose consciousness (**coma**) and remain comatose or, if not comatose, may show signs of residual confusion and disorientation, amnesia, and lethargy. The depth of the coma and the length of time that an individual remains comatose are vital items of information about the underlying severity of brain damage. Coma severity is measured clinically by the **Glasgow Coma Scale** (GCS, Teasdale and Jennett 1974, Table 18-4). It employs bedside clinical measurement of eye movement, motor activity, and verbalization to quantify coma severity. A severe or deep coma is generally denoted by GCS scores of 8 or less. Lesser reductions in consciousness are denoted by GCS scores above 8. Mild head injuries are generally denoted on the GCS by scores of 13 or higher. Because of its verbal component, others have developed several pediatric variants (e.g., Yager et al. 1990) or have modified the GCS levels themselves, e.g., substituting smiling and following objects for the verbal orientation level, (Levin et al. 1992).

Ultimate favorable recovery is less probable for patients with prolonged coma, many of whom will die or progress to a **persistent vegetative state** (i.e., a reduction in consciousness, but with sleep-wake cycling and eye opening) or show severe and disabling residual deficits. Recovery without permanent neuropsychological deficits is more probable for individuals with a coma duration of less than 24 hours (particularly those with a duration of less than 6 hours), unless there has been severe focal trauma (Shapiro 1985, Shapiro and Smith 1993). For confused individuals, the amount of time elapsed until information is remembered on a day-to-day basis (**post-traumatic amnesia, PTA**) is a vital indicator of outcome. Longer periods of PTA may correspond to greater probabilities of residual deficits. Table 18-5 shows data from the San Diego County study indicating outcome as a function of severity of the initial injury. Children with injuries of both mild and moderate severity fared well relative to those with severe injuries; mild and moderate injuries could be distinguished by whether neurological sequelae (defined in that study by such deficits as hemiparesis and aphasic features) persisted.

18.4   Long-Term and Residual Neuropsychological Sequelae in Postnatal Traumatic Damage

The long-term neuropsychological consequences of infant head injury are usually investigated within more general studies of childhood head injury. Despite the practical importance of understanding the consequences of head injuries in the first 2 years of life, studies of these consequences have been rare. Usually, examinations of early-life head injuries are limited to perinatal injuries, as discussed earlier. Otherwise, children with brain damage during this early period of life are included in wider examinations of head injury spanning the

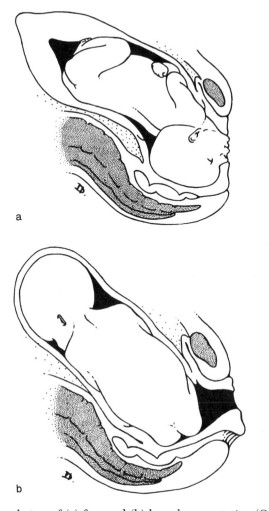

Figure 18-4.   Lateral view of (a) face and (b) breech presentation (Oxorn 1980).

entire period of childhood and early adolescence and usually without systematic attention to the age factor, both at time of injury and time of testing. In
some cases, the "pediatric sample" is actually broad enough to include individuals up to the age of 19 years. A review of the literature on the full age
range is beyond the scope of this chapter (c.f., Shapiro 1985, Ylvisaker 1986).
A major review of head injury in children was published by Parker (1990). A
detailed discussion of behavior therapy with brain-injured children is provided
by Horton (1993).

Several research collaborations have generated basic information on head injury in children. The efforts of the Levin group in Galveston, Texas, are an

Table 18-4 Glasgow Coma Scale

Response	Coma score[a]
EYE OPENING (E)	
Spontaneous	4
To speech (to any verbal approach)	3
To pain	2
Nil	1
BEST MOTOR RESPONSE (M)	
Obeys commands	6
Localizing response	5
Withdrawal response	4
Abnormal flexion	3
Extensor posturing	2
Nil	1
VERBAL RESPONSE (V)	
Oriented (aware of self, environment, and some temporal awareness)	5
Confused conversation	4
Inappropriate speech (no sustained communication)	3
Incomprehensible sounds, e.g., moaning, groaning	2
Nil	1

Source: Derived from Jennett and Teasdale (1974).
[a]Glasgow Coma Scale score = E + M + V = 3-to-15.

Table 18-5 Severity of Brain Injury and Outcome of Pediatric Population Hospitalized in the San Diego County Study (Ages 0–19 years)

Outcome[a]	Severity (%)		
	Mild (n = 1001)	Moderate (n = 95)	Severe (n = 70)
Good recovery	100.0	91.5	18.6
Moderate disability	0.0	8.4	11.6
Severe disability	0.0	0.0	21.4
Persistent vegetative state	0.0	0.0	7.1
Death	0.0	0.0	41.4
Percentage with neurological sequelae	3.0	94.0	100.0

Source: Adapted from Kraus et al. 1987.
[a]Outcome as measured by the Glasgow Outcome Scale.

288

exemplar of contemporary neuropsychological research in this area (Levin and Benton 1986, Levin and Eisenberg 1979, 1983, Levin and Grossman 1976, Levin et al. 1982, 1987, 1992).

Understanding the long-term impact of head injury on cognitive and behavioral functioning requires an assessment of what an individual's level of functioning was before the injury (i.e., premorbid functioning), as well as the general developmental level at the age at which the injury occurred. The first is unique to the individual, such as obtained school grades, whereas the second reflects normative standards. It is vital to determine whether a child's premorbid functioning was within normal parameters or was abnormal in some domain(s). To cite an example, Fletcher and colleagues (1990, Levin et al. 1992) reported that behavioral problems after mild head injury in children are similar to those seen in mildly injured adults in that they seem to reflect premorbid personality characteristics more than any acquired, organic changes. These points were also raised by Goldstein and Levin (1985) in their review of intellectual and academic outcome of pediatric brain trauma.

Also critical is information about the nature and severity of the injury itself. Levin (1983) reported, for instance, that diffuse brain insults in children are more problematic than focal brain lesions. Although children may completely recover from focal lesions, diffuse lesions may have devastating long-term effects. Studies of head injuries sustained during infancy and the preschool period point to the importance of continued neurological well-being in early life for the proper development of cognitive functioning.

We briefly discuss outcome studies in the following domains: intellectual functioning, memory, language, visuoperception, sensorimotor functioning, academic performance, and behavioral/personality changes.

General Intellectual Sequelae

A post-traumatic generalized impairment in intellectual functioning typically is a result of an injury that is severe and diffuse and/or multifocal in nature. It is usually observed after prolonged periods of coma and post-traumatic amnesia. Studies of intellectual performance after brain injury do suggest a range of deficits from the most severe (i.e., in essence, a handicapping acquired mental impairment) through less severe general impairments, specific cognitive impairments, to a return to expected (or known) levels of premorbid functioning.

An association between measured global IQ scores and the severity of brain trauma is generally accepted (Goldstein and Levin 1985). Levin and Eisenberg (1979) reported that, when examined at least 6 months post-injury, IQ scores below 85 were most common in children who had been comatose for at least 24 hours. Brink and colleagues (1970) also found a relationship between length of coma after severe head injury (i.e., coma exceeding 1 week) and IQ scores at follow-up. Measured IQs were borderline and below in 67 per cent of their sample. Children in the younger age group (ages 2 to 8 years) in the Brink study showed more severe deficits in intelligence test scores even though the length of coma was relatively shorter than in the older age group (ages 9 to 18 years). Progressive improvement in performance on IQ tests has been noted up to 5 years post-injury in children with mild or moderate head injuries.

In addition to overall performance, differences in the level of performance on the Verbal and Performance portions of the Wechsler test are known to exist. When a significant difference is observed in the absence of focal pathology, it usually reflects a poorer performance on the Performance portion of the test. This likely is due to the psychomotor loading on the Performance portion, a dimension that is typically impaired after brain trauma. In a 5-year follow-up study, Black and colleagues (1981) found that IQ test measures in these children improved slightly each year, but that the results only "approached significance." Chadwick and colleagues (1981) found that the pattern of greater Performance than Verbal IQ scores remained present at 1-year and 2½-year follow-up examinations. In contrast, Nass et al. (1989) found in a study of 28 prepubertal children statistically superior Verbal and Full-scale IQs in the left-lesioned group. They interpreted this result as an indication of the primacy of language functions in the recovery process in children with early injury.

Memory

Levin and Eisenberg (1979) have identified memory problems as being the most common impairment noted after pediatric brain trauma. They reported that verbal memory, gauged by a selective reminding test, was especially sensitive to closed head injuries in children that primarily affected the left hemisphere. When damage was restricted to the child's right hemisphere, only nonverbal tasks were performed poorly. Later performance on a measure of visual recognition memory by head-injured adolescents varied with initial injury severity (as measured by the GCS and duration of impaired consciousness) but not with lesion location or type (Hannay and Levin 1988).

Executive Functions

A study by Levin et al. (1994) examined 134 6- to 16-year-old children with pediatric closed head injury, as documented by MRI scans with a typical "executive function" test, the Tower of London reasoning test. Severity of the head injury and performance on the test were strongly related. MRI-documented volume of frontal (but not extra-frontal) lesion contributed to the prediction of performance on this task, even after severity of head injury had been taken into account.

Attention

On a vigilance task (Gordon Diagnostic System), 38 5- to 16-year-old children with traumatic brain injury had an increased number of commission errors; the authors (Timmermans and Christensen 1991) noted that vigilance task measurements correlated strongly with several hyperactivity rating scales. More frequent commission (false-positive) errors in children than in adolescents have also been reported by Levin et al. (1982). Papanicolaou et al. (1990) recorded visual and auditory ERPs in 15 children with unilateral left hemisphere lesions and found left hemisphere attenuation of the potentials during phonological detection tasks and right hemisphere attenuation during visuospatial rotation tasks. They concluded that language continued to be mediated by the right hemisphere and that visuospatial functions were not affected by the left hemisphere lesion. A study of ERPs in newborns, however, showed that abnormalities were not a reliable prognostic indicator of neurodevelopmental outcome at the age of 18 months (Beverly et al. 1990).

A related, but rarely investigated behavioral problem is fatigue after head injury. Allison (1993) found long-lasting fatigue effects that were unrelated to the length of PTA or the length of time post-injury after both minor and severe head injury.

Language

Although classical aphasia syndromes are infrequent in children, language pathology is observed quite commonly in pediatric head trauma. Infants with perinatal focal injuries are usually delayed in babbling and first-word acquisition, as well as in language comprehension (Marchman et al. 1991) and gestural communication (Landry et al. 1989). During their development up to the age of 3 years, lexical production and comprehension were delayed, and children with right hemisphere lesions produced an atypically high proportion of closed class words, suggesting a heavy reliance on well-practiced, but under analyzed speech formulas (Thal et al. 1991). Left-sided ventricular dilation was especially related to poor early language abilities (Bendersky and Lewis 1990). However, Feldman et al. (1992) found more than half of such children were able to catch up in their language development compared to non-injured peers by the age of 2 years. Comparing two twin pairs, one of whom suffered perinatal left hemisphere injury, over a 2-year period, Feldman et al. (1989) reported scores comparable to those of the uninjured twins on most neurodevelopmental measures except expressive picture vocabulary and the expressive scale of a sequenced inventory of communication development.

Object naming difficulties are a particularly common residual deficit; neologisms, literal paraphasias, and verbal paraphasias are common (Dennis 1992, van Dongen and Visch-Brink 1988). Deficits are commonly observed when the broader functional concepts of communication are employed because subtle, non-aphasic language deficits may persist (Goethe and Levin 1986). These deficits are seen, for example, in analyses of narrative discourse and the structure of information supplied in discourse (Chapman et al. 1992).

Woods and Teuber (1973, Teuber and Rudel 1967) examined children whose head injuries occurred from infancy through the preschool years (as manifested by the presence of a unilateral hemiplegia). They gave these children a set of cognitive tests in late childhood and early adolescence to determine the differential patterns of cognitive deficits that arise when the damage is located predominantly in either the right or left hemisphere. They also examined the related issue of developmental plasticity of both hemispheres. The results indicated that, when the brain injury was located in the left hemisphere, children showed subsequent deficits in tests of both verbal and nonverbal skills relative to neurologically normal children. In contrast to what is often observed in adult left hemisphere injury, however, classical aphasias were not common. Eide and Tysnes (1992) found cognitive and speech deficits primarily after focal contusions in the left temporal lobe. With right hemisphere injury, **aprosodia,** i.e., flat intonation during spontaneous speech and affective-prosodic repetition, has been reported (Bell et al. 1990). Since affective comprehension was fully intact in these children, the authors viewed the aprosodia as a motoric disorder.

Visuoperceptual Skills

In 3- to 5-year old children with focal congenital right or left hemisphere injuries, Stiles and Nass (1991) found that spontaneous grouping of blocks was delayed in both groups, but that the left hemisphere group showed difficulty with local relations within the groupings whereas the right hemisphere group had general difficulty with organizing blocks into spatial arrays. High-risk infants with intracranial hemorrhage showed, on follow-up at age 5, poor perceptual-motor skills and intermodal memory, as well as impairment across a range of verbal and preacademic abilities (Selzer et al. 1992). Two measures of visuo-perceptual skills—three-dimensional construction of block models and copying of geometric figures—were impaired at follow-up in one-third of school-aged children with acquired head injuries who were followed by Levin and Eisenberg (1979).

Sensorimotor Functioning

Bawden and colleagues (1985) noted that severely head-injured children performed specifically more poorly than children with either mild or moderate injuries on high-speed tasks, even when performances on more basic measures of motor function were relatively similar. Finger tapping and manual dexterity tasks frequently are performed poorly after closed head injury, even in the absence of gross motor impairments (Chadwick et al. 1981).

Academic Performance

Head injuries of at least moderate severity often have an impact on academic achievement. However, even children with mild head injuries (tested at least 6 months post-trauma and without any premorbid learning disorders) showed relatively poorer arithmetic than reading scores on the WRAT achievement test, which the authors suggested was accounted for by the impact of the demands of time-limited calculations on attentional and information-processing-speed resources (Johnson 1991, Levin and Benton 1986). Virtually any neuropsychological deficit, e.g., slowed visuomotor performance, visuospatial impairment, and poor attention and recall can affect academic performance (Ewing-Cobbs et al. 1986).

Behavior and Personality Changes

Behavior problems and difficulties in adaptive functioning are common after closed head injury (Asarnow et al. 1991), although after mild head injuries adaptive functioning is less affected. No particular form of brain damage has been found to predispose for a specific disorder, although a trend toward hypoactivity was observed in some children. This relationship was also found by Brown et al. (1981) and was confirmed in a study by Seidel et al. (1975), which suggested that the incidence of psychiatric disorders is twice as high in children with cerebral pathology than in children with physical handicaps without cerebral involvement. The groups in the study by Seidel and co-workers were comparable in degree of physical handicap so that both suffered the same degree of motor and sensory deficit, as well as visibility of handicap. As did Rutter et al. (1970a, Shaffer et al. 1975), these authors concluded that the increased incidence of psychopathology was clearly a function of cerebral pathology. Eide and Tysnes (1992) observed that adaptive and social functioning was most markedly impaired in subjects with multifocal bilateral lesions. Donders (1992) investigated the question of whether premorbid functioning may be related to behavioral outcome after head injury for 60 6- to 16-year-old children with TBI. Only 11 per cent seemed to have premorbid disturbances according to parent- and teacher-rating scales. He concluded that premorbid behavioral and psychosocial factors were not clearly related to behavioral outcome or to the severity or type of head injury.

As in adults, post-traumatic stress disorder (PTSD) (Grant and Alves 1987) can occur in children. However, children seem to be less prone to denial and intrusive flashbacks (Terr 1985). The components of PTSD include (1) ego disorganization caused by the event; (2) a narcissistic injury, i.e., a sense of being devalued; (3) triggering of a primitive defense mechanism; (4) a compulsion to repeat the trauma; and (5) hypervigilance to prevent its recurrence (Green 1985). However, as with adults, it is likely that transient adjustment disorders and milder reactive fears and stress can account for a sizable percentage of post-traumatic stresses, when careful differential diagnosis is performed.

Researchers agree that an understanding of the long-term effects of head injury in children requires systematic study of the age of onset and the age at testing and that such studies need to take into account the location, focal specificity, and extent of the lesion, as well as the type and developmental complexity of the behavior under study (Boll and Barth 1981, Finger and Stein 1982, Goldstein and Levin 1985, Levin et al 1982). Fletcher et al. (1987) broadened the perspective related to age by rephrasing the issue as not whether age effects are present, but why they occur. Changes in the behavioral status of the individual at any one age are considered to be useful data to obtain, but at this time only limited information on these questions is available.

Summary

This chapter described brain damage in the neonate and the young infant. Traumatic perinatal brain damage due to a mechanical source has long been associated with cerebral palsy, which is often accompanied by cognitive defects of varying degrees and with changing psychological consequences during development. Improvements in professional care and advanced technologies have led to significant decreases in its occurrence. Brain damage due to traumatic head injury throughout infancy is of increasing concern, especially with the early identification of battered babies. The neuropsychological and behavioral consequences of head injury in children vary quite dramatically, depending on age, severity of injury, and accompanying environmental conditions.

19

Focal Neurological Disorders

This chapter deals with some pediatric neurological disease processes that have not been discussed in previous chapters, such as brain tumors and cerebrovascular conditions. These conditions are not very common in infancy and early childhood, but they do pose a special challenge to the neuropsychologist, given both the tenuousness of the child's neurological condition and the seriousness of concurrent secondary medical problems. Determining the integrity of mental functioning before and after surgical intervention, the influences of radiotherapy and chemotherapy on cognitive ability, and most important, arriving at useful prognostic statements concerning mental functioning are some of the tasks confronting the neuropsychologist. Ris and Noll (1994) provide a current review of the existing studies and of the problems encountered in research.

19.1   Intracranial Neoplasms

Childhood intracranial neoplasms represent a small but important minority of pediatric neurology cases. An annual incidence rate of 2.2 to 2.5/100,000 during the first decade of life has been estimated (Dennis et al. 1991a). Table 19-1 shows some of the most frequently observed childhood intracranial neoplasms. Intracranial tumors are typically defined by their cellular nature, as indicated below. It is also common to define these tumors further by their location (e.g., hemispheric, subcortical, cerebellar) and whether they originate above or below the tentorium, i.e., **supratentorial neoplasms** or **infratentorial neoplasms.**

An early epidemiological study of childhood tumors reported on all intracranial neoplasms in the first 18 months of life that were recorded in the Connecticut Tumor Registry from 1935 to 1974 (Farwell et al. 1978). Fifty-four cases of infants with tumors occurred during that period. In all, 30 per cent were medulloblastomas, 16 per cent were ependymal growths, 13 per cent were meningeal growths, and 9 per cent were astrocytomas. In terms of location, 44

Table 19-1   Selective Listing of
Pediatric Intracranial Neoplasms

Glioma
Low-grade astrocytoma
  High-grade astrocytoma
  Ependymoma
  Choroid plexus papilloma

Primitive neuroectodermal tumor (PNET)
  Medulloblastoma

Congenital
  Craniopharyngioma
  Neurofibroma

Meningioma

per cent were in the cerebellum, 37 per cent in the cerebrum, and 17 per cent in the brainstem. More current estimates place greater weight on astrocytomas and significantly less weight on meningiomas. One contemporary estimate suggests that 10 to 20 per cent of all intracranial neoplasms are medulloblastomas, 15 to 25 per cent are low-grade and 10 to 15 per cent are high-grade supratentorial astrocytomas, 10 to 20 per cent are cerebellar astrocytomas, 6 to 9 per cent are craniopharyngiomas, 5 to 10 per cent are ependymomas, 10 to 20 per cent are brainstem gliomas, 0.5 to 2 per cent are pineal tumors, and 12 to 14 per cent are other intracranial neoplasms (Heideman et al. 1993). Infratentorial tumors are more common than supratentorial ones in childhood, the opposite of what is seen in adulthood. Neurofibromas are found mainly along peripheral and cranial nerves, as well as in the skin; they are characteristic of von Recklinghausen's disease (neurofibromatosis) and are genetically (autosomal dominant) transmitted.

Recognizing the presence of a tumor in infancy and early childhood may be difficult for several reasons. Many of the symptoms are general in nature (e.g., headache, projectile vomiting, retinal swelling) and usually offer minimal cues for localization and differential diagnosis. Common neurological signs of possible tumor growth include those of hydrocephalus, seizures, and increased intracranial pressure. Problems with balance, steadiness, and gait are frequently observed with infratentorial growths. The young child's inability to give accurate verbal information about his or her symptoms further complicates this task. These difficulties may lengthen the time before diagnosis is made and intervention is attempted, resulting in a worsening of chances for a favorable outcome. Contemporary medical diagnostics are aided by radiological (Osborn 1994) and by immunohistochemical and other cellular analyses that exceed the purview of this chapter (see Deutsch 1990).

Once a diagnosis is attained, the general treatment of intracranial neoplasms is surgical removal of as much of the tumor as is feasible, followed by radiation therapy and/or chemotherapy in an attempt to eradicate the effect of any remaining cancerous cells. Surgery is usually the initial intervention, to remove the bulk of the tumor and to decrease intracranial pressure. Heideman and colleagues (1993) provided a discussion of different surgical approaches. **Radiotherapy** (the irradiation of brain regions to destroy tissue) was enhanced in the 1980s by improved three-dimensional lesion localization using MRI and more selective radiotherapy delivery modes, such as implanting small radioactive seeds into affected tissue and the so-called gamma knife (Albright 1993). Yet, irradiation in the young child was shown to produce adverse intellectual and other cognitive sequelae; irradiation while the brain is still developing during the first 5 years of life seems to be associated with subsequent cognitive decline. Therefore, a valuable development in neuro-oncology was of feasible approaches in children under the age of 5 years (and especially under the age of 3 years) to delaying radiotherapy for up to several years through the enhanced use of chemotherapy after surgical resection (Duffner et al. 1993). A current question is whether and for which cases chemotherapy alone after surgical resection may be appropriate, without a need for later radiotherapy (e.g., White et al. 1993).

Survival and the probability of lasting deficits are determined chiefly by the histological nature of the neoplasm. The malignancy of a tumor reflects its growth potential and, to a great degree, the patient's prognosis. Benign tumors have a relatively good prognosis, whereas malignant tumors have a poor prognosis. Additional factors that may influence prognosis include risks involved in surgical removal, the site of the tumorous growth, accessibility to surgical intervention, the importance of surrounding neural tissue, growth patterns, and the child's age. Gjerris (1976), for example, found that survival rates were poor for children with tumors during the first 4 years of life compared to children with tumors in the second 4 years. Neurobehavioral morbidity in survivors also seems to be related to age at onset, age during irradiation treatment, and lesion size and location.

Astrocytoma

An **astrocytoma** is a glioma that arises from the astrocyte cells of the CNS. **Gliomas** are glial cell tumors, and they account for the majority of childhood intracranial tumors. The grading of astrocytomas is based on prognosis.

A benign astrocytoma ("low grade," grades I or II) is common among the childhood neoplasms, although its incidence is relatively infrequent in children younger than the age of 2. It is typically slow-growing and forms cysts or cavities. Grades III and IV astrocytomas are considered "high-grade" with a poor prognosis.

The predominant site for astrocytomas in childhood is in the cerebellum (DeLong and Adams 1975). However, one in five pediatric hemispheric tumors are astrocytomas (Slooff and Slooff 1975). The optic nerve and chiasm, hypothalamus, and brainstem also may be sites of growth for gliomas. The prognosis for low-grade astrocytomas is favorable, although rarer cases with rapid and widespread tumor growth have a poorer prognosis. Malignant or "high-grade" forms of astrocytoma, such as **glioblastoma multiforme,** have a poor prognosis, but are quite rare in childhood. Brainstem gliomas also have an especially poor prognosis, which relates more to localization than cellular malignancy (Cohen and Duffner 1985). An **ependymoma** is a glioma of variable malignancy that usually arises from the ependymal matrix on the floor of the fourth ventricle and extends laterally and inferiorly. Since this position makes complete surgical removal less likely, recurrence after surgical removal makes the prognosis guarded at best.

Choroid Plexus Papilloma

A **choroid plexus papilloma** is a benign neoplasm that occurs predominantly in the first 3 years of life and tends to have a favorable prognosis. A majority of these tumors grow within one of the lateral ventricles, although some occur bilaterally. They are capable of secreting cerebrospinal fluid. Hydrocephalus is frequently observed in cases of choroid plexus papillomas.

Medulloblastoma

Medulloblastoma is the most common posterior fossa tumor in children. A revision of terminological classifications of pediatric tumors proposed by the World Health Organization placed medulloblastoma under the category of "primitive neuroepithelial (or neuroectodermal) tumor (PNET)," of which it is the most common form (Rorke et al. 1985). A medulloblastoma is regarded as an embryonal tumor that usually develops from the population of cells that proliferate in the first 6 to 8 months of postnatal life to become the cerebellar granule cells. In a series of 68 children with medulloblastomas, the majority of cases were observed to occur early in the first decade of life (Ingraham and Matson 1954). The peak age of incidence was 5 years (Heideman et al. 1993).

The tumor is usually situated in the cerebellum on the lateral midline. The site of development is usually the vermis. As with most tumors, the mechanism of abnormal growth remains unknown. It infiltrates the ventricular system at the level of the fourth ventricle. Ventricular infiltration results in an obstructive hydrocephalus and permits these tumor cells to disseminate and seed throughout the entire neuraxis via the cerebrospinal fluid. This obstruction commonly leads to the tumor's first symptoms, those of increased intracranial pressure. Surgical removal of as much of the tumor as possible and subsequent radiotherapy of the entire neuraxis are vital for favorable outcome. Increased surgical advances have resulted in more aggressive removal and a lower surgical mortality rate (Heideman et al. 1993). Contemporary treatment also includes chemotherapy.

Treatment of these medulloblastoma tumors has yielded what has been considered to be the most significant "success" in survival from pediatric brain tumors (Duffner and Cohen 1992). Cushing's initial report in 1930 noted that only 1 of 61 children survived after 3 years. Through the 1960s, the long-term prognosis for medulloblastoma was generally poor, as eventual regrowth of the tumor was highly probable. In the 1954 Ingraham and Matson series, for example, only 10 per cent of children survived for 5 years. Higher survival rates were reported during the 1970s and continued to improve. McIntosh (1979), for example, reported a dramatic increase in the number of survivors 5 years after diagnosis and intervention in a 1970 to 1974 sample when compared to a 1965 to 1969 sample. His study suggested that one-third of the cases may survive 5 years without recurrent growth, and a very small minority may live for decades without any recurrence. Researchers at the Hospital for Sick Children in Toronto, Canada, reported similar improvements in survival rates in a sample of 144 children with medulloblastoma treated between 1950 and 1980 (Park et al. 1983), as shown in Figure 19-1. The Toronto researchers also reported that children with medulloblastomas before the age of 6 years had a lower 5-year survival rate than those with the tumor after age 6 (59 per cent versus 41 per cent). One factor that may have accounted for this difference was the form of the medulloblastoma. The researchers subtyped medulloblastomas by histological means and reported that a form called desmoplastic medulloblastoma, a subtype with a poorer prognosis, was observed more commonly in younger children, with 52 per cent of this form occurring in children under the age of 5 and 95 per cent in children under the age of 10. Contemporary estimates now place general survival rates at 60 per cent (Duffner and Cohen 1992), and those at lower risk (i.e., with little remaining tumor tissue after surgical resection and no evidence of seeding) have a survival rate of 75 per cent (Walker and Rosenblum 1992) or even as high as 90 per cent (Albright 1993). Poorer outcomes may be related to brainstem infiltration that is intractable to surgical resection.

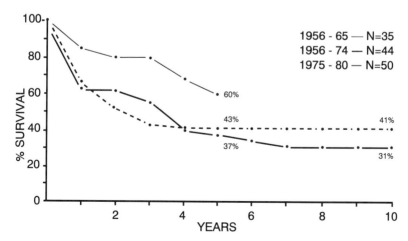

Figure 19-1.   Treatment period in relation to survival rates. N = Number of cases (Park et al. 1983).

Despite the improvement in long-term survival rates, cognitive deficits are common residual impairments among survivors. Morbidity is an important concern, given favorable survival rates, and neuropsychological studies of medulloblastoma survivors are increasing in number. Cognitive deficits may be the result of the tumor itself, but importantly, may also be a consequence of the radiotherapeutic regimen (Raimondi and Tomita 1979). Delayed complications of radiotherapy can also include short stature as a result of growth retardation and hypopituitarism (Park et al. 1983). Duffner and colleagues (1988) showed a progressive decline in IQ scores over a several-year period, with mean full-scale IQ values of 93.5 before intervention and a mean IQ value of 84.5 3 or more years later. At equivalent levels of radiation dosage, younger age in childhood has been associated with greater declines in the serial measurement of intellectual functioning (Silber et al. 1992). Ellenberg (1982) presented broader serial neuropsychological assessments of two young medulloblastoma patients. Both patients showed some recovery in cognitive skills by 15 months after surgery, but with residual deficits in attention, concentration, and in fine motor skills. Behavioral changes, when present (as reported by parents on a personality inventory), showed a tendency for psychotic symptoms in young survivors (Kun et al. 1983).

Craniopharyngioma

A **craniopharyngioma** is a supratentorial, midline cystic tumor that arises from a congenital malformation. Craniopharyngiomas and other midline tumors, such as chiasmal gliomas, are commonly found anteriorly in the brain, compressing and infringing upon the optic chiasm, the hypothalamus, and the third ventricle. This location results in the commonly observed triad of symptoms: visual problems, endocrinological disorders, and increased intracranial pressure due to the partial or total blockage of cerebrospinal fluid circulation. A bitemporal hemianopsia is a common visual field defect noted in these presentations. The endocrinological disorder may result in early growth retardation. Survival without major medical difficulties is common after successful removal of the growth; however, removal of a craniopharyngioma is sometimes hampered by its peripheral growth into poorly accessible, yet vital, surrounding regions (Shillito 1978). Advances in microsurgical techniques (Hoffman 1985), radiotherapy (Nagpal 1992), and combined treatment modalities (Wen et al. 1992) have accounted for improvements in outcomes.

Meningioma

A **meningioma** is a neoplasm that arises from any of the meningeal layers and remains well delineated from underlying brain tissue. Although it is a relatively common form of intracranial neoplasm in adulthood, less than 1 per cent of pediatric intracranial neoplasms examined at the Hospital for Sick Children in

Toronto, Canada were meningiomas (Drake et al. 1986). Pediatric meningiomas typically are benign.

Neuropsychological Outcome

Dennis and her Toronto colleagues have conducted one of the larger cognitive studies of children with brain tumors (age at onset from 15 months to 15 years), although it is limited to only some major neuropsychological domains (1991a, 1991b, 1992). They examined 46 children with a variety of tumors; the most common varieties were craniopharyngioma (50 per cent), astrocytoma (17 per cent), and medulloblastoma (13 per cent). Localization was likewise heterogeneous; notable numbers of children had diencephalic, limbic, or subcortical white matter involvement. Complicating the analysis of their findings was a 20 per cent incidence of closed head injury in the patients' premorbid history, although severity was not noted. The researchers examined intellectual and memory functioning, employing the Wechsler scales and three memory subtests (Recognition, Content, and Sequence) from the Goldman-Fristoe-Woodcock Auditory Memory Test (Goldman et al. 1974). They found memory deficits, mainly for serial order of pictures, although semantically based word-picture association memory was not affected. The memory defect was related to the length of time since tumor onset. After irradiation treatment, memory impairment was related to older age at tumor onset and to location of the tumor in the thalamic/epithalamic region. In an analysis of the brain regions that most often affect memory functions, the authors suggested that subcortical lesions do not affect word-picture association, but that associative memory (memory for the serial order of pictures) was affected mainly by lesions in the limbic system and the hypothalamic-pituitary axis, and representational memory (working memory) by lesions in the pineal-habenular region and the anterior and medial thalamic nuclei (Dennis et al. 1991b). The analysis of hormone status and radiation treatment effects (Dennis et al. 1992) suggested that verbal, but not nonverbal, intelligence varied positively with age at radiation treatment and that serial position memory defects were strongly related to hormone depletion and age at tumor onset. Working memory deficits were also related to radiation history and tumor sites in the thalamic-epithalamic region. Memory for word meanings was unrelated to radiation history or hormone levels.

Because of its scattered appearance in different parts of the CNS and the body, children with neurofibromatosis do not show consistent radiological, EEG, or brainstem auditory evoked responses (BAER) findings. Duffner et al. (1989) evaluated 47 children and found that 60 per cent had MRI abnormalities, but that these were not related to cognitive abilities or seizure activity.

Children with neoplastic disease not localized in the CNS but who nevertheless require prophylactic radiotherapy of the CNS may also present with cognitive and behavioral changes. Fletcher and Copeland (1988) provided a review of this literature.

19.2 Cerebrovascular Disease

Acute cerebrovascular accidents (CVA, "strokes") are far more characteristic of elderly populations than of infancy and childhood. Strokes do occur in childhood, however. Mayo Clinic epidemiological work suggested a post-neonatal pediatric CVA incidence rate of 2.52/100,000 per year (Schoenberg et al. 1978). Hemorrhagic strokes are more common than ischemic CVAs. Of particular concern in this section are perinatal hemorrhage, occlusive CVAs, and arteriovenous malformations (AVM) and aneurysms.

Perinatal Hemorrhage

The extravasation of blood from intracranial blood vessels is a common consequence of the perinatal mechanical injuries described in the previous chapter. The major forms of perinatal hemorrhage are subdural, subarachnoid, peri- and intraventricular, and cerebellar hemorrhage. Hemorrhages typically bleed into the spaces between the meningeal layers overlying the brain, hence their names, subdural and subarachnoid. Peri- and intraventricular hemorrhages are discussed in Chapter 17. A cerebellar hemorrhage, like a periventricular (intracerebral) hemorrhage, involves bleeding into nervous tissue itself. Perinatal intracranial hemorrhages usually arise from the large venous sinuses, as well as from venous vessels, such as the vein of Galen. Figure 19-2 shows the superficial and deep venous systems of the brain. As expected, the severity of intracranial hemorrhage as shown on MRIs correlated strongly with neurological and cognitive outcome in a follow-up of 14 children 4 to 8 years later (Ford et al. 1989).

A **subdural hemorrhage,** the discharge of blood into the subdural space, is particularly devastating to the newborn. It is usually a consequence of trauma during full-term delivery, resulting from excessive molding of the head during delivery. The molding increases stress and strain on the meningeal structures, such as the tentorium and the falx cerebri, and results in the tearing of these structures and nearby veins. Blood from a subdural hemorrhage does not readily reabsorb into the bloodstream. In survivors, obstructive membranes surround the bleeding for several weeks after the episode because of a proliferation of fibroblasts, which surround fluids, such as blood, that contain large amounts of protein (Schurr 1969). These obstructions inhibit reabsorption.

There are several types of subdural hemorrhage. One form involves bleeding from the convex, bridging veins of the cerebral hemispheres entering the superior sagittal sinus. Another form involves bleeding from deep venous structures into the posterior fossa region. A final type of subdural hemorrhage involves bleeding from small pial veins. Of the three types of subdural hemorrhage, the deep-structure bleeding into the posterior fossa is by far the most serious.

Cerebral subdural hemorrhage results in the discharge of blood over the convexity of the cerebral hemispheres. The veins that tear in this type of traumatic hemorrhage are the superficial bridging veins between the medial superior

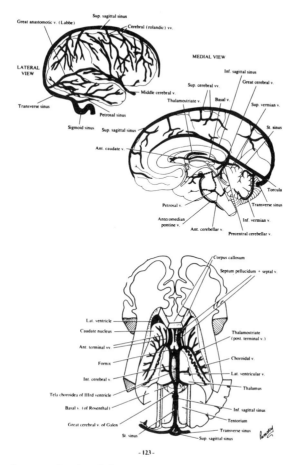

Figure 19-2. The superficial and deep venous system of the brain (Pansky and Allen 1980).

aspect of the cerebral hemispheres and the superior sagittal sinus. The bleeding results in a thin layer of blood over the entire cerebrum, but is less dramatic in consequence than a posterior fossa bleed. Fifty to eighty per cent of survivors of a cerebral subdural hemorrhage have a generally favorable neurological outcome at follow-up. The remaining survivors may be left with focal cerebral signs and hydrocephalus (Hill and Volpe 1989).

A subdural hemorrhage into the surrounding posterior fossa region of the brain results from a tear at the junction of the falx cerebri and the tentorium, near the vein of Galen. This form of bleeding is usually fatal within the first 3 days of life if it occurs at birth. The vein of Galen is particularly susceptible to tearing because it is located between the two cerebral hemispheres, which maintain some relative mobility, and the fixed and passive vascular sinuses. While the head is being molded during delivery, the vein may kink and stretch, with resultant occlusion of blood flow or rupture. In addition to the seriousness of a rupture itself, the accumulation of blood in the posterior fossa region causes compression of the brainstem and its displacement against the skull. This compression has very serious, if not fatal, immediate consequences for normal homeostatic body functioning. Since blood is not easily reabsorbed, the subdural hemorrhage remains and causes continued compression of the structures in that region of the cranium.

A skull fracture, in addition to head molding, can cause a perinatal subdural hemorrhage.

Another type of subdural hemorrhage is sometimes observed in large or postmature neonates who have suffered a traumatic birth. In these cases, continued bleeding from small pial veins is seen and results in an abrupt presentation of symptoms 2 to 5 days after birth. Occasionally, a perinatal subdural hemorrhage does not become clinically evident until sometime during the first 6 months of life and is known as a chronic subdural hemorrhage.

The overall outcome of subdural hemorrhage is very poor. Death during the early neonatal period is common. In an 8- to 13-year follow-up of 42 infants with perinatal damage, Natelson and Sayers (1973) found that 5 of 10 infants with a subdural hemorrhage died within a week of birth, 4 were mentally handicapped at follow-up, and only 1 was within the normal range of mental abilities. An additional 13 infants had a chronic subdural hemorrhage during the first 6 months of life, which the authors felt was most likely related to mechanical injury suffered at birth. All 13 suffered from accompanying seizure activity. Only 3 of the 13 had IQs in the normal range at follow-up. Whether or not the four survivors without mental handicap suffered cognitive or learning difficulties could not be ascertained from the data.

A **subarachnoid hemorrhage,** the discharge of blood into the subarachnoid space, is currently the most common form of perinatal intracranial hemorrhage (Volpe 1977b) and occurs predominantly in premature babies after breech delivery or in difficult term deliveries. Subarachnoid bleeding in preterm infants is usually related to an accompanying anoxic episode; during a full-term delivery, it is related to mechanical injury. In these cases, the bleeding arises from capillaries or from small meningeal vessels. The episodes are usually milder and less extensive than are subdural bleeds (Cartwright et al. 1979). Bleeding is usually bilateral and occurs predominantly over the temporal lobes. One major result of subarachnoid hemorrhaging is hydrocephalus.

Volpe has delineated three syndromes of subarachnoid hemorrhage (Hill and Volpe 1989). The first group is composed primarily of preterm infants with minor hemorrhaging and without major sequelae. The second group consists of full-term infants who have suffered a hemorrhage and show seizures very early in neonatal life. Finally, a smaller group of infants suffer massive bleeding with rapidly fatal consequences, probably due to the occurrence of both a traumatic injury and severe anoxia. Outcome is generally related to the severity of the initial episode and is usually good unless that episode was associated with a preceding hypoxic-ischemic event or with traumatic brain damage.

Historically, **intracerebellar hemorrhage** has been recorded as an uncommon perinatal event that is sometimes seen in difficult term deliveries. However, it has been acknowledged that this hemorrhage occurs with greater frequency in very premature (i.e., less than 28 weeks gestational age at birth) infants (Grunnet and Shields 1976). Intracerebellar hemorrhages show a variety of distributions of bleeding in the cerebellum, including total or partial bleeding into the cerebellar hemispheres. In the Grunnett and Shields sample, the intracerebellar bleeds occurred together with periventricular bleeds and respiratory distress. The prognosis is poor; most infants who have been so diagnosed died soon after the bleed. Volpe (1977b) cautioned, however, that cerebellar functioning should be monitored carefully in all small premature babies suffering any intracranial hemorrhage to determine if subfatal intracerebellar bleeds may have occurred.

Occlusive Cerebrovascular Disease

Infant and childhood occlusive disease is relatively rare; occlusions of the cerebral arteries are primarily problems of late adulthood. Occlusions may be formed by emboli blocking vessels or by thrombosis of cerebrovascular vessels. Congenital or acquired structural cardiac lesions are the most common site for embolic formation in children (Roach and Riela 1988). When occlusive disease occurs, hemiplegia is the most frequent manifestation (Dusser et al. 1986). It is often found in isolation, although it may be accompanied by an impairment in consciousness, convulsions, or (in older children) aphasia. **Acute infantile hemiplegia** is a condition that may be observed after occlusion of a segment of the anterior circulation; the term "acute hemiplegia in childhood" has gained in current usage because the condition's onset is not limited to infancy. The onset of acute hemiplegia need not be cerebrovascular in origin (see Chapter 21 on hemispherectomy). When onset is indeed cerebrovascular, there also is a diverse set of etiologies. Perhaps the most common cause is a preceding infectious disease. One study reported that half of their sample of both ischemic and hemorrhagic stroke patients had a preceding infectious disease (Eeg-Olofsson and Ringheim 1983). In the study by Dusser and colleagues (1986) of 16 youngsters with ischemic stroke aged between 6 weeks and 2 years, cardiac disease was present in 6, the cause was idiopathic in 5, cerebral infections were present in 3, and "Moya-moya syndrome" was present in 2. First described in Japan, **Moya-moya syndrome** is a progressive intracranial arterial occlusion with basal telangiectasis; the Japanese name reflects the observed nonspecific radiographic pattern of a hazy or "puff of smoke" appearance (Raimondi et al. 1992).

Children with idiopathic occlusive acute hemiplegia generally showed normal developmental levels when followed up several years later by Dusser and colleagues (1986). "Severe" retardation was noted in two of five children with involvement of both the cerebral cortex and the cerebellum. Retardation was noted more frequently in patients with the Moya-moya syndrome. As with idiopathic presentations, severe retardation was noted more frequently in patients with cardiac etiologies when both the cerebral cortex and the cerebellum were involved.

Arteriovenous Malformations and Aneurysms

Arteriovenous malformations (AVMs) are predominantly due to a failure of capillary development between arteries and veins during prenatal development. Blood vessels may become distorted and tortuous, and an atypical shunting of circulating blood may be observed. Although AVMs and aneurysms may be completely asymptomatic in childhood, large AVMs may present with focal neurological and cognitive deficits, and aneurysms, should they burst, do result in changes to brain tissue. Aneurysms of the pericallosal arteries in children are found mostly after severe head trauma, but may present postoperatively with symptoms similar to those after callosotomy (Brown et al. 1990, Nakstadt et al. 1986). Only a minority of AVMs become symptomatic in the first decade of life. After infancy, childhood AVMs are one of the more frequent causes of an intracranial bleed and, before the age of 15 years, are far more frequent causes than are aneurysms (Tamaki and Ehara 1992). When they do become symptomatic, it may be as a result of an intracranial hemorrhage, or at times, they show features of a space-occupying lesion. Vascular malformations that present clinically in early infancy are somewhat different in presentation than those in young children and adolescents. Newborns with AVMs presenting clinically usually do so with congestive heart failure, rather than hydrocephalus or subarachnoid hemorrhage (Roach and Riela 1988). Posterior fossa AVMs with aneurysmal dilation of the vein of Galen, as another example, typically present by the end of infancy, not later (Roach and Riela 1988).

Clinical identification of aneurysms in children under the age of 10 years is uncommon, although rare cases of neonatal aneurysms have been documented (Choux et al. 1992). Subarachnoid hemorrhage (in isolation or sometimes with associated coma, mass-effects, or seizures) form the clinical presentation. The majority of aneurysms are in the anterior circulation in both children and adults; however, the proportion of posterior circulation aneurysms is greater in children (Choux et al. 1992).

Summary

But for in specialty clinics, the family physician or the general clinical psychologist rarely sees children with the focal neurological disorders discussed in this chapter. The present neuropsychological literature reflects this low incidence. Although the literature on adult aneurysmal subarachnoid hemorrhage is sizeable, child neuropsychological reports are few in number. The exception to this is the growing literature on outcomes of children with medulloblastomas and on the sequelae of pediatric CNS radiotherapy. Most studies limit cognitive data to intellectual measures, and some take rather broad liberties in defining cognitive function and dysfunction. As survival becomes more likely, carefully conceived research studies and individual clinical evaluations will play an increasingly important role in examining residual sequelae and the separate contribution of initial pathology and the side effects of treatment and will help planning good management and intervention programming.

20

Convulsive Disorders

20.1 Nature of the Convulsive Disorders

A common denominator for the set of disorders discussed in this chapter is involvement of abnormal electrical activity, or discharge, of cerebral neurons. The terms "convulsions," "seizures," and "epilepsy" are sometimes used synonymously, but do not necessarily refer to the same phenomenon. For the sake of uniformity in this chapter, the term "convulsive disorder" is used when we are discussing abnormal discharges in brain cells. These electrical changes, extracellularly recorded as EEG paroxysms, are thought to be summations of synchronously developing depolarizations and hyperpolarizations in neurons (Goldensohn and Ward 1975). In simpler terms, the modulated balance of excitatory and inhibitory synaptic influences that are normally present in neurons is disturbed in an epileptogenic area of ganglion cells in the gray matter of the brain. A gigantic hyperpolarization spreads to other areas; the specific type of such spreading determines the timing, form, and distribution of epileptic discharges and hence the clinical picture (Figure 20-1).

The terms convulsion, seizure, epilepsy, and spasm have also been used to define an abnormal cerebral discharge; however, these terms have additional or different meanings as well. For example, the fact that a child has had a convulsion or a seizure does not automatically imply the presence of epilepsy. A seizure may not always present clinically as a convulsion (i.e., abnormal motor activity), nor is a seizure the sole cause of a convulsion. Convulsions may also be caused by such nonseizure factors as breath-holding spells or may be very closely mimicked, in early infancy, by an extremely jittery (though otherwise normal) baby. Seizures may be triggered by external stimuli (e.g., flickering lights, television) or even by the child's own singing or recitation (Herskowitz et al. 1984). The disease process causing a convulsive disorder need not originate in the CNS but, as in the specific case of febrile seizures, may be extracerebral.

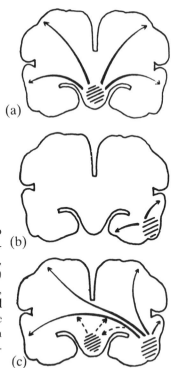

Figure 20-1. Types of epileptic seizures according to spreading of bioelectric activity: (a) primarily generalized seizures: grand mal (tonic or tonic-clonic seizures), petit mal (myclonic and astatic seizures, absences); (b) focal seizures of motor, sensory, or hypersentivity type, psychomotor seizures, adversive seizures; (c) generalized seizures of focal origin: grand mal (tonic or tonic-clonic seizures), minor seizures (not petit mal) with sudden dropping or sudden head, arm, or other body movements (Doose 1975).

Epilepsy, at this point simply defined as recurrent and persisting seizure activity, may occur at any time during the life of an individual. Most forms, however, tend to develop during the first years of life or during puberty and early adulthood. In addition to a brief description of the epilepsies, the main concern in this chapter is with their psychological correlates and sequelae in relation to time of onset and duration; the chapter also examines the type, frequency, and origin of the convulsive disorders of early life.

In contrast to the convulsive disorders of infancy and childhood, epilepsy may be viewed as a long-range disturbance of the functioning of the individual, rather than as a disorder of development. Therefore, the topic overlaps to some extent with those discussed in Part IV. However, the many commonalities between early convulsive disorders and epilepsy favor treating them jointly in this chapter.

In discussing convulsive disorders, it is important to understand that abnormal electrical discharges of neurons are symptoms, rather than causes, of a disease. As with many isolated symptoms, the presence of a convulsion does not signify the existence of a single disease. Rather, the underlying cause of a convulsion may be one of numerous entities that may or may not be readily diagnosable, e.g., traumatic, metabolic, infectious, vascular, toxic. A relatively large percentage of convulsive disorders are caused by unknown factors and are labeled idiopathic. Unless properly treated, convulsions may lead to death or to further seizures, regardless of the underlying cause. How a seizure may "kindle," or increase the likelihood for, further seizures is an active area of research. Kindling is an important issue when dealing with convulsive disorders in early life since animal research suggests that the immature brain is more susceptible to seizures than the adult brain (Moshe et al. 1982).

20.2   Convulsive Disorders in Infancy and Childhood

Convulsive disorders in infancy and childhood differ in many respects from those in adulthood. Perhaps most importantly, they occur far more frequently in individuals under the age of 15 than in adults and are considered by some authors to be a "disorder of childhood" differing in type and etiology from the adult disorders. Approximately 90 per cent of all epileptic patients develop their initial symptoms before the age of 20 (Livingston 1972). Unlike childhood convulsive disorders, the etiologies of convulsions in older individuals are more commonly symptomatic in nature, i.e., they occur after brain trauma or in response to neoplastic or cerebrovascular disease. The types of behavioral manifestations seen in convulsive disorders also change over time.

Three common convulsive disorders that are observed in infancy and early childhood are (1) neonatal seizures, (2) infantile spasms, and (3) febrile convulsions. The three (note the variability in naming) are different age-specific medical diagnoses that vary widely in etiology and prognosis. Figure 20-2 shows a schematic frequency distribution of the occurrence of each type of disorder. Neonatal seizures are bimodally distributed in the first week of life, infantile spasms are most frequent around the first half-year of life, and febrile convulsions usually occur in later infancy and early childhood.

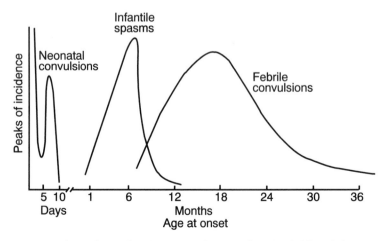

Figure 20-2.   Chronology of epilepsy in infancy and early childhood (Brett 1975).

Neonatal Seizures

This form of convulsive disorder is the most frequent neonatal neurological emergency (Rose 1977). **Neonatal seizures**—seizures occurring up to 44 weeks of conceptual age—were documented in 0.5 per cent of the babies in the NIH Perinatal study (Holden et al. 1980). Fenichel (1980) reported that premature infants have seizures 15 times more often than full-term babies and have a very high (approximately 90 per cent) mortality rate. Table 20-1 provides a list of the common neonatal seizure patterns.

Neonatal seizures usually occur as a result of serious neurological perinatal conditions, such as anoxic episodes and hemorrhaging. However, neonatal seizures related to other factors, such as cocaine use of the mother, have also been described (Kramer et al. 1990). Owing to the relative immaturity of synaptic connections and myelin coating, seizures with bilateral cortical involvement are rare in neonates because there is less capacity for spreading the electrical abnormality throughout the brain. Occasionally, **hemi-convulsions** are observed in which manifestations on one side very gradually change to the opposite side and then may or may not return to the original side. Neonatal seizures have immediate, negative effects on cerebral metabolism and on protein synthesis, which may have long-lasting consequences (Volpe 1977).

There are two peak times for the occurrence of neonatal seizures: (1) the first and second days of life and (2) toward the end of the first week. Anoxia, intracranial bleeding, and hypoglycemia are common causes for seizures during the first peak, and simple hypocalcemia is the primary etiology for the second peak (Rose 1977). In the NIH Perinatal Study, 37.9 per cent of all documented cases of neonatal seizures occurred within the first 24 hours, 65 per cent by the end

Table 20-1   Common Neonatal Seizure Patterns

Subtle (or minimal)	Abnormal eye movements; mild posturing; oral, lingual, pedaling, rowing movements; brief tremors; apneas
Clonic	
Focal	Rarely imply focal brain lesions
Multifocal	Fragmentary, anarchic; must be differentiated from jitteriness
Hemiconvulsive	Rare in newborns; more frequent in young infants
Tonic (focal or generalized)	May resemble decerebrate posturing; often accompanied by abnormal eye movements, apnea, cyanosis; more common in premature newborns
Myoclonic	Often fragments of infantile spasms that are seen in later infancy; must be differentiated from Moro reflex and startles of non-REM sleep
Tonic-clonic	Rare in newborns

Source: Lombroso 1983a.

of day 2, and 87 per cent by the end of the first week of life (Holden et al. 1982). The recurrence rate after a single unprovoked afebrile seizure is quite high (51.8 per cent); additional seizures after one recurrence were observed in 79 per cent, particularly in children with abnormal neurological findings, focal spikes in the EEG, and with complex partial seizures. The lowest recurrence rate was found after a single generalized tonic-clonic seizure in children with a normal EEG and normal neurological examination, regardless of whether anti-epileptic medication was used or not.

The common causes of neonatal seizures are (1) perinatal anoxic episodes and mechanical trauma, (2) infections and malformations, (3) miscellaneous factors, and (4) idiopathic. Each accounts for roughly 25 per cent of the total incidence (Table 20-2). Many times, seizures develop unpredictably. Lombroso (1978), for example, found that neither the Apgar score nor the history of obstetrical complications had much predictive value for seizures. In Volpe's (1977) series, anoxic episodes were responsible for the greatest single percentage of neonatal seizures; others (e.g., Brown 1973) found metabolic causes to be more prevalent. Aberrantly low levels of glucose (i.e., hypoglycemia) or calcium and inborn deficits of amino acid metabolism are particularly important in this regard.

The clinical manifestations of neonatal seizures vary (Table 20-3). In many cases, particularly those involving premature infants, clinical manifestations are

Table 20-2 Presumptive Etiologies in 239[a] Newborns with Seizures

Etiology	Number of cases
Intracranial birth injury	36
Hypocalcemia (see text)	36
Hypoxia	26
Infections	22
Congenital CNS malformations	19
Hypoglycemia	14
Dysmaturity (see text)	13
Excessive amount of blood magnesium	4
Excessive amount of blood sodium	4
Nitrogen blood deficiency (hyponatremia)	1
Miscellaneous[b]	16
Of doubtful origin	62
	253[a]

Source: Rose 1977.
[a]In 14 cases, two or more etiologies were suspected.
[b]Includes five cases with strong family history of epilepsy; four cases of systemic sepsis; one sibship and another case of pyridoxine dependency; and one case each of Leigh's disease, undetermined leukodystrophy, congenital heart disease, and hemorrhagic disease of the newborn.

Table 20-3 Classification of Neonatal Seizures

Classification of clinical seizures and relationship to EEG seizure discharge	Number of seizures recorded	Number of patients[a]
I. Seizures with close association to EEG seizure discharges		
A. Focal clonic		14
1. Unifocal	18	
2. Multifocal	23	
a. Alternating		
b. Migrating		
3. Hemiconvulsive	15	
4. Axial	2	
B. Myoclonic		4
1. Generalized	35	
2. Focal	3	
C. Focal tonic		2
1. Asymmetric truncal	6	
2. Eye deviation	2	
D. Apnea[b]	4	1
II. Seizures with inconsistent or no relationship to EEG seizure discharge		
A. Motor automatisms		22
1. Oral-buccal-lingual movements	31	
2. Ocular signs	33	
3. Progressive movements		
a. Pedalling	21	
b. Stepping	19	
c. Rotary arm movements	16	
4. Complex purposeless movements	20	
B. Generalized tonic		13
1. Extensor	51	
2. Flexor	18	
3. Mixed extensor/flexor	21	
C. Myoclonic		13
1. Generalized	23	
2. Focal	38	
3. Fragmentary	5	
III. Infantile spasms	11	2
IV. EEG seizures without clinical seizures		11

Source: Mizrahi & Kellaway 1987.

[a]The most frequent seizure type was considered primary for each patient. Twenty-two patients had more than one type.

[b]Occurred only in one patient who had been treated with phenobarbital before monitoring.

extremely difficult to observe. The most frequent form has been defined as "subtle" or "minimal" because its clinical manifestations are easily overlooked. Volpe (1977) listed horizontal eye deviation, repetitive blinking or eyelid fluttering, oral-buccal-lingual movements, apnea, and pedaling or swimming limb movements as the most common manifestations of subtle neonatal seizures. However, tonic and clonic features are usually absent. Despite these subtle behavioral manifestations, the EEG in these cases is markedly abnormal.

Focal seizures are rare during the neonatal period; when they do occur their cause is typically a traumatic focal brain injury (Volpe 1977). Multifocal or migratory convulsions are fairly common behavioral manifestations of neonatal seizures. Tonic seizures are more commonly seen in premature infants and are a sign of brain injury (Fenichel 1980). Apnea, upward eye deviation, and stiffening of the extended body are observed in these tonic seizures.

Neonates with seizures show significant developmental handicaps on all parts of the Brazelton examination (Emory et al. 1989). The prospective Boston series (e.g., Lombroso 1983a and b, Rose 1977) examined at several points during childhood 265 who, as full-term neonates, suffered from neonatal seizures. Two distinctly different prognostic groups were revealed at the 5-year examination: those who were normal and those who were severely abnormal or had died. In the series, 52 per cent were normal, 20 per cent had died, and 28 per cent showed severe abnormal development, persisting neurological deficit, or continuing seizure activity. Prognosis was influenced by etiology, seizure type, and type of EEG abnormality. In some conditions, the etiology was clearly the most important consideration: simple hypocalcemia and subarachnoid hemorrhage were causes with good outcomes, whereas structural malformations and anoxic episodes carried poor prognoses (Tables 20-4 and 20-5). Outcome was not related to either seizure duration or severity, but the type of seizure had a definite influence. An especially poor prognosis was observed in children who suffered from the subtle form of neonatal seizures. Poorly organized seizure patterns, such as myoclonic and tonic seizures, also had less favorable prognoses than focal and well-organized patterns.

Legido et al. (1991) examined the outcome at 31 months of 40 infants with EEG recorded ictal activity. Of these children, only 27 survived; 56 per cent showed continuing seizure activity, 67 per cent showed developmental delay, and 63 per cent had cerebral palsy. Predictive of outcome were frequent, brief seizures and interictal EEG background.

The NIH Perinatal study (Holden et al. 1980) provided follow-up information on 277 neonates who had suffered seizures. The mortality rate in the series was 34.7 per cent, with two-thirds dying during the neonatal period. Death was associated with birth weight (there was an excessive number of deaths of infants under 2500 g and over 4000 g in the series), gestational age, a low 5-minute Apgar score, number of days of seizure activity, and duration of seizure. When the seizure picture was complicated by apnea, the death rate rose to 60 per cent. Of the 181 survivors, 18.8 per cent were mentally retarded, and 15.2 per cent showed borderline intellectual levels. Mental retardation was associated

Table 20-4   Relation of Etiology to Abnormal Outcome

Etiologies	Abnormal clinical outcome	Seizures	Mental retardation (MR) (IQ < 80)	Others	Predict-ability of MR
		Neurological sequelae			
Hypocalcemia					
Early Onset	11	2	4	5	
Late Onset	1	0	1	1	
Anoxia	21	8	18	13	Good
Intracranial Injury					
Subarachroid hemorrhage	2	0	2	1	
Contusion	2	2	0	1	
Ventricular hemorrhage	8	2	4	4	
Infection of the CNS	14	5	8	4	
Hypoglycemia	9	7	9	5	Good
Congenital cerebral malformations	17	10	17	7	Good
Miscellaneous	14	5	2	0	
Unknown	20	14	10	11	

Source: Lombroso 1978.

with cerebral palsy. At 7 years, cerebral palsy was moderate or severe in 11.6 per cent of the sample and nonhandicapping in 2.2 per cent. Six per cent were diagnosed as having cerebral palsy, but died before the age of 7. Of the survivors, 22 per cent had subsequent afebrile seizures, and 12.7 per cent were considered to be cases of active epilepsy. Surviving children with very low birth weight and epilepsy seemed to be significantly more impaired intellectually than children with normal birth weight (Watkins et al. 1988). In another comprehensive follow-up of the 52,000 children in the Collaborative Perinatal Study (Ellenberg et al. 1986), 2635 children experienced one or more seizures between birth and age 7. The study confirmed that neurological abnormalities in the first year of life and the presence of minor motor seizures were associated with increased rates of mental retardation at age 7. However, in contrast to other studies, age of onset seemed to have little prognostic value.

Another follow-up study that examined 482 children with seizures during the first year of life over their next 5 to 10 years (Cavazutti et al. 1984) indicated normal development in 62 per cent of children with febrile seizures as compared to only 14 per cent of those with infantile spasms, 15 per cent of those with status epilepticus, and 24 per cent in the remaining children. The occurrence

Table 20-5 Relation of Etiology to Clinical Outcome at Age 5 Years

Etiologies	Number of Cases	Number dead	Clinical Outcome		Normal (%)	Predict-ability
			Abnormal	Normal		
Hypocalcemia						
Early Onset	19	4	7	8	42	
Late Onset	17	0	1	16	94	Good
Anoxia	25	3	18	4	16	Good
Intracractable Injury						
Subarachroid hemorrhage	13	0	2	11	85	Good
Contusion	7	0	2	5	71	
Ventricular hemorrhage	8	4	4	0	0	Good
Infection of the CNS	20	5	9	6	30	
Hypoglycemia	12	0	9	3	25	Good
Congenital cerebral malformations	18	8	9	1	5	Good
Miscellaneous	19	1	13	5	68	
Unknown	52	5	15	32	62	
Total	210	30	89	91	43	

Source: Lombroso 1978.
*"Good" signifies a confidence level of between 0.1 and 4 per cent and applies both to predictions of normal or of abnormal outcome at age 5 years.

of mental retardation followed a similar pattern. Epilepsy developed with equal frequency among children who had partial and generalized seizures, but the former showed mental retardation more often and most often suffered from birth asphyxia (Pratrap and Gururaj 1989). Other indicators of favorable outcome were the onset of seizures during the second half of the first year of life and normal EEG recordings between seizures.

Infantile Spasms (West Syndrome)

Infantile spasms peak in occurrence between the fourth and sixth months of life (Chevrie and Aicardi 1978). This condition is also known as West syndrome, named for a physician who, in the mid-1800s, reported a particularly severe type of seizure in his young son. **Infantile spasms** have three common clinical manifestations: the flexor spasm (the most common type, occurring in 70 per cent of the cases), the nodding spasm (involving head movements), and the "Blitzkrampf" or lightning spasm (because it occurs extremely rapidly). A typical symptom triad of spasms, severe mental retardation, and a markedly abnormal EEG was first described by Vazquez and Turner (1951). The EEG has been labeled as hypsarrhythmic and shows random high-voltage slow waves and spikes spreading to all cortical areas (Figure 20-3).

In roughly half the cases of West syndrome, the spasms are preceded by other types of seizures, an indicator of a very poor prognosis. However, in idiopathic cases of infantile spasms, normal development is observed until the spasms occur. There is a 2:1 preponderance of males who suffer from infantile spasms, but little familial incidence (Jeavons et al. 1973).

A notable relationship in female children between West syndrome and agenesis of the corpus callosum has been described (Aicardi et al. 1965, Dennis and Bower 1972, Gastaut et al. 1978). Ocular anomalies, particularly involving the fundus, have been tied to those infantile spasms with known prenatal etiologies (Curatolo et al. 1981). A CT scan study of patients with West syndrome revealed global cortical and subcortical atrophy, with particular involvement of the frontal

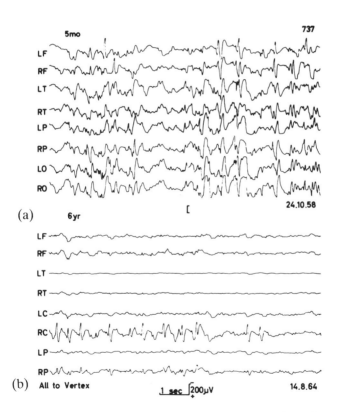

Figure 20-3. Hypsarrhythmic brain activity: (a) Five-month-old male with West syndrome and hypsarrhythmic EEG; (b) Same patient at age six years, with EEG now showing focal spike-wave activity as frequently seen in Lennox-Gestaut syndrome (Lou 1982).

and temporal lobes (Gastaut et al. 1978). Pneumoencephalography commonly reveals dilation of one or both lateral ventricles, consistent with the findings of atrophy. **Agyria** (i.e., a smooth cortical surface) is frequently observed in cases coming to autopsy (Harper 1967).

In general, infants with West syndrome have an extremely poor prognosis for mental development. In one of the best-documented follow-up series of children with West syndrome, Jeavons et al. (1973) assessed the intelligence of survivors of infantile spasms with the Griffiths scale of mental abilities. Only 3 of 112 infants performed at a normal intellectual level at follow-up, and 10 were mildly subnormal; the majority (88 per cent) remained mentally retarded. A further follow-up at 5 to 14 years of age (Jeavons et al. 1973) found that 18 of the 98 children had died, many before age 4. Thirteen of the 98 children had made a full recovery, but most continued to convulse, and 50 per cent had persistent neurodevelopmental abnormalities (most commonly, spastic diplegia and quadriplegia). Recovery was related to the etiology of the spasms, rather than to any treatment, such as steroid drug therapy. Children with spasms due to perinatal damage most commonly had persistent neurological abnormality, whereas idiopathic spasms and spasms due to early-life immunization procedures were associated with a better prognosis and mental abilities in the normal range.

A later follow-up of 150 cases (presumably the previous 98 plus additional new cases) confirmed the earlier follow-up findings (Jeavons et al. 1973, Jeavons and Harding 1975). Of 150 children who had suffered West syndrome, only 16 per cent were found to be educable in a normal school setting at follow-up 2 to 12 years after the onset of seizures; an additional 10 per cent were educable in schools for the "educationally subnormal," and 18 per cent were attending basic skill training centers. The remaining 56 per cent had either died or were considered uneducable. Children with normal development and mental function before the onset of seizures fared better in school: 37 per cent were in a regular school, and 36 per cent were educable at special schools and training centers. In sum, the Birmingham series indicated that the mental and neurological prognoses for children who suffered from infantile spasms were best either when the etiology of the infantile spasms was idiopathic or when the seizures followed from an immunization procedure. Roughly one-third of the cases with these etiologies showed full recovery. However, in children with other etiologies, particularly those involving perinatal damage, a high death rate and persisting severe mental retardation in survivors were observed, regardless of therapeutic drug regimens used. The absence of mental subnormality or other types of seizures at the time of the initial examination and spasms that occurred for less than 10 months were also indicators of good recovery. These results were confirmed in another major 6-year follow-up of 286 children by Lombroso (1983a and b). Consistent with these findings, another study (Favata et al. 1987) found developmental and/or neurological abnormalities (including poor language development) before the onset of spasms, symptomatic etiology, and abnormal CT findings to be associated with low IQ at the time of follow-up, whereas other developmental milestones (sitting, walking) were not predictive of outcome.

Another follow-up investigation reported by Chevrie and Aicardi (1977, 1978, Aicardi and Chevrie 1970) involved all forms of seizures occurring during the first year of life; the majority of the disorders (165 of 334) were infantile spasms. Of the 165, 9 per cent died by the time of follow-up, only 20 per cent were mentally normal, and 61 per cent were severely retarded. Death occurred most frequently in cases of infantile spasms with a symptomatic rather than idiopathic etiology. An investigation of the developmental histories of children with West syndrome by Ohtahara et al. (1980) found that 59.3 per cent of 108 West syndrome children continued to have seizures later in childhood; 85.9 per cent showed slow spike and wave discharge along with characteristic seizure patterns (Lennox-Gestault syndrome). The mental prognosis for cases that evolved from West into Lennox syndrome was particularly poor; this may be due to neuronal migration defects in such children recently described by Guerrini et al. (1992) and Ricci et al. (1992). Another aspect of the developmental course of surviving children is the increased prevalence of psychiatric disorders, particularly autistic and schizoid behavior patterns (Caplan et al. 1991, 1992a and b & c, Riikonen and Ammell 1981).

Febrile Seizures

Approximately 2 to 5 per cent of all children between 6 months and 5 years have one or more febrile seizures, accounting for between one-third to one-half of all the convulsive episodes in childhood. **Febrile seizures** occur soon after the onset of a febrile illness not directly affecting the CNS, usually 3 to 6 hours after the onset of the fever (Livingston 1972). However, febrile seizures can also be seen during the second or third day of an illness (Lennox-Buchtal 1973). Body temperature is usually at its peak at 39 to 40°C when the child seizes. Acute upper respiratory infection, tonsillitis, otitis media, and bronchial pneumonia are some common causes of febrile seizures. The seizure is usually generalized and of short duration, though some may last for 20 minutes or longer. Males are more susceptible to febrile seizures than females. Most investigators believe that there is an inherited susceptibility to seize above a certain threshold of body temperature, with autosomal dominant transmission (Brazier and Coceani 1978).

Children who have had a single febrile seizure have an excellent prognosis: there is little, if any, lasting neurological or mental deficit. The prognosis is less positive for children who have a febrile convulsion in conjunction with afebrile seizures, for those who have pre-existing CNS abnormalities, or if the fever-inducing infection involves the CNS (Wallace 1984).

In a long-term follow-up study, children who had febrile seizures were compared with their nearest-aged sibling on the WISC and the WRAT test of academic achievement at 7 years of age (Ellenberg and Nelson 1978, Ellenberg et al. 1986). The mean Full-scale IQ for the 431 febrile-group children, 93.0 (SD = 13.9), was not significantly different from the sibling group's mean IQ of 93.7 (SD = 12.8). WRAT performances, collected only from children with

IQs above 90, did not indicate any group differences in spelling, arithmetic, and reading abilities.

20.3 Epilepsy

Nature and Classifications

The term "**epilepsy**" refers to persistently recurrent attacks, usually of the same type of seizure, that are frequently accompanied by episodic and often chronic psychological changes and pathological activity in the EEG. It has been estimated that 0.5 per cent of the total population suffers from one of the many forms of epilepsy. The prevalence of epilepsy in children has been estimated as 1.9 per cent (Rose et al. 1973). Only about 15 per cent of children with occasional seizures develop epilepsy. In addition, epilepsy may develop later in life, usually during late adolescence or early adulthood, as well as after brain lesions acquired later in life.

Table 20-6 shows the widely accepted international classification of epileptic seizures (Gastaut 1983) based on type of seizure. Almost all forms of epilepsy

Table 20-6 International Classification of Epilepsies of Childhood

1. **Primary generalized epilepsies**
   True petit mal
   Tonic-clonic major seizures (grand mal)
   Combined petit/grand mal
   Primary myoclonic epilepsy

2. **Secondary generalized epilepsies**
   Associated with diffuse brain disease, including epilepsies secondary to specific encephalopathies and nonspecific encephalopathies (infantile spasms and Lennox-Gastaut syndrome)

3. **Primary partial epilepsies**
   With motor, sensorimotor, affective, or visual symptoms

4. **Secondary partial epilepsies ("lesional")**
   With elementary symptomatology
      with motor symptoms
      with special sensory or somatosensory symptoms
      with autonomic symptoms
   With complex symptomatology
      with impairment of consciousness only
      with cognitive symptoms
      with affective symptoms
      with psychosensory symptoms
      with psychomotor symptoms (automatisms)

Source: Gastaut 1983.

involve some type of abnormal motor activity. The classic form of a generalized seizure presents in succession both hypertonic spastic states and clonic movements of the musculature. A distinction among minor seizures (which frequently start in childhood and adolescence), focal seizures, and generalized seizures is frequently made. **Generalized seizures** include **petit mal epilepsy,** with sudden states of unresponsiveness and disruption of activity, which are occasionally accompanied by nystagmic upward eye movements; minimal jerky movements in the arms; short, sudden backward movements of the head; brief clouding of consciousness for a few seconds with dropping of the head forward; brief lifting of legs and hands. **Myoclonic seizures** are also of the generalized type. They show sudden loss of muscle tone, dropping to the floor, jerky movements of arms and face musculature, and oral automatisms. Frequent **absence seizures** (sudden loss of consciousness) with a characteristic EEG pattern are also described as generalized seizures.

Focal seizures (also known as partial seizures) are limited to parts of the body, frequently on one-half of the body, although they can spread and become secondarily generalized. Seizures of focal onset have their origin in various parts of the brain. If the precentral (motor) gyrus is involved, the symptoms of rigidity and clonic movements are confined to the opposite half of the body. Such elementary symptoms are called **focal motor seizures** or Jacksonian epilepsy. The prodromes of irritability and peculiar sensations (**auras**) frequently precede focal as well as other seizures. In psychomotor seizures (**complex partial seizures**), these auras may be simple sensations of smell and taste, but may also include more complex experiences, such as the feeling of strangeness or of stretching or condensing of time, mood changes, or outright hallucinations. These auras are sometimes followed by a limited clouding of consciousness with stereotyped movement sequences, e.g., chewing, smacking, swallowing, but also buttoning and unbuttoning the same button and similar patterns. The seizure is followed by a transient period of post-ictal confusion. Psychomotor seizures have been related specifically to temporal or frontal lobe damage and, in some cases, to specific damage in the area of the uncus (uncinate fits).

Generalized seizures often start with an initial shout, falling to the floor, turning of eyeballs upward or to the side, lack of pupil reaction, and tonic tension of the musculature. This is followed by rhythmic, clonic jerking for 1 or 2 minutes and usually a period of comatose sleep, often with subsequent disorientation ("fugue"). **Epileptic status** usually refers to grand mal seizures following each other so rapidly that consciousness does not fully return; status also may occur occasionally with psychomotor seizures.

Etiology

Although trauma has been suggested as the primary cause of epilepsy, a full variety of pre-, peri-, and postnatal disorders—including disorders of metabolism, infections, and anoxic episodes—have also been considered. In addition, a genetic continuum of degree of susceptibility to epilepsy has been proposed.

Annegers et al. (1982) found the risk of seizure disorders in relatives of patients with childhood-onset epilepsy to be 4.1 times as high as in the general population.

The developing brain is more susceptible to repeated seizure activity, with resulting cell death or at least inhibition of continuing cell enlargement and the formation of more complex connections between neurons. Hence, the effect on intelligence is more profound in children. Especially in children with uncontrollable seizures for a period of at least 2 years and with early onset, mental retardation is common (Huttenlocher and Hapke 1990).

The fundamental mechanism for triggering seizures and developing epilepsy remains unknown. Reviewing several studies of epilepsy in humans, monkeys, and cats, Wada (1964 p. 452) concluded that focal cortical epileptogenic lesions form the basis for the development of (1) an acquired epileptic tendency with heightened brain excitability and progressive lowering ("kindling") of seizure threshold, (2) an independent and irreversible epileptogenic functional alteration of deep structures and homologous cortical areas, (3) changes in spontaneous behavior between seizures and in patterns of seizures, and (4) impaired learning ability unrelated to overt electrographic seizures at the time of testing. Changes in the sodium-potassium balance, in the availability of GABA (an inhibitory neurotransmitter, Morselli et al. 1981), and in other biochemical mechanisms have been identified (National Institute of Neurological and Communicative Diseases and Stroke 1979). In animals (rats), experimentally induced epilepsy has been modulated by grafts of fetal GABAergic neurons (Fine et al. 1990).

20.4 Development During Infancy and Childhood

Intelligence and Academic Achievement

Considerable research has addressed the question of the long-term development and outcome of children with epilepsy. As shown in the previous section, even neonatal convulsive disorders have a relatively poor prognosis. Children with recurrent seizures and epilepsy would seem to run an even higher risk. In addition, deleterious effects of continuing anticonvulsant medication must be considered in connection with long-term outcome. Farwell et al. (1990), for example, found lower IQs in children with a history of febrile seizures who were long-time phenobarbital users, as compared to children who took placebo medication. Rodin et al. (1986) reported that phenobarbital, but not phenytoin, levels were inversely related to IQ, suggesting that a "therapeutic range" of this medication may be "toxic" with regard to learning abilities. The main metabolic mechanism in antiepileptic medication seems to be folate depletion (Corbett et al. 1985).

The neuropathological process underlying epilepsy is also closely related to outcome. Normal development can be expected in 10 to 20 per cent of children with hypoxic-ischemic encephalopathy, in 90 per cent of survivors of subarachnoid hemorrhage, in 10 per cent of children with intraventricular hemorrhage, in 50 per cent with hypocalcemia of early onset, in 35 to 50 per cent with hypocalcemia of late onset, in 20 to 50 per cent with bacterial meningitis, and in no children with developmental structural defect (National Institute of Neurological and Communicative Diseases and Stroke 1979).

Several studies have addressed the psychological performance, life adjustment, and numerous other characteristics of patients with epilepsy. Investigating the relation between seizure type and intelligence, Collins and Lennox (1947) found the poorest results in patients with both grand mal and psychomotor seizures and the best results in patients with petit mal only, with the second-highest IQs in children with psychomotor epilepsy (Table 20-7). Similar results were reported by Gudmundson (1966), Freudenberg (1971), and Sillanpaa (1983). In a detailed study of neuropsychological performance in children, O'Leary et al. (1983) reported that early onset, regardless of seizure type, places a child at risk for cognitive dysfunction.

Another detailed study by Freudenberg (1968) of 380 children and adolescents up to age 18 indicated that intelligence in epileptic children with prenatal damage was normal (then defined as IQ 90 to 110) only in 14.3 per cent and that 38.1 per cent of this group had severe retardation (IQ below 50). For birth trauma cases, 36.9 per cent had below-normal intelligence, but only 6.2 per cent had severe retardation. Similar results were found in children with cerebral damage during the first year of life (32.5 and 2.5 per cent, respectively); children with damage acquired later showed increasingly better intelligence, and 80 per cent of children damaged during the third year of life showed normal intelligence. Freudenberg noted that in two-thirds of the children developmental delay was present even before the occurrence of seizures, suggesting that the intellectual deficit for the most part is probably not a secondary effect of seizures per se or of environmental factors. Although there can be a latency period of up to several years between cerebral damage and the beginning of seizures, the degree and extent of intellectual retardation were smaller the later the epilepsy became manifest for all types of seizures (Freudenberg 1968).

Table 20-7   Intelligence of Epileptic Patients

	Children (Stanford)		Adults (Bellevue)	
	N	Average IQ	N	Average IQ
Petit mal only	18	113.2	38	114.0
Psychomotor only	8	108.0	21	112.2
Grand mal only	36	105.3	114	112.0
Grand mal and petit mal	25	102.7	79	112.6
Grand mal and psychomotor	11	102.2	42	105.9

Source: Collins 1951.

Harrison and Taylor (1976) reported a 25-year follow-up of 207 of an original sample of 628 children who were first seen at from birth to age 5 years because of seizures. The sample was stratified and corrected for attrition. Disregarding the reason for seizures, the authors reported that for two-thirds of the sample there were only minimal effects on academic and occupational achievement; 10 per cent of the survivors had been institutionalized, 10 per cent had died, and 6.6 per cent were invalids living with their parents. Primary risk factors for poor outcome were continuing seizures, including subsequent afebrile seizures, a history of seizures in parents and siblings, and pre-existing neurological damage. Mitchell et al. (1991) confirmed that underachievement is common, but no relation between achievement and severity or duration of seizure disorder or exposure to anticonvulsant medication was found. Older children and children from poor home environments were affected more severely. Another study of matched groups of children in the acute phase and in the chronic phase of epilepsy and of normal children found no difference on neuropsychological tests of frontal, parietal, and temporal lobe function (Rao et al. 1992). However, the type of seizure, age at onset, seizure frequency, and history of cluster attacks were associated with deficits in attention, kinetic melody, delayed response learning, and social functioning. In contrast, a more recent study by Niemann et al. (1985) found that age at onset was not predictive of the cognitive status of children with epilepsy, but that indices of EEG discharging activity and level of medication were strongly related to cognitive development. The estimated total number of major motor seizures in 10- to 14-year-old children has also been related to decrease of cognitive and neuropsychological function (Dean 1983).

A follow-up study of 100 children with temporal lobe epilepsy into adulthood (Lindsay et al. 1979) found 33 free of seizures and living independently, 32 socially and economically independent but receiving anticonvulsive medication and not necessarily seizure-free, and 30 dependent on parents or in institutions (5 had died before the age of 15).

Other Neuropsychological Sequelae

Bornstein et al. (1988) found that memory and attention were more disturbed in patients with complex partial seizures than in those with other seizure types. Even in children with subclinical epileptiform discharges, below-normal intelligence and specific deficits in verbal short-term memory have been reported (Kasteleijn-Nolst-Trenite et al. 1988, Siebelink et al. 1988). Holdsworth and Whitmore (1974) noted attentional problems in 42 per cent of epileptic children. Kasteleijn-Nolst-Trenite et al. (1990) reported that left-sided discharges are more frequently related to poor performance on verbal tasks and that right-sided discharges are more often related to visuospatial deficits. In the adult, impairment of sustained, focused attention is quite common, even when the patient has normal intelligence (McDaniels and McDaniels 1976), with the exception of psychomotor epilepsy of unknown origin (Matthews and Klove 1967).

Stores et al. (1978) examined the problems of activation, vigilance, attention, and distractibility in epileptic children by means of parent and teacher ratings, as well as vigilance tests. In their comparison of 71 epileptic and 35 healthy control children, boys tended to show more inattention, motor hyperactivity, poorer concentration, and poorer perceptual accuracy. The authors ruled out medication effects and interpreted the sex difference as a result of the higher vulnerability of boys to epileptogenic lesions. A breakdown into four groups was made: (1) 3/sec spike-and-wave pattern, (2) irregular spike-and-wave pattern, (3) right temporal focal spike discharge, and (4) left temporal focal spike discharge. Attentional function decreased in order from group 1 through 4, with boys with left temporal spike discharge showing the poorest performance. The results suggest that the left hemisphere in males is most vulnerable because of its relatively slower maturation. Hyperkinesis seems to accompany the inattention syndrome.

Freudenberg (1968) also reported poor performance on the Bender Gestalt test in epileptic children. Perceptual-motor problems were common in all epileptic groups, although again were most severe in symptomatic epilepsy. It was noted that even the least impaired petit mal group showed significant deficits relative to controls. In 96 severely impaired epileptic children between 5 and 18 years of age, three-quarters had substantial difficulties in coordination, and two-thirds showed dysarthria (Harvey et al. 1988). In relation to learning, Stores (1978) showed that epileptic boys had more reading problems than epileptic girls of the same age and socioeconomic environment. Again, children with focal epilepsy, and especially with left temporal discharge, showed the most severe reading impairment, whereas those with right temporal discharge showed no difference from controls. Children with left temporal lobe seizures performed more poorly on auditory-verbal memory tasks, whereas children with right temporal lobe seizures had more impairment on visuospatial memory tasks (Cohen 1992).

Educational and Occupational Outcome

Holdsworth and Whitmore (1974) examined the school progress of 85 epileptic children and adolescents in rural British communities. For half of the sample, the seizures started within the first 5 years of life. Eighty children were still on medication at the time of the study. Thirteen children had frequent seizure activity (defined as at least one seizure a month). Average-to-superior school progress was reported for 31.2 per cent, 53.1 per cent were "holding their own" at or below average levels, and 15.6 per cent were seriously falling behind their peers. Rates of failure were greater than among nonepileptic pupils. Six children were poor in all subjects, whereas most others showed relatively specific areas of weakness: reading (10), writing (5), speech (4), spelling (2), memory (2), and incoordination (10). Of the 21 children who were doing well academically, 5 were very good in all subjects, 3 only in arts, 6 in oral work, 2 in mathematics and science, 1 in French, and 4 in physical education.

In a study of 200 children with epilepsy, Whitehouse (1976) found that 70 per cent required special education and that even in the remaining 30 per cent "some still showed minor learning problems, enough to raise difficulties in classroom situations" (p. 23). Rodin and Rennick (1979) found a poor socioeconomic and occupational outlook for epileptics, which they ascribed partly to inadequate schooling. A 20-year prospective follow-up of 233 children in northern Finland (including those living in institutions at the time of follow-up) found that 27 per cent were unable to complete even basic education, 40 per cent completed primary education, 31 per cent completed lower or upper secondary education, and only 1.5 per cent attended college or university. Forty per cent were on permanent disability pension, 3 per cent on temporary disability or sickness leave, and 57 per cent were normally employed, mostly in manual or unskilled occupations. Only 12.6 per cent completed regular compulsory military service; 72 per cent were not married (Sillanpaa 1983). Nevertheless, 80 per cent felt that the epilepsy had only a slight or no effect on their lives and choices. Favorable social-occupational outcome was found to be related to the occurrence of one seizure type only, good short-term treatment outcome, absence of status epilepticus, and normal mental development. In the United States, Clemmons and Dodrill (1983) reported that 43 per cent of 42 epileptic adolescents were either employed or involved in continuing education, whereas 57 per cent reported no competitive employment, with 31 per cent of these receiving federal living subsidies. State vocational rehabilitation services were made available to 36 per cent, with a placement rate of 13 per cent. Vocational adjustment and living skills were strongly related to test results emphasizing language skills and less to tests of emotional adjustment (Dodrill and Clemmons 1983).

Behavior Problems

Reviewing reports of behavior problems in epileptic children, Remschmidt (1981) stressed that the type of problem is age related. During infancy and early childhood, motor restlessness, aggressiveness, intolerance of frustration, increased sibling rivalry, and disorders in play behavior and in integration in social groups are common, whereas in school-aged children cognitive deficits, problems of social integration, and isolation are predominant. These latter problems become more pronounced during puberty and adolescence, often complicated by personality alterations (lack of drive, psychomotor slowing, rigidity). Harvey et al. (1988) identified a large number of epileptic children with mood disturbances. They noted that many of the symptoms could be due at least in part to the anticonvulsant medication (e.g., motor restlessness with phenobarbital) as well as to the underlying organic damage, rather than to epilepsy itself. At times, behavior problems may disappear entirely after a change in medication. Freudenberg (1971) found many reactive disorders—especially in cases of petit mal seizures—including depression, psychosomatic and sleep disorders, and anxiety, but rarely psychomotor retardation and personality alteration. Similar findings were reported by Stores (1978), Stores et al. (1978), and Gebelt (1971).

Another reactive disorder frequently mentioned is increased emotional dependence on the mother and other important people in the child's life (Hartlage et al. 1972); such problems are mainly related to environmental stress and upbringing (Boldyrev 1987). Epileptic school-aged children make suicide attempts 15 times more often than expected in a population of that age (Brent 1986).

Whether or not there is a characteristic epileptic personality has been debated for some time (Whitman et al. 1984). Studies of children with epilepsy show that personality alterations do not become apparent until puberty and that a relatively large number of adolescents do not show a classical syndrome or, for that matter, any striking personality alteration at all. Sohns (1981), for example, did not find that personality characteristics differentiated between special school students with a history of seizures who currently had seizures and those who were seizure-free (although cognitive and performance tests did). If present, the hyperkinetic and the rigid-sticky type of personality alterations seemed to be most frequent. In addition, persistence of affect is often mentioned, i.e., such adolescents, once irritated or angry, cannot channel their emotion and may lose control. An association between temporal lobe epilepsy and aggression and violence has been reported widely, although some studies insist that it is not the temporal lobe damage but the damage or dysfunction of the basal forebrain that may be associated with such behavior (Stevens and Hermann 1981). Another report indicated that depression may be the most frequent psychopathology during adolescence (Kaminer et al. 1988). A report on 100 children with temporal lobe epilepsy indicated that, of the 13 children who underwent temporal lobe excision, all showed no further seizure activity and improved social, psychiatric, and personality functioning compared to those who did not undergo the operation (Lindsay et al. 1984). The authors noted, however, that males were more often single and sexually indifferent, particularly if seizures continued during adolescence (Lindsay et al. 1979).

Freudenberg (1968) demonstrated a relationship between personality alteration and intellectual defect (Figure 20-4). The highest number of personality alterations was found with symptomatic grand mal seizures; they were least frequent in patients with petit mal and in patients with early onset of epilepsy. It must be remembered, however, that rigidity and perseveration, as well as hyperactivity, may not be direct consequences of the disorder itself, but rather a coping mechanism developed by epileptic patients in an attempt to maintain emotional balance against increasing intellectual and social demands with which they are unable to cope. In this sense, Remschmidt (1972) viewed the behavioral changes as a balancing attempt with regression to a lower level of biological and psychosocial functioning.

In a review of psychotic disorders associated with epilepsy, Rentz (1979) found psychoses to be rare but, if present, to manifest themselves between the ages of 7 and 14. Most cases were described as delirious psychosis with paranoia and hallucinations. Lindsay et al. (1979) noted that 85 per cent of the children in their follow-up had psychiatric problems in childhood, but that in adulthood 70 per cent of this part of their population (excluding those with mental handi-

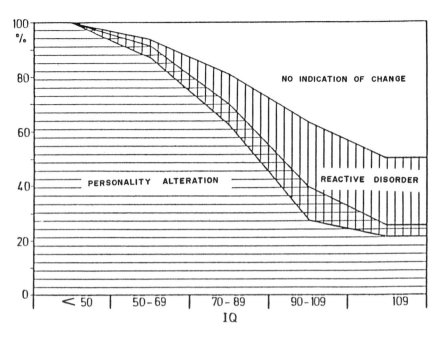

Figure 20-4. Proportion of 380 epileptic children with personality alterations and reactive disorders in relation to intelligence (Freudenberg 1968).

cap) were psychiatrically healthy. They found schizophrenia in 10 per cent of their population with continuing epilepsy with left hemisphere focus. No psychiatric disorders were found in those with right hemisphere focus. Wolf and Forsythe (1978) listed the following contributing factors for psychiatric disorders: long duration of epilepsy without seizure-free periods, psychotic episodes in the history, abnormal psychosocial factors, disorders of intellect, poor perception, poor performance in school, and the use of certain antiepileptic medications. In addition, hallucinatory phenomena before the seizure (aura) and the disorientation after the seizure (postictal fugue) may directly contribute to the appearance of psychosis or psychotic-like features in epileptics.

Summary

The convulsive disorders of infancy and childhood represent a heterogeneous set of symptoms, with varied etiologies and different prognoses for later-life neurological and mental normality. It is not possible to examine the consequences of a convulsive disorder independently of the underlying etiological condition. Why some newborn babies suffering perinatal anoxia, for example, have seizures, whereas others do not is a question of both empirical and practical importance, and the answer is presumably related to the extent and location of tissue damage. In general terms, children who suffer from infantile spasms tend to be severely mentally retarded at follow-up; those few who recover to normal-range capability seem to do so more as a function of the type of underlying etiology, rather than because of any successful therapeutic intervention. The consequences of neonatal seizures seem dichotomous: roughly half the children will recover to normal-range capabilities, whereas the other half die or suffer persistent and severe neurological and mental difficulties. On the other hand, febrile seizures are relatively benign, and recovery without lasting sequelae is the norm.

Epilepsy—recurrent and persistent seizure activity—is frequently associated with motor disorders, but may be the only major symptom of structural damage or may occur for unknown reasons (idiopathic). Of the several forms of epilepsy in children, petit mal seizures seem to have the least and focal left temporal and grand mal seizures the strongest association with intellectual and visuomotor deficit, especially in boys. Personality and behavior disorders are closely related to the degree of intellectual impairment and occur most frequently in grand mal epilepsy.

21

Hemispherectomy and Other Surgical Manipulations

Much recent neuropsychological research has been concerned with the development of different functional capabilities in each hemisphere. The extreme situation, where one hemisphere has complete control of all physiological and behavioral functioning, is very rare. This chapter reviews an example of lateral dominance where most of one cerebral hemisphere has been removed surgically. The main indications for this type of surgery are extensive invasion of the hemisphere by tumor, usually in adults, and infantile hemiplegia associated with neonatal convulsions. Hemispherectomy is more accurately called **hemidecortication,** or removal of half of the cortex, since primarily cortical tissue is removed; the thalamus and striatum, as well as brainstem connections, usually remain. Often, portions of the frontal and the occipital pole are also left in place to minimize the postoperative shift of the remaining hemisphere into the space left by the removed hemisphere (**Montreal-type hemispherectomy,** Verity et. al. 1982). However, the terms "hemidecortication" and "hemispherectomy" are used interchangeably in the literature to refer to essentially the same surgical procedure. Other relevant surgical manipulations that radically alter the functioning of the brain are also discussed in this chapter.

Hemispherectomy is important in developmental neuropsychology because it may illuminate various aspects of the development of the cerebral hemispheres and their ability to recover from surgically imposed insults during childhood. Unfortunately, the available follow-up studies have not provided definitive answers, partly because of the infrequency of the operation, partly because the data reported have often been incomplete and without standardized test results, and partly because of the paucity of long-term follow-up. Nevertheless, the available studies shed some light on the relation between hemispherectomy in adulthood and in childhood and the differential hemispheric specialization during development. Extensive reviews have been written by Dimond (1972a), Piacentini and Hynd (1988), and Smith (1974).

Hemispherectomy for the most part removes diseased tissue that is already nonfunctional. Hence, it is likely that the lesion itself has caused changes that predate surgery. Improvement of function after hemispherectomy is found mainly because of successful reduction of seizure activity.

21.1   Hemispherectomy for Tumor

Hemispherectomy for tumor is performed if one cerebral hemisphere is invaded by pathological tissue, such as by a malignant glioma, which occurs most frequently in adults and only rarely in children. The clinical picture after surgery is rather devastating. Many abilities normally subserved by the hemisphere are severely affected or lost. For example, a postoperative hemiplegia is invariably seen in adults. As with any malignant cerebral tumor, the possibility for recurrence of the tumor in other regions of the brain is high. Because of the poor survival rate, few long-term follow-up studies of adult hemispherectomy patients have been conducted. The potential for follow-up is much greater if the hemispherectomy is performed on patients with infantile hemiplegia (discussed in the next section).

The rationale for hemispherectomy in tumor cases was developed by Dandy (1928). He reasoned that, since each of the lobes of a hemisphere could be removed individually without dramatic impairment, it was logical to expect that the entire hemisphere (in his cases, the right hemisphere) could be removed with little future impairment. In his initial report of five cases of right hemispherectomy for tumor, Dandy noted no major effects on language, general intelligence, or personality. However, he did not have the results of detailed performance tests, and the patients were not followed over time.

Zollinger (1935) reported the first case of a left hemispherectomy for tumor performed on an adult. He found, surprisingly after removal of so much cerebral tissue from the patient's dominant hemisphere, that many language abilities remained intact, including an elementary vocabulary. However, the patient died 17 days after the operation, and no formal tests were given to document the findings. During the next two decades, there were only a small number of similar ablations for tumors.

More detailed studies of hemispherectomy for tumor have been conducted since the 1960s. Smith and his colleagues (Burklund and Smith 1977, Smith, 1966, 1969, Smith and Burklund 1966) presented several case reports of hemispherectomy for tumor in adults. In one case, a 47-year-old man who underwent a left (dominant) hemispherectomy for glioma was followed postoperatively and examined in detail with standardized tests. Immediately after the operation, the patient showed a right hemiplegia, a right hemianopia, and severe aphasia. During a 7-month follow-up, continuing recovery of language functions was observed. Smith (1966) concluded that the remaining right hemisphere makes some contribution to normal language performance, especially to receptive language. In 1969, Smith studied three cases of right (nondominant) hemispherectomy and found that all three patients showed specific nonlanguage deficits but no aphasia or other language disorder.

Based on these and past case reports, Smith (1969) compared the behavioral effects of right and left hemispherectomy for tumor in adults. He concluded that the left hemisphere plays a greater role than the right in speech, reading, and writing, but not verbal comprehension. He suggested that the right hemisphere is specialized primarily for nonverbal reasoning and visual ideational capacities, as evidenced by the marked impairment in these abilities after the removal of the nondominant hemisphere. Smith (1974) noted that hemispherectomy patients showed no evidence of other mental changes (psychosis, bizarre behavior, etc.) often associated with other cortical ablations.

Gott (1973a) studied one left and two right adult hemispherectomy cases. Using a general battery of neuropsychological tests, she demonstrated that after a hemispherectomy there is a memory defect, regardless of the side of operation. Specific lateralized deficits similar to those in previous reports were seen; the two right hemispherectomies showed greater nonverbal deficits, and the left hemispherectomy patient had greater verbal and language difficulties.

The systematic differences between right and left hemispherectomy reports in adults are consistent with the cerebral lateralization literature: massive removal of a cerebral hemisphere leads to hemisphere-specific deficits. Patients with a right hemispherectomy usually show left-side sensory and motor symptoms, as well as disturbed nonverbal capacities, while maintaining most language abilities. Patients with a left hemispherectomy show disturbed right-side sensory and motor functions and a severe disturbance in language. Because of the paucity of long-term follow-up studies, the issue of the "recovery" of lost abilities cannot be addressed adequately.

21.2 Hemispherectomy for Infantile Hemiplegia and Sturge-Weber Syndrome

The onset of infantile hemiplegia, i.e., unilateral paralysis in early childhood or infancy, is acute at or near birth in 75 per cent of cases, is frequently preceded or followed by convulsions, and in many cases is associated with mental retardation or some degree of personality or behavioral disturbance. Although the clinical picture is similar in most cases, the pathological disturbance can arise from one of three factors:

(1) Conditions present before or associated with birth, such as an anoxic episode, or hemorrhage during labor
(2) Conditions acquired after birth, usually a specific cerebrovascular disease, such as embolism associated with acute infectious diseases, or cortical trauma accompanied by hemorrhage
(3) **Sturge-Weber disease,** in which a slow-growing tumor affects the blood vessels (angioma) in the area of the trigeminal nerve (inner-

vating one half of the face and eye), causing inadequate blood supply to the brain, brain atrophy, and calcifications, which are often accompanied by focal or generalized seizures, hemianopia, hemiplegia, and progressively poorer mental function (Hoffman et al. 1979)

The prognosis for infantile hemiplegia without intervention depends upon the amount of injury to the nervous system. The presence of convulsions makes the outlook less favorable because deterioration often occurs in such cases, presumably related to greater hemispheric damage. Treatment of infantile hemiplegia before about 1950 was largely directed at the control of seizures and correction of the physical deformities resulting from prolonged hemiplegia and spasticity. On the whole, results of treatment were not encouraging; many patients were institutionalized because of severe intractable seizures and behavior disorders, as well as permanent hemiplegia.

After Dandy's (1928) report of cerebral hemispherectomy in adults, McKenzie (1938) performed a hemidecortication in a young woman because of intractable epilepsy associated with spastic hemiplegia. After the operation, the patient's seizures stopped, and her general health and alertness improved but her hemiplegia remained unchanged. Krynauw (1950) carried out 12 hemispherectomies for infantile hemiplegia over a 5-year period. His patients ranged in age from 8 months to 21 years and included ten left hemispherectomies and two right hemispherectomies. In all except one of the patients, the injury occurred during the first 10 months of life. Significant improvement in overall functioning was reported. None of the cases (including those with left hemispherectomy) showed impairment of speech as a consequence of the operation. No specific psychological documentation was presented. Krynauw argued that hemispheric dominance had "adjusted itself" before the operation as a result of the early neural injury (causing the hemiplegia) and that it was therefore the minor hemisphere that was removed in all cases.

Krynauw also specified that in all cases hemiplegia alone was not a sufficient indication for the operation. He insisted on the demonstration of unilateral cerebral disease by either air contrast studies or by a triad of symptoms: hemiplegia, seizures, and the presence of lowered intellectual functioning and/or uncontrolled emotional outbursts. Krynauw's favorable results established hemispherectomy as an acceptable and widely adopted form of treatment for certain cases of infantile hemiplegia.

21.3 Psychological Outcome of Hemispherectomy for Infantile Hemiplegia

The first studies of hemispherectomy to include psychological tests generally found good recovery of intellectual functions after the operation. Cairns and Davidson (1951) reported on three patients, two right-sided and one left-sided operation. All three patients showed general clinical improvement and an increase in intelligence test scores after the operation, with an average increase of about 20 IQ points. Munz and Tolor (1955) summarized the psychological test findings on four cases of hemispherectomy performed on patients between the ages of 14 and 24 years, emphasizing several important limitations of their findings: there were unequal intervals between the time of operation and psychological testing of the patients, there was a lack of controls, and postoperative follow-up periods were short. However, Munz and Tolor did consider the operations a success; the seizures stopped, and there was no permanent increase in motor weakness. The patients were generally more pleasant and manageable, but did show some personality changes, namely, increased feelings of morbidity and inadequacy. Munz and Tolor offered no reason for these personality changes. Although there were generally postoperative increases in IQ, Munz and Tolor stressed the importance of the premorbid intelligence level of the patient; only in cases with near-average preoperative intelligence, and presumably with one hemisphere functioning normally, can significant increases in IQ be expected. Hence, the previous psychological make-up of the individual must be considered when evaluating the effects of hemispherectomy.

During the 1960s and early 1970s, reviews and reports of larger series of hemispherectomy patients were presented, possible surgical pitfalls of the operation pointed out, and the long-term results of the operation questioned. A review by White (1961) of 269 cases from the world literature demonstrated an operative mortality of 6.6 per cent and a high rate of complications. White's review suggested that in the majority of cases overall improvement in functioning did result, including reduction of antisocial behavior. Carmichael (1966) expressed his disillusionment with results of the operation because of the inexplicable late complications occurring in otherwise healthy patients after surgery. Ignelzi and Bucy (1968), on the other hand, suggested that "practically all children suffering from this condition should have a cerebral hemidecortication" (p. 15) because of the remarkable clinical and psychological improvement.

Verity et al. (1982) reported a follow-up study of 8 infantile hemiplegics reviewed 3 to 16 years after hemispherectomy. The authors found that, although postoperative complications were frequent, the operation was followed by a marked reduction in seizure frequency and improvement in behavior; there was little overall change in intellect or hemiplegia. Four of the patients showed borderline intelligence.

Wilson (1970) and Goodman (1986) attempted to reconcile the various postoperative findings and concluded that cerebral hemispherectomy in infantile cerebral disorder has a low operative mortality; the improvement in seizures and behavior disorder occurred in from 70 to 90 per cent of patients. However, late complications occurred in as many as 33 per cent of hemispherectomy patients and as early as one year and as late as 20 years after surgery (Tinuper et al. 1988); the cardinal complication in 30 to 40 per cent of the cases is subdural hemorrhage, resulting in obstructive hydrocephalus of the remaining hemisphere. Goodman (1986) pointed out that surgical procedures, including subtotal hemispherectomy, **Oxford-type hemispherectomy** (Adams 1983, Beardsworth and Adams 1988) with dural closure of the cavity, and commissurotomy, to correct or minimize the complications were available, and therefore long-term postoperative complications were remediable if not avoidable. For example, fatal late complications with the Montreal-type hemispherectomy have been reported in only 5 per cent of cases (Rasmussen 1983). Good outcome on long-term follow-up (up to 36 years) was also reported by Lindsay et al. (1987).

In a review of large-scale psychological studies, McFie (1961) criticized the failure to obtain pre- and post-hemispherectomy indices of intellectual ability. He made repeated IQ measures of 34 hemispherectomized hemiplegic patients, ranging in age from birth to 5 years at the time of onset of hemiplegia and from one to 31 years old at the time of hemispherectomy. Twenty-one cases had a right and 13 cases a left hemispherectomy. McFie compared the test scores of 28 of the cases with those of 9 patients with partial hemispheric removal and found that the hemispherectomy patients displayed a greater increase in test scores after the operation. The IQ increase was found exclusively in patients with onset of infantile hemiplegia during the first year of life. He found no significant difference in the postoperative increase in scores between cases of left and right hemispherectomy in the infantile hemiplegia group and argued for a "critical period" for hemispherectomy recovery up to one year of age during which the two hemispheres were still equipotential. McFie found that the greatest improvement occurred in patients with normal EEGs in the remaining hemisphere.

In contrast to earlier studies, McFie noted that the majority of patients showed a verbal intellectual deficit, in some cases dysphasia, irrespective of the hemisphere damaged. He attributed the results to a limit on the capacity of the remaining hemisphere to take on the normal function of both hemispheres, i.e., an overloading of the remaining hemisphere. St. James-Roberts (1979, 1981) reviewed McFie's classic study and noted several shortcomings: confounding of interage comparisons by differential status of the residual hemisphere, overdependence on unreliable IQ scores from young children, unequal distribution of three different psychometric tests across age groups, and inadequate control of recovery-period characteristics.

Basser (1962) investigated hemispherectomy with special reference to speech in 102 cases of hemiplegia of early onset; 48 cases had left hemisphere lesions, 54 had right hemisphere lesions, and hemispherectomy was performed in 35 cases. In 17 the left hemisphere was removed, and in 18 cases the right. Basser considered whether the cerebral lesion was sustained before or after the onset of speech. He found that with regard to speech, hemispherectomy was beneficial in some cases, but in the majority speech was unchanged. Basser concluded that speech was developed and maintained in the intact hemisphere and that in this respect the left and right hemispheres were "equipotential." One of Basser's major conclusions was that the verbal IQ of his patients remained unchanged, regardless of which hemisphere was removed. However, as St. James-

Roberts (1979) pointed out, only 20 hemispherectomies were reported in detail, and no verbal IQ scores were provided. In addition, the IQs that were reported were generally low, indicating severe mental handicap and probably damage to the residual hemisphere. Basser did not use formal quantitative tests, but merely provided short descriptive phrases, such as "speech improved" or "dysphasic."

Griffith and Davidson (1966) presented the results of three patients with right hemispherectomy and 8 patients with left hemispherectomy for infantile hemiplegia who were tested preoperatively, postoperatively, and 4 to 15 years later on standardized IQ tests. They found systematic differences in the effects of hemispherectomy on language functions, but not on nonlanguage functions. Two right hemispherectomy patients had higher verbal than nonverbal abilities, and two left hemispherectomy patients had higher nonverbal than verbal skills. The authors suggested that the transfer of an ability from one hemisphere to the other after early brain damage may be incomplete and questioned whether the hemisphere removed was actually the nondominant hemisphere, as Krynauw had suggested.

More recent hemispherectomy research includes detailed neuropsychological procedures and more careful case descriptions and controls. Several long-term follow-up studies have been published. However, even recent studies provide only limited information. For example, Caplan et al. (1992) reported only that nonverbal communication had improved postsurgically in 10 children with a mean age of 3½ years.

A series of studies by Dennis and colleagues (Dennis 1977, 1980a, Dennis and Kohn 1975, Dennis and Whitaker 1976, Dennis et al. 1981, Kohn and Dennis 1974) focused on differences in the information processing skills of left and right hemidecorticated infantile hemiplegics and Sturge-Weber patients, carefully matched for age at hemiplegia, age at hemidecortication, and verbal IQ. The authors demonstrated that right and left hemisphere differences cannot simply be attributed to gross verbal-nonverbal distinctions. Their tests compared specific linguistic capacities, such as syntax, between the two groups. Right hemidecorticates tend to be significantly better in the understanding of syntax than left hemidecorticates. Conversely, using right hemisphere visuospatial tasks, Dennis and collaborators found that left hemidecorticates are markedly superior in performance. These findings have been supported by other hemispherectomy studies (Damasio et al. 1975, Gott 1973b, Zaidel 1979, 1978) and imply that previous studies relied too much on single, gross measures of hemispheric performance, such as verbal IQ.

Another detailed report by Netley (1972) compared the dichotic listening performance of 12 patients who were hemispherectomized for infantile hemiplegia and 12 matched controls. He found that congenitally injured patients performed differently than patients injured in infancy: the infantile injuries group recalled less material presented to the ear ipsilateral to the remaining hemisphere than the congenitally injured patients. Netley suggested that injury during the infantile period has a more permanent effect on the dichotic performance. Damasio et al. (1975) reported a case of right hemispherectomy performed on a 20-year-old woman who had suffered head trauma at age 5. They found improvement in left-sided sensory and motor performances over time, suggesting significant "adaptation" even in a mature brain. Zulch (1974) has noted, however, that much recovery may be due to strengthening of ipsilateral connections before the hemispherectomy.

Hemispherectomy is invariably followed by hemianopia because of the removal of the respective occipital lobe. Ptito et al. (1987) studied visual discrimination in four hemispherectomized patients matched with two control subjects, requiring them to indicate whether two stimuli, presented simultaneously in the two hemifields, were the same or different. Hemispherectomized patients failed on this task when it was presented two-dimensionally (patterns), but performed significantly above chance level with three-dimensional object presentation. The authors concluded that alternate visual structures, such as the superior colliculi, and the abilities of the remaining hemisphere, were responsible for these residual visual capacities.

A study of considerable import by Smith and Sugar (1975) dealt with the long-term follow-up of a boy who showed cyanotic difficulties at birth, right hemiparesis at 5 months, and right-sided seizures at age 3.8 years. A left hemispherectomy was performed at age 5.5. Postoperatively, EEG abnormalities disappeared from the remaining right hemisphere, and the seizures ceased entirely. Before the operation the patient's mental age was reported to be 4.0 years with a marked speech defect, but with normal verbal comprehension. Four months after surgery he showed marked improvement; his mental age had risen to a value approximate to his chronological age, and his speech had rapidly become normal. When tested 3 years later, his mental age was 7 years, 10 months, only slightly below his chronological age of 8 years, 8 months. In a first follow-up report, 15.5 years after the operation at the age of 21, a comprehensive battery of neuropsychological tests was given. On most of the tests, the patient scored in the average range. The WAIS Verbal IQ (113; in the bright normal range) was 15 points higher than the Performance IQ of 98. During re-examination with the same battery 5.5 years later at the age of 26.5, Smith and Sugar found that the patient had made even more remarkable progress—he was completing college and was working in an executive position. The development of his intellectual and language capabilities was also reflected in his test scores: a WAIS Full-scale IQ increase from 107 to 116, a slight increase in his Performance IQ from 98 to 102, and a large increase in his Verbal IQ from 113 to 126. Other tests documented similar above-average findings. Considering the demonstrated superior verbal abilities and average nonverbal, visuospatial capacities, it is difficult to conceive that this patient received a *left* hemispherectomy 21 years earlier! In a more recent report, Smith et al. (1988) confirmed the rapid improvement of cerebral functions after right hemispherectomy in a 6-year-old boy and ascribed it to the effect of diaschisis, i.e., that removal of the diseased tissue allows undamaged portions of the brain to resume normal functioning (see Chapter 8).

In contrast, Byrne and Gates (1987) described a 5-year follow-up of a boy who underwent left hemispherectomy at the age of 6 months. Preoperatively, he showed normal development; postoperatively, he showed delayed development with normal maturation of functions, similar to that reported after early brain trauma. No specific impairment of either linguistic-communicative or visuo-motor-spatial functions was apparent.

To summarize, detailed recent reports of hemispherectomy for infantile hemiplegia, with the exception of Smith's case, seem to coincide more closely with the reports of hemispherectomy for tumor in adults than with the earlier child hemispherectomy reports indicating highly optimistic functional "recovery" in children. It seems that these earlier reports did not use sensitive enough tests to detect hemisphere-specific deficits. It should also be remembered that successful elimination of seizure activity itself and the subsequent withdrawal of sedative anticonvulsant medication may contribute to better performance.

21.4 Implications of Hemispherectomy Research

Data from hemispherectomy reports have a bearing on two issues. First, assuming that lateralization is present in the young brain, recovery in infantile hemiplegics undergoing hemispherectomy has been interpreted as indicating the plasticity of the young brain, since some type of radical reorganization appears more likely than after adult hemispherectomy. Second, given that there is some recovery after a hemispherectomy performed early in life, what is the effect of the removal of a cerebral hemisphere on the lateralized abilities represented in that hemisphere? Assuming no shift in function from the removed to the remaining hemisphere, hemispherectomy seems to indicate that lateralization is not present early in infancy and that functions are represented in both hemispheres. This finding would support the concept of "equipotentiality" discussed in Chapter 5. We consider these two issues separately.

Plasticity

Isaacson (1975, 1976) has emphasized that hemispherectomy studies provide the only human experimental cases analogous to animal lesion studies, in that both the tissue ablated and the substrate of remaining function are known. Hemispherectomy reports have been interpreted to show that the immature brain is "functionally plastic" (Smith 1974) in the sense that a function normally subserved by one cortical hemisphere may be transferred or relearned by the other hemisphere as long as damage to the original hemisphere occurs early in life. The adult-child comparisons seen in the early hemispherectomy reports tended to support this view as they indicated greater recoverability and less vulnerability in the child's brain because fewer deficits were observed after the operation.

As discussed in Chapter 8, the groundwork for the belief in the diminished vulnerability of the immature brain was laid in animal work by Kennard in the late 1930s and early 1940s. Many experiments with animals confirmed that, when the behavioral effects of lesions differ according to the age at which they are inflicted, the difference is one of greater sparing of function for the earlier lesion (Teuber and Rudel 1971); this has been termed the "Kennard principle" (Schneider 1979). Many of the early hemispherectomy studies were interpreted as following this principle; for example, McFie's (1961) conclusions about juvenile versus congenital lesions. Differential recovery after hemispherectomy has even been used to to determine the critical period of infant cortical plasticity. Based almost solely on hemispherectomy reports, this period has variously been set at 12 months (McFie 1961), 17 months (Netley 1972), 5 years (Krashen 1973), 12 years (Lenneberg 1967, based on Basser 1962), and 15 years (Obrador 1964) of age.

Most of the recent hemispherectomy studies, however, have not directly supported the Kennard principle; some, such as the studies of Isaacson (1975) and Fletcher and Satz (1983), have rejected it completely. Dennis and colleagues in particular have argued that with appropriate testing procedures deficits similar to, though less severe than, those seen in adult tumor cases can be described in children. A comprehensive review by St. James-Roberts (1981) concluded that the hemispherectomy data fail to support the differential plasticity model. Although some cases, notably Smith and Sugar's (1975) left hemispherectomy case, seem to provide direct evidence for the greater functional plasticity of the young brain, the bulk of the studies provide no evidence of greater recovery from childhood lesions (indeed, there may be *less* recovery; see Kolb 1989 and Robinson 1981).

Lateralization and Equipotentiality

The data reviewed in Chapter 5 suggest that differential lateralization between the hemispheres may be genetically determined and that it develops at an early age. The opposite concept, equipotentiality, maintains that both hemispheres are equally capable of carrying out all cognitive functions in early life and that progressive lateralization occurs as the child grows older. During the equipotential period, variously estimated to end sometime between age one year and puberty, one hemisphere can fully compensate for the loss of function in the other. Hemispherectomy data showing greater functional recovery in children were once thought to support the equipotentiality concept; however, recent hemispherectomy studies and the critique of the plasticity concept described above indicate just the opposite; namely, that differential specialization of the hemispheres is present very early in life. Thus, a left hemispherectomy in childhood will result in some type of linguistic impairment, and a right hemispherectomy will result in some visuospatial deficit. The theory of equipotentiality, or the similar concept of "safety (or duplication) in the nervous system" expressed by Campbell (1960), therefore does not seem to be supported by the effects of hemispherectomy.

In an attempt to reconcile the earlier reports of nervous system plasticity with the evidence suggesting specific deficits similar to the adult pattern of reciprocal specialization of the hemispheres, Teuber and Rudel (1967, 1971) discussed the "necessary cost" of early brain damage; by this term they implied that, after the removal of large amounts of tissue, there is necessarily a diminished developmental capacity. As a specific example, Teuber suggested that, when language develops in the right hemisphere of children with left hemisphere lesions, it does so at the expense of the development of nonlanguage functions. Presumably, in a case of left hemispherectomy, language functions move into the intact right hemisphere, which results in a **crowding effect** in which a limit is imposed on the development of nonverbal functions. This crowding effect is very similar to McFie's (1961) notion of "overloading" a hemisphere. Smith (1974, Smith and Sugar 1975) noted, however, that the crowding effect can be explained more parsimoniously by assuming that the presence or absence of damage to the remaining hemisphere is the critical factor determining the extent of development for language and nonlanguage functions. Instead of the crowding concept, Smith et al (1972) proposed a developmental hierarchy in which language functions take precedence over reasoning functions. Language is therefore considered a more necessary ability in humans and is preserved first. A case report by Ogden (1988a and b) offered a similar interpretation. Two cases of late left hemispherectomy showed only minimal comprehension deficits, suggesting that the right hemisphere can mediate verbal memory and more subtle aspects of language; however, the patients were severely impaired in nonverbal memory, cognitive visuospatial skills, and complex extrapersonal orientation, usually considered as right hemisphere functions; other "right hemisphere functions," such as simple visuospatial and orientation abilities, emotional expression, and face recognition, were normal. The author interpreted these findings as supporting the hierarchical takeover of functions, i.e., that the right hemisphere assumes those functions most essential for independent survival while those least required are crowded out. Other case studies by Bigler and Naugle (1985) accepted the same hierarchical process of plasticity. Recently, Satz et al. (1994) presented data on epileptic patients whose speech dominance had been determined by carotid amytal tests. They found that all patients with left- or bilateral language dominance had onset of epilepsy before the age of 12 months, suggesting interhemispheric transfer of language. In early-onset patients, however, not only nonverbal, but also verbal abilities were more impaired than in late-onset patients, suggesting that crowding effects are most pronounced if damage occurs in infancy.

The timing of the "shift" in functions may or may not be related to the time of hemispherectomy. Since the operation is performed to remove diseased, largely nonfunctional tissue, a functional reorganization of the brain may occur well before surgery. In fact, no shift in functions need be assumed in congenital defects. In cases of perinatal or early infantile damage, it has been assumed that the diseased hemisphere may continue to function and in fact hinder the shift to the other hemisphere and that only through hemispherectomy will the healthy part of the brain be "released" to assume full functioning and to develop all the abilities of which it is capable. Such considerations of timing do not affect the notions of crowding and developmental hierarchy discussed above, but may explain the remarkable recovery in many cases after a considerable amount of cortical tissue has been removed.

Piacenti and Hynd (1988) disagreed with the strict hierarchical plasticity concept and argued, as do Fletcher and Satz, that more recent studies, especially the work of Dennis, provide support for a genetically predetermined linguistic system and an age-independent model of recovery from brain damage. They state that "any early damage affecting the central speech zones will have a variable but nonetheless important impact on linguistic development in the majority of infants and children" (p. 595).

21.5   Other Surgical Manipulations in Childhood

Other surgical manipulations in childhood of interest to neuropsychologists include temporal lobectomy, surgical removal of tissue because of tumor (Pizzo and Poplack 1993), and the repair of cerebrovascular malformations and aneurysm. These latter disorders were discussed in Chapter 19. Temporal lobectomy is frequently performed in adults for the control of severe seizure activity originating in that area (Chapter 20) and less frequently in children. Anterior callosotomy is used to prevent the spreading of seizure activity and to treat otherwise intractable seizures; M. J. Cohen et al. (1991), Nordgren et al. (1991), and Oguni et al. (1991) all reported that cognitive functioning remained unchanged after surgery and that no new memory or speech problems were found postoperatively. Green (1988) and Dochowny (1989) provided an overview of surgical interventions in children with seizures, including focal resection, callosotomy, and hemispherectomy; they reported that early surgical intervention improves later psychosocial status and adaptive function. Commissurotomy is also performed to prevent the spreading of unilateral seizure activity across the midline of the cortex. The neuropsychological consequences of commissurotomy have been described in some detail in Chapter 9.

Lobectomy

Anterior temporal lobectomy (removal of part of the temporal lobe but with sparing of the posterior language areas of the temporal lobe) and other cortical resections in children are carried out to control focal seizures that are resistant to medication (Wyllie et al. 1989). Caplan et al. (1992c) reported no significant social or communicative deficits postoperatively and during a 15-month follow-up they found the expected normal developmental changes. Galin and Nachman (1990) reported that binaural story recall is not affected by this procedure, although interference with binaural hearing by the diseased temporal lobe had been suspected. Smith and Milner (1988) found recognition deficits for abstract designs in a large-scale study of patients with right temporal lobe excisions; in contrast, patients with primarily right frontal lobe excisions were impaired in recalling the frequency of occurrence of the designs. They attributed the deficit after frontal excisions to a disorderly search process in memory and in cognitive estimation, specific to frontal lobe functioning. Dennis et al. (1988) reported on 26 temporal lobectomy patients and described recognition defects also for verbal tasks, a functional dissociation between judging the familiarity of an event and identifying its attributes. In this study, patients with right lobectomy made better judgments than those with left resections. The difference between the Smith and Dennis findings may be explained by the use of abstract designs in one and of verbal material in the other study. A 20- to 30-year follow-up of 14 patients by Stevens (1990) found that 9 remained seizure-free, but that psychoses occurred in several subjects, especially if lobectomy was performed at later ages.

Surgery for Tumor

Childhood tumors were discussed in Chapter 19. The occurrence and removal of tumors may reveal considerable information about the neuropsychological functioning of the affected area. However, the scattered reports of tumor surgery in children do not provide the opportunity for systematic study as yet, particularly since tumors often invade areas surrounding the location of surgery and intracranial pressure affects other brain areas. Dennis et al. (1991a) found the diencephalic, the subcortical white matter, and the limbic lobes to be most frequently involved. Because of these locations endocrine dysfunctions, such as hypopituitarism, are frequent and require hormone therapy. Brown and Slobogin (1987) reported on 26 children who had surgery for tumors in the fourth ventricle and brainstem area. Twenty-one of these children showed marked personality changes, in addition to neurological signs of brainstem dysfunction: emotional incontinence, fear, and aggressive behavior were prominent with preserved intellect. The authors interpreted these findings as an indication of the disconnection of the brainstem reticular activating system from cortical control or modulation. In contrast, removal of benign astrocystic and oligodendrocytic tumors in one of the cortical hemispheres had little effect on personality and intelligence; 70 per cent of 42 consecutive cases had no problems in school on follow-up (Hirsch et al. 1989). A multivariate study of risk factors for intellectual outcome (Ellenberg et al. 1987) found that age at treatment, tumor site, the interaction between age and site, whole brain radiation, and the interaction between age and radiation were predictive of intellectual outcome, whereas chemotherapy, hydrocephalus, and extent of surgical resection were not.

In children with Sturge-Weber disease, occipital lobectomy has been carried out successfully. Ogunmekan et al. (1989) provided case reports indicating that intellectual deterioration did not occur if surgery was done as early as 6 months; however, surgery later in life did lead to intellectual decline.

Summary

Hemispherectomy has proved to be a valuable and potentially life-saving surgical intervention for many patients. The theoretical interpretation of hemispherectomy reports has illuminated the interrelated notions of plasticity and differential lateralization of cerebral functions in childhood. Although one may conclude that the plasticity of the child's brain has been over-rated in the past, that the Kennard principle no longer holds in these cases, and that the more specific experiments after hemispherectomy for infantile hemiplegia demonstrate early lateralization of the human brain, many deficiencies in our understanding of the effects of hemispherectomy still remain. Other surgical interventions, especially temporal lobectomy and tumor surgery in children, have provided valuable information on the role of specific brain areas in language, personality development, and various aspects of memory in childhood.

IV

Disturbances of Function

This part of the book deals with childhood disorders of function that are frequently encountered in clinical practice, such as minimal brain dysfunction; motor disorders; attentional, visual, auditory and language disorders; deficits of cognition and learning; and emotional disorders.

Thompson and O'Quinn's (1979) developmental disabilities cube (Figure IV-1) illustrates well the relationships among the major factors involved in disturbances of function. Whereas the first and second parts of this book dealt with normal development (i.e., the time dimension of the cube) and the third part is concerned with etiological factors, Part IV addresses what Thompson and O'Quinn call interdependent systems. This term is well chosen because any division into auditory, motor, visual, language, and other disorders must remain arbitrary to some extent. There is considerable overlap in the condition of almost every individual afflicted with such disorders; pure disorders in any area are rare. Nevertheless, it seems desirable to deal with each area individually first, describing the disorders of that function and their relationship to neurological status and only then pointing out their commonality with other disorders.

Functional disorders resulting from perinatal and early-life events do not develop along rigid lines determined by etiology. The dysfunctional child is constantly interacting with other children and with adults in an environment that may help him or her learn to compensate and at least partially overcome the disabilities. Alternately, the child may lack the support needed, and hence any deficit in functional abilities is compounded. Numerous failures where other children succeed easily, being excluded where peers happily play together, being viewed as deviant, and so on seem almost unavoidable for even the mildly handicapped child. Periods in hospitals and institutions not only disrupt normal development and the stimulation needed for growing up but may also create

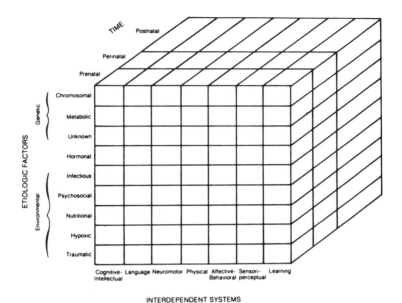

Figure IV-1. Developmental disabilities cube depicting the interaction of etiologic factors occurring during a time period of development resulting in manifestations in various systems (Thompson and O'Quinn 1979).

anxieties and frustrations far more severe than those experienced by the healthy child. For these reasons, emotional disorders are quite common in children with functional disabilities and are not necessarily related specifically to the etiology of the handicap.

22

Soft Neurological Signs and Their Significance

Neurological **soft signs** are minimal and difficult-to-assess impairments of neurological functions. Historically, they have been described as indicators of minimal brain damage (MBD) in children with a variety of different problems of behavior, emotion, and learning. The term was discarded in response to various investigations that showed that actual brain damage could not be demonstrated in a majority of these children (MacKeith and Bax 1963). However, the substitute term "minimal brain dysfunction" still survives; hundreds of publications on the subject, many of them critical, appear almost every year. The term has been used to refer to a syndrome that includes behavioral manifestations, such as fluctuations in behavior, intellect, attention, activity level, impulse control, and affect. Both the unitary nature and the meaningfulness of such a syndrome have been questioned seriously. Whether or not the term MBD is used, the significance of soft signs remains a major issue in child neuropsychology. This chapter reviews the concept of minimal brain dysfunction, the nature of soft neurological signs, the subgrouping of such signs, their possible etiology and measurement, and their meaning in the context of the neuropsychological evaluation of the child.

22.1 Minimal Brain Dysfunction

Minimal brain dysfunction (**MBD,** originally referring to "minimal brain damage") has been called a wastebasket category (Ross 1973), and the use of the term has been deprecated as not a diagnosis but an escape from making one (Ingram 1973, Touwen 1978a). MBD children often might otherwise be labeled as learning disabled (LD), dyslexic, or hyperkinetic or as suffering from attention-deficit disorder or a specific developmental disorder. Clements (1966) presented a list of as many as 99 different signs and symptoms of MBD in children; Small (1982) listed almost as many symptoms that have been attributed

347

to MBD of unspecified origin. It is this overinclusiveness of signs and symptoms that has clouded the issue of the diagnosis of MBD and has led to the uncritical diagnostic use of this label (Weiss 1980). Much of the looseness of definition has been encompassed in the phrase "minimal cerebral damage (maximal neurologic confusion)" proposed by Gomez (1967, p. 589).

The term MBD came into popular use as a result of a study of 500 premature and 492 full-term infants at the age of 40 weeks by Knobloch and Pasamanick (1959). In the premature sample, cerebral damage of a wide range of severity was demonstrated, ranging from cerebral palsy to "minor but clearly defined deviations from the neurological and behavioral developmental pattern" (p. 1384). The authors also noted that such minor deviations were frequently compensated for by the age of 15 to 18 months, although some of them persisted well into the preschool period. Knobloch and Pasamanick proposed that such minor neurological deviations represented the least impaired end of a "continuum of reproductive casualty." Fuller et al. (1983) reported significant neuropathological findings in the white and gray matter in the superficial cortical and deep basal structure of the brain of 16 premature infants who died within the first month of life; the authors argued that with the increasing survival rate for prematurely born children such lesions may be precursors of later MBD and LD-type developmental disabilities. Similar findings were reported by Badalyan and co-workers (1981) for children born under conditions of anoxia.

It is apparent that there is a large group of children who show minor deviations from the norm on neuropsychological or neurological measures, but who show no other signs of definite brain damage. The use of the category MBD has traditionally been based on behavioral, rather than neurological, criteria (Benton 1974, MacKeith and Bax 1963), which has undoubtedly contributed to the confusion. The continuing inclusion of behavioral findings in lists of "neurological" signs of MBD has led to further confusion and, in fact, to complete rejection of the MBD concept by many psychologists. Although the neurologist's report typically includes a mental status examination, psychologists often express dissatisfaction with the limits of this measure. Moreover, a large number of studies, mainly from the Gestalt theory camp (e.g., Ayres 1966, Cruickshank et al. 1976a and b, Frostig 1975, Kephart 1975), relied primarily or even exclusively on the behavioral aspects of the MBD syndrome. This reliance left such studies open to the criticism that MBD is merely inferred and that the concept is based on circular reasoning. As a result, general use of the term MBD as a cause of childhood abnormalities and the inference of brain damage from behavioral symptoms have been abandoned by many authors and criticized as "empty and superfluous" (Satz and Fletcher 1980). Indeed, Satz and Fletcher suggested that the term "should be discarded as illusory." Instead, they preferred to study specific syndromes of abnormalities (e.g., dyslexia, arithmetic disabilities, etc.) and their subcategories without any inference of cause-effect relationships.

However, one fact that is often ignored is the heterogeneity of this group of children (see Shaffer 1978 for a discussion of this issue as related to hyperkinesis). In recent decades, there has been an increased awareness of this heterogeneity, and the term MBD has been modified to refer to "minimal brain dysfunctions" to include the diversity of children within this group (Rie and Rie 1980, Small 1982). The term, however, still refers most commonly to groups of behavioral, not neurological disorders, and the inference of minimal damage to neurological structures is only an assumption (Taylor 1983).

Using this more restricted definition of MBD makes it possible to describe these children more adequately and to see that they require more careful diagnosis than just the label MBD. If discussion of MBD children is restricted to those with clear evidence of mild damage to the nervous system, we obviate many of the behavioral classification problems and see that MBD is not a primary diagnosis of a unitary disorder at all, but at best an accessory diagnosis that does not imply a specific etiology nor homogeneity of cause, course, or treatment. This is a conclusion that Schmidt et al. (1987) also reached in a study of 399 8-year-old children.

22.2   Soft Neurological Signs

Clinical Manifestations

The identification of a sign of neurological dysfunction is based on objective evidence of the underlying disturbance. Such is the case for obvious or hard signs of neurological disturbance, such as an abnormal **Babinski sign** (extensor plantar reflex), which indicates significant corticospinal disease. These traditional signs of neurological disturbance are considered pathognomonic of (i.e., invariably associated with) CNS dysfunction and are an important method of inference making used in comprehensive neuropsychological assessment. Pathognomonic signs include such signs as a markedly asymmetrical motor or sensory pattern on half of the body (e.g., hemiplegia), dysarthria, abnormal reflexes, changes in pupillary size, and some visual field deficits. Evidence for these pathognomonic signs has accumulated over the years and has been documented extensively.

In the neurological assessment of children with minor behavioral disturbances or of children with learning disabilities and without obvious neurological impairment, however, there has been some variability or uncertainty about these traditional hard signs. Clearly, the signs are not found with the same frequency or severity as in children with definite brain damage; instead, more subtle findings are apparent on the neurological examination. Not willing to give up the notion altogether that they reflect something about the status of the brain, clinicians and researchers have called these uncertain signs "soft neurological signs" to distinguish them from the hard or pathognomonic signs (Tupper 1991). They have also been called minor signs by some authors (Touwen 1979). These soft signs include associated movements of other limbs or digits than the one intended, motor incoordination, right-left confusion, mild hemiparesis, and so forth and are described below in more detail.

Bender (1947) was the first to use the term "soft neurological signs" in her description of 100 schizophrenic children who were examined neurologically. However, the existence of soft signs was known since about the turn of the century, but they were often considered to be equivocal, which emphasizes the fact that clinicians did not know how to fully interpret these signs (Kennard 1960). Yet, it was Bender's use of the term "soft signs" and the growing climate of interest in the neuropsychological bases of childhood disorders that highlighted the importance of soft neurological signs.

Most influential was the two-volume book by Strauss, Lethinen, and Kephart, *Psychopathology and Education of the brain-injured Child* (Strauss and Kephart 1955, Strauss and Lethinen 1947). In these books, the authors defined what subsequent authors termed the **Strauss syndrome:** difficulty of figure-ground perception, abnormal distractibility, perseverative tendencies, conceptual rigidity, emotional lability, hyperactivity, and motor awkwardness. They literally viewed this collection of disorders as a unitary syndrome in children resulting from brain damage of unspecified origin: "all brain lesions, wherever localized, are followed by a similar kind of disordered behavior" (Strauss and Lethinen 1947, p. 20). The hypothesis of the unitary nature of the syndrome fuelled controversy because of the inclusion of purely behavioral anomalies and because localized lesions in the adult brain usually lead to highly distinctive and specific syndromes. Their hypothesis referred, of course, to the fetal or infant brain with its very different capacity for compensation during the course of development; hence, the effects of at least some forms of congenital damage may be viewed as more general compared to adults and as leading to maturational delay or to a more generalized defect of unspecified range. However, even this reasoning to justify this hypothesis has been refuted in light of the fact that some children show highly specific deficits, e.g., in language development, in auditory discrimination. Moreover, in the course of further development, many children with highly specific learning problems, especially in learning to read, have been identified who show few or none of the facets of the Strauss syndrome. Birch and others have argued that even the child with only minimal indications of brain damage does not present the syndrome with any degree of regularity. "A whole group of people came to define brain-damaged individuals as a stereotype of hyperactive, distractable, perceptually disturbed children. Nothing could be farther from the truth" (Birch 1959, p. 413). It was this historical background that led to soft signs becoming a common means for documenting MBD or other neurologically based learning disorders (Gaddes and Edgell 1993, Small 1982).

The acceptance of soft signs as evidence for MBD is not without contention, however. At the time of the Oxford International Study Group on Child Neurology in 1962, it was realized that the inference of brain damage from an essentially behavioral description of the child represented a logical error, and the term "minimal brain dysfunction" was proposed as a substitute (MacKeith and Bax 1963). In the United States, a national task force was formed to clarify the concept of MBD; in retrospect, the task force did not meet its objective, but it did criticize the diagnostic use of soft signs (Clements 1966). One of the most outspoken critics of the use of soft signs was Ingram (1973), who stated that reference to soft signs was "diagnostic of soft thinking" (p. 529). Thus, Ingram stated what many clinicians and researchers had felt all along: the use of soft neurological signs as direct evidence of minimal cerebral damage was faulty.

Many studies have since taken a critical look at the measurement, diagnostic utility, and meaning of these signs. One of the earliest attempts to decipher the meaning of soft signs was made by Rutter et al. (1970a) in the Isle of Wight study. They proposed that we are dealing not with equally valid signs of disturbance, but rather with three different groups of soft signs:

1. Signs that indicate developmental delay and disappear with age.
2. Signs that are difficult to elicit and have poor reliability in the neurological examination; these are generally considered difficult to test, irreproducible, or unreliable signs. They are the ones typically considered soft signs and suggest the presence of minor degrees of CNS damage, as contrasted with hard signs suggesting the definite presence of brain damage.
3. Signs that result not from pathological neurological conditions but from causes other than neurological damage; for example, such symptoms as nystagmus or strabismus.

Other investigators followed Rutter et al.'s (1970a) lead and began subgrouping soft signs. Subgrouping does have several advantages, even though at present there is little empirical justification for it. The major advantage of subgrouping is that it allows for the exclusion of signs that are unreliable or due to nonneurological factors. A second advantage is that, due to our lack of research knowledge concerning soft signs, it may be useful to investigate the classes of soft signs separately; for example, signs that would indicate developmental delay might be correlated with developmental disorders, signs that indicate abnormality might be examined in other abnormal populations, etc.

Clinically, subgroups of soft signs seem to make sense, at least on the surface. Most clinicians currently divide soft signs into two categories. One category consists of those signs that would be considered normal in a younger child and that, because they persist, are abnormal in the older child. This category has been called "developmental-only" by Denckla (1979) and the "soft-developmental type of soft sign" by Gardner (1979). It corresponds to Rutter et al.'s (1970a) Category 1. The second category of soft signs consists of those that are pathological at any age, but are more subtle manifestations of hard signs. These belong to Rutter et al.'s (1970a) Category 2 and are what Denckla (1978) referred to as "pastel classics" from the neurological exam or what Gardner (1979) has called the "soft neurological type" of soft sign. Unfortunately, not all studies of soft signs make such a division, and the literature is replete with many studies and tests that lump all soft signs together. This chapter makes this division of soft signs, using the terms *developmental soft signs* and *soft signs of abnormality*.

Developmental Soft Signs

Developmental soft signs include only those signs that are considered abnormal if they persist beyond the age at which they are traditionally seen. This category makes the assumption that there are certain behaviors that the child outgrows, and that are problems only if they continue. A second type of developmental soft sign is the delayed appearance of a developmental soft sign that suggests some type of neurological disturbance.

A further point needs to be made concerning developmental soft signs. Because these signs are related to the child's development, it is expected that he or she can outgrow the problem, and thus the difficulty represents a delay, rather than a deficit, which would occur if the delay persisted indefinitely. Hence, if a child not walking at 24 months were still not walking at 6 years of age, one would probably consider the child motorically impaired or cerebral palsied or would use some other diagnostic term. Thus, it is possible for a child's developmental soft sign to turn into a hard sign just by persisting as the child gets older. Even though such authors as Kinsbourne (1973) and Friedlander et al. (1982) consider soft signs to represent a delay or maturational lag, there is no guarantee that the child will outgrow the problem. Longitudinal studies suggest that the difficulties experienced by the MBD child (including so-called developmental soft signs) do not go away, but rather change form as the child grows older (Spreen 1989b, Satz and Fletcher 1980). Since soft signs at preschool age seem to relate more to concurrent perceptual-motor ability, Satz et al. (1978) proposed that these are indicators of deficits in areas that are "in primary ascendance" at that time and that the meaning of such signs changes to other areas as the child grows older and responds to the demands of school. Gillberg (1985, Gillberg and Gillberg 1989b) followed a group of 10-year-olds with soft signs to the age of 13 and noted that in almost half of these children soft signs no longer persisted on follow-up; however, behavioral and educational problems showed only a minimal decrease.

Table 22-1 lists most of the developmental soft signs that have been described in the literature. They include such traditional neurological signs as associated or overflow movements and motor impersistence, as well as such vague developmental changes as maturity of pencil grasp, clumsiness, and difficulty on constructional tasks. This table is based mostly on clinical anecdotal experience; more refined measures are not yet available.

Finally, another point needs to be made concerning the assessment of developmental soft signs. Few studies have yet evaluated soft signs with regard to developmental differences (Connolly and Stratton 1968, Fog and Fog 1963, Rudel et al. 1984). It would be expected that different developmental soft signs would be more important at different ages, but we have little evidence of this hypothesis. Developmental norms are sorely needed in this area of clinical assessment if one is to make valid inferences concerning "delays" or "lags" (Spreen and Gaddes 1969).

Table 22-1   Developmental Soft Signs

Associated movements (overflow or mirror movements)
Difficulty building with blocks
Immature grasp of pencil
Inability to catch a ball
Lateness in developmental milestones, e.g., standing, talking, walking
Lateness in suppressing primitive reflexes, e.g., Babinski, tonic neck reflex
Motor awkwardness; clumsiness for age
Motor impersistence
Poor gait, posture, stance
Slowness of gait, hand movements, opposing the fingers to thumb, tapping
Speech articulation problems
Tactile extinction on double simultaneous stimulation

Soft Signs of Abnormality

Soft signs of abnormality are those that would be considered abnormal at any age, although they are minor compared with hard signs. Table 22-2 presents a fairly comprehensive listing of these signs. Soft signs of abnormality are mild abnormalities that one would find when conducting a traditional neurological examination, and they include such abnormalities as reflex asymmetries, hypo- and hyperreflexia, nystagmus, dysarthria, tremors, or hypokinesis. An example of a child with such signs would be the right-handed, average-IQ child with

Table 22-2   Soft Signs of Abnormality

Astereognosis
Asymmetries of associated movements
Auditory-visual integration difficulties
Choreiform movements
Diffuse EEG abnormalities
Dysarthria
Dysdiadochokinesis
Dysgraphaesthesia
Hypokinesis
Labile affect
Motor impersistence
Nystagmus
Oromotor apraxia, drooling, active jaw jerk
Pathological reflex
Postural and gait abnormalities
Posturing of hands while walking
Reflex asymmetries
Reflex increase or decrease from normal
Significant incoordination
Tone increase or decrease from normal
Tremors
Word-finding difficulties

significant, independently assessed reading disability who showed some asymmetrical right-sided incoordination, bilateral associated movements, and very mild word-finding difficulty and who had an EEG record of diffuse, nonlocalizing abnormalities, judged as borderline by the electroencephalographer.

These soft signs of abnormality are not the usual pathognomonic signs encountered by the neurologist. The etiological or localizing significance of these signs is most often not apparent. CT scans usually are normal (Thompson et al. 1980), as is skeletal maturation (bone age) (Schlager 1979). Thus, some authors have referred to these signs as nonfocal neurologic signs, in contrast to soft or equivocal signs (Hertzig and Shapiro 1987, Shapiro et al. 1978).

22.3   Etiology

Minimal neurological abnormalities represent, by definition, the least extreme end of the distribution of potentially damaging events and overlap with the distribution of the normal, healthy child. In theory, any of the causal factors described in Part III of this book may be regarded as possible etiologies. The impact of such damage remains small enough to remain clinically obscure in the newborn and therefore even more elusive at a later age.

In most reports, the MBD child is not recognized until school age, and the diagnosis is based on the neurological status at the time of assessment. Etiology remains inferred and is often described simply as "congenital," covering a wide variety of possible pre-, peri-, and postnatal events. Kaffman et al. (1981) and Sobotkova et al. (1983) found significant differences in the retrospectively obtained obstetrical history (complications of pregnancy and delivery, medications in labor and delivery, low birth weight, shorter gestational age, chronic illnesses of mothers) between children with soft signs and normal children. However, Schain (1968) already pointed out that even the influential Kawi and Pasamanick (1958) study showed evidence of perinatal complications in only 37.6 per cent of their disabled sample as opposed to 21.5 per cent in controls: "No single etiology is sufficient to explain causation in MBD children" (p. 353). She pointed out that a disease entity of MBD could only be supported if a common etiological factor were found. However, behavioral studies as well as etiological studies suggest that no such entity exists.

Schain (1968) argued that two different genetic factors should be taken into consideration when the etiology of soft signs is discussed: (1) an autosomal mode of inheritance of defects and (2) a genetically determined predisposition to MBD, i.e., an enhanced vulnerability to perinatal stress. Rutter (1982) described the genetic syndrome notion as a "possibility," but added that the claims so far "outrun the empirical findings that could justify them" (p. 21). Stewart (1980) also referred to the interaction among genetic, perinatal, and constitutional factors, whereas Martin (1980) stressed the effects of nutrition, injury, and illness. Wender (1977) proposed a genetic biochemical basis of MBD (irregularities of amine metabolism), especially with respect to hyperactivity. In a study of 399

8-year-old children, Schmidt et al. (1987) rejected the notion of a homogeneous syndrome based on the presence of soft signs. Weiss (1980) in her review of the various potential etiological factors concluded that the etiology of soft signs is presently unknown and likely to be multifactorial and heterogenous.

Dykman and Ackerman (1976) attributed at least one form of the MBD/ hyperactive syndrome to a possible frontal lobe dysfunction, namely the impulsive type who cannot sustain attention and is unable to evaluate and weigh different alternatives. Such frontal lobe dysfunction has been related to antisocial behavior (Kandel and Freed 1989). The opposite type would be a "posterior" defect; in these children a sensory processing deficit in visual, auditory, or other sensory areas leads to an inability to differentiate, and input is constantly overloaded and confused. Focusing and scanning as two separate abilities would support a breakdown into subtypes. In addition, the authors distinguished dimensions of arousal and attention to arrive at a fourfold typology based on an information processing model (including the "frontal lobe" types). Arousal is viewed as related to the reticular formation. A similar discussion of specific subtypes related to location of lesion has been presented by Prechtl (1978). These and other suggested subtypes remain, however, speculative at this time.

22.4 Measurement of Soft Signs

Both types of soft signs, developmental and abnormal, present many methodological and measurement problems. In addition to general measurement concerns, such as reliability and validity, which are important for any assessment measure, Taylor (1983) emphasized the necessity of demonstrating several types of validity for soft signs. Construct validity is crucial because any neuropsychological or neurological assessment technique needs to be demonstrated to be related specifically to (1) other measures of neural functioning, such as tests of the structural integrity of the brain (radiological measures, such as a CT scan); (2) indices of insults to the brain, such as an abnormal perinatal history or postnatal head trauma; or (3) the presence of other minor congenital abnormalities (Paulsen and O'Donnell 1979). Taylor (1983) also suggested the use of criterion-referenced tests that emphasize discriminant as well as convergent validation; thus, a good evaluation for soft signs not only indicates relationships to abnormality in brain functioning but also does not show associations to other factors that confound the assessment, such as social class, parental education, or even low IQ.

Shafer et al. (1983) concluded that, although there are a multitude of methodological concerns in soft sign measurement, many measures of soft signs are in fact reliable. In their review of past reports by Rutter et al. (1970a), Werry and Aman (1976), Nichols and Chen (1981), and Quitkin et al. (1976), they found a fair amount of interrater agreement, ranging from about 57 per cent to greater than 80 per cent. Good agreement was also found by Vitiello et al.

(1989). Some studies have avoided the interrater agreement difficulty by using only a single examiner (Kennard 1960, Peters et al. 1975).

Another methodological issue addressed by Shafer et al. (1983) is the stability of measures of soft signs over time—intraobserver variability. Conflicting reports on this issue are found in the literature. Denckla (1985) found high levels of agreement for fine motor coordination items when retesting the same subjects after 3 weeks; Peters et al. (1975) found adequate agreement up to 6 months later, and Shapiro et al. (1978, 1979), although without statistical evidence, demonstrated consistency of their nonfocal neurological signs on follow-up at either 1, 2, or 7 days. Quitkin et al. (1976) also showed a test-retest correlation of .96 on retesting within 2 days of the initial examination. McMahon and Greenberg (1977), on the other hand, reported repeat examinations over an 8-week period, but with only 12 of 44 subjects receiving consistent scores on their soft signs measure. Reliability is also confirmed in studies showing good long-term stability after 4 years (Hertzig 1982). Another follow-up from age 6 to 15 years showed strong persistence of soft signs (Tautermannova et al. 1990). Thus the majority of studies that have addressed this issue have reported adequate stability (Shafer et al. 1983, Stokman et al. 1986).

In another study long-term stability of soft signs over a period of 15 years into adulthood was mixed with considerable changes (Spreen 1988b). With the same neurologist as the examiner, learning-disabled students were examined at the ages of 10 and 25 years. Of 203 students, 67 who presented with both hard and soft signs at age 10 showed hard signs at age 25 in only 55 per cent of cases and soft signs in 95 per cent; of 73 students who presented with soft signs only at age 10, 85 per cent still showed soft signs at age 25, but 24 per cent also had developed hard signs; of 35 learning-disabled students with normal neurological findings at age 10, 12 per cent had developed hard signs and 73 per cent had developed soft signs at age 25. There was also a significant shift in signs. The signs found at age 10 frequently turned into different signs at age 25, although they almost invariably belonged to the same area of the CNS (e.g., motor, sensory, motor/speech, and visual) as indicated by a factor analysis. Such fairly dramatic shifts suggest that the nature of both soft and hard signs changes with development into adulthood, but that the indicators of a neurologically compromised nervous system remain present (Spreen 1989b).

Another methodological concern is the possible confounding effect of including subjects with evidence of a focal neuroanatomical abnormality in a study of children with soft neurological signs. Past research is mixed on this issue. Hertzig (1981, 1982) followed up on 66 low-birth-weight children, including 13 with localizing and 20 with soft neurological signs. As a group, children with soft signs had sustained more complications at birth, whereas children with focal signs suffered more postnatal complications. At 8 years of age, children with soft signs were more often found in special education settings or had been referred for psychiatric evaluation than neurologically normal peers, although the difference between groups in IQ and reading and arithmetic tests was not significant. Most researchers, however, do not specifically define any exclusionary criteria for neurological conditions, although some indicate that they have used them (Lerer and Lerer 1976, Peters et al. 1975, Prechtl and Stemmer 1962, Werry et al. 1972). Clearly, the presence of focal neurological deficit is a potentially confounding problem in the measurement of soft signs that can affect construct validation and needs to be accorded appropriate attention. Other confounding effects in soft sign studies include errors of inference due to inappropriate multiple statistical comparisons, selection bias—also referred to as Berkson's paradox—operating in clinical settings, and examiner bias (Shafer et al. 1983).

Other measurement issues have not been addressed adequately in the literature and affect clinical practice more directly. Such issues as the reliability of individual soft signs, as compared to aggregate measures or batteries, have been addressed for short periods in children by Vitiello et al. (1989), in adolescents by Stokman et al. (1986), and over a 15-year period by Spreen (1989b). The results have isolated some of the more reliable signs (e.g., nystagmus, dyspraxia of tongue movement, anaesthesia, simultanagnosia) and could potentially be useful in eliminating unreliable or problematic items. The development of reliable items would probably increase the likelihood that individual investigators would adopt them as part of their battery, thereby increasing the comparability and communication of results across studies.

A second issue, thus far alluded to but not addressed adequately, is the lack of normative age-related data to support the items themselves. Only Gardner (1979) and Spreen (1989b) have made a concerted attempt to provide normative data on measures used for neurological soft-sign measurement. Such data are especially crucial for the measurement of developmental soft signs, as they may provide the only criteria against which to base the interpretation. Finally, scaling of soft-sign measures also deserves attention. Many soft-sign items are scored on an all-or-none basis (presence-absence); for example, the Neurological Dysfunctions of Children (NDOC) (Kaufman and Kaufman 1981). Yet, some items, such as those in Gardner's (1979) series of tests, on the Physical and Neurological Examination for Soft Signs (PANESS, Holden et al. 1982), or on the Quick Neurological Screening Test (QNST), include scaling for these measures. Scaled items generally have obtained better reliability in the studies mentioned above.

22.5   Clinical Significance of Soft Signs

If one assumes that soft signs can be assessed reliably, then one is still left with the question of whether they bear any direct relationship to neurological status or whether they can be used to identify neurobehavioral difficulties during routine clinical examination. Unfortunately, the literature on this topic is still heterogeneous and vague at best. Except for the reported increased incidence of soft signs in children with various learning and behavior disorders, the evidence to establish a direct relationship between soft signs and present and future neurological status is still sparse (Schmitt 1975, Touwen and Sporrell 1979).

One is left with only presumptive evidence (Taylor 1983, Taylor and Fletcher 1983) regarding the association. The investigation of soft-signs-neurological-status correlations in a well-designed study is a major research necessity in this area.

Investigators supportive of soft-sign research who have looked for indirect evidence suggestive of biological factors in behavioral disorders contend that children with behavioral or learning disorders tend to have a greater number of soft signs than do normal children. However, soft signs in some cases may merely represent nonpathological variations of the normal (Wender 1971). Thus, a great many studies have compared normal children with hyperactive, delinquent, learning-disabled, language-disordered, or motor-disordered children, all in search of the indirect link between neurological and behavioral status. One of the overlooked factors in this association, however, is that even if there is an increased frequency of soft signs in developmentally or neurologically impaired children, it is unclear what exactly this increase would imply or whether it would aid in distinguishing neurologically impaired children from the broader classification of other childhood behavioral disorders (Satz and Fletcher 1980, Taylor and Fletcher 1983).

The above-mentioned study by Spreen and collaborators (Denbigh 1979, Spreen 1981, 1989b, Spreen and Lawriw 1980) that involved a 15-year follow-up of 203 children with learning problems and of 52 normal learners showed significant differences between the four groups (normal learners, LD with hard neurological signs, LD with soft signs, and LD without neurological signs) for the majority of outcome variables. These differences were typically present in linear fashion; that is, the learning-disabled children without neurological findings fared worse than the controls, the normal children with soft signs showed poorer outcome than those without neurological impairment, and the hard-sign group showed the poorest outcome of all four groups (see Chapter 29).

This study seems to confirm the impact of neurological signs on long-term outcome and suggests that neurological impairment may be meaningfully treated as a continuum. However, the relationship between neurological signs and behavioral outcome remains complex and depends on interactions with many other variables. For example, Spreen (1981) did not find a relationship between soft signs and delinquency in his sample, but McManus et al. (1985) claimed such a relationship based on a study of 71 incarcerated delinquent youth without comparison groups. Soft signs, therefore, can be seen as a nonspecific factor in the assessment of these children.

Hertzig et al. (1969) compared 90 learning-disabled children with controls and found that 69 per cent of the learning-disabled children showed soft signs compared with only 6 per cent of the controls. It should be noted, however, that admission to the facility where these children were located was based on a confirmed diagnosis of brain damage. By contrast, Kenny and Clemmens (1971) concluded on the basis of evaluations of 100 children with learning and/or behavioral problems that there was no significant relationship between neurological examination, including soft signs, and final diagnosis. Landman et al.

(1986) found that, at preschool age, soft signs were related to visuoperceptual, fine motor, and gross motor performance on the Pediatric Exam of Educational Readiness and on the McCarthy Scales, but that there was no relationship between soft signs and performance on the linguistic, memory, sequencing, verbal or pre-academic sections of these examinations. Nevertheless, Page-El and Grossman (1973) argued that involvement of the CNS is a common denominator in learning disabilities and recommended neurological examination as a prime assessment procedure.

Adams and collaborators (1974), in a screening of 368 children, compared 9- and 10-year-old learning-disabled and normal control children with soft signs and found that graphaesthesia and dysdiadochokinesis were lower in the disabled group than in controls, but that the magnitude of the differences was not sufficient for clinical usefulness. Peters et al. (1975) compared two groups of boys, learning-disabled and normal controls, on 80 special neurological signs. They reported statistical significance for 44 of the signs; these were mostly motor coordination items. On this basis, these authors argued for the validity of the neurological examination of children with minimal CNS deviations and developed their special neurological examination. Rie et al. (1978) identified, in a group of 80 children with learning difficulties, 6 different factors in a soft-sign battery: a general broad range ability factor, verbal-motor and visuomotor integration factors, and age, sex, and hyperactivity factors.

Similar results have been reported for children with other developmental neurological abnormalities, specifically hyperactivity, language or reading disorders, and psychosis and other psychiatric disorders (Shaffer 1985). In an early investigation, Prechtl and Stemmer (1962) found a high incidence of reading difficulties in children with excessive clumsiness and choreiform movements. Wolff and Hurwitz (1973) also compared a group of normal boys with boys who showed choreiform movements and found that the choreiform group (measured with soft signs) showed more reading, spelling, and behavioral difficulties than the control children. Werry et al. (1972) also found a greater frequency of soft signs in a group of hyperactive children compared to a group of neurotic children without hyperactivity. The most differentiating signs included those reflecting sensorimotor incoordination. Twelve children with soft signs who showed anxiety-withdrawal disorders at age 17 were followed up to age 27 (Hollander et al. 1991). Subjects who as adults continued to have soft signs also showed adult anxiety or affective disorders, whereas subjects who had no anxiety disorder during adolescence had fewer soft signs as adults and no adult anxiety or affective disorders.

Other non-longitudinal studies have addressed the association of MBD neurological symptoms with clumsiness and other motor problems (Gubbay et al. 1965, Paine 1968, Prechtl and Stemmer 1962), visuomotor disability (Brenner et al. 1967), and behavior problems (Mordock and Bogan 1968). In the comparison of carefully preselected clinic-referred groups, typically moderate group differences on all these variables can be found. Even when 31 6- to 8-year-old learning-disabled children with "questionable brain disorder" (as inferred merely on the basis of a history of serious illness and trauma) were compared to a learning-disabled control group without such a history, significant differences, especially in motor and sensory test performance, were found (Tsushima and Towne 1977); the two groups could be discriminated on the basis of five such tests with an accuracy of 72.6 per cent. In a study of temperament, Carey et al. (1979) found among 61 children with soft signs a higher number of less adapted, less persistent, and more active children with negativistic behavior when compared to a control population. However, children in a hyperactive and in a learning disability control group were somewhat similar in temperament, suggesting that these behaviors are not unique or even characteristic for children with soft signs. In contrast, negative results were reported by Kenny and Clemmens (1971) and Stine et al. (1975): in their large studies of children, neurological signs were not predictive of any particular form of behavior.

Most studies of soft signs start with the school-aged child. Information about the origin of these signs is often inferred retrospectively and based on questioning of the mother. This methodology leaves unanswered the question of how many children underwent the same type of stress, but did not show developmental problems. Hertzig (1981) addressed this issue in a study of a group of low-birth-weight children, which found an increased incidence of soft (nonfocal) signs in that group. Kalverboer (1976, Kalverboer et al. 1975) addressed this question by exploring the effect of pre- and perinatal problems and of neurological findings in the neonatal period on neurological and behavioral characteristics of 147 preschool children. Fifty per cent of these children had a normal newborn optimality score; the other half had a nonoptimal score (minor brain dysfunction risk). The global measure of integrity of the CNS in the neonate did not correlate significantly with the same measure at preschool age, although a subgroup of boys without complications during the interval between neonatal and preschool examination did show a small, but significant correlation of .28, explaining approximately 9 per cent of the variance. Although this study suggests that these risk indicators in the neonatal period are relatively unstable and have little predictive significance, it also showed a significant difference between preschool optimal and nonoptimal children in a free-field behavior observation, especially for boys and in nonstimulating situations. Therefore, the Kalberboer study confirms a rather tenous association between early signs and later childhood status.

From the data of the Collaborative Perinatal Study, Nichols (1987) reviewed 10 soft signs and 16 other behavioral, cognitive, perceptual-motor, and academic problems in the 29,000 participants. Reviewing these variables in relation to antecedent perinatal and early infancy factors and familial patterns, he found an association with poor performance on the Bayley scale at the age of 8 months and with maternal smoking during pregnancy; a weak genetic component was also suggested by data from twins, siblings, and cousins of the participants. However, the many weak associations between antecedent variables and soft signs at age 7 confirm that soft signs have multiple etiologies. In addition, Yu-Cun et al. (1985) found an inverse relationship between soft signs and familial education level, as well as with location, i.e., soft signs were more frequently found in children from suburban and mountain areas as compared to children raised in a Beijing urban environment, suggesting that perhaps social-environmental factors contribute to the occurrence of soft signs. In a Swedish follow-up study of 141 children from preschool to age 7, Gillberg and Rasmussen (1982) also confirmed that nonoptimal pre-, peri-, and postnatal events and hereditary factors were related to the presence of soft signs, but psychosocial disadvantage in itself did not seem to be a major etiological factor. Gillberg (Gillberg et al. 1984, Matousek et al. 1984) also noted an increased frequency of EEG abnormalities (low frequency and paroxysmal activity) in children with soft signs at ages 7 and 10 years as compared to normal controls. Head circumference was not related except for five children with gross micro- or macrocephaly (Gillberg and Rasmussen 1982), and Denckla et al. (1985a) found that CT scan abnormalities were extremely rare. Paulsen and O'Donnell (1980) and Willems et al. (1979) reported an increased number of minor physical anomalies in children with soft signs.

In sum, most studies show an increased incidence of soft signs among a variety of exceptional children, although there have been some conflicting reports. Still, this finding does not provide concrete information about the utility or meaning of soft signs. Rather, we have presumptive evidence of the soft signs-neurological status and soft signs-behavioral status relationships, and soft signs become another nonspecific measure of neuropsychological functioning.

Another persistent factor influencing outcome is the general intellectual level of the child. This factor has been de-emphasized in many studies. When it is included, however, children with lower IQ levels (though not mentally retarded) almost invariably tend to show poorer response to treatment and poorer long-term outcome. Why such an interaction between treatment and intelligence exists has not been explained adequately.

Barlow (1974) questioned the usefulness of soft signs in the prediction of individual performance (diagnosis) and raised the issue of guilt by statistical association. In contrast, Helper's review (1980) concluded that neurological soft signs elevate the "risk of psychopathy, lowered SES, antisocial behavior and psychiatric contact, but total social and vocational incapacitation are evidently not the rule" (pg. 110). Small (1982) also concluded that such children carry "an enormous negative prognostic burden" (p. 33). However, the overlap of soft signs in both abnormal and normal groups remains a significant cause for concern (Helper 1980).

In clinical practice the measurement of soft signs can be used only as part of a more extensive evaluation of suspect children and does not lead to firm diagnostic statements about neurological status. Proper weighing and interpretation of soft signs must depend on the examiner's knowledge and expertise in the context of other information about the child to be truly useful for long-term management or planning.

Summary

After a history of lengthy debate and numerous investigations, the concept of soft signs and the inference of minimal brain dysfunction still remain poorly defined and elusive in their consequences. Insofar as the term refers to a group defined only by behavioral abnormalities, the MBD term seems unnecessary, implying causality that cannot be demonstrated. A more recent series of studies using more strictly defined neurological signs suggests a moderate association between the presence of MBD signs and outcome. However, the outcome in early and middle childhood or adulthood of children with MBD does not suggest a unitary syndrome, but rather a wide range of behavioral, educational, psychiatric, and occupational problems. Attempted subdivisions of the MBD groups—Clements and Peter (1981) describe a total of seven "syndromes of MBD"—have so far remained speculative. A few long-term studies of children with MBD in middle childhood suggest that persisting MBD signs may frequently produce a lifelong handicap; if the MBD term is retained for a well-defined group of children, it should be confined to the least impaired end of a continuum of neurological dysfunction with a wide range of possible consequences. No single etiological factor can be identified; most likely, MBD is the result of an interaction of genetic, nutritional, and pre- and perinatal stress factors.

23

Attention Disorders and Hyperactivity

Attentional deficits characterize a number of childhood syndromes. However, attempts to delineate these deficits have been confounded by confusion in terminology. For example, the terms "MBD," "conduct disorder," and "hyperactivity" were often used interchangeably in earlier studies. MBD children are defined as having neurochemical and neurophysiological dysfunction and perceptual or learning disabilities, although these features are not always associated with the hyperactive syndrome. In contrast, hyperactivity has often been treated as part of the MBD syndrome despite statistical evidence to the contrary. The *Diagnostic and Statistical Manual of Mental Disorders* (DSM-III-R, American Psychiatric Association 1987) used the term "Attention-Deficit Hyperactivity Disorder (ADHD), Table 23-1) but allowed for attention deficit disorder with or without hyperactivity in the previous edition and again in the current edition (DSM-IV, American Psychiatric Association 1994). Co-morbidity of ADHD with conduct disorders, oppositional-defiant behavior, mood disorders, anxiety disorders, learning disabilities, speech and language disorders, and mental retardation is extremely high, e.g., 50 per cent with conduct disorders (Biederman et al. 1991); 41 per cent with learning difficulties (Holborow and Berry 1986); and 78 per cent with speech and language disorders (Baker and Cantwell 1992), which can make differential diagnosis difficult.

23.1   Definition

Attention-Deficit Hyperactivity Disorder (ADHD) refers to a constellation of symptoms including inattention, difficulty in delaying gratification, overactivity or motor restlessness, distractibility, impulsivity, and short attention span. It is often accompanied by emotional immaturity, aggressiveness, and poor academic performance (Barkley 1981). The term "**hyperactivity**" is also used to refer to excessive restlessness and should be differentiated from ADHD, which incorporates the constellation of symptoms described above.

363

Table 23-1 Diagnostic Criteria for Attention-Deficit Hyperactivity Disorder

A disturbance of at least 6 months during which at least eight of the following are present:

Often fidgets with hands or feet or squirms in seat (in adolescents, may be limited to subjective feelings of restlessness)

Has difficulty remaining seated when required to do so

Is easily distracted by extraneous stimuli

Has difficulty awaiting turn in games or group situations

Often blurts out answers to questions before they have been completed

Has difficulty following through on instructions from others (not due to oppositional behavior or failure of comprehension), e.g., fails to finish chores

Has difficulty sustaining attention in tasks or play activities

Often shifts from one uncompleted activity to another

Has difficulty playing quietly

Often talks excessively

Often interrupts or intrudes on others, e.g., butts into other children's games

Often does not seem to listen to what is being said to him or her

Often loses things necessary for tasks or activities at school or at home, e.g., toys, pencils, books, assignments

Often engages in physically dangerous activities without considering possible consequences (not for the purpose of thrill-seeking), e.g., runs into street without looking

Onset before the age of 7

Does not meet the criteria for a pervasive developmental disorder

Severity:

Mild: Few, if any, symptoms in excess of those required to make the diagnosis and only minimal or no inpairment in school and social functioning

Moderate: Symptoms or functional impairment intermediate between "mild" and "severe"

Severe: Many symptoms in excess of those required to make the diagnosis and significant and pervasive impairment in functioning at home and school and with peers

Source: American Psychiatric Association 1987.

Earlier thinking focused on overactivity as the primary symptom. Then attentional deficits were viewed as the central component of the syndrome (Douglas and Peters 1979). The DSM III-R renaming of the hyperactive syndrome as ADHD reflected another shift in emphasis, returning hyperactivity as a central part of the disorder. Barkley (1981, p. 14) defined the hyperactive syndrome as "a developmental disorder of age-inappropriate attention span, impulse control, restlessness, and rule-governed behavior that develops in late infancy or early childhood (before the age of 6), is pervasive in nature, and is not accounted for on the basis of gross neurological, sensory, or motor impairment, or severe emotional disturbance." The variance in definition across the last 40 years makes comparison of the numerous studies of the syndrome difficult. In this chapter, we refer to older studies with the terms used in those studies, whereas discussions of more recent studies use the term "ADHD."

The characteristics of the syndrome have been poorly differentiated from normal behavior. Traits of high activity, distractibility, and short attention span exist in the general population. If 49 per cent of the population is by definition more active than the mean, how active must a child be to be considered hyperactive (Carey and McDevitt 1980)? Barkley suggested the following criteria in addition to those of DSM III-R in making the diagnosis: parental and/or teacher complaints of inattentiveness, impulsivity, and restlessness; deviation from age norms on a standardized parent or teacher rating scale of hyperactive behavior of at least two standard deviations (i.e., 98th percentile or higher); and problem behaviors identified in 8 of the 16 types described in Table 22-1 in discussions with the parent, or at least 12 of the 16 types in discussions with the teacher. These criteria also provide objective guidelines for judgment of the severity of ADHD.

Studies using statistical clustering techniques suggest that ADHD is not a unitary syndrome but rather a loose association of symptoms affecting alertness or arousal, selective or focused attention, distractibility, sustained attention, and span of apprehension. To clarify matters, many researchers have chosen to describe particular core-symptom patterns and to avoid global labeling (Ross and Pelham 1981). Subtyping on the basis of degree of attention deficit, hyperactivity, aggression, internalizing symptoms, and the situational nature of symptomatology, as well as on drug responsiveness (Barkley 1990) and co-morbidity for anxiety (Pliszka 1989), has been attempted, but no generally accepted subtype classification has been developed to date. Bryhn (1991) and other authors have argued that ADHD represents a set of interrelated subprocesses with distinct neural substrates, rather than a single entity. However, careful diagnosis of the ADHD syndrome does have utility in pediatric treatment.

23.2   Incidence

Paine et al. (1968) reported that the syndrome occurs predominantly in boys, at an estimated male:female ratio of 4:1 (Ross and Ross 1982). Steinhausen (1982) even reported a 9:1 ratio. The higher ratio of males in clinic samples may be related to selective referral, rather than actual incidence: expectations for males and the fact that males are more likely to be aggressive and antisocial may trigger more referrals. Females are more likely to present with problems in mood, affect, and emotion. McGee et al. (1987) calculated that the occurrence of ADHD may be equal in males and females if controls are used for these differences in expression. Estimates of the incidence in school-aged children in North America range from 3 to 5 per cent (Barklay 1990, Shaywitz and Shaywitz 1991). In an attempt to reconcile the varying estimates of ADHD, a sample of 14,000 children encompassing different socioeconomic and ethnic groups in Ontario, Canada, was tested with the Conners rating scales for teachers and parents. Approximately 1.6 per cent were considered to be hyperactive, whereas 8.3 per cent had hyperactivity in combination with other symptoms (Trites 1986). Figure 23–1 shows the hypothetical overlap of ADHD with other disorders.

British estimates of the incidence of ADHD are much lower. The Isle of Wight study identified only two cases among 2199 children aged 10 and 11 years (Rutter et al. 1970b), whereas a much larger proportion was diagnosed as

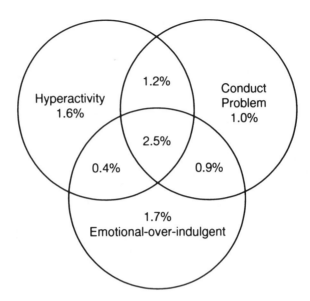

Figure 23-1. Venn diagram of hyperactivity, conduct problem, emotional overindulgence (per cent of subjects above criterion factors on Conners Teacher Rating Scale). Essentially pure hyperactivity (ICD-9): 1.6%; essentially ADD (DSM-III): 8.3%. (Trites 1986).

restless or overactive in association with a conduct or neurotic disorder. Such discrepancies underline the nonspecificity and variability in classification.

23.3   Behavioral Characteristics

Attention and motor activity will be discussed. Other related behavioral characteristics of ADHD children are academic problems, social immaturity, and physical problems, e.g., physical immaturity, motor incoordination, mildly abnormal reflexes. These are discussed later in this chapter.

Attention

The neural basis of attention and its role in information processing have been described in detail by Cohen (1993). In studying attentional deficits in hyperactive children, Douglas and Peters (1979) hypothesized that "the major disability of hyperactive children is the inability to sustain attention and inhibit impulsive responding on tasks or in social situations that require focused, reflective, organized, and self-directed effort" (p. 173). They characterized the attentional deficit on the basis of distractibility and vigilance tasks (Sykes et al. 1971, 1973).

Experimental studies (Posner and Rafal 1987) have shown that components of attention itself—namely, the ability to shift attention and the ability to focus attention selectively on a specific stimulus—are separable. Classical studies of distractibility that investigated whether children could screen out task-irrelevant stimulation or potential distractors indicated that hyperactive children are no more vulnerable to extraneous stimuli than normal children. In addition, tests of incidental learning showed no evidence that hyperactive children are more likely to process and remember task-irrelevant information than normal children (Douglas and Peters 1979).

The performance of hyperactive children on vigilance or sustained-attention tasks has been evaluated using a **continuous performance task** (**CPT**) format. This test requires the subject to monitor a screen on which letters appear at regular intervals and to respond whenever a previously specified stimulus appears. Hyperactive children make more errors of omission (fewer correct detections) and of commission (more incorrect responses), show more rapid deterioration in performance than controls, and are less able to inhibit premature or repetitive responding, indicating poor impulse control (M.L. Grant et al. 1990, Fischer et al. 1990). Impairment in sustained attention is specific to tasks requiring prolonged attention; no impairment was observed on a Choice Reaction Time Test, which requires sustained attention only for brief periods. On one version of the simple reaction time tasks, a warning signal is followed by a preparatory interval that is terminated by the onset of the reaction signal. The results indicated that hyperactive children showed longer response latencies than normal children (Douglas and Peters 1979). When performance on a self-paced attention task (Serial Reaction Test) was compared with that on an experimenter-paced or controlled task (CPT), hyperactive children were impaired on both tasks relative to controls; however, they did more poorly on the latter.

A study by Ullman et al. (1978) showed shorter attention span during free play; hyperactive children tended to be more inattentive and impulsive on vigilance tasks. Attentional deficits generalized across a variety of experimental tasks.

ADHD children detected fewer signals than controls in a CPT format with infrequently occurring signals (Kasper et al. 1971). Kaspar and his collaborators interpreted this finding as an indication that the level of stimulation in such children is too low and that therefore they tend to seek out other sources of stimulation. Similarly, Conte and co-workers (1986, Conte et al. 1991) found that ADHD children learn less efficiently on a paired associate learning task if the information is presented at slow rates. Weinberg and McLean (1986) also saw ADHD as a "primary disorder of vigilance . . . a more subtle form of narcolepsy" (p. 165) that they include among the subtypes of specific developmental learning disorders. This notion of a low stimulation level in ADHD children provides one model to explain the effect of stimulant drug therapy, to be discussed later.

Further support for this model comes from electrophysiological studies. Slower reaction time in children with a poor ability to concentrate is accompanied by poor orientation and preparation response on the EEG (Gruenewald-Zuberbier et al. 1978). The EEG activity level in hyperactive children showed a lower degree of activation than that of controls (Gruenewald-Zuberbier et al. 1975). The arousal response to tone became comparatively weaker in the course of the experiment. Similar results were obtained in studies of cortical-evoked potentials (reviewed by Stamm and Kreder 1979). These findings have been interpreted as evidence of underarousal (Hastings and Barkley 1978) in ADHD children. Clinical EEG findings, on the other hand, have remained ambiguous. In a long-term follow-up study, Weiss and collaborators (1971) found a somewhat increased number of abnormal EEGs (42 per cent) in 6- to 13-year-old hyperactive children. Approximately the same number of abnormal EEGs was found at follow-up 5 years later. However, test-retest reliability of the EEG for the individual subject was low, and EEG findings at age 10 and 15 were not related to measures of adult outcome (Hechtman et al. 1978). Steinhausen (1982) also reported 42.9 per cent abnormal EEGs in his sample, most of which were characterized as "maturation deficit." In a sample of 73 hyperkinetic children, the same author found 38.9 per cent abnormal EEGs (versus 29 per cent in normal controls, 26.9 per cent in children with conduct disorders, and 29 per cent in children with emotional disorders).

In conclusion, there is evidence of increased impulsivity, problems with sustained attention, and physiological underarousal in hyperactive children. Douglas and Peters (1979) suggested that hyperactive children have a constitutional predisposition for poor impulse control and attentional problems, which in turn may contribute to impaired higher cognitive functions, such as problem-solving ability.

Motor Activity

The second major symptom of the ADHD syndrome is increased motor activity. Ullman et al. (1978) used devices for measuring activity levels included grid-marked playrooms, wrist and ankle actometers (motion recorders), and stabilimetric chairs that record the child's movements while seated. Although conclusions were somewhat clouded by a short drug-washout period and the small number of subjects, group comparisons indicated that all measures of activity tended to discriminate the hyperactive from the control children. Hyperactive children showed generalized restlessness; increased activity was less noticeable in free-play situations, but was recorded more frequently during restricted play, movie-viewing, and structured tasks (Sykes et al. 1971).

It should be noted that measures of activity levels failed to correlate with measures of attention in the hyperactive group; children who were inattentive did not necessarily show excessive restlessness. This finding indicates that the children were not homogeneous in their expression of behavioral symptoms.

23.4   Etiology

Brain Damage

Historically, hyperactivity was thought to be caused by brain damage because many children were diagnosed with the syndrome following the epidemic of encephalitis lethargica after World War I (Kessler 1980). Popularization of the Strauss syndrome (Strauss and Kephart 1955) further contributed to the assumption of cerebral dysfunction. However, comparison of the incidence of neurological soft signs in hyperactive and control children has generally failed to support an association between brain damage and hyperactivity (Rutter et al. 1970a, Werry et al. 1972), although positive findings have been reported in some recent studies (Luk et al. 1991, Mikkelsen 1982, Nichols 1987). Soft signs (Chapter 22) may not be specific to ADHD, but tend to occur more frequently in many deviant populations and are inversely related to IQ and age (Rapoport and Ferguson 1982, Taylor 1987).

Congenital risk factors have been cited as a possible etiology for childhood hyperactivity (Johnson 1981, Rapoport and Ferguson 1981). However, further research failed to confirm that hyperactive children experience pre- and perinatal complications more frequently than normal children (Johnson 1981, McGee et al. 1984b). An exception to this is the continuing controversy over the incidence of hyperactivity among low-birth-weight and premature infants discussed in Chapter 13. Some studies have reported an increased incidence (Alden et al. 1972, Francis-Williams and Davies 1974, Steinhausen 1982), whereas others suggest that the incidence in both populations is approximately the same (Simonds and Aston 1980).

Attempts have also been made to predict behavioral outcome from prenatal and perinatal events. The Kauai study (Werner and Smith 1977, Werner et al. 1971) followed more than 1000 pregnancies prospectively for almost two decades, and the Collaborative Perinatal Study followed more than 50,000 pregnancies until age 7 years. The Kauai study revealed that perinatal stress by itself successfully predicted only severe disabilities, e.g., mental retardation or physical handicaps. The Perinatal Study suggested that prenatal variables (e.g., maternal smoking or proteinuria during pregnancy) have some relationship to hyperactivity, low academic achievement, and neurological soft signs. However, the likelihood of these problems in the presence of these presumed damaging prenatal events increased only from 2 to 5 per cent (Nichols and Chen 1981). Anastopoulos and Barkley (1988) also reported that mothers of ADHD children were more exposed to nicotine and alcohol and that the children showed increased exposure to lead and anticonvulsant medication. These three and other studies suggest a weak relationship with congenital risk factors (Hartsough and Lambert 1985). Spreen (1988a) also found more ADHD symptoms at the time of referral in groups of learning-disabled children with definite and with soft neurological signs as compared to a group without such signs and with controls; however, this difference was only marginally significant when these subjects were neurologically re-examined in adulthood.

Several studies have found an association between minor physical anomalies of hands, feet, ears, face, and mouth and hyperactivity (Firestone et al. 1978, Rapoport and Quinn 1975, Waldrop and Halverson 1971). However, a follow-up study at the age of 3 years using teacher and parent questionnaires suggested that the relationship between anomalies and behavioral problems is weak and that the use of anomalies in isolation has only limited predictive usefulness (Burg et al. 1980).

Genetics

An underlying genetic component of the hyperactive syndrome, based on findings from both twin and adoption studies, has also been suggested (McMahon 1980, Stewart 1980). Monozygotic twins showed a higher concordance rate than dizygotic twins (Goodman and Stevenson 1989, Willerman 1973). Safer (1973) reported a higher incidence of hyperactivity among full siblings of hyperactive children than among half-siblings. Biological parents of hyperactive children have been found to show an increased prevalence of psychiatric illness, including antisocial behavior, neurosis, suicide, alcoholism, sociopathy, and hysteria, than biological parents of controls (Morrison and Stewart 1971, Wender 1971). Cantwell (1972, 1975) reported similar findings based on the psychiatric examination of a group of nonbiological parents of adopted hyperactive children and a group of biological parents of hyperactive children. The finding that hyperactive behavior in adoptees was associated with psychiatric problems in biological parents has since been confirmed by other investigators (Cadoret et al. 1975, Morrison and Stewart 1973). Cantwell (1975) and Alberts-Corush et al. (1986) both observed that hyperactivity occurred more often in biological first- and second-degree male relatives of hyperactive children than in relatives of control children. This increased incidence of hyperactivity in male biological relatives was seen as support for the genetic transmission of the hyperactive syndrome.

Unfortunately, many of the studies are limited by the small number of subjects involved or are flawed in design and do not support the notion of the hyperactive syndrome as a "genetic entity" (Rutter 1982a).

Toxins

Environmental agents, such as lead poisoning (David et al. 1972, Weiner 1970) and radiation from television and fluorescent lights, have been suggested as causes of hyperactivity (Ott 1974), although the role of these agents has not been elucidated fully.

Feingold (1975) proposed that hyperactivity may result from the toxic effect of certain food additives or natural components of foods. To eliminate the disorder, he advocated a diet consisting of fresh meats and vegetables, milk, and homemade products devoid of artificial colors and flavors. Early reports on the efficacy of this treatment were mainly anecdotal and suggested improvement in behavioral symptoms in some patients (Brenner 1977). However, controlled investigations have generally been unable to demonstrate any such improvement (Conners 1980, Johnson 1981, Mattes and Gittelman 1981, Williams and Cram 1978). Challenge doses of food coloring administered to children who were on the so-called Feingold diet have produced only the occasional positive finding attributable to chance (Mattes and Gittelman 1981). A carefully designed double-blind study using two types of challenge doses with a group of children who were on an additive-free diet and another group who were on a strict phosphate-free diet showed completely negative results (Walther 1982). The relationship between food additives and hyperactivity cannot be confirmed. Similarly, the effect of ingestion of refined sugar, fancifully described as "the most ubiquitous toxin" (Buchanan 1984), has not been been confirmed in several challenge studies (Milich et al. 1986).

Among other environmental factors, inadequate environmental stimulation (Tizard 1968), large family size and density, and social disadvantage were more frequent in families of hyperactive children (Rutter et al. 1970b). Miller (1978) studied family interaction patterns and proposed that hyperactivity is a reaction of the child to psychological disturbance in the family, including alcoholism, chronic anxiety, and recurrent maternal depression. However, it is unlikely that a majority of children from troubled families can be characterized by an ADHD diagnosis.

Biochemical Dysfunction

Several theories of biochemical dysfunction in hyperactive children have emerged. Wender (1971) proposed that hyperactivity is the behavioral correlate of an imbalance in the functioning of two systems mediated by the catecholamine neurotransmitters, which determine the state of arousal and the level of activity and responsiveness. He suggested that the inhibitory mechanisms in the CNS are impaired in hyperactive children, resulting in domination by the excitatory system (Roth et al. 1991, Silbergeld 1977). Bond (1981) suggested that a biochemical release from response inhibition as found in the fetal alcohol syndrome in animals may serve as a model for the causation of hyperkinetic behavior. It has also been proposed that hyperactivity results from delays in biochemical development (Silbergeld 1977). Depletion of norepinephrine in pathways that maintain alertness by acting on the posterior attention system of the right hemisphere has been identified as one such cause (Posner and Peterson 1988, Shaywitz and Shaywitz 1991). In support of this hypothesis, oculomotor responses showed no asymmetry in ADHD children as compared to the faster movement controlled by the right hemisphere in normals (Rothlind et al. 1991). Further evidence for decreased dopaminergic activity in ADHD children has been reported by Rogeness et al. (1989) and Shekim et al. (1987). Marshall

(1989) developed a model for ADHD of cholinergic/adrenergic imbalance that leads to poorly regulated arousal levels.

Zametkin and Rappaport (1987), however, concluded that the neurochemical mechanisms in ADHD are more complex and that no single neurotransmitter is involved exclusively. Animal experiments and biochemical studies of hyperactive children provide insufficient evidence to confirm or reject the proposed theories of neurochemical dysfunction in hyperactive children (Garfinkel 1986).

Frontal Lobe Dysfunction

Stamm and Kreder (1979) suggested immaturity or late maturation of the frontal lobes as the etiological basis of hyperactivity. This immaturity or developmental lag results in an apparent motor, attentional, and behavioral dyscontrol observed in hyperactive children and is similar to the explanation proposed by Kinsbourne (1973) and by Satz (1977) for MBD. Frontal lobe dysfunction is also proposed as one of six neuropsychological subtypes of ADHD by Conners and Wells (1986): two groups without cognitive disabilities and with overactivity as a result of anxiety, a group with ADHD symptoms secondary to learning disability, a group with isolated motor impulsivity that is unresponsive to treatment, a group with visuospatial difficulties, and a group with deficits typical of frontal lobe dysfunction that were responsive to drug treatment.

The evidence for frontal lobe developmental delay is inferred primarily from behavioral patterns and tests, such as CPT, card sorting, and planning tasks (Boucagnani and Jones 1989, Chelune et al. 1986). This "argument by analogy" approach—if frontal lobe lesions produce a certain type of behavior in brain-damaged children and adults, similar behavior in other children is the result of frontal lobe lesions—is often used in neuropsychology, but poses many problems (Taylor and Fletcher 1983). Two of these restrictions are that evidence from lesion studies cannot necessarily be generalized to other populations showing similar behavior, especially if based on findings with animals or adults, and that similar patterns of test results may be due to a variety of different causes due to a lack of specificity ("multidetermination" of errors).

For the reasons outlined above, radiological studies of ADHD children supporting the frontal lobe hypothesis and studies with children with acquired frontal lobe lesions are of critical importance. Shaywitz et al. (1983) found no difference between children with attention deficit disorder and normal children on a variety of CT scan measures, but Hynd et al. (1990a and b) reported that ADHD is related to the lack of asymmetry in the frontal region and smaller right frontal width in MRI studies, as well as to a smaller corpus callosum, especially in the region of the genu and splenium. Further support for this view comes from cerebral blood flow studies by Lou et al. (1984, 1989), which showed that ADHD children exhibited hypoprofusion in the central areas of the frontal lobes and the caudate-striatal region as compared to normal sibling controls and non-ADHD dysphasic children. Methylphenidate medication increased cerebral blood flow in the central regions, including the basal ganglia and mesencephalon. Johnson and Roetig-Johnson (1989) also reviewed findings from children with diffuse frontal lobe lesions who displayed pronounced difficulties in maintaining attention when faced with competing stimuli and in shifting attention. In a PET scan study Zametkin et al. (1990) reported that ADHD children, with parents who had residual ADHD features, showed reduced cerebral glucose utilization, especially in the frontal lobes thus providing some indirect support for the frontal lobe hypothesis. This metabolic change persisted into adulthood. Finally, Bornstein et al. (1990) found reduced levels of plasma amino acids (e.g., phenylalanine, tyrosine) in ADHD subjects. Data by Fischer and her colleagues (1990), however, argue against a frontal lobe hypothesis or, at least, indicate that a more discrete frontal lobe contribution should be specified.

Hynd and Willis (1988) connected the frontal lobe and the dopaminergic theories in postulating that a critical system controlling the inhibition and regulation of behavior is impaired in ADHD because dopaminergic neurons originate in the midbrain and pass through the central frontal regions to the prefrontal areas.

Multiple Etiologies

More recently, attempts have been made to devise models that incorporate a multiplicity of etiological factors underlying hyperactivity. Kenny (1980) proposed an encompassing model containing seven interacting components: genetic predisposition, developmental lag, below-average intellectual and social skills, specific learning problems, disadvantaged environment (premature birth, nutritional deficiency, and poor social support and resources), emotional problems, and poor family relations. By combining some or all factors, different interactive etiological models of hyperactivity can be formed, each with different implications for diagnosis, treatment, and management.

In summary, a number of etiologies have been proposed for the hyperactive syndrome. Historically, a tendency toward a unitary concept of the syndrome has prevailed. Researchers have sought genetic, biochemical, neuroanatomical, or environmental explanations for the disorder. However, more recent research suggests that many diverse factors may interact to produce ADHD. A multifactorial approach reflects more adequately the complexity of the syndrome.

23.5   Development of the ADHD Child

Childhood

Studies of infants and young children reveal a series of typical behavioral symptoms thought to precede the ADHD syndrome. Infants who consistently exhibit these behaviors are more likely to be diagnosed eventually as hyperactive than those who do not. A composite of these behaviors during development was presented by Ross and Ross (1976). The infant's behavior is unpredictable; he or she may be crying or screaming one moment and calm the next. Crying is typically shrill and piercing, described as sounding like a siren or an animal in distress. The infant's personality is described as hypertonic, querulous, irritable, demanding, and unsatisfied. The infant is often very active and may exhibit advanced motor activity in the presence of normal growth and general development. Sleep patterns are reminiscent of the premature infant, with predominantly active or transitional sleep and only brief periods of quiet sleep.

The preschool child eventually diagnosed with ADHD often shows similar patterns of behavior: motor restlessness, lability in mood at times characterized by tantrums, poor sleep patterns, decreased frustration tolerance, and a short attention span. Development of walking and speech may be slow, and clumsiness is common (Szatmari et al. 1989). Behavior in group settings is often aggressive or destructive. Rejection in peer social interactions may lead to poor self-esteem.

Schleifer et al. (1975) observed nursery school behavior and found that hyperactive children were not differentiated from normal children on measures of motor activity and social behavior during free-play situations. However, during structured play periods, when children were required to remain seated and participate in activities supervised by the teacher, hyperactive children were more often out of their chairs and more aggressive toward peers.

By school age, family and peer relations and school progress are all affected. Disruptive behavior, distractibility, poor sleep patterns, and low self-esteem are often in evidence. Camman and Miehlke (1989) also measured a linear increase in non-target body movement during 45-minute lessons far in excess of those observed in control subjects. Between 20 and 50 per cent of ADHD children also meet the criteria for a diagnosis of conduct disorder (Barkley 1990). In addition, the hyperactive child often shows inadequate social skills. In school, poor work habits and problems with impulsivity and aggressiveness may be observed. Compared to children rated as aggressive only, children with hyperactivity and hyperactivity/aggressiveness showed more inattention and impulsivity on the continuous performance test (Halperin et al. 1991).

Most research has focused on boys. Only one study addressed sex differences and claimed that ADHD girls show the same poor concentration and attention span as boys, but that they do not show the impulsive response style and presented fewer conduct problems to their teachers (de Haas and Young 1984).

Assessment of the academic performance and cognitive abilities of hyperactive children in primary school reveals comparable IQ scores for hyperactive and control groups (Bohline 1985, Loney 1980). However, beginning in grade three, intelligence test scores of hyperactive children are usually lower and more variable than those of control children (Miller et al. 1973, Palkes and Stewart 1972, Wikler et al. 1970). Nussbaum et al. (1990) showed that this decrease is mainly due to a drop in WISC-R arithmetic scores. The authors found that older ADHD children are more likely than younger ADHD children to experience academic difficulties, as well as emotional problems of withdrawal and uncommunicativeness; in addition, significantly more depression has also been reported (Bohline 1985). McGee et al. (1984a) found more specific reading retardation in aggressive-hyperactive boys than in boys who showed only aggressiveness or only hyperactivity.

Adolescence

ADHD children in adolescence generally have cognitive, emotional, and social problems. In an 8- to 10-year follow-up study of 84 hyperactive children, Huessy et al. (1974) reported an increased risk for academic, emotional, and social problems. In this group, the school dropout rate was 5 times that of the general population and the institutionalization rate was 20 times greater. At the same time, overt hyperactivity seemed to decrease in a portion of these children. Mendelson et al. (1971) reported from a 2- to 5-year follow-up into adolescence that half the children showed moderate improvement of hyperactive behavior, one-quarter showed definite improvement, and one-quarter remained unchanged.

The prospective follow-up studies at the Montreal Children's Hospital by Weiss and colleagues (1979) included children with long-term and sustained hyperactivity described by both parents and teachers. The initial age ranged from 6 to 13 years. All children in the study had a WISC IQ of more than 84, no major brain damage, no evidence of psychosis, and were living at home with at least one parent. Referrals came from pediatric and psychiatric outpatient departments and from private pediatricians.

In a preliminary study psychiatric referrals were excluded, and the hyperactive group was matched with a control group. The mean ages were 8.8 years for the study group and 8.5 years for the controls. The hyperactive children showed increased motor activity, distractibility, poor frustration tolerance, sleep disturbances, motor incoordination, and social maladjustment (Werry et al. 1964). Sixty-four children were seen at an initial follow-up 4 to 6 years later (Weiss et al. 1971), at a mean age of 13.3 years (range 10 to 18 years). Behavioral symptoms, social adaptation, academic achievement, and cognitive and motor performance were evaluated.

Overall, the authors concluded that the prognosis of this group as they matured into adolescence was relatively poor. Behavioral symptoms assessed with parent and teacher ratings showed that hyperactivity was no longer considered the chief complaint at follow-up. However, an analysis of the activity patterns of the hyperactive subjects revealed increased organized behavior unrelated to classroom activity; for example, they showed restlessness characterized by such activities as playing with pencils, rather than increased locomotion observed in younger hyperactive subjects. Distractibility remained a significant problem, although some improvement in concentration was observed. A similar pattern was found for aggressiveness.

The most common abnormal traits were emotional immaturity, lack of ambition, and inability to maintain goals. Low self-esteem was commonly observed and may have been related to the experience of school failure (Weiss et al. 1978). Many showed poor social adjustment: 30 per cent were reported by their mothers to have no steady friends, 25 per cent showed acting-out behavior, and 10 per cent had been referred to courts. Twenty-five per cent had a history of antisocial or delinquent behavior, an increase over the previous assessment (Weiss et al. 1971). The authors concluded that, at a 5-year follow-up, hyperactive subjects showed an inferior social and behavioral adjustment relative to normal adolescents.

Cognitive functioning assessed with the WISC showed a small increase in Full-Scale IQ from the initial evaluation to follow-up, which was attributed to practice effects (pretest IQ = 103.6, follow-up = 106.9). At the initial assessment, the hyperactive adolescents showed poorer performance on both the Lincoln-Oseretsky Motor Development Scale and the Goodenough Draw-a-Person Test. At follow-up, no change was observed in the Goodenough test, but motor development scores were worse compared to age norms. In a later study of a subset of the hyperactive patients (n = 15) and matched controls (Hoy et al. 1978), the hyperactive group showed significantly lower scores on test of visuo-motor function, including the Bender Gestalt test. The analysis of individual Oseretsky items also indicated that the hyperactive group showed poorer performance on items measuring fine motor coordination.

Poor academic performance was experienced by 80 per cent of the hyperactive subjects. Only 20 per cent were in the school grade appropriate for their age or were achieving at an average or above-average level. Seventy per cent had repeated at least one grade (versus 15 per cent of the controls), and 30 per cent had repeated two or more grades. Ten per cent had been placed in special classes for varying periods, and 5 per cent had been expelled from school. Children who were successful in school at follow-up showed an initial mean IQ that was ten points higher than the rest of the group and a trend toward lower hyperactivity and distractibility scores at the initial assessment. However, poor intelligence was not the main factor involved in the academic failure of hyperactive children. Rather, uneven cognitive patterns, verbal difficulties, and poor self-esteem were considered to be important factors contributing to poor academic performance (Minde et al. 1971).

In a test of sustained attention, subjects tried to identify the letters in a series of orally presented words. A series of tests of stimulus processing included visual scanning (Matching Figures Test), continuous auditory monitoring, and simultaneous monitoring of several information sources. Performance on all tests of sustained attention and stimulus processing was significantly lower for the hyperactive group (Hoy et al. 1978). This group had more errors on multiple-choice tasks and more errors of commission on sustained attention tasks. Hynd et al. (1989) confirmed this finding in a speeded classification task, but also found that ADHD children without hyperactivity did not show such a deficit. Hoy et al. (1978) suggested that the hyperactive group analyzed stimuli at a more superficial level. Because no group differences on measures of distractibility were noted, the deficit on sustained attention tasks was attributed to attentional blocks or momentary lapses of attention (Sykes et al. 1971, 1973). It was also suggested that attentional and stimulus processing deficits may translate into social problems because successful social interaction requires simultaneous monitoring of several information sources and in-depth processing of relevant stimuli, followed by selection and use of an appropriate social strategy. The authors concluded that attention and stimulus processing deficits, rather than overactivity and distractibility, most clearly differentiate hyperactive subjects from controls during adolescence (Hoy et al. 1978).

Morrison (1980) studied the relationship between hyperactivity and delinquency in adolescents previously diagnosed as hyperactive and reported that a history of violence was four times as prevalent and arrests and convictions twice as frequent than in adolescents not previously diagnosed as hyperactive. Offord et al. (1979) divided a group of delinquent children into those with evidence of hyperactivity and those without. The hyperactive children displayed more antisocial symptoms, including recklessness, irresponsibility, fighting, and drug use. These behaviors also emerged at an earlier age than in other delinquents. The authors suggested that this subgroup of hyperactive delinquents is likely to have a poor prognosis for adulthood. It should be noted, however, that both studies were retrospective. Hence, the relationship between hyperactive behavior in infancy and childhood and later delinquency remains ill defined.

Adulthood

In an early study of the outcome of hyperactivity in adulthood, Laufer and Denhoff (1957) concluded from clinical observations that these children do not outgrow their symptoms, but manifest increased incidence of psychopathology later in life. In a 25-year follow-up study by Menkes et al. (1967), 18 subjects were selected because of a childhood diagnosis of hyperactivity. Three subjects of this sample were still considered to be hyperactive at follow-up, and four had been institutionalized as psychotic. Of the 11 subjects examined neurologically, 8 showed definite findings, 1 showed borderline results, and 2 were neurologically normal.

Borlund and Heckman (1976) compared a group of men diagnosed as hyperactive 20 to 25 years earlier with their brothers. At follow-up, those diagnosed as hyperactive showed an excess of symptoms of hyperactivity, including restlessness, nervousness, impulsivity, and difficulty with temper. Despite similar levels of intelligence and education, the hyperactive group had a lower socioeconomic status and more psychiatric problems, characterized by increased sociopathy, and social and marital problems. In a retrospective study, Morrison (1979) also reported that psychiatric patients who were formerly diagnosed as hyperactive showed significantly more personality disorder, schizophrenia, sociopathy, alcoholism, and drug abuse than controls. A relationship between alcoholism and childhood hyperactivity has also been reported by Goodwin and collaborators (1975).

In a prospective study of the adjustment of hyperactive children in adulthood, G. Weiss and her colleagues reassessed their group of hyperactive children 10 years later at a mean age of 18.5, ranging from 17 to 24 years (Hechtman et al. 1976, Weiss et al. 1979). Seventy-five hyperactive subjects and 44 controls were contacted and agreed to participate. Thirty-five of the control subjects had also participated in the earlier 5-year follow-up study. The results of biographical data, a psychiatric assessment, and a Brief Psychiatric Rating Scale suggested that many of the hyperactive subjects continued to have some adjustment difficulties as young adults. One major characteristic of the group was impulsiveness, as demonstrated by an increased incidence of car accidents and change of residence, as well as by impulsive responses during cognitive testing. A second enduring characteristic was restlessness; significantly more hyperactive subjects reported feeling restless during the interview and were observed as being restless.

Personality trait disorders were diagnosed significantly more often in the hyperactive group than in controls; the most frequent traits were impulsive and immature-dependent personality disorders. These disorders were considered to be "characterological" (versus clinical states) and did not prevent the subjects from functioning socially, attending school, or holding a job (Weiss et al. 1979). Two additional hyperactive subjects were diagnosed as borderline psychotic.

Significantly more hyperactive subjects than controls rated their childhood as unhappy. This finding may relate to the previous observation of low self-esteem among hyperactive children. The hyperactive adults completed significantly fewer years of education than controls (10.5 versus 11.3), and the mean academic grade in high school was lower; significantly more subjects quit school because of poor achievement. Subjects in the hyperactive group also failed grades significantly more often and were more often expelled from school.

With regard to court referrals, there was a statistical trend ($p < .07$) for more hyperactive young adults to have had more court referrals in the previous 5 years, but no differences were found in the number and the seriousness of offenses. Since there was no difference between groups during the last year of the follow-up, the authors interpreted this finding as suggesting a reduction in court appearances over time (Weiss et al. 1979). There was a similar trend for an increased percentage of hyperactive subjects to use nonmedical drugs (mainly marijuana or hashish) in the previous 5 years, but no difference between groups during the last year of the follow-up. There was no difference between groups regarding the severity of drug use.

Job status and satisfaction of hyperactive young adults did not differ from that of controls. In a concurrent study (Weiss et al. 1978), rating scales to assess competence were sent to secondary schools and employers of the hyperactive and control subjects. Teachers rated hyperactive subjects to be inferior to controls on all items of the scale. However, no group difference on the employers' questionnaires was found. This discrepancy in findings may be explained by the many choices of work available and the increased freedom to change jobs and to select a satisfactory work environment at the time of the study. In a later study, Spreen (1988b) found significant differences in the job and employment situation between formerly learning-disabled adults with symptoms of ADHD and those without.

The follow-up by Weiss et al. (1985) into adulthood (age 25) indicated that half of the 63 subjects in their study continued to have mild to severely disabling symptoms of the syndrome (impulsivity, irritability, restlessness, emotional lability), whereas the other half seemed to have lost their symptoms as they grew older; 23 per cent had an antisocial personality disorder, but schizophrenia and alcoholism were not found more commonly in their group. In general, there was more overall psychopathology and less ability to function than in normal controls. These results were confirmed in another follow-up study by Wender et al. (1981). Stimulant drug treatment did not eliminate educational and daily-living difficulties, but seemed to result in less social ostracism and improved feelings toward themselves and others (Hechtman et al. 1984).

In summary, the findings suggest that the ADHD syndrome does not disappear over time, as shown by the presence of academic, emotional, and social problems on follow-up. Some symptoms observed in infancy and childhood persist; namely, restlessness, aggressiveness, emotional lability, and antisocial behavior. Impulsivity, distractibility, and attentional problems were also observed consistently over time (Ross and Ross 1976, Weiss et al. 1971). Academic underachievement and low self-esteem emerged during adolescence and often persisted into adulthood. Increased delinquency, psychiatric disorders, and alcoholism were found in retrospective studies, but the major prospective studies found only marginal evidence for such an increase. The finding of comparable job status and job satisfaction among hyperactive adults and controls and of fewer court referrals than during adolescence may be interpreted as providing some evidence for improved long-term outcome.

23.6   Drug Therapy

Pharmacological treatment of hyperactivity has relied most heavily on stimulant drugs, most often Ritalin (methylphenidate hydrochloride) and Dexadrine (dextroamphetamine). Cylert (magnesium pemoline) was introduced because it shows fewer side effects (Singh and Ling 1979). Stimulant medication was first used in the 1930s for children with behavior and learning problems (Bradley 1937). By the 1950s, stimulants were widely used as the treatment for hyperactivity. Approximately 2 per cent of all elementary school children in the United States received stimulant medication for treatment of hyperactivity in the 1970s (Singh and Ling 1979); it is still the preferred treatment.

Treatment studies indicate improvement of symptoms in about 75 per cent of hyperactive children (Steinberg et al. 1971, Weiss et al. 1979). Studies incorporating a placebo control, however, show up to 60 per cent improvement with placebo only. Cohen et al. (1981) also reported that, at kindergarten age, similar improvement in hyperactivity could be found in children treated with methylphenidate with and without behavior modification, as well as in a group that received no treatment at all. These findings underline the importance of adequate experimental controls in drug research (Ullman and Sleator 1986).

Only a subgroup of hyperactive children seems to be responsive to stimulants. Several significant psychological and physiological indicators of subjects who are drug responsive have been described in more than 40 studies (Barkley 1990, Thomson 1992), but none of them accounts for a large, clinically meaningful amount of variance. It seems that greater severity of ADHD and the presence of neurological signs indicate better responsiveness to drug treatment, whereas the presence of emotional problems may be linked to poor responsiveness. A combination of drug therapy with various forms of child psychotherapy and parent training has shown considerable merit (Barkley 1990, Dubey et al. 1983, Smith 1986). Treatment with EEG biofeedback techniques has also shown promising results (Loubar 1991).

Research indicates that stimulant drugs cause the following behavioral effects in hyperactive children (Barkley 1981): decreased activity level, decreased aggressive behavior and disruptiveness, decreased impulsivity, increased attention span and concentration, and improved compliance to adult demands.

Activity

Stimulants reduce measured activity levels in hyperactive children, but results may depend upon the environmental setting in which the measures are taken (e.g., free play versus structured settings), the type of activity measured (wrist, ankle, locomotor), and the type of instrument used (actometers, pedometers, ultrasonic generators, grid-marked playrooms).

Seat restlessness and arm and ankle activity in structured settings were significantly reduced by stimulant medications (Barkley 1977). However, Barkley and Cunningham (1979) reported that gross motor activity (as measured by ankle and locomotor activity) was reduced only in structured situations; in large, free-field informal settings, gross motor activity does not seem to change. Medication does not alter the amount of running, jumping, and climbing in hyperactive children.

Attention

Results from studies measuring different indices of attention support the role of stimulant treatment in improving attention in hyperactive children (Barkley and Cunningham 1979). Improvement in performance on a wide variety of measures of attention is attributed to an improved concentration span and inhibition of impulsive responding.

Behavioral Symptoms

Studies with rating scales administered to parents, teachers, and physicians, such as the Conners Symptom Questionnaire (Conners 1972), in general have shown improvement. For example Conners et al. (1972) administered either stimulant medication or placebos to 81 children diagnosed as hyperactive. Parent, teacher, and clinician ratings obtained before treatment and at weekly intervals during treatment for 8 weeks indicated significant improvement in behavioral symptoms after 4 and 8 weeks, particularly in defiance, inattention, and hyperactivity as judged by teachers. Results with the Parent Rating Scale suggested improvement in conduct disorder, impulsivity, immaturity, and antisocial behavior. Other studies indicate that, although all five sections of the Teacher Rating Scale are sensitive to stimulant drug treatment, the hyperactivity section shows the most reliable improvement (Barkley 1977).

Intelligence and Academic Performance

Barkley and Cunningham (1979) reviewed 17 short-term studies of the effect of stimulant drugs on academic performance in hyperactive children. When the results of the studies were combined, a crude estimate of the effects of stimulants on academic performance was obtained. Of the 52 dependent measures of achievement, 43 were not significantly improved by the stimulants. In cases where performance did improve, results were scattered and inconsistent. It was therefore concluded that improvements in performance were more related to enhanced attention resulting from drug treatment. One recent study, however, did report that ADHD children under treatment worked more efficiently and accurately on mathematical problems (Pelham 1986).

Studies using the WISC to assess the effect of stimulant medication on intellectual ability in hyperactive children found equivocal results; some studies reported improvement in Full Scale IQ, and others reported changes in either Verbal or Performance IQ. Some authors reported no significant changes in IQ. The inconsistency of findings suggests that basic intellectual or cognitive processes probably do not change significantly and that fluctuations in performance are related to improvement in concentration and attention (Barkley 1977).

In summary, the literature to date suggests that stimulant drugs have no effect on intelligence or academic achievement, but that the primary benefit of drug therapy is decreased activity and improved attention and concentration. The drugs' usefulness is limited to short-term behavioral management, e.g., decreasing disruptiveness and impulsivity and improving compliance with adult demands. A combination of drug and behavioral therapy is not necessarily successful in long-term management (DuPaul et al. 1991).

Summary

The concept of "attention disorder with hyperactivity," or ADHD, like that of MBD, has been rather poorly defined over time. In recent years, the focus has been on attentional deficits, rather than on motor restlessness and other behavioral manifestations. Etiology remains unclear, although a multifactorial causation based on genetic susceptibility, biochemical alterations, and environmental interactions has been proposed. The distinction between primary and secondary symptoms (i.e., the reaction to academic failure and to disciplinary measures) is difficult. Although hyperactivity does not seem to affect IQ per se, children tend to fall behind in school and to show numerous behavioral symptoms, including delinquency during adolescence. Adjustment as adults, as far as can be seen from the few existing studies, shows job status and job satisfaction comparable to nonhyperactive controls and a diminishing incidence of delinquency. Treatment with stimulant drugs has no direct effect on intelligence or achievement, but does reduce activity, disruptiveness, and impulsivity and improves attention, concentration, and compliance with adult demands.

24

Motor, Sensorimotor, and Praxis Disorders

Human behavior and all activity of the CNS can ultimately be expressed only by means of muscle actions guided by the sensory systems. In this chapter, we provide a description of the gross motor disorders, the fine motor disorders, and the more complex disorders associated with the motor system, i.e., sensorimotor disorders and the apraxias. The motor system was described in Chapter 3.

24.1 Motor Disorders

Cerebral palsy (CP) is a general term referring to the full variety of motor disorders after lesions at any level of motor control except those secondary to mental retardation or caused by progressive diseases. Anoxic episodes (Chapter 17) and prematurity (Chapter 13) are important considerations. A first description was published by Little (1862, Denhoff and Robinault 1960), whose paper led to general acceptance of the origin of the disorder (also described as Little's disease). Although the term originally referred only to disorders of the cerebrum, lesions at other levels are frequently included. Since the cause and type of impairment are not specified in the term, it is currently used only in the generic sense. A division into pyramidal (spastic), extrapyramidal (rigid, athetoid, or ataxic), mixed, and dystonic type of CP is frequently made.

Spasticity and Spastic Diplegia

Lesions at the cortical level or in its projections into the corticospinal tracts leave the appropriate muscles without voluntary control. The muscles remain resistant to active or passive movement, are often initially hypotonic, and show abnormally increased reflexes. The condition is usually described as **spasticity.** Mild or moderate forms of the disorder produce clumsiness and weakness. The condition can be unilateral or bilateral, depending on the lesion. **Spastic diplegia,** a frequent form of CP, results from bilateral lesions of the cortex, but is more likely to occur with lesions in the subcortical white matter near the lateral ventricles (periventricular leukomalacia), affecting primarily the lower extremities, but usually with some milder involvement of the arms.

Rigidity

In contrast to spasticity, **rigidity** (which is also associated with lesions in the area of the globus pallidus) involves increased muscle tone. Both agonist and antagonist muscles contract simultaneously, producing stiffness. Rigid muscles are electrically active at rest, whereas spastic muscles are not.

Paralysis

Paralysis (paresis) which is a loss of voluntary movement in a muscle and muscle weakness can occur with lesions at any level of the motor system. With lower-level lesions, strength and muscle tone are more affected than dexterity; the opposite is the case with upper motor neuron lesions, when fine motor ability in particular is affected, muscle tone and reflex activity are increased, but atrophy of the muscles is less pronounced.

Dystonia and Athetosis

Dystonia and athetosis are closely related. These terms refer to disordered tonicity of the muscles (**dystonia**) and to involuntary, slow movements of the trunk and/or limbs (**athetosis**). There is usually a slow, spasmodic twisting that interferes with voluntary movements and may result in fixed body postures. These postures may involve a foot or hand, the back, or the lips or eyes in some cases. The lesion is usually in the basal ganglia, which shows evidence of atrophy, cavitation, or marbling.

Chorea

Chorea (Greek: dance) refers to involuntary irregular, jerky, and brisk movements, primarily affecting the limbs, face, jaw, and tongue. Choreiform movements often occur together with athetosis (**choreoathetosis**). The lesion is probably in the area of the basal ganglia (lateral to the motor pathways). In athetosis after kernicterus, the lesion is often more marked in the globus pallidus. However, for both chorea and athetosis the exact site of the lesion is controversial. Both motor disorders are frequently symptoms of an imbalance of the relative activities of cholinergic and dopaminergic neurons and their receptors (Brain 1985).

Ataxia

Ataxia refers to the inability to control the rate, range, force, and direction of movement adequately and is usually an indicator of dysfunction of the cerebellum and its afferent pathways. Balancing problems and difficulty in performing precise movements are common.

Tremor

Rhythmic oscillations of part of the body at rest or during activity are referred to as **tremor.** Physiological (normal) tremor occurs as result of oscillations intrinsic to the motor system (Goodman and Kelso 1983). Pathological tremor may seriously interfere with the ability to perform precise movements and is the result of lesions at various levels of the CNS. At the level of the pallidum, lesions may produce tremor at rest, primarily in the fingers and the head muscles; this is known as **resting tremor** or passive tremor. Tremor associated primarily with intentional movement indicates cerebellar lesions; this is known as **intention tremor** or action tremor.

24.2   Causes of Motor Disorders

Numerous possible causes for motor disorders have been identified, although in the individual case the etiology may remain speculative. "Premature delivery is the single most important antecedent of CP" (Paneth 1993). Paneth lists as causes, in order of importance: birth asphyxia; low birth weight; congenital anomalies of the brain; white matter damage (periventricular leukomalacia); prenatal strokes; metabolic disorders, toxins, and infections of the mother; and abnormal thyroid function of the mother. According to Volpe (1976), one neurological consequence of periventricular leukomalacia frequently is spastic diplegia. Fewer negative outcomes are observed in periventricular leukomalacia when lesions are limited to the area surrounding the frontal horns of the lateral ventricles than when they extend posteriorly. Fazzi and colleagues (1991) indicated a poor outcome for children with periventricular leukomalacia when the lesions, as noted on ultrasonography, show a posterior distribution or are greater than 1 cm in diameter. Extrapyramidal disturbances, particularly choreoathetosis and rigidity, have been associated with the basal ganglia damage that can occur in status marmoratus (Chapter 17). Motor deficits and seizures, as well as mental retardation, are possible sequelae of cerebral necrosis, depending upon the locus and extent of cell death.

Neonates with 5-minute Apgar scores consistently 3 or lower had a risk of developing CP that was 162 times greater than that of infants with 5-minute Apgar scores between 7 and 10 in the Perinatal Project. More than one-third of the surviving children with Apgar scores 3 or below at 20 minutes showed a motor disability at follow-up (Nelson and Ellenberg 1979). In the study by

Mulligan and colleagues (1980), 18.5 per cent of survivors suffered from major neurological disorders at follow-up (e.g., spastic di-, quadri-, and hemi-plegia); 9 per cent had milder neurological sequelae. Bilateral spastic paresis was the most common form of CP observed by Nelson and Ellenberg (1981). Neonatal seizures occurred in all eight of the surviving children who had 20-minute Apgar scores of 3 or lower.

Risk factors were studied by Nelson and Ellenberg (1986) as part of the Collaborative Perinatal Study of 54,000 pregnancies. In a group of 189 children with CP, 21 per cent had clinical indications of asphyxia. Leading prenatal predictors of CP were mental retardation of the mother, birth weight below 2001 g, and fetal malformations (Table 24–1). Breech presentation was also a predictor, but breech delivery was not. Low birth weight remains the most important predisposing factor since it is frequently associated with subdural hemorrhage in the posterior fossa area or with epidural hemorrhage in the spinal cord and brainstem as a result of malpositioning during birth.

Spasticity has also been associated with structural malformations, such as microgyria, porencephaly, and atrophy of one hemisphere, and with sclerotic lesions in one or more lobes of a hemisphere. Drillien (1974) found that indications of arrest or distortion of brain development during the prenatal period were frequent in CP neonates; 15 per cent of low-birth-weight children had

Table 24-1   Sequential Stage Analysis According to Birth Weight, Using Stepwise Multiple Regression Analysis

Stage	Total	Birth weight group below 2001 g
Before and during pregnancy	Maternal mental retardation, severe proteinuria, motor deficit of sibling, third-trimester bleeding	Maternal mental retardation, severe proteinuria, prenatal maternal seizures, prenatal hyperthyroidism
Before and during pregnancy, during labor and delivery	Gestational age <32 weeks, breech presentation, placental complication, maternal mental retardation, chorionitis	Maternal mental retardation, breech presentation, severe proteinuria, prenatal maternal seizures, prenatal hyperthyroidism
Before and during pregnancy, during labor and delivery, postpartum	Birth weight <2001 g, time to cry >5 min, Moro reflex asymmetrical, white race	Time to cry >5 min, prenatal maternal seizures, severe proteinuria, breech presentation
Before and during pregnancy, during labor and delivery, immediately postpartum, neonatal period	Neonatal seizures, birth weight <2001 g, time to cry >5 min, major non-CNS malformation	Neonatal seizures, time to cry >5 min, major non-CNS malformation

Source: Nelson and Ellenberg 1986.

either a major brain malformation or three or more minor ones. Half of these children showed moderate or severe neurological deficit at 1 to 3 years of age.

Although the association between motor disorders and malformations, including those outside the CNS, is clearly demonstrated, the etiology remains speculative. In elucidating the cause of brain structure abnormalities that occur prenatally, it is important to distinguish between an arrest or deviation of development and destructive lesions. The former might occur in relation to maternal exposure to drugs, such infections as rubella, and some viruses. The latter is more likely with cytomegalovirus, bacterial infections, and maternal blood loss causing a drop in fetal blood pressure. The nature of the structural abnormality may be related to the stage of development of the embryo or fetus at which the disrupting influence occurs. Some forms of motor disorders in children (e.g., Friedreich's ataxia) are hereditary (Jabbari et al. 1983). Monreal (1985) even found a family background of neurological impairment in 60 to 70 per cent of 62 children with CP as compared with three control groups and therefore suspected a variably expressed dominant genetic transmission. In others, the etiology may be described as multifactorial, including an interaction with such factors as socioeconomic status and maternal weight.

Although many motor disorders are evident at birth and leave little room for diagnostic speculation, signs of spasticity may not show up until the end of the first year and minor weaknesses may not be evident until later. Dystonia, athetosis, and choreoathetosis are often not recognized until the second year of life. In contrast, motor disorders of the newborn often improve markedly with age, suggesting that the developing nervous system is capable of compensating for small CNS lesions. Less obvious signs of motor disorder are a generally slow motor development, asymmetrical postures and limb movements (including even an early strong hand preference), and the persistence of grasp, tonic neck, and Moro reflexes beyond a developmentally appropriate age. The **Moro reflex** is elicited when the infant is left unsupported in the supine position and consists of flexing of the thighs and knees, fanning and clenching of fingers, and outward spreading and then bringing together of the arms. These instinctive reflexes normally disappear after the age of 6 months.

Hypotonia and overly active reflexes may also suggest persisting motor defects. Prechtl and Stemmer (1962) described the child's inability to hold its fingers quiet while stretching out its arms and keeping its eyes closed as a choreiform syndrome that may suggest minor damage to the basal ganglia or the cerebellum. Little information is available about early evidence for complex sensorimotor integration defects, dyspraxia, and similar problems found in early or late childhood.

24.3 Animal Studies

In systematic studies about the effects of selective ablation of the motor areas in animals, unilateral and bilateral removal of motor and premotor areas in monkeys less than 4 weeks old did not immediately produce paresis. When paresis developed later, it was much less severe than with similar lesions in adult animals (Kennard 1942). When neighboring areas were also ablated, the motor deficit in the young animal was aggravated, but this did not seem to affect the adult animals. Kennard interpreted this finding as a capacity for CNS reorganization, a capacity that slowly and progressively diminishes as the animal completes the second year of life. Sectioning the pyramidal tract (Lawrence and Hopkins 1972) and hemispherectomy in rats (Hicks and D'Amato 1970) resulted in similar findings. Functional recovery after thalamic lesions in cats due to reorganization of projections from the sensory to the motor cortex has also been demonstrated (Asanuma et al. 1985); lesions of both the sensory cortex and the dorsal column leading to the thalamus did not allow such recovery (Asanuma and Arissian 1984).

Hecaen and Albert (1978) speculated about the potential mechanisms of compensation for lesions in the immature brain. They listed regeneration of tissue (including hypertrophy of the ipsilateral pyramid), formation of new connections, generation of abnormal axons provoked by chemical changes resulting from the lesion, and vicarious takeover of function; all of these contribute to the plasticity of the immature brain. The studies leave no question, however, that in spite of these compensatory mechanisms, recovery of motor function remains limited and more subtle forms of motor impairment persist.

24.4   Studies with Children

The incidence rate of motor disorders of any type in children has been estimated to range from 1 to 2 per 1000. However, incidence is inversely related to birth weight. The overall incidence rate has declined during recent decades, but remains unchanged at 12 per 1000 for surviving newborns with a birth weight of less than 2500 g (Kudrjavcev et al. 1983). Rutter et al. (1970a) reported an incidence of 2.0 to 2.5 per 1000 in school-aged children in Great Britain, and van Wendt et al. (1985) reported a rate of 5.7 per 1000 in Northern Finland. Survival of severely or profoundly mentally retarded children was 68 per cent at age 5 and 54 per cent at age 10; children with better intellectual outcome (and presumably fewer associated deficits) showed normal survival rates over this period (see also Alexander and Bauer 1988). Of children with known intracranial hemorrhage, only 40 per cent appeared normal at an 11- to 20-month follow-up, 20 per cent had mild motor defects, and 40 per cent had moderate to severe motor defects (Krishnamoorthy 1977). The same study also showed intracranial hemorrhage in 65 to 75 per cent of autopsied babies who had respiratory distress at birth. In a study by Brown et al. (1974) about half of the 94 infants with such complications either died or suffered significant handicap. A study of 74 neonatal intensive care unit survivors with CP, with a follow-up at 2 and 8 years of age, showed that the majority of those who were sitting at 2 years (47 children) were ambulatory at age 8. At 2 years of age, the tonic labyrinthine, asymmetrical, and symmetrical tonic neck and Moro reflexes related negatively to ambulation. Children who did not walk at age 8 also showed poor foot placement and/or parachute reactions at age 2 (Watt et al. 1989). Even in children who appear normal during the first year of life, however, subtle defects may show up on long-term follow-up.

The estimated frequency of various types of cerebral palsy among affected children is shown in Table 24-2. In a more recent retrospective study of children with CP in the Rochester, Minnesota area, Kudrjavcev et al. (1985) also found the spastic form to be predominant (70 per cent).

Postnatal motor disorders are frequently the result of head trauma, including child abuse. Mealey (1975) reported that over 80 per cent of subdural hematomas occur during the first year of life. In a study of 80 infants suffering head trauma, 36 per cent were a consequence of child abuse, 28 per cent resulted from "falls and blows," and 4 per cent were related to car accidents. Motor disorders have also been reported after bacterial meningitis, *Hemophilus influenzae* infection, immunization reaction, and other infections. A follow-up study by Feigin and Dodge (1976) showed that, of 88 preschool children with bacterial meningitis, 9 had hemiplegia or quadriplegia (although the paralysis persisted in only 3 children after 1 year), and two showed persisting ataxia. Again, it remains an open question whether more subtle motor sequelae persist in children who apparently recovered by the 1-year follow-up. Costeff et al. (1988) reviewed the eye-sighting preference of hemiplegic children and adults; they found that, unlike dominance for speech and hearing, eye-sighting dominance is not irreversible after a critical period of development.

Associated intellectual loss has frequently been observed; 50 to 70 per cent of children with CP are mentally retarded. The distribution of IQs in a group of 401 children with CP (Figure 24-1) shows the expected shift toward the low end, although some children with superior intelligence were also present (Cruickshank et al. 1976a). Mean IQs were around 55 for quadriplegic and

Table 24-2   Classification By Sex and Type of Cerebral Palsy as Reported in the 1951 New Jersey Study

Type	Boys		Girls	
	Number	Per cent	Number	Per cent
Spastic	374	46.6	271	44.8
Athetoid	192	23.7	141	23.3
Rigidity	96	11.9	81	13.4
Ataxia	95	11.8	57	9.4
Tremor	10	1.2	17	2.8
Mixed cases	24	2.9	24	3.9
Rare cases	11	1.3	13	2.1
Total (1406)	802	100.0	604	100.00

Source: Hopkins et al. 1954.

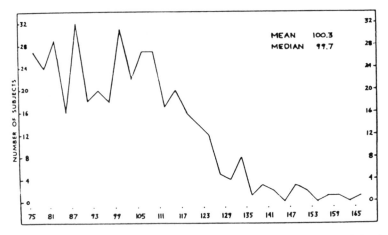

Figure 24-1. Distribution of IQ scores in 401 children with CP (Cruickshank et al. 1965).

around 75 for hemi- and paraplegic children and vary also with the type of motor disorder (Table 24-3). Even if subjects with an IQ lower than 80 are excluded, adult CP patients still show a significantly poorer performance on tests of nonverbal intelligence, dysarthria, reproduction from memory, and visual memory, but not in other tests of abstraction and retention. Sensorineural hearing loss and visual defects are frequently present (Alexander and Bauer 1988, van Wendt 1985).

Gordon et al. (1972) studied the learning styles used in two basic educational tasks by children attending metropolitan preschools. The neurologically impaired children (n = 85) were either children with myelomeningocele and accompanying hydrocephalus or children with CP. A group of 124 socioeconomically middle-class children and a group of 75 lower-class children of the same age but without neurological impairment were also examined. Although a statistical analysis and important sample attributes (such as IQ levels) were not

Table 24-3 Comparison of Mean IQ and Standard Deviation, Birmingham and New Jersey Group, Birmingham Mixed Cases Omitted

	Spastic		Athetoid		Ataxic	
	Birmingham	New Jersey	Birmingham	New Jersey	Birmingham	New Jersey
Mean	67.9	71.94	67.6	72.60	63.3	54.96
SD	27.7	29.73	25.5	30.41	19.3	27.06
n	277	522	41	249	4	129
Not yet assessable	9	0	4	0	0	0

Source: Cruickshank et al. 1976a.

reported, clear-cut quantitative and qualitative differences between the neuro-logically intact and the neurologically handicapped groups were evident. Teachers had to remain available for the brain-damaged children in order to obtain optimal performance. Even their optimal performance, however, was be-low that of control groups. The neurologically intact groups usually requested specific aid from the teacher on specific parts of the test, the middle-class group more directly than the lower-class group. For the brain-damaged chil-dren, the teacher's assistance was required to maintain attention, restructure the task, reduce frustration, and prevent illogical mistakes. The neurologically intact children, over the short-term, benefitted from occasional teacher assis-tance; however, fewer errors were made even when the teacher was not as-sisting. The brain-damaged group did not show independent gains in perfor-mance, but usually returned to their initial haphazard, trial-and-error approach to the tasks.

In a detailed retrospective study, Annett (1973) used a British version of the Wechsler Intelligence Scale for Children to examine 106 early-onset hemiplegia children after they were 5 years old. The group was heterogeneous with regard to onset and cause. The mean IQ was approximately 80, with more than 60 per cent of the children scoring in the borderline or average range (IQ greater than 70). Looking for correlates of general cognitive deficit, the author found lower IQs in children with greater physical disability, recurrent seizure disorders, and early onset of hemiplegia. Speech problems were found more often in children with late-onset hemiplegia (i.e., after the age of 44 months), but this finding obtained only for right hemiplegia. For left hemiplegia early onset was more often related to speech problems. In cases of unilateral hemiplegia, the authors found no difference between Verbal and Performance IQ related to the side of hemiplegia, but in bilateral hemiplegia the Performance IQ tended to be lower, a finding confirmed by Pavlokin (1985, Glos and Pavlokin 1985). Eagle (1985) suspected that, because of the severe deprivation of early sensorimotor experi-ence in CP children, Piagetian milestones of cognitive development might be delayed. Her results showed, however, that reaching these milestones depended mainly on the degree of mental handicap, rather than the type and severity of physical handicap. Brown et al. (1989) found that children with unilateral hem-iplegia did more poorly than normal children on tasks requiring pointing move-ments to visual targets; they concluded that unilateral lesions can result in bi-lateral visuomotor impairment. Similar conclusions were reached by Lenti et al. (1991) who found tactile extinction levels raised on both sides of the body in 39 hemiplegics.

Anarthria or dysarthria in CP children does not impair short-term memory and rhyme judgments, suggesting that "articulatory coding" (or "covert re-hearsal") is not essential for these skills (Bishop et al. 1989, 1990, White et al. 1994). Bishop and colleagues found, however, that subjects of these studies were impaired in receptive vocabulary, but not in comprehension of grammar. The authors concluded that retention of unfamiliar words is facilitated by overt or covert repetition of novel phonological strings.

One study explored the role of familial left-handedness. Annett (1973) found that in right hemiplegics without familial left-handedness, the Verbal and Performance IQs were more highly correlated with the motor speed of the affected hand than with the speed of the nonaffected hand; the opposite was true for other handedness groups. The author concluded that children without familial sinistrality are more dependent on the left hemisphere. In children with familial left-handedness, Annett found more physical and intellectual disability except in left hemiplegic females, suggesting that perhaps cerebral organization and capability for compensation are different for this group.

Several studies have addressed the question of subtle motor disorders and other associated deficits in relation to clinical neurological findings. Teuber and Rudel (1967), in particular, examined the long-term progress of lesion effects and found that immediate and definite clinical deficits in infancy tend to recede with time. For example, mirror movements after childhood hemiparesis tend to become less frequent between the ages of 6 and 16 years (Woods and Teuber 1978); the synkinesis consisted of unintentional movements with the other hand when the child was required to tap one finger against the thumb with one hand only. That different types of motor activity and especially of fine motor skills are relatively independent of each other has been known for some time (Seashore et al. 1940). In a detailed study with ten brain-damaged and ten normal children for each age group between 6 and 12 years, Schilling (1970) confirmed that this diversity of relationships also holds in children for the six sets of tasks measured with the Oseretsky Test of Motor Development. The finding should be considered as a warning not to treat motor deficits as a unitary phenomenon. Instead, each type of motor activity should be measured individually for a fuller assessment of the child's abilities. Wyke (1968) showed specific deficits for an arm-hand precision task. Steinwachs and Barmeyer (1952) found deficits in several measures of writing grip pressure and writing time in adolescents with motor retardation. A study by Klawans et al. (1982) speculated that a progressive writing tremor in six patients that began between the ages of 8 and 54 years could be ascribed to hypoxia at birth.

Although several studies of disorders of relatively simple motor activity found little or no association with intellectual deficit, this dissociation does not hold for more complex motor tasks. Groden (1969), in a study that included mentally retarded children, found correlations ranging from .51 to .68 between mental age and motor skills, coordination, and complex reaction time tasks, even when chronological age was partialled out. This finding is understandable since complex motor activity involves a considerable cognitive component. Levine et al. (1987) found a strong correlation between CT measures of lesion size, degree of hemiplegia, EEG abnormalities, and intelligence. In patients with left hemisphere lesions, receptive vocabulary was selectively impaired, and the sequential performance on the Kaufman intelligence test (K-ABC) was also poorer than the simultaneous performance (Lewandowski and deRienzo 1985).

Sensorimotor Disorders

Motor disorders rarely occur in isolation. Movements have to be guided not only by vision but by touch and sensory and kinesthetic feedback from the body itself. Various submodalities of somatosensory perception, such as touch, vibration, temperature, and pain; tactile recognition (stereognosis); and somatospatial perception of the limbs and body have been recognized as having different types of receptor cells (Casey and Rourke 1992). Touch, pressure, and kinesthetic perception proceed via lateral dorsal columns and the ventrobasal thalamus (the epicritic system), pain and temperature via lateral columns, the ventral basal pulvinar, and the lateral posterior thalamus (protopathic system) to the somatosensory cortex (Kolb and Wishaw 1990, see Chapter 3).

Lesions can occur at any level from the sensory receptors to the cortex, and their effect can range from raised thresholds to complete loss of one or more modalities unilaterally or bilaterally. Mildly raised unilateral thresholds may be detected only by testing for **sensory "extinction,"** a term coined by Bender (1945). Applying two tactile stimuli simultaneously to homologous parts on both sides of the body results in extinction, i.e., lack of recognition of the stimulus on the affected side. Similar types of extinction can be observed in other senses through the techniques of dichotic listening, already discussed in the section on disconnection syndromes, or dichaptic form perception (see Chapter 5). Hugdahl and Carlsson (1994) tested dichotic listening in children with right and left hemiplegia and compared them to healthy children. When instruction called for the recall of words only from one ear (focused attention), normal children showed a strong right-ear advantage under right-ear and a minimal left-ear advantage under left-ear instructions. In contrast, both right and left hemiplegic children showed the same ear advantage irrespective of attentional instructions. The authors interpreted their findings as evidence of hemi-inattention and hypoarousal of the lesioned hemisphere.

Tactile sensory loss is frequently present in CP children and is highly correlated with cortical motor deficit, as shown by Laget et al. (1976) in a study of the somatosensory evoked potential in 43 infants and children. The loss is most pronounced if the lesion encroaches on the parietal area, especially the postcentral gyrus. Similar lesions are likely with somatosensory disorders such as **astereognosis,** the inability to recognize objects by touch, and **dysgraphesthesia,** the inability to recognize symbols drawn onto parts of the body, e.g., the palm of the hand. Stereognosis is well developed in early childhood, whereas graphesthesia develops fully between 6 and 7 years of age (Maiuro et al. 1984). Another somatosensory ability impaired by parietal lobe lesions is **finger recognition,** i.e., the ability to indicate which finger was touched by the examiner. This ability develops gradually during childhood and reaches optimal levels at age 10 (Benton et al. 1983).

Boll and Reitan (1972) reported significant differences between congenitally brain-damaged and normal children on a variety of measures, including motor strength and speed, psychomotor skills, and more perceptually based somatosensory skills, such as finger localization, fingertip number writing, and tactile form recognition.

Motor impersistence (the inability to maintain a motoric action, such as maintaining eyes closed, tongue protruding, mouth open, lateral eye fixation on gaze, or fixation on the examiner's nose during confrontation testing) was also present in brain-damaged children, although no increase or decrease with age has been reported (Garfield 1964). Teuber and Rudel (1967) stressed that some of the effects of hemiplegic lesions sustained in childhood are not manifested until adulthood. An example is the Aubert task, for which the comparison of brain-damaged and normal subjects showed no differences in children, but only in adults. The **Aubert task** requires the adjustment of a luminous line to a vertical position while the body is tilted at various angles from horizontal. It was also noted that this task was not related to the intelligence level. Brown et al. (1989) confirmed these findings and concluded that in children with unilateral lesions bilateral visuomotor impairment may result.

Tourette Syndrome

A relatively rare (1 per 2000, Bruun 1984) movement disorder, not generally recognized until 1954, Gilles de la Tourette syndrome has attracted much attention in recent years (Cohen et al. 1988). **Tourette syndrome (TS)** characterized by facial, body, and vocal tics with onset between 2 and 15 years of age (DSM-III-R). **Tics** are involuntary muscular contractions or habitual movements. Examples can include facial grimacing or explosive grunts or barks. In children, ADHD is often a precursor of TS (Matthews 1988). About one-third of affected children also show **coprolalia** (shouting of obscenities), and one-quarter manifest imitative gestures (**echopraxia**) and **copropraxia** (vulgar gestures). Uncomfortable sensory tics are often present (Kurlan et al. 1989). Self-multilations have also been reported (Eisenhauer and Woody 1987, Robertson et al. 1989). Associated features of sleep disorder, somnambulism, night terrors, migraine, and various forms of psychopathology, including obsessional ideas and depression (Caine et al. 1988), obsessive-compulsive symptomatology (Grad et al. 1987), and childhood schizophrenia (Kerbeshian and Burd 1988) have been noted, but incidence rates for these features are probably inflated because they are based on clinic populations and the features, rather than TS itself, may have led to the referral. No specific form of psychopathology has been found, and MMPI personality profiles tend to show general rather than specific elevations (Shapiro and Shapiro 1982). However, Burd et al. (1987) suggested that the development of TS in children with autism and other pervasive developmental disorders may constitute a distinct subgroup of autism with relatively favorable outcome.

Although TS was originally considered a psychiatric disorder, recent work suggests that subcortical impairment secondary to a neurochemical disturbance (dopaminergic overactivity, Riddle et al. 1988, Schelkunov et al. 1986) and autosomal dominant genetic transmission with incomplete penetrance (Robertson

1989, Robertson and Gourdie 1990) are involved. The exact etiology, however, remains unknown (Barkley 1986, King and Ollendick 1984). Nonspecific abnormalities (Caparulo et al. 1982) or no abnormalities (Harcherik 1985) in CT scans have been reported. In 21 of 45 cases EEGs showed sharp waves and slowing (Volkmar 1984). Perinatal trauma was ruled out as an etiology in one study (Incagnoli and Kane 1983). Response to treatment with clonidine, haloperidol, pimozide, or similar drugs is favorable in 70 to 80 per cent of the cases (Kerbeshian 1985, Shapiro et al. 1989). Poor attention span in TS children suggests a relationship, possibly genetic, to attention deficit disorder in 50 to 60 per cent of TS boys (Comings and Comings 1984, Sverd et al. 1988), although detailed testing did not confirm specific central processing deficits in these children (Harcherik et al. 1982, Joschko and Rourke 1982). Robertson (1989) and Bornstein et al. (1983) reported that language skills were largely unimpaired, whereas deficits in visuopractic performance and learning problems, especially in written arithmetic, were fairly frequent. Such deficits tend to worsen as the child grows older (Bornstein et al. 1985).

Praxis Disorders

The term "**praxis**" refers to the performance of skilled motor acts or sequences of purposeful motor movements, such as hair combing and tooth brushing, and includes such symbolic acts as saluting and other gestures. **Apraxia** is the acquired inability to carry out purposeful movements in the absence of motor, sensory, or comprehension deficits that would explain such disabilities. Apraxia has been studied extensively in adult patients (Adams and Victor 1993, Friedman and Heilman 1993). A distinction between **ideomotor apraxia,** limited to simple, single gestures (waving good-bye, blowing a kiss), and **ideational apraxia,** alterations in the ability to perform a sequence of complex gestures (drawing, construction, complex gestures), is usually made. Further distinctions based on the locus of the movement (whole body, limb-kinetic, oral-facial movements, dressing) have also been made, and specific cerebral lesions, including specific disconnection syndromes, rather than direct lesions of the motor system, have been demonstrated (Heilman 1979a and b, Kimura 1993).

Few studies of apraxic children have been published (De Negri 1967, Robaye 1967). Classical apraxias are rare in children and are primarily the result of head trauma or disconnection syndromes, whereas clumsiness may be the result of extrapyramidal and cerebellar lesions, i.e., may not meet the definition of apraxia. Lehmkuhl (1984) reported cases of ideomotor and ideational apraxia in children after head trauma between the ages of 5 and 8½ years. Brenner et al. (1967) described a group of agnosic-apraxic children with significant impairments in manual skills and spatial judgment, but also in spelling, arithmetic, and social adjustment. However, Lamm and Epstein (1992) showed a clear dissociation of severe developmental constructional apraxia and visual agnosia with normal reading, writing, and arithmetic.

Some authors, however, have used the term "apraxia" loosely (Ayres 1965, Gaddes and Edgell 1993, Rappaport et al. 1987) and have included deficits in eye-hand (ocular-motor) accuracy, oral-motor planning, gross motor planning, and finger identification as part of a developmental dyspraxia syndrome. Such disorders are usually investigated in studies of the clumsy child (Gubbay 1979) and are labeled "developmental dyspraxias" or simply "dyspraxia." Smyth and Glencross (1986) found that such children process proprioceptive information more slowly than normal children, although they process visual input normally. They proposed that abnormal clumsiness is associated with a dysfunction in proprioceptive information processing but not in the response selection process. This finding was confirmed by Haron and Henderson (1985), who showed that dyspraxic children were also impaired in both passive and active touch object recognition. Clumsiness has also been associated with neurological soft signs (Landman et al. 1986, Schellekens et al. 1983) and with asymmetrical trophic limb changes (Iloeje 1988). An association between dyspraxia and the developmental Gerstmann syndrome (dysgraphia, dyscalculia, finger agnosia, right-left disorientation, to be discussed in Chapter 29) has also been reported (PeBenito et al. 1988).

Dewey et al. (1988) studied children with impaired articulation and found that those with impaired verbal sequences of consonant-vowel syllables were also impaired in other motor sequences, such as limb and oral gestures. They interpreted this finding as an indication of a more generalized motor disorder. Bridgeman and Snowling (1988) found that such children also had difficulties in discriminating the segmentation and coding of phonemes. This topic is discussed in more detail in Chapter 27. Congenital asymmetrical ocular-motor apraxia has been associated with various other CNS disorders (Catalano et al. 1988, PeBenito and Cracco 1988).

Summary

A great variety of motor disorders can be found in children, and they are sometimes referred to by the generic term "cerebral palsy." Although perinatal intracranial hemorrhage is the most frequently cited cause, numerous other causes (including infections and intoxications) must be considered. Intellectual deficit is frequently associated with the degree of motor impairment, but normal intelligence is present in some cases, suggesting a wide variability in cognitive and other psychological functions. Tourette syndrome consists of a well-defined group of facial, body, and vocal tics that have been studied in detail, although the definite etiology still remains elusive. Apraxia is rare in children, but some minor motor problems, such as "clumsiness" and sensorimotor feedback problems, have been described as developmental apraxia by some authors. Symptoms may not be obvious until later childhood and may, in fact, extend into the continuum described earlier as "minimal brain dysfunction" (MBD).

25

Visual Disorders

Many hereditary and developmental disorders may affect the developing visual system. Depending on the site and extent of the damage, the resulting disorder may vary from absolute blindness, when there is not even light perception, to visual impairments only identifiable under special conditions, e.g., nightblindness.

Visual impairment may refer to any incapacitating loss or distortion of vision. The term "blindness" implies that the individual has no useful vision. The legal definition of **blindness** requires that visual acuity in both eyes with proper corrective lenses is 20/200 (6/60) or worse as measured with the Snellen Chart or an equivalent test, or that the field of vision in both eyes is restricted to less than 20 degrees. The prevalence of congenital blindness, including blindness acquired during the immediate postnatal period, has been reported to range from 1 to 8 per 10,000 (Jan et al. 1977). Acquired blindness occurs at approximately one-quarter the rate of congenital blindness. Visual impairment occurs most often in combination with other handicaps. In a survey by W.D. Williamson et al. (1987), 17 per cent of visually impaired children also had hearing loss, 46 per cent had seizures, and 78 per cent had severe developmental delay. Similar figures were reported by Gardner et al. (1986).

Pathology in various parts of the visual system may be manifested in similar ways; for example, visual field disturbances may result from lesions anywhere in the visual system, from the outer eye to the visual cortex. It has been estimated that about one-third of cases of blindness are the result of CNS damage, whereas the remaining two-thirds are caused by ocular problems. The main causes of visual dysfunction in children are (1) very low birth weight/prematurity; (2) family history of a visual defect; (3) infection during pregnancy, especially rubella and *Toxoplasma gondii* (Langset et al. 1989); and (4) difficult or assisted labor (Morse and Trief 1985).

Since impaired visual processing may result from damage to any part of the visual system, the discussion of visual disorders follows the pathway taken by the visual image. Figure 3-4 illustrates the primary visual system. Animal research has established the existence of a secondary visual system that projects from the retina to the pulvinar nucleus of the thalamus via the superior colliculus and terminates in the circumstriate, or visual association areas (Chapter 3). This secondary visual system seems to be involved in movements related to vision, such as orienting toward objects or obtaining information about space by moving the head, eyes, and body. The superior colliculus has been described as the primary area that correlates vestibular and proprioceptive inputs (Rapin 1982, Shebilske 1976). The two visual systems interact in visual functions, and damage to one system may potentially modify the activity of the other (Hecaen and Albert 1978). Jan et al. (1977) postulated that cortically impaired children may have use of the second visual system since they are able to ambulate and avoid obstacles in a familiar environment. Evidence that the brainstem contributes to visual perception in humans has been found in adult commissurotomized patients (Trevarthen 1970). Although the processing in the right and left visual fields becomes independent after this type of surgery, separate moving visual stimuli presented to each visual half-field can be integrated by these "split brain" patients.

25.1 Damage in the Primary Visual System

Cornea and Lens

As outlined in Chapter 3, the visual image enters the eye via the cornea and lens and is received by receptors in the retina. The cornea and lens act as refractory mechanisms that focus the image clearly on the retina. If the focus of the image is behind the retina, **hyperopia** occurs; if the focus of the image lies in front of the retina, the term "**myopia**" applies. Infants are usually hyperoptic and attain a normal focus with growth of the eye (Biglan et al. 1988). If normal focus is not reached when the eye ceases to grow, the image projected onto the retina will be unclear. However, corrective lenses can usually provide normal or near-normal acuity. Intelligence and academic achievement are typically normal in such children (Stewart-Brown et al. 1985).

Damage to the cornea or lens results in the obstruction or distortion of image formation and diminished vision. Such damage may be the result of a variety of congenital or infantile disorders, but is particularly associated with certain prenatal infections and nutritional deficiencies. For example, the eye may harbor live rubella virus for months or even years. Infection in the lens may result in unilateral or bilateral cataracts (Martyn 1975). Congenital **glaucoma** (increased intraocular pressure that results in clouding of the cornea) and transient nonglaucomatous corneal clouding also occur with congenital rubella syndrome. Inflammation of the cornea frequently occurs in congenital syphilis, which can persist in the eye for decades. Most ocular manifestations of congenital syphilis appear after the age of 5 or 6 years, although they may occur at any age (Chan 1975a).

Vitamin A deficiencies, whether caused by malnutrition or by diseases of the child or mother during pregnancy, may result in lesions of the cornea. Vitamin B deficiencies also lead to severe corneal vascularization. Children suffering from kwashiorkor may manifest lens lesions. Corneal damage is evident just before death (Chan 1975b).

Retina

The **retina,** the ocular site of the focused image, may be divided into the peripheral and the macular, or central, portion, which differ both structurally and functionally from each other. Peripheral vision and **scotopic vision**—the ability to perceive light, dark, and motion—are a function of the peripheral retina. **Rod cells** are the predominant visual receptors serving these abilities. **Central vision,** or sight directed at an object, and **photopic vision,** the ability to discriminate color, are functions of the macular retina. The **cone cells** are the predominant visual receptors for these functions.

Damage to the retina may reduce the ability to receive and transmit visual information, depending upon the site and magnitude of the retinal damage. Congenital and developmental disorders that result in damage to the retina include prenatal infections (e.g., rubella, syphilis), hypoxia (Van Hof Van Duin and Mohn 1984), and nutritional deficits. An early symptom of retinal damage due to vitamin A deficiency is **nightblindness,** or nyctalopia, which is an inability to see normally at night or in very dim light and which implies impaired rod cell function. **Retrolental fibroplasia** (now frequently called retinopathy of prematurity) refers to an overgrowth of immature blood vessels from the retina into the vitreous humor behind the lens. These vessels outgrow the capacity to nourish themselves; scar tissue develops and impairs retinal functioning. Retrolental fibroplasia has been linked to the administration of high concentrations of oxygen to low-birth-weight or premature infants (O'Neill 1980).

Optic Nerve

The **optic nerve** carries visual information from the retina to the brain. Any damage to the nerve will result in impaired vision. The exact nature of the deficit depends on the extent of the damage. The outer fibers of the optic nerve carry information from the peripheral retina, and the inner fibers carry information from the macular retina. When only the outer fibers of the optic nerve are damaged, peripheral vision is affected. This limitation of vision has been termed peripheral field restriction. When the central portion of the nerve is affected, only central vision is affected, manifested as a central **scotoma** (blind spot). When the entire nerve is affected, the eye is blind. Optic nerve disorders may occur as a consequence of prenatal malformations, optic neuritis, optic atrophy, increased intraocular pressure, or tumorous growth.

Optic nerve aplasia refers to a prenatal malformation in which the optic nerve and retinal vessels are completely absent. The eye is, of course, blind. A less severe form of optic nerve malformation is **optic nerve hypoplasia** (Hoyt 1986). This congenital deficiency of the retina and optic nerves is generally attributed to a primary failure of the development of the retinal ganglion cells and their axons. This process begins approximately 6 weeks after conception, normally reaching the optic chiasm by the seventh week and the lateral geniculate body by the eighth week. Cranial defects, including defects of the midline structures (corpus callosum, septum pellucidum, pituitary body) may lead to endocrine disturbances, such as growth hormone deficiency, adrenal insufficiency, hypothyroidism, and antidiuretic hormone production disturbance, which are frequently found in children with hypoplasia (Ouvrier and Billson 1986, Tait 1989). The occurrence of optic nerve hypoplasia has also been related to age of the mother, i.e., mothers of children with hypoplasia were younger than those of children with cerebral palsy or fetal alcohol syndrome, although the cause remains unknown (Robinson and Conry 1986). Complete, unilateral, or partial failure of the development of retinal ganglion cells results in varying degrees of optic nerve hypoplasia. Typically the consequence is an attendant abnormality of vision, ranging from complete blindness to peripheral field defects with spared central vision, depending on the severity, laterality, and symmetry of the condition. Because of the endocrine disturbances, precocious puberty and hypogonadism have been observed.

Optic neuritis (inflammation of the optic nerve) and **optic nerve atrophy** (degeneration of the optic nerve fibers) are a consequence of many congenital and infantile developmental syndromes, including prenatal infections, nutritional deficiencies, toxicity, or increased intracranial pressure. Optic neuritis may result in temporary reduction of vision if the inflammation subsides or in the permanent loss of vision if the inflammation leads to optic nerve atrophy. For example, with congenital syphilis, the arachnoid sheath surrounding the optic nerve may be infiltrated by the virus and cause optic nerve edema in the acute stage and optic atrophy in the chronic stage. A variety of administered drugs may induce optic neuritis and/or optic nerve atrophy (chloramphenicol, phenothiazines, quinine, Atoxyl), as may exposure to various toxins or poisons, such as lead, methyl alcohol, and carbon disulfide (Biglan et al. 1988).

Optic Chiasm

The optic nerve continues on toward the posterior areas of the brain and emerges on the floor of the middle fossa of the cranial cavity. At this point, anterior to the pituitary gland, the two optic nerves, one from each eye, meet and form the **optic chiasm,** which is the crossing-over point for the fibers of the optic nerve. Half of the fibers from each optic nerve cross over and project to the opposite hemisphere. Damage to the optic chiasm typically creates symmetrical and usually binocular visual field defects, depending on the extent and exact position of the damage. For example, a bitemporal hemianopia (Figure

3-4) occurs with lesions affecting the medial aspects of the chiasm. The most frequent cause of this type of chiasmal damage in children is a craniopharyngioma or optic glioma, although occasionally a dilated third ventricle may result in similar damage (Martyn 1975).

Optic Tract

The **optic tracts** include fibers from the temporal half of the visual field of the eye on the same side (uncrossed fibers) and the nasal half of the visual field of the eye on the opposite side (crossed fibers). Damage to the optic tract usually results in **hemianopia** (half-field blindness), which is irregular unless the damage is total. With total damage, the result is a **homonymous hemianopia** affecting the same half-field of vision (either left or right) from both eyes (Figure 3-4). Usually, central vision is spared, but the entire peripheral visual field is lost. Many degenerative and demyelinating diseases (e.g., Tay-Sachs) affect the optic tracts, as well as other portions of the visual system.

Lateral Geniculate Nucleus

The optic tracts terminate in the **lateral geniculate nuclei.** These bodies are relay stations that send visual information to the occipital cortex and to reflex centers in the brain that control eye movements and muscles in the eye (Biglan et al. 1988).

Ocular Motility

An important aspect of vision is ocular motility. Normal binocular vision depends on each eye sending slightly different images to the higher cortical centers, where they are fused into a single percept. This fusion requires the coordinated simultaneous movement of the two eyes. Each extraocular muscle responsible for moving the eye must have the strength to contract and relax in conjunction with muscles of the other eye and other muscles of the same eye. The motor centers of the brain are involved in both reflexive (via the third, fourth, and sixth cranial nerves) and voluntary (via the left and right motor cortex of the frontal lobes) eye movements. When the position of the body changes, involuntary reflex stimuli elicit movement of the eye muscles and thereby hold the perception of the world steady. Teuber (1966) used the term "**corollary discharge**" to identify this involuntary outflow of stimulation that prepares the visual systems for changes in the visual image that are the expected consequences of an intended movement. In the absence of corollary discharge, the external world would be experienced as unstable. No conclusive physiological mechanism responsible for this hypothesized reflex action has been identified (Hecaen and Albert 1978).

Impairments of ocular motility may be manifested in various ways. **Extraocular muscle palsies** are defects in individual ocular muscles resulting from impairment of the nuclear or infranuclear portion of the cranial nerves (in the subcortical structures of the brain, e.g., pons), of the neuromuscular junction, or of the muscle itself. Paired movements of the two eyes upward, downward, laterally, and in convergence and divergence are called **conjugate eye movements.** These movements may be impaired because of disorders of the supranuclear (i.e., cortical) centers or other pathways that govern the direction of both eyes in unison. **Nystagmus** is an involuntary rhythmical oscillation of one or both eyes in any or all fields of gaze. It may be defined further in terms of plane, amplitude, rate, or severity of prevalence in various directions of gaze. The oscillations may be of equal speed in each direction (pendular) or slow in one direction and rapid in the opposite (biphasic). **Strabismus** ("crosseyedness" or heterotropia) is an abnormality in which one eye fixates its macula on the object of gaze while the other eye is directed elsewhere. It may be classified further as paralytic or nonparalytic and according to position (convergent versus divergent).

Impaired eye movement may result either in a lack of stereoscopic vision because the two images cannot be fused properly into a single percept or in **diplopia** (double vision). Diplopia, however, is not usually a problem in infants or very young children, as they tend to consciously suppress one image in order to avoid confusion.

Disorders of ocular motility may be a result of weak extraocular muscles or CNS abnormalities caused by trauma, anoxic episodes, inflammation of the brain after various infections, compression of the cranial nerves by increased intracranial pressure, or the toxic effect of drugs. For example, lead poisoning may result in strabismus, and ingestion of some hormonal compounds, such as progesteronal steroids, may cause paralysis of the extraocular muscles. Abnormal eye movement may be seen in blind children, not because of muscle or CNS disorders per se but as a function of their blindness, i.e., lack of learned muscle control. For example, Martyn (1975) suggested that the pendular ocular nystagmus and strabismus present with congenital rubella are more commonly due to cataracts, glaucoma, optic nerve damage, or high refractive error than a direct consequence of CNS disease. It has also been suggested that strabismus in infants, which sometimes goes unnoticed during the early months or years, may lead to reduced visual acuity that may be prevented by treatment (Lewerenz 1978).

Optic Radiation

The **optic radiation** emerges from the lateral geniculate nuclei, spreads in a fanlike fashion through the temporal lobes, and terminates in the middle layers of the primary visual cortex (area 17) of the two occipital lobes. Damage in the optic radiation may lead to visual field defects. The entire visual half-field is not always affected, but a symmetrical quadrant loss may be evident for both eyes (Figure 3-4). For example, damage to the lower geniculocalcarine fibers, which course forward into the temporal lobe (Meyer's loop), usually produces an upper quadrantanopia, a small upper sector defect. Lesions of the optic radiation within the parietal lobe usually produce lower-quadrant field defects (Figure 3-4). Visual hallucinations may occur with damage to this area.

Occipital Lobes

Damage to the occipital lobes also produces contralateral visual field defects. Depending on the site and extent of damage, the field defects may vary from small blind spots adjacent to central vision in both eyes (**homonymous para-central scotoma**) to complete hemianopia. Such defects are usually caused by trauma or cerebrovascular disorders and were described in 1917 in the classical work by Poppelreuter (1990).

Damage to the occipital cortex may result in cerebral or **cortical blindness,** a loss of vision in the presence of normal pupillary reflexes and without significant eye disease. Since pupillary responses are affected by pregeniculate lesions but not by postgeniculate lesions (Martyn 1975), the term "cortical blindness" refers to blindness resulting from any postgeniculate damage. Although cortical blindness in adults occurs mainly because of thrombosis of the vertebral and/or basilar arteries, which affects the blood flow to the visual cortex, cortical blindness in children is often a consequence of hydrocephalus, meningitis, toxic or hypertensive encephalopathy, trauma, or diffuse demyelinating degenerative disease (Barnet et al. 1970, Duchowny et al. 1974).

Cortical blindness remains permanent more often in adults than in children. Almost all children with cortical blindness recover at least some visual function (Duchowny et al. 1974). Suggested underlying mechanisms contributing to cortical blindness include cellular ischemia (temporary deficiency of blood flow) as a result of hypotension, vasospasm, cerebral edema, thrombosis of cortical veins (Barnet et al. 1970), and focal ischemia of white matter (Tyler 1968).

The onset of recovery from cortical blindness may vary from hours to months. The typical course of recovery progresses from perception and tracking of light stimuli to perception of moving objects close to the eyes. Next, large, particularly brightly colored objects can be seen. Barnet et al. (1970) noted that at this stage visual hallucinations occasionally occur. Finally, visual acuity progressively improves, although visual cognitive and perceptual deficits may persist for a long time or remain permanently. Often, the blindness is only one sign of more generalized structural brain damage, and refined visual-perceptual testing may be hampered by profound mental retardation (Barnet et al. 1970, Jan et al. 1977).

Two of the six children with cortical blindness examined by Barnet et al. (1970) denied their inability to see. In adults this denial of cortical blindness is termed Anton's syndrome or **anosognosia.**

Since visual evoked responses (VERs) originate in the occipital cortex, this electrophysiological technique may be of value for identifying visual disorders with a central origin. In addition, since this technique requires little active participation of the patient, it has proved useful for the study of the development of visual behavior in infants and preschoolers (Barnet et al. 1980).

The VER is the summed cortical response (sum of postsynaptic potentials) induced in occipital lobe neurons as a result of stimulus change. Both transient VERs, resulting from an isolated and abrupt stimulus change, such as a light flash, and steady-state VERs—regular, steady cyclical responses elicited by rapidly repeating stimuli—have been investigated. Short-latency VER components are thought to reflect activity of the primary visual pathway (Ciganek 1961, Rose 1971), whereas long-latency components reach the neocortex via the second visual system and terminate in the secondary visual centers with more diffuse cortical representation.

Abnormal electrocortical development has been noted in infants during the acute phase of severe protein malnutrition (Bartel, reported in Coursin 1974) and after kwashiorkor (Bartel et al. 1978). The VER deficit manifested in children 5 to 10 years after hospitalization for kwashiorkor was restricted to the right hemisphere; this suggests either that permanent damage to the right hemisphere may be the consequence of early kwashiorkor or that the left hemisphere may overcome its maturational lag before the right hemisphere.

Reports on VERs in cases of cortical blindness, implying postgeniculate involvement, range from lack of response to completely normal responses (Bodis-Wollner et al. 1977, Frank and Torres 1979, Spehlmann et al. 1977). Some studies (Chisholm 1975, Medina et al. 1977) found a correlation between VERs and recovery of vision: both show gradual and parallel improvement during the recovery phase. However, Barnet et al. (1970) described two children who, despite their blindness, showed well-developed VERs. It is possible that this difference in findings may be related to the age of the patients involved since the previously reported cases were adults.

Persistence of VERs has been reported in two blind patients despite extensive bilateral damage to the visual areas of the brain (Spehlmann et al. 1977). Bodis-Wollner et al. (1977) examined a 6-year-old boy who was left blind after an acute febrile illness at 2 years of age. CT showed complete destruction of areas 18 and 19 in the right hemisphere, but some preservation of tissue in these areas in the left hemisphere. Tissue corresponding to area 17 (striate cortex) and part of the optic radiation were also spared. VERs to both transient and steady-state stimuli were normal. It has been suggested that VERs may be present as long as the primary visual cortex is relatively intact, but that functional vision may, at least in children, require the additional integrity of the secondary visual centers and their connections (Frank and Torres 1979).

Frank and Torres (1979) also noted that the presence of abnormal VERs is not incompatible with normal vision. Comparing a group of "cortically blind" children to an etiologically similar group of children with CNS disease but without visual symptoms, they found no significant differences in latencies for any component of the VER.

Since the study of VERs in these clinical cases has not been useful in determining the status of visual functioning in children, the relationship between

VERs and the level of nervous system functioning remains unclear. However, it is possible that differences in etiology, extent of damage, and age of onset, if viewed in relation to the normal development of the visual system, may help explain these inconsistent results. More recently, computer-based electrodiagnostic topographic brain mapping techniques ("visual evoked potential mapping") have been developed that allow the study of light or pattern responses simultaneously over large areas of the brain in a dynamic manner. The electrical activity is displayed as a multicolored moving picture on the screen, each color corresponding to the degree of electrical activity in that area (Whiting et al. 1985).

25.2   Other Visual Disorders

Other visual disorders may arise as a consequence of CNS disorder without a specific locus. For example, transient episodes of vision loss or blurring may indicate CNS involvement. **Amblyopia** refers to temporary or permanent subnormal visual acuity ("dim vision") without ophthalmoscopically detectable retinal abnormality or afferent visual pathway disease, although it can occur secondary to insufficiency of the blood supply from the basilar artery or secondary to pressure on the chiasm by a tumor (Poeck 1974). Generally, amblyopia implies a vision deficit due to sensory deprivation or inhibition occurring early in life (Martyn 1975). Intelligence scores of amblyopic children have been reported to be lower than average (Stewart-Brown et al. 1985).

Distortions of visual perception in terms of object form, contour, size, and movement (**metamorphopsias**) may occur. In adults, both localization and lateralization of lesions influence the form of the disturbance (Hecaen and Albert 1978). With lesions in the visual pathway, color vision may be impaired before form vision. True color vision impairment must be distinguished from **color agnosia** (the loss of the ability to recognize color) and **amnestic color aphasia** (the inability to recall or name colors), two conditions that may reflect cerebral damage that does not involve the perception of color radiations at all. Diplopia, although more often associated with eye movement disorders, may occur with increased intracranial pressure (e.g., tumors) or other neurological diseases such as meningitis or neurodegenerative diseases.

25.3   Assessment of the Developing Visual System in Infants

Although assessment of visual functioning during infancy has been limited by the lack of suitable assessment procedures, some research has been conducted involving both optokinetic nystagmus and preferential looking. The **optokinetic nystagmus technique** (**OKN**) refers to involuntary eye movements that occur when a succession of similar objects passes across the visual field. The eye movements consist of a slow phase in the same direction as the moving objects and a fast phase, or jerk movement, back to the straight-ahead position. The latter occurs when the slow phase brings the eyes to the edge of the orbit. The objects moving across the field and the separation between them must be within the visual resolution capacity of the visual system or no OKN response will be elicited. The basic procedure (Gorman et al. 1957) involves placing the infant under a canopy-like apparatus that passes moving stripes 15 cm above the eyes. The narrowest stripe width that elicits an OKN response is then noted as an indicator of visual discrimination ability.

The **preferential looking technique (PL)** was developed by Fantz and Ordy (1959) for assessing vision in infants. A patterned and an unpatterned stimulus are placed in front of the infant for 20 seconds, and then the stimulation is repeated with the right-left positions of the stimuli reversed. The estimate of visual acuity is based on how long the eyes fixate on the stimuli and is defined as the narrowest stripe width at which 75 per cent or more of the infants at that age show longer pattern than nonpattern fixations (Fantz et al. 1962). An age-related increase from birth is evident (Figure 25-1). The basic procedure has also been modified for the study of differential responses to stimuli, such as color (Bornstein 1978, Teller 1981), complexity (Miranda 1970), size, and number (Fantz and Fagan 1975).

Studies using these techniques on preterm infants indicate that the visual system is functional at birth (Dubowitz 1979, Kiff and Lepard 1966). Even though some differential response to patterned visual stimuli can be elicited in all infants, including premature ones, the age from conception seems to be associated with responses to the number and size of detail of stimuli; younger

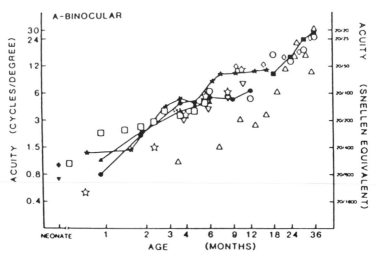

Figure 25-1. Compilation of behavioral data showing the development of grating acuity in humans over the first 3 postnatal years (Teller and Morshon 1986).

infants do not respond as well to patterns that differ only in small degrees along a given dimension (Miranda 1970).

The value of the PL procedure as a predictor of later neurological or mental deficits has been investigated. High-risk infants, many of them severely impaired, were rated as normal, suspect, or abnormal on the basis of their visual fixation performance in infancy. The results suggest that early deficits in visual processing are related to later mental status (Miranda et al. 1977). However, whether early deficits that are manifest in a less impaired group are an adequate predictor of later subtle visual processing disorders remains to be explored.

It is not yet known how performance on visually oriented tasks in infants reflects involvement of different levels of the visual system. Fantz and Ordy (1959) suggested that the OKN is a subcortical reflex and does not involve cortical processing. Fantz et al. (1962) concluded that the capacity for complex pattern perception is present from birth, since infants attend more frequently to patterned than to nonpatterned stimuli. However, Bronson (1974) suggested that these findings may be merely basic retinal processes mediated by a subcortical network, at least during the first month of life. More sophisticated neocortical-mediated mechanisms would be expected to contribute to the infant's reactions from the second month onward. Bronson (1974) proposed that "rather than conceiving of postnatal change as reflecting a general improvement in the efficiency of a total system all of whose components are to some degree functional from birth, it seems more nearly correct to posit the emergence of a series of new capabilities corresponding to the progressive development of increasingly more sophisticated neural networks" (p. 887).

As discussed earlier, Bronson (1974) ascribed the visual responses elicited within the first month of life directly to the phylogenetically older second visual system. This system responds to directional loci of salient peripherally located stimuli and does not seem to be capable of complex pattern analysis. During the second and third months of life, more sophisticated responses begin to appear, reflecting the increased participation of the primary visual system. As memories accrue, visual behavior is no longer limited to the most salient aspects of a configuration, and the infant becomes an internally directed, pattern-organizing individual. The process of postnatal visual development is viewed as the progressive encoding of increasingly complex aspects of the visual stimulus. This position implies that earlier visually oriented behaviors may differ qualitatively from later ones, rather than differ merely in relative efficiency.

Maurer and Terrill (1979) similarly suggested that two separate visual mechanisms explain the rapid improvement of the visual functions in infants. The X pathway, which mediates fine acuity, maintains fixation, and analyzes patterns, relies on special types of cells in the retina and relays via the geniculate bodies to the cortex; the second, or Y, pathway mediates peripheral detection and perception of movement and flicker and contributes to scanning. Based on animal experiments, the authors proposed that the X pathway is functional at birth and the Y pathway operates only to the superior colliculus level; the connection to the visual cortex is not functional until the second month of life.

25.4   Visual Processing and its Disorders

Visual processing, in addition to detection and active scanning of the stimulus, involves identification and analysis of salient visual cues, integration of these cues into a recognizable whole, tentative classification of the visual percept, and evaluation of the correctness of classification (which may entail alterations of classification). Disorders in visual processing are usually related to dysfunction of higher cortical centers. A variety of visually oriented tasks may be used for the assessment of these more complex visual information processing abilities. They are subdivided into (1) spatial orientation, (2) visual discrimination, and (3) object recognition tasks (Chalfant and Scheffelin 1969) and differ with respect to degree of analysis, integration, and evaluation; they may include motor components as well.

Spatial Orientation

Spatial orientation disorders may include left-right discrimination difficulty; reversal errors, such as in confusing the letters "b" and "d"; rotation errors, such as the inability to distinguish the letters "p" from "d"; directional confusion in plotting a route or map from one place to another; poor recognition of familiar or unfamiliar shapes; poor tracing of mazes; difficulty in perceiving one's own body in space; or lack of attention to part of the spatial field. This last deficit, which has been termed **hemi-inattention** or hemispatial neglect, occurs independent of visual field defects and may be manifest in a variety of ways, including failure to read words on one-half of a page or to dress one-half of the body. Ferro and Martins (1990) described three children with spatial orientation disorders: one had transient left-sided post-ictal neglect, one showed pure motor neglect after a thalamic lesion, and one developed visual neglect after the rupture of a right parietal arteriovenous malformation and recovered within 14 days. The report indicates that hemispatial attention is established early in life and can be disrupted by a variety of cortical and subcortical lesions.

Visual Discrimination

Tasks of visual discrimination may involve selecting items on the basis of some salient characteristic, such as color or shape; distinguishing an object presented in the context of a complex visual array; or identifying an object despite the fact that the total visual stimulus is not present. The rate, duration, and order of presentation of these tasks may influence performance and suggest different underlying visual processing disorders.

Object Recognition

The failure to recognize objects despite an intact visual capacity and the inability to discriminate parts of the object is called **visual agnosia.** Even if visual recognition of an object is impaired, the object may be recognized through one of the other senses. The underlying disorder seems to involve visually synthesizing or integrating the discrete aspects of the stimulus into a unified whole. In adults, both occipital and frontal lobe lesions may lead to disorders of object recognition. With frontal lobe disorders a dysfunction of active investigation activity is more likely, whereas occipital lesions may produce deficits in the synthesis and integration of visual stimuli (Luria 1966).

Failure to recognize familiar faces has been singled out as **prosopagnosia,** which may refer to a highly specific process. Young infants tend to scan faces longer than any other visual object (Haith et al. 1977); distinct developmental changes in these scanning habits have been described (Maurer and Salapatek 1976). Scanning habits may not be limited to humans. Preferential responding to birdlike shapes has also been described in finches. Although the preference for scanning of faces is determined by the relatively fixed focus of the newborn's eyes at 40 cm, this preference may also be of biological importance and may serve social interaction. The encoding of such information may be a somewhat different neural process than the processing of visual information at a later age. The importance of the right occipitotemporal area for face recognition has been suggested by studies of patients with sectioning of the corpus callosum. Prosopagnosia seems to be resistant to intensive training efforts (Ellis and Young 1988). A follow-up case study of a girl to the age of 11 by Young and Ellis (1989) suggested that prosopagnosia can occur in the presence of only minor basic impairment of other visual functions (visual object recognition) and that the child could perceive and imitate facial expressions and perform matching tasks. She also learned to read normally.

Alexia (the acquired inability to appreciate the meaning of written words or musical or mathematical symbols) and **dyslexia** (denoting a partial rather than total impairment) are usually included among the visual processing disorders, even though they are not directly related to damage in the visual system. The term "developmental dyslexia" is used to denote a congenital developmental disorder as opposed to the loss of ability resulting from injury to the nervous system. This topic is dealt with in Chapter 29.

Many developmental disorders without gross CNS damage may exert subtle effects on CNS functioning that are reflected in disturbances of visual processing. For example, Taub et al. (1977), in a prospective study, noted that children who were born prematurely had significantly lower Performance IQs in mid-childhood on the Wechsler Intelligence Scale for Children than full-term children. Tests requiring visually mediated behavior were particularly affected. In addition, performance on the Bender Gestalt Test, which involves copying a variety of geometric shapes, was also poorer for prematurely born children. Taub et al. (1977) suggested that the visual system deficit associated with prematurity is based on subtle brain dysfunction or perhaps on a limitation of brain cell growth to which the visual system may be more susceptible than other parts of the nervous system.

25.5 Hemispheric Asymmetry in Blind Children

Larsen and Hakonsen (1983) advanced a new hypothesis regarding cerebral asymmetry in blind children. They noted that Braille is read more accurately by the left hand (Hermelin and O'Connor 1971), presumably because of the higher demands of Braille on the recognition of spatial patterns, a function that relies on right hemispheric specialization. The authors argued that blind children would be more bilaterally organized because of the special cognitive strategies needed "to operate in their invisible surroundings" (p. 197); namely, the need to develop detailed cognitive maps. In an investigation of 36 congenitally blind children between the ages of 8 and 17 years, they found a lack of ear asymmetry on dichotic listening, whereas a matched control group showed the expected right-ear advantage. This finding seems to support the notion of a bilateral organization of cognitive processing in blind children. The superior processing of Braille with the left hand is similar to the advantage of the left visual field in dot pattern perception (Kimura 1969) and in the perception of pictographic Kanji signs in Japanese as opposed to the more alphabetic Kana symbols (Hatta 1977, Sasanuma and Monoi 1975). The latter advantage also seems to relate to the development of a more bilateral organization in Japanese subjects than in English-speaking subjects for dichotic listening under special interference conditions (Hatta and Dimond 1981).

25.6 Development of the Blind Child

Unless specially stimulated, blind children are likely to be delayed in motor, social, and sensory development. For example, the blind child frequently begins to smile late, at 5 to 6 months of age instead of 6 weeks (Freeman 1964). Sitting unaided, crawling, and walking all occur with some delay unless the parents encourage and stimulate the child to perform these activities. If physical activity is not stimulated, muscle tone tends to be poor, and musculature may develop improperly. The blind infant usually responds to sounds with inactivity and silence, rather than with the anticipatory responses of the sighted infant. Elonen and Zwarensteyn (1964) suggested that this inactivity is the result of heightened attention needed to hear more effectively. Toilet training may be delayed, and feeding problems are common, especially in the child with additional impairment.

The blind child is usually more introverted, shows less facial expression, has less eye contact, and tends to use sensory exploration on its own body, rather than on external objects and people. As a result, lack of social interaction and stereotyped behaviors of an autistic nature may develop. Fine (1968) found that 45 per cent of his sample of 2000 blind children displayed repetitive mannerisms, especially eye pressing, rocking, head nodding, hand flapping, and twirling movements. Ten per cent of partially sighted children also showed these tendencies. Head movements toward stimuli are poor in children without useful vision, but better in those with partial vision (Jan et al. 1987). Jan et al. (1990a) also reported head shaking in many visually impaired children, i.e., rapid horizontal and pendular head oscillations, resembling spasms, which the authors interpreted as voluntary, neurovisual adaptations to improve visual acuity. Eye pressing is found only in children with retinal disorders, never in those with bilateral optic nerve defects (Minde et al. 1983); the authors suggested that eye pressing occurs when the demand of the brain for meaningful visual information is not met adequately. In contrast, 60 per cent of cortically visually impaired children tend to show frequent light-gazing (Jan et al. 1990b). As the child learns to walk, is encouraged to explore objects, and is stimulated to engage in different activities, these autistic activities decrease.

Inactivity in the infant, delayed development, poor muscle tone, and persisting stereotyped behaviors in older children not infrequently lead to the false diagnosis of infantile autism or mental retardation. Unlike in the autistic or retarded child, these signs are reversible in blind children, provided the children are given additional stimulation. Jan et al. (1990) stressed the importance of developing the blind child's body image as a prerequisite to movement and mobility.

The congenitally blind child is limited in some aspects of concept formation that depend on visual perception and in abstract concepts that make use of visual metaphors or analogies. Results of intelligence testing are mixed, with some children showing normal and others impaired performance [see Scharf and Adams (1984) for children with retrolental fibroplasia]. The reason for this variance is that many children with visual dysfunction have multiple handicaps that may compound the effects of blindness on cognitive development; few studies distinguish between the multihandicapped and the visual dysfunction only populations. A survey by Hill et al. (1986) found that only 49 per cent of children in the Liverpool area had isolated visual handicaps. Cognitive testing of blind children must be made with specifically designed tests, e.g., the Perkins Binet Test or the Blind Learning Aptitude Test. The current Wechsler Scales for Children may only be used if items dependent upon vision are eliminated and verbal scores are prorated. When compared with sighted children matched for the total Verbal IQ, blind children tested low-average on Comprehension and Similarities and high-average on Digit Span and Information on the verbal section of the WISC (Jan et al. 1977). A study by McConachie (1990) showed that a few visually impaired children without other impairments had advanced verbal expressive abilities, but that the majority of these children lagged in expressive speech relative to comprehension. A similar intelligence profile was reported by Groenveld and Jan (1992). Langset et al. (1989) reported progressive intellectual impairment in a 5-year follow-up of children with visual impairment due to *Toxoplasma gondii* infection. A meta-analysis of 47 studies also confirmed that spatial task performance was poorer, especially in children with early-onset visual impairment (McLinden 1988). Right-left discrimination on objects or persons other than the self tended to be significantly poorer in blind as compared to sighted children (Watemberg et al. 1986).

At school age, children with visual dysfunction may have to be placed in special schools for the visually handicapped. However, in recent years mainstreaming—placement in regular schools that provide special assistance—has become the preferred method of instruction. In 1986, Hill et al. reported that 56 per cent of visually handicapped children with average ability attended regular school, whereas only 34 per cent attended schools for the visually handicapped. Of the remaining 10 per cent, 3 per cent attended special school, and the remaining subjects left school or continued schooling in other institutions. In North American communities, the percentage of children placed in regular schools is likely to be even higher.

Although the blind child is thought to be more attentive to hearing and touch, there is no evidence that acuity in these senses actually is better. However, better speech perception (e.g., better recognition of articulatory error) has been reported in blind children (Lucas 1984). The use of echo to detect the proximity of objects (echo location) develops naturally in some blind children and can be taught to older intelligent ones. Young blind children occasionally make a sharp, repetitive sound spontaneously in order to judge distances, another behavior that may be erroneously interpreted as a sign of infantile autism or other psychopathology (Jan et al. 1977).

25.7   Visual Impairment and Psychopathology

Two factors tend to be related to emotional or behavior problems in children with sensory handicap. First, any cerebral pathology responsible for the sensory impairment may itself increase the incidence of psychopathology. This relationship would be expected to exist for children with central rather than peripheral causes of sensory loss. Second, the reaction of the child to the handicap that impairs communication and social relationships may cause secondary emotional problems.

The congenitally blind child frequently has additional handicaps. In a 30-year survey of all congenitally blind children in British Columbia, Jan et al. (1977) found that 74 per cent had other handicaps, such as mental retardation, hearing loss, congenital heart defects, epilepsy, and cerebral palsy. Half of the children with acquired blindness also suffered from an additional handicap. In general, a child is less likely to have additional impairment if the cause is limited to the eye. Among cortically blind children, however, severe mental retardation is common. Blindness from infections and toxins is usually associated with other impairments, e.g., excessive arterial oxygen resulting from the high incubator oxygen concentrations used in the 1950s. Congenital rubella affects the embryo more severely in the earlier stages of development; retardation, deafness, and heart defects are the most common accompanying deficits.

Blind infants do not respond to the face of the mother and are delayed in responding to her voice. This may lead to the mistaken diagnosis of autism in such children, especially since blind children tend habitually to explore their environment and their own body by pressing their eyeballs; waving their head from side to side; smelling food, objects, and people; gazing at a light source, and waving their hand in front of the eyes. This behavior has been described as "blindism" (Thomas and Chess 1980).

Few studies have compared the incidence of psychopathology in blind and sighted children. The Isle of Wight study by Rutter et al. (1970a) found only 15 blind children; it is difficult to generalize from this number about the comparative incidence of psychiatric disorder. The study reported an incidence of emotional disorders of 16.6 per cent; four of the children were retarded.

In 1968, Magleby and Farley reported that blind children seem to be better adjusted when attending schools for the blind than when integrated into regular schools. They argued that in regular schools with sighted children, the blind child tends to be isolated and often rejected by peers and constantly has to cope with the disability in a setting designed for the sighted. In a school with other blind children, good friendships develop, and fewer behavioral or emotional problems are noted. As mainstreaming has progressed over the past two decades, this argument may no longer be entirely valid since regular schools have improved their facilities and services for the handicapped, although some specialized facilities for blind children are still needed.

Summary

Visual disorders resulting from damage within the primary visual system may range from complete blindness to subtle disorders that are only identifiable under special conditions. Other visual disorders not related to a specific locus of brain damage may be indicative of CNS dysfunction. Subtle disturbances of visual perception assumed to reflect subtle forms of brain dysfunction may manifest in a variety of ways as late as mid-childhood. Although little information is available about the role of the second visual system in humans and its disorders, it has been suggested that visual behavior of infants up to 1 month of age may reflect primary involvement of this system, whereas participation of the primary visual system increases from the second month on. The development of the blind or partially-sighted child of necessity shows some handicap-specific impairment, but general cognitive impairment is mostly found in children with multiple handicaps and cortical damage.

26

Auditory Disorders

The auditory system in lower mammals primarily serves as a protective sense and is reflexive. The reflex action is controlled and coordinated by various centers in the brainstem (Barr 1972). The human cortex has larger association areas for storage and processing of information arriving from the sensory organs, which allows differential recognition, interpretation, and association of sounds with meanings. Most importantly, an intact auditory system permits the reception, sorting, and codifying of speech and thus verbal communication with others.

Auditory processing may be divided into levels of functioning, each potentially influencing the others (Wood 1975). These functional levels include the ability to (1) detect auditory stimuli; (2) attend, both in terms of reflex action to sound and in terms of conscious focusing on the content and source of incoming stimuli; (3) discriminate between sounds and distinguish characteristics of sounds, such as frequency, intensity, and temporal sequence; (4) identify sounds previously heard so that meaning may be associated with them; (5) comprehend sounds by sorting and integrating them with other information in order to store and retain information; and (6) retrieve and restore the sounds for the formation of appropriate responses.

Detection of stimuli (auditory acuity) is a prerequisite for further auditory analysis. Rapid habituation to detected stimuli and the inability to suppress other incoming stimuli, from other senses or irrelevant auditory stimuli, may limit the ability to detect relevant auditory stimuli and interfere with further analysis. In addition, the inability to respond appropriately to a previously heard stimulus, although possibly reflecting a detection problem, may in actuality reflect a problem of more complex forms of auditory analysis, e.g., storage or retrieval.

The anatomy and physiology of the auditory system (Figure 3-1), from the receptor mechanisms of the inner ear to the auditory cortex, are highly complex, with numerous possibilities for feedback controls and an abundance of synaptic connections within and among the neuronal groups. The role of many of the

414

neuronal groups is poorly understood, and the ways in which these channels interact with each other and other areas of the brain are not clearly delineated (Eisenberg 1976). Extensive differences in structure and organization in individual nuclei exist, and transmission through the nuclei is associated with alterations of the signal parameters that reduce the correspondence between signals at successive levels. Above the level of the cochlear nucleus, all synapses are interconnected across the midline; hence, information from each ear is projected to both sides of the brain. At the cortical level, a stronger signal is received from the contralateral ear and neural pathway, and a weaker signal is received from the ipsilateral ear and neural pathway (Rosenzweig 1951). In addition, information from the cochlea may also reach the cortex by routes lying outside the classical auditory pathway (Eisenberg 1976).

26.1   Damage in the Auditory System

In general, the ability to detect sound is primarily related to the integrity of the peripheral hearing mechanisms, whereas the more complex forms of auditory analysis are accomplished by more central areas of the auditory system. Many developmental disorders may affect the developing auditory system. Since auditory acuity and the more complex forms of auditory analysis develop at different rates (Fior 1972), auditory disorders related to damage within the auditory system during the course of development may be manifest at different ages and in different forms. The focus of study has been primarily on the many developmental disorders that result in profound auditory deficits. Subtle auditory disorders manifest at an early age usually come to clinical attention because of the resulting language disorders; until recently, evaluation techniques have not provided specific information concerning the nature of the underlying auditory deficits.

It is beyond the scope of this chapter to cover comprehensively all forms of developmental auditory pathology and related etiologies. Textbooks of otology, otolaryngology, and audiology (e.g., Gottlieb and Krasnegor 1985, Keith 1981, Lutman and Haggard 1983, Northern and Downs 1988, Stein 1988) describe all the forms of developmental auditory pathology and the etiological factors involved. Some of the auditory disorders associated with pathology in the three major anatomical divisions of the auditory system are described below.

Outer and Middle Ear

Sound waves from the external world are received by specialized sensory receptors that perceive fine, rapid movements in the inner ear (cochlea) via the outer (pinna) and middle ear. The outer ear collects the sound, and the middle ear primarily transmits and attenuates it. Abnormalities of the outer or middle ear that interfere with the conduction of sound into the cochlea may lead to conductive hearing losses. Most conductive hearing losses (acuity deficits) do not exceed 60 decibels and can be treated readily with a hearing aid.

Conductive hearing loss may result from blocking of the external meatus (channel into the ear) due to congenital malformations, accumulation of ear wax, or tympanic membrane abnormalities (e.g., pressure or perforation) or from middle ear abnormalities due to congenital malformations or fractures at the base of the skull. However, the most common cause of conductive hearing loss in children is dysfunction or obstruction of the Eustachian tube, which may result in **otitis media** (middle ear infections). If the infection is brief, the auditory consequences are trivial (Rapin 1975). However, recurrent or chronic otitis media is always accompanied by some degree of conductive hearing loss, which may be variable or episodic and results in a long-standing form of fluctuating auditory deprivation (Howie 1980). In addition to acuity deficits, related sequalae of chronic otitis media may include (1) delays in the development of speech and language (Schlieper et al. 1985, Wallace et al. 1988), (2) difficulty in the production of adequate speech, (3) deficits in auditory processing and receptive language skills, and (4) depressed IQ scores and academic skills (see Chapter 27).

Inner Ear and Eighth Cranial Nerve

Damage to the receptor apparatus of the cochlea (the organ of Corti) alters the sensory processes and reduces sound transmission to the auditory nervous system. Serious impairments of cochlear processes can lead secondarily to dysfunction of the auditory nerve (Gulick 1971). Abnormalities of the inner ear or the auditory nerve may result in **sensorineural hearing loss**. The severity of the acuity deficit may range from profound deafness to mild hearing loss, present in both ears or unilaterally, and manifest as a sudden or fluctuating loss. The degree and extent of the hearing loss determine the presence of additional auditory processing deficits. For example, a child with a moderate hearing impairment may develop speech but with poor pronunciation of consonants, whereas a child with a mild hearing impairment will have normal or only slightly impaired speech. Many acquired disorders, including those caused by viral infections, intoxications, demyelinating diseases, or trauma, may result in hearing loss as a consequence of cochlear or eighth nerve damage. For example, rubella infection during pregnancy frequently results in sensorineural hearing loss of the child, most often if the infection occurs during the first trimester and least often if the infection occurs during the last trimester (Strauss and Davis 1973).

Ototoxic drugs (e.g., streptomycin, quinine, and chloroquine phosphate) ingested during pregnancy are drugs that may cause deafness in the fetus by destroying neural elements of the inner ear or by causing extensive damage to the auricle and bone structures of the middle and inner ear, e.g., thalidomide. In addition, several sulfa drugs, phenothiazines, methamphetamines, tranquilizers, and a wide array of other drugs (e.g., antidepressants, general anesthetics, nonbarbiturate anticonvulsants, and antihypertension agents) ingested during pregnancy have been linked to increased risks for sensorineural hearing loss in children (La Benz 1980, Lassman et al. 1980).

Retrospective studies of deaf children indicate that hearing impairments may be related to prematurity (Vernon 1976). However, preterm birth as such does not seem to affect the development of the hearing apparatus since differentiation of the cochlea is complete before the end of the second trimester. The assumption that duration of exposure to incubator noise is responsible for hearing loss in preterm infants has not been corroborated; rather, research indicates a strong correlation between the sum of perinatal risk factors and hearing loss (Schulte and Stennert 1978). Both anoxic episodes (Wolfson et al. 1980) and intrapartum hemorrhage into the inner ear (Wong and Shah 1979) have been suggested as specific perinatal risk factors. Intrapartum hemorrhage into the inner ear may occur as a result of intrapartum injury or physical stress, e.g., forceps delivery. Blood released into the inner ear has toxic effects on the organ of Corti, resulting in irreversible damage.

Postnatal infections (e.g., measles, mumps, bacterial meningitis) may also cause cochlear damage. The otological manifestations of congenital syphilis may occur early in childhood and result in severe bilateral hearing loss, although mild losses may occur later and even as late as the fifth decade of life (Wolfson et al. 1980). Tubercular meningitis may infiltrate and damage the sheath of the auditory nerve and the organ of Corti. In addition, drugs used in the treatment of tubercular meningitis (e.g., streptomycin, dihydrostreptomycin) and other drugs administered postnatally (e.g., neomycin, kanamycin) may be ototoxic. The effects of such drugs seem to be additive, and delayed hearing losses can occur (Strome 1977).

Subcortical Structures

Damage to the auditory system above the auditory nerve, including subcortical structures (i.e., cochlear nucleus, superior olivary complex, inferior colliculus, and medial geniculate body) and the auditory cortex, may also result in subtle to profound auditory impairments. Impairment may be temporary, as in a post-concussion syndrome or after irradiation of the temporal lobes, or it may be permanent.

Although it has been possible to distinguish between conductive and sensorineural hearing impairments in children over 3 years of age, the assessment of hearing in the infant and the differentiation of hearing impairments with central origin have proved difficult. Developments in assessment have supplemented behavioral observations in the assessment of hearing in the infant and young child. The Crib-o-gram (Simmons 1975, Simmons and Russ 1974) is an automated response unit that records the infants' startle responses to noise bursts, automatically samples activity level, and scores it with reference to internally programmed criteria and complex algorithms. Electrophysiological recording of cochlear and eighth nerve activity (electrocochleography) and middle ear mechanisms (impedance measurements) with electrodes placed in the ear are also valuable additions to assessment. Heart rate audiometry (Schulman-Galambos and Galambos 1979), auditory evoked responses (AERs), and brainstem auditory evoked responses (BAERs) have been studied in human infants (Goldie 1985, Kaga and Tanaka 1980). However, Schneider et al. (1979) have pointed out that autonomic and electrophysiological measurements record attentional rather than hearing thresholds. The authors stressed the need for using a variety of behavioral measures in infants and young children.

Auditory evoked potentials (scalp-electrode recordings of the cortical responses) induced by auditory stimuli have been described earlier in the discussion of hemispheric asymmetry (Chapter 5). Brainstem auditory evoked responses, in contrast, are thought to measure sensory function in subcortical portions of the auditory pathway. BAERs are also recorded from scalp electrodes and consist of seven waves produced in the initial 10 milliseconds after a click or tone signal. The seven components presumably derive from sequential activation of the nuclei and pathways of the auditory system. Waves I, II, and III represent activity of the auditory nerve, cochlear nucleus, and superior oliva, respectively, and waves IV and V represent activity of the inferior colliculus as shown in animal experimentation (Arezzo et al. 1985). The origins of waves VI and VII may be related to the medial geniculate body and the auditory radiations (Chiappa 1985). Auditory brainstem responses can yield information about the status and development of auditory and neurological functioning in infants, as well as the location of damage in the auditory system. For example, when used in conjunction with behavioral audiometry in infants, BAERs can aid in determining whether or not an abnormally elevated behavioral response sensitivity reflects dysfunction above the level of the brainstem. If the deficit is above the level of the brainstem, BAERs will be normal. If the BAERs are abnormal, then a brainstem or peripheral lesion would be implicated, although central pathology cannot be ruled out (Goldie 1985, Kaga and Tanaka 1980).

Information derived from both animal and human studies of preterm infants and infants with kernicterus (Wolfson et al. 1980) suggests that intrapartum asphyxia and anoxia may cause damage to the cochlear nucleus (Dublin 1978). However, BAER research on kernicterus infants indicates that peripheral lesions are likely to be present, although concomitant brainstem and cortical pathology cannot be ruled out. Other reports on cases of kernicterus also support the notion that the hearing impairment is sensorineural (Schuknecht 1974).

Animal research has suggested that auditory deprivation induced by a lack of environmental stimulation or by conductive hearing loss results in incomplete maturation of most auditory neurons of the brainstem: "There is a critical period for development of auditory brainstem nuclei. . . . Without adequate sound stimulation during this period, most brainstem auditory neurons do not fully develop" (Webster and Webster 1979, p. 687). In light of BAER research that indicated that brainstem maturation in the human may continue into the second or third year of life (Kaga and Tanaka 1980), auditory deprivation during this period, regardless of the cause, may have devastating consequences for the development of normal auditory processing. This finding is consistent with studies of the effects of chronic otitis media, indicating that early hearing deficits adversely affect later central auditory functioning, and supports the sensitive period hypothesis of language acquisition.

Cortical Structures

The term "**congenital auditory imperception**" has been used to describe deafness originating from central as opposed to peripheral pathology. Although in some instances children with congenital auditory imperception do not respond to any sound consistently (Ward and McCartney 1978), more often some sounds do elicit responses but the child does not respond to spoken language. This disturbance of language appreciation is discussed further in Chapter 27.

Most research on the effects of pathological processes at various sites in the central auditory system has involved adult patients. Lesions of subcortical and cortical areas of the auditory system in adults and children rarely affect acuity (Thatcher 1980), but the effects on complex auditory processing are a function of the nature of the auditory stimulus (speech, environmental sounds, melodies, rhythm), the temporal and spectral characteristics of the sounds (sound sequences, pitch), and aspects of the listening situation, e.g., monaural or binaural presentation, extraneous influences, such as noise and competing sounds, speaker characteristics.

In children, these more subtle disturbances of auditory processing have been referred to as auditory perceptual problems or auditory imperception, but are best described as central auditory processing disorders (Keith 1981). Techniques available for the assessment of auditory processing in children include speech and sound discrimination tasks varying in one or more dimensions, auditory figure-ground selection, and sound localization (Chalfant and Scheffelin 1969, Sidtis 1984). Techniques that involve modifications of the acoustic signal (e.g., frequency filtering of the speech signal, binaural fusion, competing messages, dichotic listening, synthetic sentences) have been developed (Beasley and Rintelmann 1979, Katz 1972). Most of these procedures are derived from methods for the assessment of medically related pathologies of the auditory system in adults. Since peripheral hearing impairments may affect central processing, these measures are most useful when peripheral hearing is normal.

Musiek and Geurkink (1980) described five children with learning difficulties referred for hearing assessments. In spite of normal audiograms, various types and degrees of auditory processing problems were detected on tests that included rapidly alternating speech, binaural fusion, low-pass filtered speech, competing sentences, staggered spondaic words, dichotic digits, and frequency patterns. One child exhibited a marked deficit of the left ear on the majority of the measures, in addition to problems of space perception noted by teachers, parents, and the examiner during testing. Diffuse right hemisphere dysfunction was suspected.

The major causes of damage to the central auditory system are trauma (perinatal or postnatal), cerebrovascular disorders, and demyelinating or degenerative diseases. Abnormal cortical functioning as indicated by AERs have also been reported in malnourished infants for as long as 1 year after intervention. The greater abnormality of AERs in malnourished infants of short stature may represent the more devastating effects of chronic malnutrition (Barnet et al. 1978).

26.2   Developmental Problems Associated with Auditory Disorders

Dependent on the nature of the lesion, auditory disorders are often accompanied by other sensory and motor deficits of varying degree and by cognitive impairment. Figure 26-1 shows the high rate of association with other handicaps found in 861 children with hearing loss in a total sample of 2988 children (CEC Report 1980). The long-term effect of auditory disorders must therefore be viewed in the context of other accompanying deficits. Balance and subtle motor skills may be affected (Butterfield 1986, Butterfield and Ersing 1986) and handedness is often less pronounced (Bonvillian et al. 1982).

Even auditory impairment without apparent accompanying disorders tends to have extensive consequences for the child not limited to hearing and auditory processing alone but extending to other senses. Mayberry (1992) presented a detailed review of studies of the development of children with congenital deafness. A study by Vargha-Khadem (1982) noted a deficit in tactile recognition of letters and nonverbal shapes in a group of 16 prelingually deaf as compared to normal-hearing schoolchildren. A recent study by Szelag et al. (1992) studied

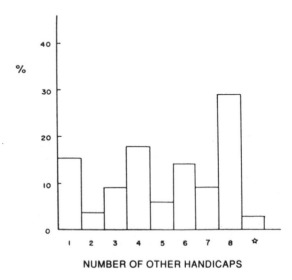

Figure 26-1.   Distribution of additional disabilities in 861 out of 2988 children with hearing loss (CEC Report 1980).

word reading and face recognition in the two hemifields of congenitally deaf children; they found, in contrast to the findings in normal children, a right hemisphere advantage for reading and no field advantage for faces. The authors concluded that the lack of auditory experiences affects the functional organization of the two hemispheres, including right hemisphere dominance for verbal tasks. Marcotte and LaBarba (1987) came to similar conclusions. This theory deserves further exploration.

The most severe limitation imposed by deafness is the inability to acquire a formal verbal language (Rapin 1979). Although lip reading may be of some help and sign language can be learned with great proficiency, communication with the majority of normal-hearing peers remains seriously disrupted. Formal language is frequently learned only when the child learns to read and write and remains less than perfect. Schlesinger and Meadows (1972) showed that academic and language performance is aided by the early acquisition of a basic communication system, i.e., sign language. Deaf children of deaf parents who communicated with signs and gestures from infancy were found to be far superior to congenitally deaf children of hearing parents who did not use sign language. However, a study by Kimura (1981) noted that, in several cases of deafness with CNS damage, signing ability was also impaired in cases of left-hemisphere-lesioned right-handers (interpreted as "manual apraxia"). Chess et al. (1980) also reported rapid acceleration of academic and social functioning in children involved in a "total communication" program. IQ scores of deaf students on nonverbal intelligence tests, such as the Raven Matrices (Marschark 1993) and the performance part of the WISC (Vonderhaar and Chambers 1975), are not significantly different from those of hearing children. As Furth (1966) and others have shown, "thinking without language" is quite adequate in deaf children.

Deaf children also learn to read and to communicate by written language, as well as other communication systems. Although a detailed review of these studies is not appropriate in the present context, it should be mentioned that concept formation in deaf children has been found to be approximately at the level expected on the basis of their age as long as it involves new concepts (e.g. symmetry or sameness), whereas for other concepts, those that are overlearned by the use of language (e.g., opposites, learned by the frequent use of such verbal examples as high-low, up-down, big-small), normal-hearing children showed a distinct advantage. In fact, Furth and Youniss (1964) showed that deaf children learned better than normal-hearing children on tasks in which interference by implicit verbal responses was likely to occur. Deaf children also learned the temporal sequence of faces better than controls, but controls were better in remembering the temporal order of nonsense syllables (O'Connor and Hermelin 1973).

The emotional development of hearing-impaired children tends to be more normal than, for example, blind children (Lou 1982). However, the incidence of emotional disorders is still higher than in normal children. This topic is discussed further in Chapter 30. After completing school, employment opportunities for deaf young adults are severely limited.

Children with central processing disorders face more subtle problems in their cognitive development (Aten and Davis 1968, Bracken and Cato 1986). In particular, school problems are common, and communication with others often remains impaired to some degree.

26.3 Psychopathology and Hearing Impairment

Few studies have compared groups of deaf and normal children in order to describe differences of adjustment, personality, and psychopathology. Rutter et al. (1970a) found psychiatric disturbance in blind and deaf children at an incidence rate of 15.4 per cent for all ages. This figure is not substantially higher than the 5 to 15 per cent incidence of psychiatric disorder for children of all ages in the general population. However, the deaf children were not divided into groups of central and peripheral, or primary or secondary deafness; the small number of children involved may have precluded such an analysis.

Vernon (1967) examined 117 prematurely born, congenitally deaf children. Thirty-four were considered emotionally maladjusted to the extent that they were unable to function adequately in school. He noted that hyperactivity was more noticeable in children with overt neurological abnormalities. A second pattern found in other children was a schizoid type of disorder with hallucinations and homosexual behavior.

A descriptive study by Norden (1981) of deaf children in a kindergarten for the deaf addressed personality development. Based on clinical judgment, the author found that personality development was good if the children were allowed to use sign language freely and formal oral speech training was avoided. The author observed that the children raised by deaf parents developed emotional strengths that were unlikely to be gained if they had been reared by hearing parents. Further support for this position is provided by Meadow (1968), who found that deaf children raised by deaf parents showed more maturity in terms of personality adjustment than children reared by hearing parents. Deaf children raised by deaf parents were better adjusted in terms of sociability, popularity, emotional responses, willingness to communicate with strangers, and lack of communicative frustration; they also showed better scholastic achievement.

Summary

This chapter presented some of the disorders associated with damage to the auditory system. Auditory deficits may range from profound hearing losses to subtle disturbances of auditory processing abilities. Although relatively little information is available about specific functional-physiological correlates of the auditory system or the effects of early damage on discrete elements within the auditory system, hearing loss seems to be related primarily to dysfunction of the peripheral hearing mechanisms, whereas more complex disorders of auditory analysis are due to damage to the more central areas. Early auditory deprivation may result in later auditory processing deficits and perhaps actual structural abnormalities. Since the more complex forms of auditory processing continue to develop into mid-childhood, subtle damage to the central auditory processing mechanisms may not be manifest for several years.

27

Language Disorders

Language, or verbal communication, is a crucial part of human behavior in society. Language permits the individual to communicate with others, a basic mechanism for social interaction. In addition, language provides the individual with a tool for thinking. Inadequate or failing language development may have far-reaching implications for a child's overall development, as well as for specific behaviors involved in communicative transactions. In this chapter, several disorders of language are addressed and the broader implications of language disorders in relation to cognitive functioning discussed.

To appreciate the manifestations of impaired language functioning in children, an understanding of normal language acquisition is helpful in identifying and quantifying specific aspects of language disorders. Although a full discussion of normal language acquisition is beyond the scope of this chapter, it should be noted that several theories and approaches to its study are available. Some emphasize the linguistic aspects (e.g., phonemic, morphemic, syntactic, semantic), some emphasize perceptual and cognitive bases of language acquisition (e.g., Vygotsky, Piaget), and others seek to explain linguistic development in terms of the development of more general cognitive structures (developmental psycholinguistics). In addition, differing emphasis has been placed on organismic and environmental factors involved in language acquisition. Studies of very young infants (between 4 days and 4 months) suggest that the infant has the ability to discriminate both prosodic and suprasegmental aspects (fundamental frequency, amplitude, and duration) of polysyllabic sequences without prior experience soon after birth, but that this ability declines during the first year of life for non-native speech sounds while discrimination in the language spoken by the caregiver increases (Karzon 1985, Mehler et al. 1988, Miller and Eimas 1983, Werker and Tees 1984). Molfese and Betz (1987) stressed, however, that lateralization of specific language and motor behavior is not necessarily present at birth, but that both mature rapidly, first in parallel and later in interaction.

424

As yet, no definitive or complete model of language development has emerged. However, it is important to realize that processes underlying the development of language depend on the existence and maintenance of anatomical and physiological factors on the one hand and environmental ones (e.g., quality of early linguistic environment, parental and peer-group speech, amount and type of social interaction) on the other.

Table 27-1 gives an outline of normal language development in children, including questions that the examiner may use to determine deviations from the normal development of communication skills.

27.1   Forms and Frequency of Language Disorders

Disturbances of language functioning may come to the attention of the clinician in a variety of forms. A child may show a marked delay in beginning to speak. Difficulty with speech comprehension may be noted. Very restricted speech, persistent echolalia, or bizarre and inappropriate speech may be present. Poor articulation and dysfluency (stuttering) are even more frequent reasons for referral; however, these often temporary disorders of speech are usually not included in a discussion of disorders of language. Although there is no generally accepted terminology and classification system for language disorders, a basic distinction has been made based on whether the disorder represents a (1) failure or (2) delay in acquiring language or a (3) complete loss or reduction in language capacity occurring subsequent to language acquisition. Marge (1972) defined these three categories and obtained estimated prevalences of language difficulties among various handicapped populations, as follows:

1. *Failure to acquire language:* children who at 4 years of age years have not shown any sign of acquiring language (0.68 per cent)
2. *Delayed language acquisition:* children whose language acquisition is below that attained by peers of the same age; the delay may occur in all components of language, in only one, or in a combination of the phonological, semantic, and syntactic aspects (6.2 per cent)
3. *Acquired language disorder:* children who had at some point in development acquired language and who subsequently suffered a complete loss or reduction of their capacity to use language (0.25 per cent)

The overall prevalence among children in the United States in 1972 of 7.13 per cent of oral language disorders agreed closely with that reported by MacKeith and Rutter (1972) for the United Kingdom (6.7 per cent). Included in this estimate are mentally retarded children, children with emotional disorders, deaf and hard-of-hearing children, speech-handicapped children, and children with specific learning disabilities. Children who speak either a dialect or a foreign language and have experienced difficulties are not included. Category 2, the largest group, represents a wide range of difficulties, from mild articulation problems to serious difficulties with syntactic formulation.

Table 27-1 Milestones in the Development of Communication

Age	Milestone	Questions for parent
0–2 months	Responsiveness to sounds in the speech frequency range	Does the child turn head or look up at the sound of voices?
	Preference for speech over other rhythmic sounds	Can the child be soothed or made to smile by the sound of voices? Does the child seem to like listening to people talk?
	Tendency to synchronize movements to breaks in speech	Does the child seem to be aware when you stopped talking? Does the child wait for a pause to reach or move?
	Categorical perception for speech sounds	
	Preference for human faces over other visual stimuli	Does the child attend to your face? Does the child seem to look at you more often than at other things when you are in the room?
2–8 months	Mother-child "dialogue" in mutual gaze, joint action, babbling	Does the child "talk back" to you when you use baby talk? Can you direct the child's attention to objects? Does the child seem to enjoy playing with you using toys and playing games, such as pattycake or "so-big"?
9–12 months	Expression of nonverbal communicative intents to requests, reject, call attention to self and object	Does the child make wants and needs known by gesturing and making sounds? Does the child attempt to get your attention this way? Does the child attempt to get you to play games or comments on his or her activities?
	Understanding a few words in outline contexts	Does the child eventually recognize a few words from games, such as peek-a-boo, and act spontaneously when he or she hears the word?
12–18 months	Use of first recognizable word	Does the child use any words to express wants or needs?
	Understanding of words outside routine contexts	Does the child understand any words without gestures or facial cues? For example, if you said, "Where's Daddy?," would the child turn and look for him?

Table 27-1 Continued

Age	Milestone	Questions for parent
18–24 months	Two words combined to form telegraphic sentences expressing a limited range of meanings	Does the child put words together in two-word sentences?
	Understanding of words for absent objects	If you ask for an object in another room, can the child fetch the correct item without gestural cues?
	Understanding of conversational obligation to respond to speech with speech	Does the child attempt to answer questions or respond to your comments in some way, verbal or nonverbal?
	Use of language to request information	Does the child ever, either verbally or nonverbally, try to get you to say the names of objects?
2–5 years	Increase in average sentence length from 2.0 to 4.5 words or more	Does the child gradually add more words to sentences?
	Over-generalization of rules for forming plurals, past tense, etc.	Does the child ever say words wrong, such as "comed, goed, foots"?
	Mastery of morphological and syntactic rules for simple sentences; emergence of complex sentences	Do the child's sentences eventually sound more like those of an adult?
	Use of linguistic rules for understanding sentences	Does the child ever misunderstand things you say, especially when you use long and complicated sentences?
	Use of language to talk about events remote in time and space	Does the child tell you about things that happened away from home? In the past?
	Use of language for diverse purposes, e.g., imaging, predicting, interpreting	Does the child talk about things that will happen later? Could happen? Does the child talk about make-believe things?
	Increased conversational skills, topic maintenance	Can the child stick to a subject in conversation, say something new about the subject?
	Clarification	If the child does not understand you, does he or she ask you to repeat? Can the child repeat or repair a sentence you misunderstand?

Table continued

427

Table 27-1 Continued

Age	Milestone	Questions for parent
	Polite, indirect requests	Can the child use language to "wheedle" things out of you? Can the child say it nicer in other ways than just adding "please"?
	Choice of appropriate speech style for the social situation	Does the child talk differently to younger children? Is the child more polite to grownups than peers?
5–12 years	Use of devices to elaborate and condense information to sentences	Can the child tell stories without stringing sentences together only with an "and"?
	Ability to use and understand unusual sentence types in the language, e.g., passives	Does the child sometimes use complex sentence forms in speaking? Writing?
	Development of metalinguistic awareness	Does the child ever make up words, play games with words, or make up puns? Could the child tell you his or her favorite word?

Source: Paul and Cohen 1982.

These prevalence figures are probably conservative estimates. In screening 237 children who were referred with another primary problem (i.e., psychological problems), Cohen and Lipsett (1991) found that 38 per cent had a previously unrecognized language impairment. A representative sample of 1665 kindergarten children in Ottawa, Canada, had an incidence of speech or language impairment of 15.5 to 25.1 per cent—slightly higher for girls than for boys (Beitchman et al. 1986). The discrepancy in reported incidence rates is probably due to the inclusion of all minor speech and language defects (e.g., mild articulatory and stuttering problems in the Ottawa study, which may not require treatment and may disappear on follow-up. Satz (1982) reported that language delay and most other language disorders occur approximately three to four times as often in boys as in girls, suggesting a further discrepancy.

27.2 Differential Diagnosis

Several considerations help clarify the nature of language disorders and aid differential diagnosis (Table 27-2). If the disorder occurs in the absence of intellectual deficit and serious environmental deprivation, it is referred to as either dysphasia or aphasia, although dysphasia remains the preferred term for congenital disorders. Frequently, however, the language disorder occurs in the context of other, more pervasive disorders. For example, significant retardation of

Table 27-2 Differential Diagnosis of Language
Disorders in Childhood

Hearing loss
Oral-area sensory deficit
Aphasia, acquired
Dysphasia, congenital
Dysphasia, developmental
Dyslexia
   Acquired
   Developmental
Minimal brain dysfunction (MBD)
Psychosis of childhood (including early infantile autism)
Nonpsychotic mental and personality disorders
Epilepsy
Mental retardation
Environmental deficits (sensory, emotional, and cultural
   deprivation; inadequate or incompetent instruction)
Normal variation

speech development is often seen in conjunction with deafness, mental retardation, and pervasive psychiatric disorders, e.g., infantile autism. Children who are intellectually subnormal often manifest retardation of a similar degree in motor, adaptive, and social aspects of development, as well as in language development. Language acquisition by the retarded child tends to be delayed, but follows basically the same pattern as in children of normal intelligence. However, it is usually accepted that some mentally retarded children also suffer from more specific forms of language disorders that could be classified as dysphasia (Benton 1978, Cromer 1978, Richardson 1972).

The language development of autistic children differs from that of normal children in several ways. Autistic children may show delayed or deviant language development, in addition to impaired social development, which is well below their intellectual level, and an insistence on sameness, as shown by stereotyped play patterns, abnormal preoccupations, or resistance to change (for a more detailed discussion see Chapter 30).

A special case of language delay (deprivation) is the **Kasper Hauser syndrome,** most recently studied in the case of Genie (Curtiss 1977). In this case, gross environmental neglect and deprivation of language stimulation led to severe language delay. A somewhat similar situation was reported by Luria and Yudovich (1971) for twins who "did not experience the necessity of using language to communicate with each other" (p. 105) and instead developed a substitute activity of practical pointing that the authors described as "synpraxic speech." From a neuropsychological perspective, such cases are of interest mainly in that they contribute to our knowledge about sensitive periods for language development discussed in Chapter 8. Both Kasper Hauser and Genie gained a considerable amount of language after deprivation ended as late as age 10 or 12, and an active language training program was started. The same applied to the twins after the age of 5. These cases suggest that language acquisition during the first years of life may not be quite as critical as some authors contend (Lenneberg 1967), although in both case studies there were serious limitations in the development of more complex use of language. Regarding Genie: "Her spontaneous speech was almost devoid of syntax, and communication was primarily single word production" (Curtiss et al. 1975).

Another consideration in clarifying the nature of language disorders is whether the primary problem is one of reception (understanding speech, decoding) or expression (encoding). The traditional clinical approach to the classification of language disorders on these dimensions is illustrated in Table 27-3. In practice, considerable overlap between problems of comprehension and expression is found, as shown in a study of 315 children with difficulty in language learning by J.A.M. Martin (1981, Table 27-4).

27.3 Receptive Disorders

Three types of receptive disorders or disorders of input (Rapin and Wilson 1978) may occur, depending on the level of receptive functions: (1) the auditory signal may not be detected (i.e., hearing loss); (2) discrimination between auditory signals (i.e., of duration, pattern, or serial order) may not be made; and (3) semantic significance (or the decoding of the meaning of the phonological aspects of speech) of auditory symbols may not be established, especially under rapid presentation conditions (DeMarco et al. 1989).

Discrimination ability may be affected differentially depending on the type of auditory stimuli. For example, discrimination of speech may be impaired, although the ability to discriminate environmental sounds remains intact. This condition has been described as congenital word deafness (Worster-Drought and Allen 1929a and b) or **verbal auditory agnosia.** The term "**auditory agnosia**" has been applied to the total inability to differentiate all varieties of sound. In contrast, the term "**auditory imperception**," as used by Worster-Drought and Allen (1929a), denotes an inability to differentiate speech sounds and some environmental sounds, with an impaired ability to imitate sounds, sing a tune, or show any natural response to rhythm. Receptive disorders are frequently accompanied by distorted speech since the speech-monitoring mechanism remains inadequate. Worster-Drought and Allen also noted the frequent occurrence of speech containing **neologisms** (words created in a patient's speech that are idiosyncratic and meaningless); the authors described as "**idioglossia**" speech that remains largely unintelligible because of the large amount of idiosyncratic elements.

27.4 Expressive Disorders

Three types of disorders of expression may be distinguished in accordance with the three types of production functions: (1) defects in the production of lan-

Table 27-3 Classification of Organically Based Language Deficits

| Channel | Decoding | | | | Encoding | | |
	Acuity	Discrimination	Association	Central processing	Association	Motor	Discrete movements
Auditory	Deafness and hearing loss	Auditory agnosia	Auditory dysphasia	Categorizing, problem solving, learning storage and retrieval, language acquisition etc.	Oral dysphasia	Oral apraxia	Oral paralysis
Visual	Blindness and visual loss	Visual agnosia	Visual dysphasia		Manual dysphasia	Manual apraxia	Manual paralyses

Source: Irwin et al. 1972.

Table 27-4 Overall Distribution of Verbal Comprehension and Expression in 315 Language-Impaired Children

Level of ability	Verbal comprehension	Verbal expression
Normal (N)	108	54
Moderate impairment (M)	60	58
Severe impairment (S)	147	203
Total	315	315

Source: J.A.M. Martin 1981.

guage occurring at the semantic level (with lexical and syntactic impoverishment) are referred to as expressive dysphasias; (2) defects at the motor level are referred to as apraxias; and (3) defects in discrete movements of the peripheral muscles (neuromotor control and coordination) are referred to as dysarthrias. Rapin and Wilson (1978) made an additional distinction between defective programming at the syntactic and the phonemic level. Although the two levels of programming may not always be clearly separable, Yoss and Darley (1974) stressed that in some children syntax can be adequate and only the phonological output disturbed.

Motor pattern disorders affect the ability to speak in the absence of overt paralysis and have been termed verbal dyspraxias (Ferry et al. 1975, Yoss and Darley 1974) or articulatory apraxias, apraxias of speech, apraxic dysarthrias, or cortical dysarthrias. They occur in conjunction with an intact ability to perform other purposeful movements of the oral musculature (e.g., blow out a match, whistle) or other apraxias (Aram and Horwitz 1983, see also Chapter 23). In some studies, the distinction between verbal dyspraxia and dysphasia becomes blurred. For example, Ekelman and Aram (1983) and Stackhouse (1982) reported a large variety of syntactic problems in such children. Inability to perform purposeful movements of the mouth and lower face in the absence of paralysis has been termed oral or buccofacial apraxia. A study of 60 patients with developmental verbal dyspraxia (Ferry et al. 1975) indicated absent or poorly intelligible ("dilapidated") speech that became worse when tested by increasingly more complex phonetic combinations. The authors reported associated oral dyspraxia in more than half of their patients and noted that conventional speech therapy had been unsuccessful; spontaneous improvement occurred only up to the age of 6 years. In severe cases, augmentative or alternative communication may have to be used (Culp 1989).

27.5 Application of the Classification System

The approach to the traditional classification of language disorders described in the previous section—and followed in a survey by Benton (1978)—is based to some extent on the study of disturbances of language in adult brain-damaged populations where relatively discrete forms of language impairment, as implied by the various dissociations, and no impairment of basic intelligence have been observed. Dissociations between these discrete forms of language impairment in adults have been related to the clinical basis of the difficulty, i.e., specific focal brain lesions.

The application of this classification system to disturbances of language in children for the purpose of identifying specific groups of language disorders has not always been successful. In the adult, brain damage interferes with well-established, organized functions, whereas in children functions are in the process of developing in a rapidly changing system. For example, it is expected that in children, reception necessarily influences expressive output. In order to vocalize language sounds, it is necessary to receive both auditory input and feedback of one's own vocalizations. Lack of comprehension and feedback may reduce verbal output, thus interfering with the development of articulation skills.

The fundamental differences between language disorders of adults with acquired brain damage and those seen in children have led to a proliferation of terms designed to describe more adequately the childhood disorders, e.g., congenital or developmental dysphasia, word deafness with verbal apraxia, developmental or congenital auditory imperception. More neutral terms, such as specific developmental language disorder and developmental language retardation, have been used to describe inadequate language development without an obvious cause and to avoid unintended implications regarding the nature of the underlying pathology as seen in adults. Some brain-behavior correlates have been discussed. Stewart (1983), for example, speculated that with new imaging technology, children with specific developmental language disorder may show otherwise undetectable damage to the germinal layer or the periventricular areas. Bendersky and Lewis (1990) found ventricular dilation associated with intraventricular hemorrhage in children with delayed early language development.

Wallace et al. (1988) found that children with otitis media during the first year of life exhibited significantly lower expressive language scores, although receptive language scores were normal; however, the role of chronic otitis media in the etiology of long-term language delay was not confirmed in several other studies (Roberts et al. 1988, Roland et al. 1989, Tallal et al. 1991, Wright et al. 1988). Friel-Patti and Finitzo (1990) and Wright et al. (1988) reported a temporary decrease in hearing sensitivity at age 2 that resolved subsequently. A carefully controlled prospective study of 207 children from birth to 7 years, however, found a significant association between time spent with middle ear effusion during the first 3 years of life and both Verbal and Performance IQ scores and scores in mathematics and reading, as well as articulation and the use of phonological markers. Length of time with otitis media after age 3 was not related to outcome at age 7.

Some authors (Ingram 1976, Zangwill 1978) have stressed the commonalities among childhood language disorders and the overlap between types. Eisenson (1968a) even emphasized in his "unitary explanation" that a "basic impairment in the necessary capacity for the analysis of speech signals and for the sequencing of temporal events" (p.12) is an essential part of all developmental language disorders, especially dysphasia. On the other hand, some systematic breakdown into specific types is usually attempted. Menyuk (1978) emphasized that many language-disturbed children nevertheless follow a normal developmental sequence of language acquisition, although at a significantly slower pace. Deviant developmental patterns are rare. Menyuk stated that the nature of the basic problem changes with changes in developmental needs over time; what may begin as a segmental and suprasegmental problem later appears as semantic and syntactic problems. She documented this developmental lag-change theory with experimental and observational evidence. Kerschensteiner and Huber's (1975) case of a 23-year-old developmental dysphasic also confirms the notion as far as acquisition of grammar is concerned; their patient showed language "quite comparable to the language of children from 3 to 6 (years old)" (p. 281), although his nonverbal (Raven test) IQ was 90. The authors describe the language handicap as "incomplete maturation," especially for linguistic generalizations.

Rapin and Wilson (1978) proposed "multiple syndromes of developmental language disability," stressing that a single deficit cannot possibly account for the variety of observed disorders, although current classification systems are insufficient or inadequate.

Although the value of adapting the adult classification system for children in order to ascertain the neurological locus of impairment in children is limited, the analysis and elucidation of receptive and expressive functions have proved useful for clarifying the nature of language disorders in children. For example, impaired auditory processing of normal speech has been hypothesized to be the underlying cognitive deficit in children whose failure to acquire language is discordant with their nonverbal intelligence and peripheral hearing acuity (Eisenson 1968b). Several types of auditory processing deficits have been implicated in this regard: (1) impairment of storage capacity, especially in relation to grammatical complexity (Bliss and Peterson 1975); (2) impairment of speech sound discrimination; and (3) auditory inattention (Eisenson 1968a). In addition, other nonverbal aspects of auditory processing, such as impairment of sound localization, auditory rhythmical ability (Griffiths 1972, Kracke 1975), sequential perception (Eisenson 1968a), and discrimination of rapidly changing acoustic information (Tallal 1978, Tallal and Piercy 1978, Tallal et al. 1980) play a part in defining the exact nature of the language disorder. The assumption of a defect in serial order behavior in Lashley's (1951) sense has often been made. Tallal et al. (1985) reported that in developmentally dysphasic children "auditory perceptual variables, specifically those requiring rapid temporal analysis were most highly correlated with the degree of receptive language deficit," whereas other perceptual and motor tasks showed no such relationship. However, whether auditory processing deficits are to be viewed as (1) necessary causes of developmental language disorders, (2) sufficient but not necessary causes of developmental language disorders, (3) secondary to a primary defect of the linguistic system itself ("hierarchical structuring deficit," Cromer 1978) or even to a more general cognitive deficit (Rees 1973), or (4) concomitant with a linguistic deficit, but not causally related to it (Tallal and Piercy 1978) is open to debate. As a case in point, a study by Ludlow et al. (1980) indicated that impairment of perception of temporal order may also be found in groups of children—patients with early Huntington's disease and hyperactive children—with normal language functions. The authors suggested that the deficit in temporal sequential perception may be better understood as reflecting general cognitive dysfunction.

On the basis of observations of "several hundred 6-year-old children described as dysphasic or with specific language disorders," Cooper and Griffiths (1978) developed a descriptive grouping in five categories that makes few assumptions about underlying deficits and concomitant disorders, but instead concentrates on the evident forms of impairment:

1. Children without hearing loss but with little comprehension or use of speech. This group is described as bright and alert; they can express themselves in drawing, mime, and gesture.
2. Children with hearing loss. They may also show visual handicaps, may have a history of spasticity, and use mime and gestural communication; they are described as hyperactive and grossly immature.
3. Children with normal verbal comprehension, but with severely impoverished or absent verbal expression. Speech consists of short, simple, active declaratives. Often gross articulatory impairment, as well as other motor impairment, is present.
4. A group similar to group 3, but with late onset of relatively rapid speech development. Learning to read is often a problem, as is fine motor coordination, although the overall cognitive level is average or better.
5. Children who develop speech, but use imitative, stereotyped, and irrelevant speech. Learning ability is affected even more severely. Behavior may frequently be obsessional or eccentric, although not necessarily disruptive. Relations with other children are poor, but children in this group do relate to adults.

27.6   The Origin of Childhood Dysphasia

Most language disorders related to hearing impairment are caused by pre- and postnatal infections affecting the auditory nerve, rather than the brain itself. Language disorders of a higher level of auditory and central processing, on the other hand, have evoked much speculation about their origin, although few actual studies are available. Some authors have suggested that abnormal hemispheric dominance and interhemispheric interaction or left hemisphere dysfunction may be responsible (Lebrun and Zangwill 1981, Zaidel 1979, Zangwill 1978). Hauser et al. (1975) reported an enlargement of the left temporal horn in the pneumoencephalogram of 15 of 18 autistic children with a language defect.

The effect of sex chromosome trisomies on language lateralization has already been discussed in Chapter 11. Garvey and Mutton (1973) and Mutton and Lea (1980) reported (1) an increased occurrence of male sex chromosome trisomies (XXY and XYY) among children with specific speech and language delay and (2) depressed verbal and normal nonverbal IQ scores among Klinefelter syndrome (XXY) boys. The higher incidence in males compared to females has been explained in a polygenic reverse model by Decker and DeFries (1980, Decker 1982) that postulates that males have a lower threshold of liability to risk factors than girls. It follows from this model that affected females would be carrying more "risk genes" than males and that relatives of affected females would show a higher incidence of disorder than would be expected in the general population. This genetic risk model is of course not limited to language disorders, but can be applied to other disorders (e.g., autism, developmental dyslexia) as well. The model is partially supported in the San Diego longitudinal study (Tallal et al. 1989 a and b, 1991b) which found that 70 per cent of language-impaired children showed a positive family history, with fathers reporting a language or learning problem history 11 times more frequently than mothers. Affected mothers had five times as many sons with language or learning impairment than daughters. A twin study also showed that 3- to 5-year-old monozygotic twin pairs misproduced the same sounds on an articulation test significantly more often than dizygotic twins or unrelated children (Locke and Mather 1989).

Another series of related hypotheses about the causes of language disorders was first mentioned by Gellner (1959), who stated that subcortical lesions may be responsible for the lack of both language and cognitive development in retarded children. Subcortical lesions are also central to Matzker's (1958) theory of a binaural integration deficit in patients with a variety of disorders affecting language and to Rimland's (1964) notion of damage to the reticular activating system, proposed primarily as an explanation of autism. This notion was further elaborated by DesLauriers and Carlson (1969), based on Routtenberg's (1968) notion of two arousal systems (reticular and limbic). Support for this notion also came from studies of evoked responses to rapid-frequency-modulated tones, suggesting a fundamental auditory problem (Stefanotos et al. 1989). However, brainstem auditory evoked responses have been reported as normal (Akshoomoff et al. 1991).

Bilateral lesions of the central auditory system are most often postulated, both on the basis of the evidence concerning the normal plasticity of the infant brain (Rutter 1978) and the fact that the auditory pathways are crossed. H. Cohen et al. (1991) also reported difficulties in acoustic integration in the discrimination of consonant-vowel syllables in 7- to 10-year-old language-impaired children, suggesting bihemispheric dysfunction; such auditory processing deficits persist into adolescence and young adulthood (Lincoln et al. 1992).

In support of the bilateral lesion hypothesis, Dalby (1975) presented the results of 87 pneumoencephalograms of children with developmental dysphasia and reported that within this group 26 children showed an enlarged left temporal horn, 6 an enlarged right temporal horn, and 14 an enlargement on both sides. He concluded that medial temporal lobe structures are the most likely site of defect. In addition, there is some evidence to support the suggestion that bilateral involvement may be necessary to produce the severe receptive-expressive forms of language disorders seen in children.

Rapin et al. (1977) examined five children with "dense" deficits for decoding acoustic speech and profound impairments of oral speech. Three of these children exhibited bilateral cerebral dysfunction as inferred from bilateral epileptogenic discharges in the EEG. The other two were brothers, with similar language difficulties. The onset of language deterioration in the older brother coincided with classic brief absences that were compatible with temporal-lobe discharge. The younger brother showed no seizure or EEG abnormality, but exhibited a similar language deficit. It was suggested that the language disorders may not always reflect adventitious brain abnormality, but may be genetic in some children. The authors also suggested that bilateral dysfunction must be suspected in children with a severe receptive language difficulty, whether congenital or acquired.

The only case reported in the literature of a child with a developmental language disorder who came to autopsy (Landau et al. 1960) also showed bilateral involvement. This boy had severe receptive and expressive language deficits and was initially thought to be deaf, although later audiograms indicated auditory acuity within the normal range. He learned to speak and understand within limits, but understanding was possible only if speech was presented to him slowly and with pauses between words. On autopsy, it was noted that he had old cystic infarcts involving the superior temporal gyrus bilaterally and severe retrograde degeneration on both medial geniculate bodies.

Although bilateral damage to the adult cochlea, eighth nerve, or the cortical part of the auditory system would require rare and complicated combinations of lesions, several pre-, peri-, and postnatal diseases are capable of producing bilateral auditory system lesions: asphyxia neonatorum (Windle 1971), kernicterus (Carhart 1967, Gerrard 1952, Matkin and Carhart 1966), and maternal virus infections that involve the fetus, most notably rubella (Hardy 1968; Monif et al. 1966). Many of these diseases have been implicated as playing a role in the etiology of language disorders. For example, Goldstein et al. (1960), in a retrospective study, identified several etiological factors common to deaf and dysphasic children (Table 27-5). In Table 27-6, the etiological factors have been reorganized to indicate which factors were predominantly associated with deafness or dysphasia in children. Only rubella and complications during pregnancy were associated in approximately the same proportions with both deafness and dysphasia. Mental retardation and early infantile autism also tended to be associated more frequently with these factors (Chase 1972).

Athetosis has long been known to be strongly associated with language disorders in cerebral palsy (Achilles 1956). A study by Flower et al. (1966a and b) compared groups of children with athetosis and hearing impairment (including kernicterus children) to those with athetosis but without hearing impairment. Although language development was slowest in the hearing-impaired ath-

Table 27-5 Etiological Classification of Deaf and Dysphasic Children

Etiological classification	Number of deaf children	Number of dysphasic children
Unknown	60	26
Prenatal		
Heredity		
Hearing loss	12	3
Speech disorder, CNS disorder	0	6
Rubella of first trimester of pregnancy	10	7
Other congenital complications		
Historical data	9	4
Inferred from clinical evidence of brain damage	2	5
Rh, severe jaundice shortly after birth	0	4
Perinatal		
Complications of labor and birth	1	6
Postnatal		
Meningitis	9	1
Severe infection in infancy	11	1
Convulsive disorder	0	6

Source: Goldstein et al. 1960.

etosis group, the authors failed to find a specific association between dysphasia and kernicterus.

It should be noted, however, that the plasticity hypothesis has been challenged, both on theoretical grounds of early hemispheric structural asymmetries assumed to be fundamental to language development and on the basis of the

Table 27-6 Condensed Etiological Classification of Deaf and Dysphasic Children

Condensed etiological classification	Number of deaf children	Number of dysphasic children
Meningitis, severe infection in infancy, family history of hearing loss	32	5
Maternal rubella, complications during pregnancy	19	11
Rh, complications of labor and birth, convulsive disorders, congenital brain abnormality, family history of speech or neurological disorder	3	27

Source: Goldstein et al. 1960.

findings by Annett (1973), Rankin et al. (1981), and Kiessling et al. (1983) that right hemiplegic children are inferior in speech production, vocabulary, comprehension, and syntax comprehension and formulation to a carefully matched group of left hemiplegic children. Inferior speech perception in 28 children with congenital hemiplegia was also confirmed by Bergman et al. (1984), who emphasized that in early childhood and perhaps up to age 3 hemispheric dominance for speech processing is transferred to the alternate hemisphere, but that this does not occur in later life.

With lesions acquired later, a reorganization of language is more likely. Dennis (1980b) demonstrated the rapid recovery of language in a 9-year-old girl who suffered a stroke involving the left anterior cerebral artery. On the basis of a detailed linguistic analysis, she stressed that major reorganizations had taken place that "change the fundamental organization, not just of the output mechanics, but of her language" (p. 66).

A review by Bishop (1987) concluded that verifiable localized lesions remain relatively rare in children with developmental dysphasia, that CT scans frequently are normal, and that an interaction of genetic influences, slowness or abnormalities of brain maturation, poor verbal home environment, recurrent otitis media, and localized lesions should be considered in the study of the etiology of developmental language disorders. Abnormal hand preference, however, has not proved to be more common in language-impaired children (Bishop 1990a). Jernigan (1988) reported "frank parenchymal abnormalities, possibly related to myelin deficiencies" in 17 per cent of developmentally dysphasic children, using MRI techniques. Plante et al. (1991, Plante 1991) found atypical perisylvian asymmetries in most of eight language-impaired boys, but not in controls; these asymmetries were not the result of lesions and were interpreted as prenatal alterations of brain development. Atypical perisylvian asymmetries were also found in a majority of parents and siblings, suggesting that they were due to a transmittable biological factor.

No long-term follow-up studies of children with various forms of congenital lesions that would further clarify the etiology of childhood dysphasia have been published. Among the many basic environmental influences during pregnancy investigated in the Collaborative Perinatal Study (La Benz 1980), higher risks for sensorineural hearing loss in infants born to mothers who took ototoxic drugs were noted, but most other environmental factors played only a minimal role in the prediction of speech, hearing, and language deficit at age 3 or 8 years. Even weighted measures of these factors in a multiple regression analysis accounted for less than 8 per cent of the variance.

27.7 Acquired Language Disorders

Although acquired language disorders represent the smallest proportion of cases of affected children, these children have provided perhaps the most striking evidence concerning the complexities inherent in the study of the developing nervous system. The effects of cerebral lesions acquired during infancy and childhood on language functioning may differ markedly from those of lesions acquired during adulthood. For example, one notable clinical feature of the language of children with acquired aphasia, in contrast to adult aphasics, is the reduction in the amount of speech produced, regardless of the locus of lesion (Alajouanine and Lhermitte 1965, Guttman 1942, Rapin et al. 1977). In fact, it has been observed that the aphasic child may not only have reduced verbal output but may also be reluctant to communicate or exchange information by writing or using gestures (Alajouanine and Lhermitte 1965). Basso and Scarpa (1990) also found that nonfluent aphasia was more common in children than in adults, but that the incidence of apraxia and acalculia was equal. Whereas dominant hemisphere involvement generally precipitates language disorders in adults, large brain lesions sustained early in life, even if treated by hemispherectomy, do not produce profound language impairment, regardless of the side of the brain involved. These findings and the observation that children recover language functions more rapidly than adults have formed the basis for theories about the ontogeny of cerebral dominance and of plasticity and critical periods for the development of brain functions, two key issues in developmental neuropsychology (Chapter 5 and 7).

Dennis and Whitaker (1977) and Satz and Bullard-Bates (1981) reviewed the evidence on acquired aphasia in children and confirmed earlier suggestions for an initial equipotentiality of the two hemispheres for language. They concluded that this assumption holds only up to an age of approximately 1 year. Although before this age, right hemiplegia was associated with a 2:1 risk for language impairment, the frequency of aphasia associated with right hemiplegia increases dramatically after this age and by age 5 approximates the ratios found in adults. Satz et al. (1988) confirmed this finding in an analysis of four large-scale studies, and Vargha-Kadem et al. (1985) drew similar conclusions from a study of 28 children with left hemisphere and 25 with right hemisphere lesions; age and side of the lesion, rather than its severity stood out as the critical variables in this study. A detailed single-case follow-up of a 3½-year-old boy with a congenital left hemisphere lesion showed normal development, especially in syntax and inflectional morphology (Levy et al. 1992).

These findings are somewhat modified by studies of hemispherectomy reviewed by Ludlow (1979), which suggest that, although phonemic discrimination and lexicon may have an equal potential in the right and left hemisphere, the discrimination of complex syntactic material may be more seriously impaired by left hemispherectomy. This finding seems to suggest that the left hemisphere may "retain a nonredundant language behavior—syntactic complexity" (p. 185). Dennis (1980a), in a review of hemispherectomy studies, stressed that the left hemisphere also "allows for the development of a set of semantic abilities not available to the right" (p. 183).

In later childhood, however, aphasic syndromes similar to those found in adults are more common. Visch-Brink and Van de Sandt-Koenderman (1984) described the cases of two 11- and 9-year-old boys who showed neologisms, verbal paraphasias, and literal paraphasias; of a 5-year-old boy with phonemic jargon aphasia; and of an 11-year-old girl with fluent aphasia and empty speech. In all cases, the appearance of aphasic symptomatology was observed only during the early stage of recovery. Neologisms also disappeared early in the case of a 9-year-old girl (van de Sandt-Koenderman et al. 1984). Acquired conduction aphasia has been reported in a 10-year-old who underwent aneurysm surgery; recovery was dramatic (Tanabe et al. 1989). Even crossed aphasia (i.e., aphasia after right hemisphere tumor in a right-handed 15-year-old), suggesting atypical initial lateralization of language in the right hemisphere, has been demonstrated and surgically verified (Martins et al. 1987). Atypical forms including mutism after closed head injury were reported for nine patients (Levin 1983); Cole et al. (1988) described two children with acquired verbal auditory agnosia and mutism, as well as epilepsy. Muteness can also be the result of acute cerebellar lesions (Rekate 1985).

Children with hydrocephalus in the first year of life have been found to show a limited resilience of language. In a study of 75 such children compared to 50 control subjects, Dennis et al. (1987) concluded that "for the most part, hydrocephalics and normals show commensurate age increments of performance," but that with increasing age hydrocephalic children fall behind, especially in word-finding and in higher levels of language-related academic skills. Language and intelligence shared a common variance of only 18 to 39 per cent, suggesting that language tests tapped functions other than those involved in intelligence.

The effect of milder injuries in children has been studied by Ewing-Cobbs et al. (1987), Dennis and Lovett (1990), and others. Dennis and Barnes (1990) found that after closed head injury three-quarters of their sample of 33 children and adolescents between the ages of 5 and 19 years remained impaired after 3 years in at least one of four discourse tests: knowing the alternate meaning of ambiguous words in context, getting the point of figurative or metaphoric expressions, bridging inferential gaps between events in stereotyped situations, and producing speech acts expressing the apparent intention of others.

27.8   Language Disorders in Relation to Cognition

Although many language disorders in children occur together with cognitive deficits of similar severity, specific language disorders, by definition, assume normal intelligence and nonexceptional home background. Many of the children suffering from such disorders tend to remain language-handicapped; they are frequently resistant to speech therapy and also tend to be handicapped in reading and other school subjects (Zangwill 1978). However, the assumption of normal intelligence can be confirmed only by nonverbal intelligence tests. In studies with such tests, it has been found that, although nonverbal intelligence is in the normal range, it is usually lower than similar test scores for siblings and parents. If both expressive and receptive language are disturbed, a certain amount of deprivation even in a normal home environment is likely to occur. For example, the dysphasic boy described by Landau et al. (1960) showed a Performance IQ of 78 at age 6; after 3 years of intensive training, the measured Performance IQ was 98. Hence, Benton (1978) interpreted the finding at age 6 as "pseudoretardation."

De Ajuriaguerra et al. (1976) conducted a cross-sectional study of 40 and a longitudinal study of 17 developmentally dysphasic children. In their cross-sectional study, the authors made a distinction between children with "re-strained" expression, marked by the use of simple sentences, enumerative and descriptive narration, and little discrepancy between expression and compre-hension, and a second group of "unrestrained" subjects whose speech was more voluble and who used complex sentences, variant word order, and generally incoherent narration and showed a large discrepancy between expression and comprehension. The majority of the children were normal in intelligence on the WISC, including its verbal part, but inadequate on the information, vocabulary, and arithmetic subtests. They also showed a deficit in spatial reasoning. Affective disorders tended to delay the onset of expressive language, but were not related to the severity of expressive or receptive deficits at a later age. The development of the 17 children followed longitudinally over a 2-year period suggested that the most progress was made by children who had the highest need to com-municate and showed the least degree of affective disorder; primarily, these children belonged to the "restrained" group. The authors concluded that de-velopmental dysphasia is not the same as a developmental language delay, but that other factors must be taken into account and that such dysphasia represents a particular form of disorganization of language during development, with the specific inability to acquire the structural or syntactic logic of language.

The relationship between language and cognition has been a subject of spec-ulation, study, and theory formulation for many investigators. At first glance, the comparison with deaf children seems attractive. As are children with specific language deficit, deaf children are deprived of verbal stimulation and tend to develop largely without oral speech; hence, their intellectual development must proceed without the constant aid of verbal mediation that normal hearing chil-dren are able to use.

Unfortunately, the parallel with deaf children is suited only for a portion of children with specific language disability; namely, the types of disability listed in Table 27-3 as decoding problems. Presumably, the deaf child maintains the central processing ability for symbolic material, as witnessed by the acquisition of alternate means of communication and even lip reading. Hence, the discus-sion about the relationship between language and cognition focuses on the abil-ity to use central processing of language for cognition. If, as Table 27-3 implies, central processing is basic to categorizing, problem solving, learning, storage and retrieval, then a disorder at this level must be considered as a pervasive deficit of cognitive function. On the other hand, if the manipulating and pro-cessing of symbolic material are abilities that may be involved in, but are not basic to, all cognitive skills, then we would expect some, but not all cognitive skills to be affected.

Luria (1966, Luria and Yudovich 1971) followed Pavlov in viewing the speech system as the highest regulator of human behavior, the "second signal system": "no single complex form of human mental activity can take place without the direct or indirect participation of speech" (p. 85). Bay (1962), consistent with his unitary view of brain function, also viewed the process of concept formation as inseparably interwoven with language. In contrast, a modifying role of language was assumed by Milgram (1973) and others who viewed language as a "verbal mediator," rather than as central to all cognitive activity. Verbal mediation assists and facilitates learning, problem solving, and concept formation, but is not identical with them.

More recent experiments have shown a defect in sequential perception and related cognitive activity in dysphasics (Kracke 1975), although an earlier study by Furth (1964) had shown that sequence learning was not significantly more impaired in dysphasic than in deaf children. Moore and Law (1990) also found poor copying performance on the Griffiths Mental Development Scale in 96 3-year-old language-delayed children compared to 100 controls, and Bottos et al. (1989) found delayed locomotor development. Spellacy and Black (1972) reported a mean Leiter Scale (nonverbal) IQ of 99.4 for their younger language-impaired children (age 41 to 71 months) as contrasted with a Peabody Picture Vocabulary Test (PPVT) IQ of 75.8. The older groups (72–95 and 96–120 months), however, showed IQs of 75.8 and 73.9 on the Leiter Scale, whereas their PPVT IQs were 67.5 and 58.1, respectively. The findings suggest a deficiency even in nonverbal intelligence for the older children, but less for the younger children. This conclusion remains tentative because the study was not longitudinal in nature and did not use matched samples.

A mild inferiority of dysphasic subjects in visuospatial functioning (Doehring 1960) and less habituation of the visual orienting response to new visual stimuli (Mackworth et al. 1973) have been observed. Children who at age 3 still showed severe echolalia were found 1 year later to be significantly lower in IQ than those who had only mitigated echolalia, even though the echolalia stage had disappeared at follow-up and the two groups were originally matched for IQ (Fay and Butler 1968).

In other words, the question whether a central processing deficit is crucial to cognitive activity still is unresolved. Menyuk (1978), after a review of the experimental evidence, concluded that "the nature of the specific task requirements may render language useful, nonuseful, or interfering in carrying out these tasks" (p. 69). Benton (1978) noted that several studies showed a strikingly large range of scores in dysphasic children. This suggests that perhaps a more detailed breakdown into types of language dysfunction may clarify the question in future experimentations. A study by McFie (1975) noted that, although the effects of lesions in children younger than age 10 on intelligence and scholastic achievement were quite variable, left hemisphere lesions at any age tended to affect verbal long-term memory and span of apprehension quite consistently.

27.9   Language Disorders and Psychopathology

Cantwell and Baker (1987) examined 202 children between 2½ and 16 years of age consecutively referred to a speech and hearing clinic and found that 46 per cent met DSM-III criteria for a psychiatric diagnosis (Table 27-7). The two most common disorders were Attention Deficit Disorder and Oppositional Conduct Disorders. In children with pure speech disorders, the incidence of psychiatric disorders was 3 per cent, of speech and language disorders 59 per cent, and of language disorders only 7 per cent. Language disorders were associated with psychiatric disorder, especially in the form of behavior problems. There was a trend of an increased prevalence of psychiatric disorder in children with low IQ and a low educational level of father. Psychiatric disorder was also associated with other developmental disorders, such as enuresis. However, the clinical neurological examination showed no differences between the psychiatric and nonpsychiatric groups of language-disordered children, nor did family background, maternal or paternal age, nonlanguage developmental milestones, and other pre- and perinatal factors distinguish the psychiatrically well from the abnormal group. On follow-up 3 to 4 years later, more than half of the children with pure speech disorder or with pure language disorder showed psychiatric recovery, whereas only 30 per cent of children with both speech and language disorders recovered; 20 per cent were well initially, but showed psychiatric disturbance at follow-up. Attention deficit disorder with hyperactivity was also found more frequently in 188 5-year-olds with general linguistic impairment (Beitchman et al. 1989), although Tallal et al. (1989b) reported that in 56 male and 25 female language-impaired children, no increased incidence of emotional disturbance was found if items pertaining to speech and language development or to neurodevelopmental delays were excluded from the analysis of the Child Behavior Checklist.

The contribution of environmental factors is indicated by differences in behavior according to the type of school placement. Griffiths (1969) found that

Table 27-7   Psychiatric Diagnoses in 202 Children
Referred to a Speech and Hearing Clinic

Diagnosis	Percentage of occurrences
No mental disorder	54
Attention deficit disorder, with hyperactivity	17
Oppositional or conduct disorder	8
Affective disorder	4
Anxiety disorder	6
Adjustment disorder	5
Pervasive developmental disorder	1
Other psychiatric disorder	5

Source: Cantwell and Baker 1987.

children with severe language disorders developed behavior problems after being transferred from special to regular schools. Seidel et al. (1975) noted that both psychiatric disorder and reading retardation were less frequent among crippled children attending special schools rather than regular schools. Rutter et al. (1976) reported that, when educationally handicapped children were placed in special schools, secondary behavior problems were less likely to develop.

27.10   The Outcome of Childhood Language Disorders

For children who fail to develop language or who show severe delay in language acquisition, often accompanied by general cognitive handicap, language development usually remains in step with general mental development. Although specific training procedures have been shown to be effective within a limited setting, generalization and long-term maintenance of responses acquired during training remain persistent problems (Ruder and Smith 1974) and show large variability among individuals. Such variability may represent the confounding of several factors, such as type and severity of brain damage, as well as motivational, attentional, and general activity levels.

Children with specific language delay tend to show even more variability. Tallal et al. (1991b) followed 100 children with language impairment from age 4 to 8 years and compared them to an IQ-matched control group. In 85 per cent of these children, learning disabilities were found while their language abilities improved. Five children with more severe congenital auditory imperception at age 1.4 to 3.4 years did not benefit from early guidance with amplification perceptual training nor from a synthetic approach; they showed, if anything, less, not more, interest in sound as they grew older (Ward and McCartney 1978). The authors reviewed other follow-up studies and confirmed that the long-term outlook for children with receptive language problems (but without deafness) is quite poor. Vetter et al. (1980) reported from the large population of the Collaborative Perinatal Study that correlations between language measures at age 3 and at age 8 were between .00 and .43 for language comprehension, sentence complexity, and word identification. The same study (Darley and Fay 1980) also attempted an examination of the long-term predictive value of several perinatal stress measures, of family factors, of physical signs in newborns, and of 8-month Bayley Developmental Scale measures for speech and language status at age 8 years. The at-birth variables contributed only 0.6 per cent of the variance (0.8 per cent if combined with the 8-month follow-up variables); adding the 3-year indices to the prediction formula accounted as much as 11.5 per cent of the variance. In a study reported by Caputo et al. (1981) of a group of preterm infants followed up to the age of 7 to 9.5 years, there were only marginal relationships between measures of birth stress and language development unless the mother's IQ was added to the multiple regression equation. These findings provide a good indication of the large variability described by many authors in the past: some children show unexpected spurts in language development, whereas others remain stagnant, and a majority show a gradual increase in language capability. Especially for children with severe comprehension deficit and autism, prognosis has to be considered extremely guarded.

More is known about the long-term outcome of acquired aphasia in childhood. Figure 27-1 shows the recovery rate for understanding of sentences (Token Test) and for picture naming in several 10- to 17-year-olds, indicating that even during late childhood and adolescence an exponential function of initial recovery during the first 100 days can be expected (Niebergall et al. 1976). However, such rapid recovery does not necessarily result in a normal-for-age level of performance. In a follow-up of 15 children 1 to 10 years after the onset of acquired aphasia, Cooper and Flowers (1987) found persistent poor performance on language measures, such as word, sentence, and paragraph comprehension; naming; oral syntactic construction; and word fluency compared to controls, although all were oral and grammatical in their communications. They were also impaired in school learning, especially in arithmetic. The course and prognosis of acquired aphasia are of course dependent on etiology. Poor prognostic indicators are inflammatory disease, widespread damage, presence of epilepsy (Cooper and Ferry 1978), and severe EEG changes, whereas traumatic aphasia is usually considered to be prognostically favorable (Remschmidt et al. 1980). Woods and Teuber (1978b) reported that, of 25 aphasic children aged 2 to 15 years at onset, 21 showed full recovery after 4 years. In the four remaining cases, vascular etiology and epilepsy with hemiparesis were reported, although several of the younger children also had vascular lesions. Although frequently claimed, no clear-cut relationship between the age at onset and the degree of recovery can as yet be documented because of the confounding etiological variables (Satz and Bullard-Bates 1981).

Summary

In clarifying the nature of language disorders in children, several factors must be considered: whether the language disorder is part of a more pervasive disturbance, whether the primary problem is one of reception (necessarily also affecting expression) or expression per se and which aspects of each are affected, whether the disorder reflects a failure or delay in language acquisition and if so whether it is congenital or developmental in nature, or whether it is a loss or reduction of language capacity. In addition, a distinction must be made between the ability to communicate, which includes not only speech but also sign language, communication by gesture, writing or any other means, and verbal language ability. It is often extremely difficult to distinguish among the various conditions. Overlapping deficits may also be expected. Children with receptive auditory discrimination problems may also have a sensorineural hearing loss or may demonstrate autistic traits. Mentally retarded children may exhibit general language delay, as well as specific language disorders.

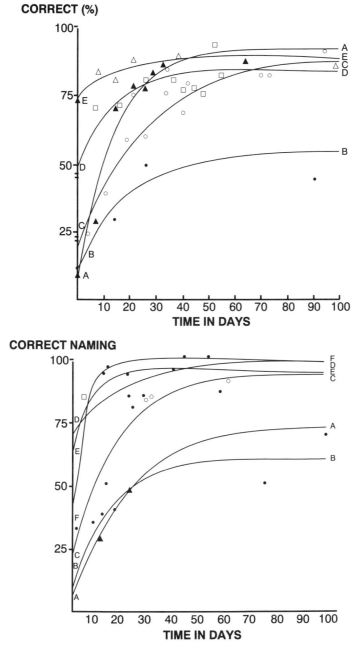

Figure 27-1: Exponential function of initial recovery from traumatic aphasia on the Token Test (above) and on Picture Naming (below) for individual patients between the age of 10 and 17 years (Niebergall et al. 1976).

Although the contribution of several prenatal and perinatal factors to language disorders has been established, the individual contribution of each factor to the specific forms of language disorder requires further elucidation. Dysphasia acquired during childhood is perhaps the best understood form of language disorder, and it also carries good prognostic implications; prognosis for most other language disorders is poor, and response to treatment tends to be limited.

28

Developmental Handicap

The term "developmental handicap" (DH) has gradually replaced a series of now outdated historical equivalents (idiot, moron, imbecile, oligophrenia, mental deficiency) although "mental retardation" is still the term preferred by many researchers and associations. The long-standing popularity of such general designations of unspecified cognitive deficit rests on their assumed value for describing a section of the population that has difficulty coping with the educational, social, and economic demands of society. As a result, the population so designated varies in size with changes in society itself. However, in most Western societies it is estimated to involve a considerable proportion of the population. For this reason, neuropsychologists and other clinicians almost invariably have to deal with developmentally handicapped persons in their regular practice.

Other forms of specific cognitive deficit are discussed separately in this book. The focus in this chapter is on the development of pervasive cognitive disabilities and intellectual handicap, as well as on the development and characteristics of other cognitive features of DH children, e.g., learning, memory, problem solving, reasoning, and concept formation. The development of the Down syndrome child is used as an example.

28.1 Intelligence

Although explorations of the dimensions of intelligent behavior have extended into numerous abilities, conceptualized as factors of primary mental abilities by Thurstone (1938) or as a large number of factors in the famous cube model of Guilford (1956) with operations-content-product dimensions, most studies still treat intelligence as unitary, or at least as a complex that can be described by one general factor, as first suggested by Spearman (1927). One widely used breakdown into fluid and crystallized intelligence (Cattell 1971) distinguishes between the capacity to find relationships (e.g., word fluency and psychomotor speed) and the sum of acquired abilities, e.g., space and verbal meaning (Table 28-1). In clinical practice, Wechsler utilized the dichotomy of distinguishing verbal intellectual functioning and non-verbal or visuomotor based performance intellectual functioning. Halstead (1947) and Hebb (1949) developed the concept of biological intelligence based on neuropsychological theory. Hebb also suggested a breakdown into two types of intelligence, similar to Cattell's fluid and crystallized intelligence: (a) problem solving and learning of new and unfamiliar material and (b) stored knowledge and experience. Hebb believed that type (a) intelligence would be more likely compromised by brain damage than type (b). Das et al. (1979) divided intelligence into factors of simultaneous and successive processing, based on Luria's neuropsychological theory, and suggested that simultaneous processing is more closely related to right hemisphere function, whereas successive processing is more closely related to left hemisphere function. This notion was also adopted by Kaufman and Kaufman (1983) when they developed a specific intelligence test battery for children.

Most of these and similar breakdowns of cognitive abilities into major components based on empirical data and factor analytical studies, however, are rarely used in clinical practice. Instead, neuropsychological studies tend to have a

Table 28-1 Major Differences between Cattell's Factors of Intelligence

Fluid	Crystallized
Reaches its maximum early (age 14) and drops after age 20	Reaches maximum later (age 20?) and shows no decline with age
High correlation with rate of learning in new situations	Less correlated with rate of learning
Primarily constitutional and related to brain processes; varies with physiological conditions	Variance mainly related to cultural and environmental factors; consists of acquired habit systems and some specific cerebral substrates
Capacity reduced by brain damage	Total capacity reduced less by brain damage, but specific functions (language, symbolic, or mechanical abilities) may be differentially affected
Difficult to distinguish in the structure of primary abilities	Leads to increasing development of primary abilities
In factor analysis, loadings on this factor decrease only marginally during adulthood	Test loadings decrease in adulthood, especially with heterogeneous groups who specialize in different areas
Best measured in tests requiring speed in finding a response	Better measured with power tests, without time limit and largely avoiding error of response factors

pragmatic orientation toward cognition, one based on available tests with demonstrated usefulness in neurological populations. A breakdown into performance and verbal intelligence based on common sense and practical division of parts of a test, such as the Wechsler tests, rather than empirical demonstration, is readily adopted if the available methods suggest it.

28.2 Incidence and Description

General IQ values are still frequently used to define DH in research practice. One reason for their popularity is the global and seemingly unitary concept of developmental handicap (DH), which suggests a general deficit of cognitive functions without specification of range and area of deficit, mechanism, or cause. Approximately 3 to 4 per cent of the population of Western societies today is usually described as DH (McLaren and Bryson 1987, Spreen 1978a), although the size of the substantially developmentally disabled population, as defined by state disability plans in the United States, is only 1.73 per cent of the general population (Jacobson and Janicki 1983). However, this figure may almost double if the cut-off point for DH is raised to 75, as described below.

Subdivisions of DH are usually made on the basis of deviations from the average IQ and Adaptive Behavior Quotient (ABQ) of 100, with mildly handicapped being 2 standard deviations below, or IQs between 69 and 55 on the Wechsler Intelligence Scale for Children; moderately handicapped being 3 standard deviations below (IQs between 54 and 40); severely handicapped being 4 standard deviations below (IQs between 39 and 25); and profoundly handicapped being 5 or more standard deviations below (IQs below 25). The American Association on Mental Retardation prefers terms indicating the need for support ("intermittent, limited, extensive, pervasive needed supports" 1992) and an extension of the "intermittent support" group up to an IQ and ABQ "standard score of 70 to 75 or less." Both the ambiguity of this cut-off point and its increase to 75 have been criticized as impractical for legislators, politically motivated, and an unnecessary extension into the low range of the learning disabled population with IQs between 70 and 75 who now receive services as learning disabled persons.

For educational purposes, a division into slow learners (IQ 75 to 85), educable (IQ 55 to 74), trainable (IQ 25 to 54), and custodial (IQ below 25) has frequently been applied. Although these subdivisions seem to have some merit for classification and general practical purposes, considerable variability in many cognitive skills exists within these subpopulations. Arguments against the use of the IQ measure as the sole indicator of an individual's capabilities have been raised for some time. Current definitions of DH include social adjustment as a second criterion: "significantly subaverage intellectual functioning existing concurrently with related limitations in two or more of the following applicable adaptive skill areas: communication, self-care, home living, social skills, community use, self-direction, health and safety, functional academics, leisure, and work. Mental retardation manifests before age 18" (American Association on Mental Retardation 1992). However, since adequate measures of adaptive behavior usually rely on reports from persons familiar with the daily behavior of the individual, this second criterion is still frequently neglected.

Both theorists of intelligence and developers of intelligence tests have been relatively unconcerned about neuropsychological issues, and neuropathological considerations have had little influence on their thinking. For example, Wechsler (1958) stated, "It is probable that factors of the mind are to some extent physiologically and anatomically determined, but this is not a necessary condition for their acceptance."

28.3   Etiology

The etiology of 30 per cent of severe, and 50 per cent of cases of mild DH remains unknown (McLaren and Bryson 1987). Investigations into the etiology of the other half of DH persons show that the full range of disorders described in Part III of this volume, particularly the prenatal influences, can be involved. For DH with unknown etiology, mental development may be impaired as a result of sociocultural and psychological influences, although Coulter (1987) and Huttenlocher (1991) suggested that in such cases "hypoconnectivity," a developmental disturbance in neural connectivity mediated by dendritic, axonal, synaptic, or glial mechanisms, may be involved. The American Association on Mental Retardation (1992) has embraced this highly hypothetical construct and included hypoconnectivity in its etiological classification system (Table 10-1).

It has been estimated that violent abuse and neglect contribute to DH in 3 and 24 per cent of this population respectively (Buchanan and Oliver 1977). Hence, the cognitive status of the DH individual may represent a mixture of influences in all these spheres. Moreover, the psychometric properties of any IQ measure follow a normal Gaussian distribution so that a certain proportion of DH may result from genetic variability of the trait. Dingman and Tarjan (1960) plotted the expected frequencies at the low end of the distribution against incidence statistics; the comparison yielded an apparent excess at the low end of the distribution (Figure 28-1). A similar kind of excess was, incidentally, reported independently by Yule et al. (1974) for the distribution of measures of reading, i.e., an excess at the dyslexic end. Although such comparisons of incidence and expected distribution statistics may be somewhat speculative and fraught with problems of sampling and the questionable validity of IQ measures in the low range, Dingman and Tarjan's explanation that the excess represents an additional distribution curve of pathological DH underlying the normal variability makes intuitive sense. Such an explanation is also supported by the fact that profoundly intellectually handicapped persons almost invariably show evidence of severe neurological damage. Dingman and Tarjan's graph suggests, in fact, that pathological cognitive deficit not only has its highest prevalence at the low end of the distribution but that it also ranges well into the normal IQ area.

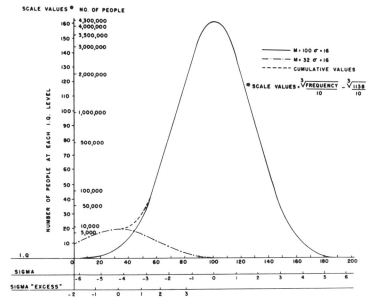

Figure 28-1. Frequency distribution of IQs assuming a total population of 210 million (Dingman and Tarjan 1960).

That neuropathology may be involved in a large number of children with DH has been confirmed in a number of studies. Caviness and Williams (1979) and Salam and Adams (1975) reviewed advances in research on the pathology of DH with a traditional breakdown into areas of disorders of the germinal, embryonal, fetal, late uterine, parturitional, and postnatal periods. Neurological examinations show that among moderately and severely handicapped children, only about 2.5 percent are free of neurological findings, i.e., of structural malformations and other indications of CNS pathology. In contrast, mildly DH children have fewer indications of neuropathology. Support for this two-group distinction comes from the Collaborative Perinatal Study (Broman et al. 1987). In a follow-up study of 36,800 children up to age 7 in 12 CPS collaborating centers in the United States, most DH subjects with IQs less than 50 had major CNS disorders, and for those who did not, the authors found a high frequency of maternal urinary tract infection during pregnancy, another potential contributing cause. For the mildly, but not the severely DH group, socioeconomic status was a major correlating factor, even though for the group under study "heroic efforts" were made to use the excellent prenatal medical care provided for participants in the study. However, even for this group, organic risk factors, such as maternal short stature, late age at menarche, urinary tract infections, anemia, and toxemia during pregnancy were frequent. Rao (1990) found obstetrical complications in 69 per cent of 8- to 12-year-old mildly handicapped children. Autopsy findings of severely DH patients show a high incidence of malformations and other CNS pathology. Dekaban (1967) found that only 12.5 per cent of his series of autopsies were free of structural abnormalities. Davison (1977) reported that microcephaly is common in DH persons and that the cholinergic synaptic density may be low. Leisti and Iivanainen (1978) called attention to hypothalamic dysfunction in 12 of 15 DH subjects.

Moreover, as shown in Table 28-2, the incidence of devastating motor, sensory, and physical handicaps in profoundly handicapped children is extremely high, as is the incidence rate of abnormal EEGs and seizure activity (Cleland 1979). With lesser degrees of DH, the number of neuropathological findings diminishes, and among the mildly DH up to 70 per cent have been described as suffering from a psychosocial disadvantage (previously also called cultural-familial retardation), suggesting that in these cases DH exists as the result of poor environmental conditions and genetic endowment. It is also recognized that DH may follow psychiatric disorders, sensory deprivation, and sensory defect. Nevertheless, neuropathology can be and has been found in a fair proportion even of mildly handicapped individuals, and so the current discussion need not remain restricted to the severe and profound range of DH. Callaway (1973) has mustered an impressive summary of studies demonstrating the relationship between averaged evoked potentials and measures of intelligence. Other electrophysiological correlates are discussed by Kerrer (1976).

The two-group distinction between organic and psychosocial DH takes up much space in the DH literature and repeats to some extent the arguments for and against the notion of minimal brain dysfunction discussed in Chapter 22. Kohen-Raz (1977) listed retardation of more than 4 months in the development of gross motor function and an increasing discrepancy between actual and expected mental level during the first 15 months of life as indicators of organic cognitive impairment. Such differences in developmental milestones, however, remain only superficial demarcations in the field, which was artificially created by the umbrella concept of DH itself. Hooper et al. (1993) argued for a different approach that would view mental handicap as a heterogeneous disorder with various neuropsychologically defined subgroups; such subgroups, in turn, may correspond to different neurobiological findings in these children. From the point of view of our current discussion, it would be more meaningful to follow the cognitive handicap of such individual subgroups of children with specific psychological disorders. However, because of the traditional subdivision, a brief discussion of some general findings for DH children is presented.

28.4 Cognitive Characteristics of the Organically Impaired DH Child

Numerous attempts have been made to characterize the brain-damaged child as being distinct from children whose cognitive development is unimpaired or whose impairment is ascribed to sociocultural factors. The most advantageous research design includes the use of dual control groups: the brain-damaged DH

Table 28-2 Observed Frequencies of Disability

	Number and per cent of cases						Est. cases in 100 M general population
	Age birth–21		Age 22+		All cases		
Combinations of conditions	n	%[a]	n	%	n	%	
Specific combinations of conditions							
Autism (AUT) only	348	0.024	36	0.001	384	0.009	9
Cerebral palsy (CP) only	602	0.048	383	0.013	985	0.023	24
Epilepsy (EP) only	307	0.021	384	0.013	691	0.016	17
Mental retardation (MR) only	8574	0.590	21 305	0.731	29 879	0.684	720
AUT, CP	5	0.001	0	0.000	5	0.000	0
AUT, EP	16	0.001	5	0.000	21	0.000	1
AUT, MR	532	0.037	174	0.006	706	0.016	17
CP, EP	83	0.006	55	0.002	138	0.003	3
CP, MR	1085	0.075	1531	0.053	2616	0.060	63
EP, MR	1897	0.128	4609	0.158	6506	0.149	157
AUT, CP, EP	0	0.000	0	0.000	0	0.000	0
AUT, CP, MR	13	0.001	5	0.000	18	0.000	0
AUT, EP, MR	81	0.006	35	0.001	116	0.003	3
CP, EP, MR	979	0.067	630	0.022	1609	0.037	39
AUT, CP, EP, MR	10	0.001	8	0.000	18	0.000	0
All cases	14 532		29 160		43 692		1053
Total instances of each condition							
Cases with AUT	1005	0.069	263	0.009	1268	0.029	31
Cases with CP	3400	0.233	2612	0.090	6012	0.138	145
Cases with EP	3373	0.232	5726	0.196	9099	0.208	219
Cases with MR	13 171	0.906	28 297	0.969	41 484	0.949	1000
Total conditions	20 949		36 898		57 863		1395
Conditions/case	1.44		1.29		1.32		

Source: Jacobson and Janicki 1983.

[a]Column per cent of cases for specific combination reflects joint probability for occurrence within the survey population.

group is compared not only to a matched group of non-organic DH individuals, but also to a group of normal children matched for mental age. This design permits the search for differences between the two target DH groups and contrasts both with a group of normal children at a similar stage of development.

Basic to such research are assumptions that disturbed or altered brain function would produce a reduced, or in some specified fashion altered cognitive performance. One earlier theory of this type, the Strauss syndrome, proposed by a group of Gestalt psychology researchers, has already been discussed (Chapter 22). Another major theorist, Birch, proposed a less general notion of a child's cognitive change with brain damage, distinguishing between subtractive dysfunctions (i.e., the simple loss or deficiency in one or more cognitive areas) and additive dysfunctions, which are accompanied by seizures, spasticity, perseveration, or perceptual distortion. Such behavioral changes were perceived as being the result of active, ongoing distortions of the CNS processes (Birch and Diller 1959). A series of studies attempted to pinpoint the behavioral difficulties, proposing that the integration of input from more than one source was specifically impaired (Birch and Belmont 1965, Cravioto et al. 1967).

Another difference between brain-damaged and non-organically handicapped children was the prolongation of critical inhibition after a response (Birch et al. 1965). A somewhat similar emphasis on the importance of the "stimulus trace" can be found in the earlier work of Ellis (1963). Ellis proposed that such a trace would be both shorter in duration and lower in intensity in the DH child, a condition that would result in deficits in learning and retention. Birch's and Ellis' concepts are to some extent compatible: whereas Birch's notion of prolonged inhibition was aimed at an explanation of perseverative behavior, poor cross-modal association, and sluggishness in thinking, Ellis' theory attempted to account for failures of short-term memory. Weak and short traces do not necessarily exclude the notion of prolonged inhibition after stimulation has taken place.

Research into both theories has not provided sufficient confirmation for the continued usefulness of either. In fact, cross-modal integration has only rarely been found to be specifically impaired in brain-damaged children if their ability to do unimodal tasks is taken into account. The brain-damaged child with DH does not reflect a simple diagnostic entity, but may, as Birch's notion of subtractive and additive deficits suggests, show considerable variability from one individual to another. However, generalizations, such as those by MacMillan (1982), that "there is now considerable skepticism as to the usefulness of classifying mental retardation by form, due primarily to our current inability to separate biological and psychological forces" (p. 60) or Fisher and Zeaman's (1970) statement that "it does not appear to make any difference how one gets to be a retardate, whether through bad genes, brain pathology, or seizures, the maturational results are the same" (p. 164), tend to reflect a premature pessimism.

For example, in a detailed study using several types of memory tasks, Burack and Zigler (1990) found clear evidence that in the brain-damaged DH group at age 13 intentional learning (central recall and memory span) was more impaired than in the non-organic DH group whereas there were no differences in incidental learning. Both groups were inferior in learning compared to a matched group of non-retarded children. This finding was confirmed in a meta-analysis of 24 studies in this area by Weiss et al. (1986), suggesting that the cognitive structure of brain-damaged DH individuals may be different from that of the non-organically handicapped.

More sophisticated studies have applied factor analysis to the investigation of differences between DH and normal children and between organically impaired DH children and those without indications of brain damage. Such studies usually extend the well-investigated notion of the developmental differentiation of factor structure as originally formulated by Garrett (1946): "abstract or symbol intelligence changes its organization as age increases from a fairly unified and general ability to a more loosely organized group of abilities or factors."

The differentiation hypothesis has been investigated and at least partially confirmed mainly in the 6- to 18-year age range, although no agreement seems to exist about the exact nature of these changes (Reinert 1970). Differences in level of intelligence have been postulated to produce a delay in differentiation (Lienert 1961, Reinert et al. 1966) or, more likely, a different, not a more simplified factor structure in DH persons (Baumeister and Bartlett 1962, Belmont et al. 1967, Ellis 1963, Lienert and Faber 1963). Such differences in structure have been described as the occurrence of additional factors, variously labeled as "speed" (Das et al. 1979), "trace" (Ellis 1963), or "freedom from distractibility" (Leckliter et al. 1986) with loadings on such tests as Arithmetic, Digit Span, Coding, and Block Design of the Wechsler tests; these findings lend at least partial support to the postulated stimulus trace or prolonged inhibition theories of changes in cognition. The same factors were also identified in a study of a population with traumatic brain injury (Moore et al. 1993).

Hebb's (1949) theory suggested that children depend much more on type (a) intelligence, but adults can rely more on type (b)—stored knowledge and experience—for daily living. Wewetzer (1958) and Lienert (1961) proposed a "genetic divergency hypothesis" (Reinert et al. 1965) about changes in the factor structure of intelligence between groups of subjects with the same age and increasing intelligence level that are analogous to changes in factor structure found with increasing age. The changes consist not only of the appearance of additional factors, as described above, but also in the degree of intercorrelations: low-IQ subjects show higher correlations, more loadings on a general factor, higher commonalities, and higher intercorrelations between centroid factors. It should be remembered, however, that except for the work of Das, all these studies used the commonly available tests and hence are restricted in generalizations to the range of cognitive abilities sampled by such tests.

Ideas about the lateralization of cerebral lesions in at least some portion of organic DH children led to the speculation that either verbal or visuospatial abilities should be relatively more impaired. Hence a Verbal IQ—Performance IQ "split" on the Wechsler tests has been postulated for organically impaired

DH children. The evidence for such a split in group studies, however, has remained unsatisfactory and contradictory (Filskov and Leli 1981). At least one study found no difference between 46 carefully matched pairs of brain-damaged and cultural-familial DH persons in measures of level and dispersion for the WISC subtests (Spreen and Anderson 1966).

Halstead (1947) attempted to move away from the traditional intelligence concept by using the term "biological intelligence" for the basic coping and adaptive abilities of the organism; this concept was based on his studies of patients suffering primarily from frontal brain lesions. Halstead included measurements of time estimation, finger tapping, flicker frequency, and other tests that were not typically included in traditional intelligence testing. His theory of intelligence exerted little influence on the thinking of his contemporaries or on our current thinking. However, most of his tests became widely used because of the neurodiagnostic work of his student Reitan.

Several studies with the Halstead-Reitan battery of tests have been published to describe the difference between brain-damaged and normal children. Consistent with Halstead's and Hebb's theory, vocabulary was found to be the most sensitive test in separating brain-damaged children from matched normal controls (Boll 1974, Reed et al. 1965, Reitan 1974). The groups also differed in concept formation, recognition of rhythms, and block design, but not on tests of finger tapping, tactile form recognition, and other perceptual and motor tasks. Boll (1972) concluded that brain-damaged children are conceptually rather than perceptually impaired, but this conclusion would seem to be a generalization of limited value since the differences on which it was based were relatively small and the variability in the brain-damaged group quite high. Denckla et al. (1980) reported a strong association between degree of neurological impairment and spatial orientation skills in 6- to 12-year-old children as tested with route-drawing and route-walking tasks. A study by Meyer-Probst (1974) showed less effective strategies, decreased verbalization ability, reduced learning advances, and poorer transfer of practice in concept-formation tasks for 60 children with mild cerebral lesions and normal intelligence. However, the study failed to show qualitative differences in the actual solutions or in the process of concept formation between subjects and controls. As Kinsbourne (1976) pointed out, "Children at a given mental age are really quite similar in the way they think, excluding only those at the lowest extreme of intelligence" (p. 563).

Wewetzer (1975) attempted to go beyond the broad genetic divergency hypothesis by investigating the factor structure of 132 brain-damaged and 186 control subjects matched for IQ. His results suggest an almost identical seven-factor solution for the two groups on the WISC and on a variety of additional tests similar to the ones used by Strauss and by Reitan. Although this study fails to confirm a divergency hypothesis (probably as a result of the restricted range of IQ, excluding the low range because of matching requirements), Wewetzer raised the question whether the lack of homogeneity may also be the result of including subjects with widely differing etiologies. He then proceeded to compare three types of brain-damaged children (postnatal traumatic cortical, diffuse infection, perinatal diffuse hypoxia) and two types of controls (neurotics and normals) with 15 subjects in each group. A 17-variable discriminant function analysis produced 70 per cent correct classifications (Figure 28-2). The F value was significant between all groups except between the traumatic and the hypoxic and between the traumatic and neurotic groups. The best discriminating variables were spatial motor performance (Bender Gestalt Test) and figure-ground recognition, suggesting that perceptual components or disorders of depth and space perception were most crucial. Developmentally, however, it is possible that this deficit found in children of elementary and high school age may be preceded by a motor deficit at a younger age that affects perceptual functions later on.

Sohns (1980) found what seems to be a more simplified factor structure in DH schoolchildren with seizures. In his study, a three-factor solution for a series of tests was found for that group, as opposed to a four-factor solution for a comparison group of generally DH subjects without seizures. His test battery included many visuoperceptual, as well as nonverbal cognitive tests. Whether

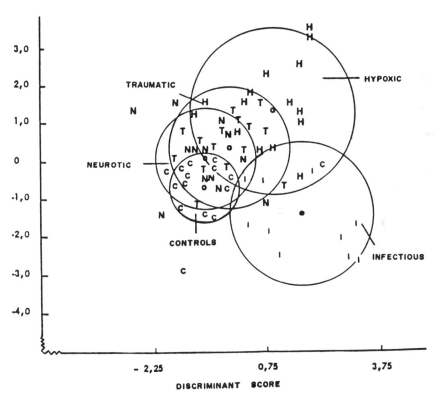

Figure 28-2. Graphic representation of a discriminant function analysis with 17 variables between DH children with traumatic hypoxic and infectious etiology, and neurotic and normal children (Wewetzer 1975).

they had clinical seizures or not, children with indications of seizure activity in the EEG fared significantly worse on cognitive testing than children without EEG signs.

Das et al. (1979) also failed to find differences in factor structure between normal and DH children; all three groups showed a simultaneous and a successive processing factor, as well as a speed factor. Snart et al. (1982) attempted a breakdown into groups with different etiologies and again did not demonstrate differences in factor structure comparing brain-damaged, Down syndrome children, and children with uncertain etiology who were moderately impaired and not institutionalized.

Yet another approach was taken by Silverstein et al. (1989), who separated three groups of institutionalized DH adults by means of cluster analysis of a Client Development Evaluation Report that generated five factors. The three clusters shown in Figure 28-3 and their characteristics (Table 28-3) indicate with high stability (as demonstrated by using split samples) three groups: one with poor motor development, highly maladaptive behavior, and a high incidence of neurological and sensory handicap; a second group that was described as a "modal cluster" with average impairment on all characteristics; and a third group that was relatively high functioning and non-organic.

In summary, investigations into the cognitive characteristics of the child with DH provide some support for a divergency of the factor structure of intelligence, although other studies fail to confirm this theory. The nature of the divergency has been postulated to lie primarily in a lack of fluid or biological

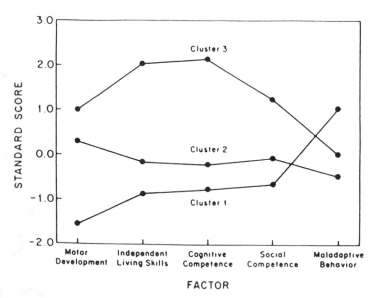

Figure 28-3. Mean profiles of the three clusters of DH subjects on the Client Developmental Evaluation Report (Silverstein et al. 1989).

Table 28-3 Demographic and Other Characteristics of Developmentally Handicapped Adults by Cluster[a]

Variable[b]	Cluster 1	Cluster 2	Cluster 3	All clusters	Strength of association
Mean age	24.4	29.3	34.6	28.9	.07
Male	43.3	59.6	50.0	54.3	.02
Profoundly retarded	97.9	80.0	6.9	73.8	.42
Cerebral palsied	60.8	21.2	12.1	29.5	.16
Epileptic	68.0	39.6	31.0	45.3	.07
Vision problems	42.3	24.9	15.5	19.3	.04
Hearing problems	24.7	18.4	13.8	19.3	.01

Source: Silverstein et al. 1989.
[a]All three clusters differ significantly at $p < .01$.
[b]All variables except age in per cent.

intelligence, more specifically in deficits of complex information processing and of strategies for learning and retrieval. For brain-damaged children, sensory, perceptual, and concept formation deficits, as well as a larger scatter between verbal and performance tasks, seem to be pre-eminent. Only one study (Wewetzer 1975) has successfully differentiated the cognitive structure of children with differing etiology. Further studies of this question would seem to be a potentially useful and meaningful approach to the study of cognition in brain-damaged children.

28.5 Development of Cognitive Functions in DH Children

The hierarchical development of behavioral and cognitive functions (e.g., moving from concrete to abstract thinking) during infancy and childhood is biologically determined to a large degree. Little evidence has been found to indicate that this development can be accelerated unless the individual has the biological endowment to perform at that higher level (NINCDS 1979). However, the progression of the individual depends on many factors, and detailed studies of specific forms of impairment and specific environmental conditions are needed to explore them. Few truly longitudinal studies of the long-term cognitive development of DH children are available.

During infancy and early childhood, a tendency toward a decrease in cognitive ability has been noted, followed by a stabilization during puberty. A follow-up from age 2 to 7 showed more diversification after 4 years, with 25 per cent of the children retaining the same level of functioning, 30 per cent showing improvement, and almost 50 per cent showing decreased intellectual levels (Roesler 1971). A later study of 222 mildly handicapped children with early brain damage followed from the age of 10 to 20 showed a reduction by ten IQ points in 11, an improvement by ten IQ points in 45, and no change in 15 subjects

(Roesler 1976). Goodman and Cameron (1978) reported a relatively high IQ constancy for the Bayley and the Stanford-Binet Scales for DH children between the age of 2 and 7. Only the initial test score was related to etiology (perinatal, chromosomal, metabolic problems, congenital anomalies, environmental neglect), but the "developmental rate, once determined, remains fairly constant" (Goodman 1977a, p. 209). Hence, the author concluded that etiology has no bearing on the course of development. Goodman and Cameron noted that the greatest amount of fluctuation can be found in the relatively high-IQ (51–80) range. This fluctuation is similar to that of normal children and suggests a considerably higher growth potential for this range of DH. In general, the family environment is crucial in contributing to such changes and often determines whether the individual will be able to live independently as an adult. Institutional care has often been shown to have a detrimental effect, except for those DH persons who come from a very poor parental environment. Similarly, children of well-to-do parents who attend private school have shown better cognitive development (Helper 1980).

The Seattle study (Barnard and Douglas 1974) explored predictors of later cognitive development in DH children in a long-term follow-up project. Individual clinical factors obtained before the age of 2 years were generally unsuccessful as predictors. However, a combination of various perinatal variables, including weeks of gestation, age of mother at birth, normal labor, diseases of pregnancy, infections during the second and third trimester of pregnancy, time at first breath, time at first cry, birth weight, 5-minute Apgar score, and highest level of bilirubin measured, provided a modest predictive accuracy when used in a multivariate formula. In addition, maternal IQ and education, nutritional status of mother, and numerous environmental factors observed throughout childhood provided a modest improvement of the predictive formula. This study and the Collaborative Perinatal Study on the same topic suggested that single specific predictor variables cannot be related to cognitive development with any degree of confidence. One study from the Collaborative Perinatal Study, however, attempted to relate neurological findings at 8 months and at 8 years of age with cognitive development (Gold 1979). Children who were neurologically abnormal at the age of 8 months but normal at 8 years tended to have specific difficulties with verbal cognitive tasks, whereas children who were neurologically normal at 8 months but neurologically deviant at age 8 years tended to show a global pattern of depressed cognitive competence.

Life-span developmental studies suggest that cognitive growth continues into the early twenties and, for higher IQ-level DH persons, even into the late thirties (Fisher and Zeaman 1970). In fact, Butcher (1968) maintained that mental growth continues in DH subjects for a longer period than in normal individuals if continued training is provided. However, different limitations may apply to subjects with differing etiologies, and early decline has also been reported, at least in an institutionalized population. Growth curves (Figure 28-4) suggest that a trend of higher initial growth and more pronounced decline is particularly evident at the mild and moderate levels of DH (Fisher and Zeaman 1970,

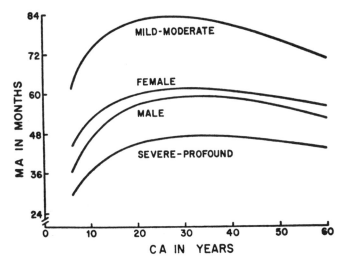

Figure 28-4.   Fitted semi-longitudinal growth curves of intelligence for four groups of institutionalized mentally retarded subjects. MA = Mental age; CA = Chronological age. (Silverstein 1979).

Silverstein 1979), although Goodman (1977b) warned that this "early decline" may be an artifact of cross-sectional studies of institutionalized populations; those leaving the institution at any age tend to be the brightest. In a semi-longitudinal approach the presumed decline changes to "regular increments, particularly in performance scores" (p. 203).

For many years, exceptional abilities in a limited area, such as chess, piano playing, painting, mechanical skills, memorization, or arithmetic in otherwise generally developmentally handicapped persons have aroused interest (Tredgold 1914). Such persons have been described as "**idiot savant**." The incidence is extremely rare (54/90,000, Hill 1977). Calendar calculation has been most frequently reported, but multiple skills have also been observed. Hill (1975) reported a 50-year-old man with an IQ of 54 who was able to play 11 musical instruments by ear, drew elaborate pictures of houses, and was able to remember important dates, such as birthdays; most exceptionally, he was able to determine the day of the week for any given date (day/month/year) within an 8-year period with 80 per cent accuracy and with a reaction time between 6 and 14 seconds. Testing showed no exceptional abilities in eidetic imagery, high-speed calculation, or a substitute compensation for normal learning, three possible explanations proposed by other researchers (Horwitz et al. 1965). Another unsatisfactory explanation is that such exceptional giftedness is the result of relative isolation, training, and encouragement of special skills in institutionalized DH persons, and the ability to sustain attention for such tasks over prolonged periods. Neuropsychological explanations include the notion that outliers may be expected at both the extremely poor but also the extremely gifted end of the spectrum for any specific trait on the basis of genetic variability. Palo and Kivalo (1980) proposed that the CNS may be severely damaged by organic processes, but that narrow areas may not only be spared but may even function extremely well. Burling et al. (1983) showed that exceptional ability in the perpetual calendar task was related to left hemisphere activation, based on eye movements to the right during this task, but not during mathematical, spatial, and music tasks. The most likely explanation for the exceptional skills of some DH persons is probably a combination of genetic variation, sparing of relevant parts of the brain, and environmental factors (Lester 1977).

Several authors have speculated about the importance of the finding that DH populations tend to have a relatively high proportion of left-handers (Gesell and Ames 1947, Touwen 1972). However, this finding does not imply cognitive impairment for left-handers in general. As Hildreth (1949) already noted, "Left-handers are not duller in general than the right-handed, but left-handedness is found more frequently among the dull when that section of the population is studied" (p. 245). In recent research, ambiguous handedness rather than left-handedness has been found to be most frequent in DH populations. Hartlage and Lucas (1973) reported that right-handers in an MBD population tend to fare prognostically better than mixed- or left-handed subjects; their study relied on a retrospective follow-up of nearly 2000 third-grade children. The authors noted that strongly left-handed children also tended to fare better than children with mixed handedness. The finding supports the notion of "pathological handedness" introduced by Satz (1977), which suggests that a relatively higher proportion of mixed handedness and left-handedness can be expected as a result of switched or ambiguous brain lateralization because of early insult to the brain (see Chapter 5). Satz's research group found that as many as 45 per cent of a retarded population had ambiguous handedness (Soper et al. 1987). Language deficits have also been found more frequently among left-handed mentally handicapped persons, which supports the pathological left-handedness model (Lucas et al. 1989).

A series of studies at Duke University (Thompson 1984) demonstrated a higher activity level and more aggressive, withdrawn-inhibited, and mixed behavior disorders in DH preschool and school-aged children. This topic is addressed in more detail in Chapter 30.

28.6. Cognitive Development of the Down Syndrome Child

The cognitive development of the Down syndrome (DS) child is used as an example of one relatively homogeneous group of children that has been studied perhaps more than any other group. The syndrome itself was described in Chapter 11 and represents a lack of both physical and psychological differentiation, a "pre-Gestalt" development (Wunderlich 1970). Gibson (1978) and Nadel (1988) reviewed the numerous studies on the psychological development of the DS child.

Several theories about the cerebral deficit of Down syndrome children have been proposed. Wiesniewski et al. (1986) confirmed earlier studies by Benda (1960) and Crome et al. (1966), who found reduced weight of brain, brainstem, pons, medulla, and cerebellum in DS children. This finding led Frith and Frith (1974) to the hypothesis of a cerebellar deficit in Down syndrome. They suggested that such a deficit would explain problems characteristic of DS children, such as muscle hypotonia and poor motor coordination and motor sequencing, expressive language, and articulation (Dodd 1976, Hanson et al. 1987). Although the articulatory problems are well established (Smith 1975), studies of the cerebellar deficit hypothesis for language have so far produced contradictory results (Seyfort 1977). The finding by O'Connor and Hermelin (1962) that DS children have a specific retardation in tactile recognition does not directly support a theory of specific deficit in cerebellar functions, although partial support was provided by Seyfort and Spreen (1979), who found that DS children did more poorly on a two-plate tapping task than an IQ-matched group of non-DS subjects.

Another hypothesis about the cerebral deficit in Down syndrome, mentioned in Chapter 11, suggests that there is delayed myelination, primarily in the development of the association cortex, i.e., in the frontal and superior temporal areas (Owens et al. 1971, Salam and Adams 1975). A shortened anterioposterior diameter of the brain, exposed insula, irregular sulci, a decreased number of convolutions, and narrow temporal and prefrontal gyri have been described (Lott 1986). A proposed relationship of such growth retardations to several mineral and vitamin deficiencies (Sylvester 1984, Williams et al. 1985) remains speculative, and treatment with supplements of these substances has been inconclusive so far. The delayed myelination of the association cortex fits in with Hebb's (1949) notion that the greater the proportion of "associative" tissue to sensorimotor tissue in the brain, the greater the potential for cognitive complexity in the individual. The notion of an impairment of growth of associative tissue in DS is also supported by behavioral studies (Cunningham 1979) and provides an attractive model for explaining the cognitive deficit of these children. From a psychometric point of view, Gibson (1978) concluded:

> The most favored psychometric abilities picture depicts Down syndrome children as relatively high-scoring on tests loaded for rote memory, psychomotor, visual-motor, and nonconceptual components. Difficulty is experienced for Mental Age-equated test material having significant abstract, symbolic, verbal and recognition vocabulary content. The profile might be reliable for Down syndrome, but is not necessarily distinctive among the mental retardations (p. 184).

The conclusion was further supported by a study of 377 Down syndrome subjects of a wide age range (4 to 56 years) by Silverstein and collaborators (1982). The authors found that five items of the Stanford-Binet Intelligence Scale were typically performed better by DS subjects; all five required figural content and visuomotor abilities. On the other hand, DS children tended to be poorer on five items involving semantic content, social intelligence, general comprehension, judgment, and reasoning. Snart et al. (1982) also reported a deficit in an auditory sequential factor, including high-level auditory and verbal abilities. Cunningham and Mittler (1981) tested these conclusions in their study of 46 DS children with the Bayley scale of mental development; their findings suggest two relatively independent blocks of variables that the authors interpreted as representing "reaching and manipulation" (Piaget's primary circular reactions) and "relating objects, imitation, causality" (Piaget's coordination of secondary circular reactions). The authors concluded that the notion of an impairment of basic stages of development leading to deficits in the associative cognitive activity of the DS child must be tempered with caution because both impairments seem to have been represented in their sample, at least at the age of testing (102 weeks). In addition, Bihrle et al. (1989) reported more global than focal visuospatial processing in DS children as compared to another group of DH children with chromosomal disorders. Gareware (1990) found that DS children can be differentiated from other DH children on the basis of sensory integration, but not by attentional skills. DS children attended as well or better than non-DS matched controls when taught to use new toys. However, DS children used investigative strategies that were more like those used by younger children, e.g., slapping and banging of the toy, rather than feeling and exploring it. The author interpreted this behavior as failure to acquire and integrate sensory information, which may reflect a deficit related to the association cortex. Poor or slow processing and retention of auditory information have also been described as characteristic for DS children (Lincoln et al. 1985, Marcell and Weeks 1988, Varnhagen et al. 1987). In addition, Thompson et al. (1985) described less intense separation anxiety, longer latencies of onset, briefer recovery periods, and a diminished range and lability of emotional responding in a study of 26 DS infants compared to age-matched controls.

Developmental delay in the Down syndrome child is usually noticed fairly early; developmental milestones, such as sitting, standing, walking, and speaking the first word tend to be delayed. Most DS children do not exceed an IQ of 70, and the average is 40. However, cognitive development generally correlates to some degree with intellectual status of the parents if the child remains at home during the first 2 years of life (Figure 28-5, Fraser and Sadovnik 1976). The highest levels of intelligence are reported for DS girls with mosaicism, although even this finding has not remained without contradiction. Whether the level of cognitive development is related to the number of physical abnormalities commonly found in Down syndrome remains an unsettled question in spite of several investigations. Zeaman and House (1962) followed the cognitive development of Down syndrome children in a semi-longitudinal study and noted that the IQ tends to drop by a few points each year until puberty (Figure 28-6). Because of the relative constancy of this drop, they suggested that intelligence in Down syndrome can be described by the formula

$$IQ = IQ / \log (\text{age in years})$$

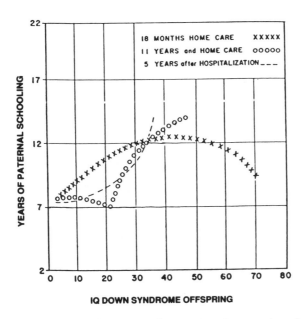

Figure 28-5. Distribution of Down syndrome IQ and paternal academic achievement (n=141, Gibson 1967).

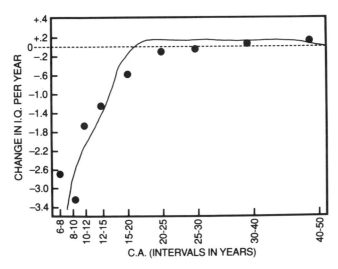

Figure 28-6. Change in IQ at different levels of chronological age in Down syndrome. Note that most of the plotted points have negative values, indicating a decrease in IQ (Zeaman and House 1962).

Fisher and Zeaman (1970) extended this finding to DH generally. The shortest growth periods of intelligence were found in the severe and profound levels of DH.

This finding was confirmed in a study by Cunningham and Mittler (1981), who reported that their group of DS children started with a near-average Bayley scale IQ that dropped rapidly during the first 2 years of life. Cardozo-Martins et al. (1985) also reported that Bayley scale scores were near normal up to the beginning of language development. Saxon and Witriol (1976) pinpointed the onset of developmental delay to the age of 4 to 6 months, "where most infants shift from subcortical to cortical control of behavior" (p. 45).

It should be remembered that studies of cognitive development in Down syndrome children are based on groups of survivors, since mortality is high and tends to affect selectively the most seriously impaired children. Warner (1935) reported that, by age 12.5 years, half of her sample had died, mostly because of congenital heart defects frequently associated with DS, as well as upper respiratory infections. Despite improved medical care, shortened life expectancy is still reported in more recent studies (Thase 1982). The selective mortality should, in theory, favor an improving intellectual outcome for the group of survivors. These considerations underline even more the decline of intelligence described above. Connolly (1978), however, warned that the decrease in cognitive abilities may in part reflect the effect of lack of extended educational opportunities and assumed deficit inferred from chromosomal and physical characteristics that could be compensated for with the introduction of special school programs. For the 3- to 5-year age range, Wishart (1987) also warned that single-test sessions may be misleading since DS children improved with practice on Piagetian infant search tasks over six sessions during a 2.5-month period, whereas non-DS children did not improve.

Schroth (1975) noted that DS children tend to show different levels of performance depending on the task demands. In mechanical learning and primary retention tasks of the level 1 type according to Jensen's theory, these children do fairly well, but on level 2 tasks requiring cognitive manipulations and insight they do worse than suggested by their overall IQ. This finding contrasts with the results in a group of DH children with a similar degree of intelligence but without organic deficit, where no such difference was found. Such comparisons cannot be made with groups of severely DH children since tasks for measuring intelligence at that level are primarily of the level 1 type. Although DS children have been described as being exceptionally good at imitation and as having a good sense of rhythm and music, little evidence has been found to support such notions (Belmont 1971).

Hartley (1981) first suggested anomalous cerebral asymmetry in DS children based on dichotic listening test results, an idea confirmed by Gienke and Lewandowski (1989) and Mosley and Vrbancic (1990). Based on studies of sequential movements and transfer of training, Elliot (1985, Elliot et al. 1986, 1987) speculated that "the sequential language problems exhibited by individuals with DS are related to the dissociation of language and sequential processing mechanisms, i.e., the right hemisphere of persons with DS is dominant for language, whereas sequential processing mechanisms are controlled by the left hemisphere" (Elliot 1985, p. 96). This notion was supported by Bain (1990, Bain and Spreen 1991), who found that, in contrast to a matched non-DS group, DS adults showed a left-ear advantage on a fused rhymed dichotic test, no ear advantage on a regular dichotic listening test, and decreased tapping scores for the left hand during verbalization (dual task paradigm). Bain concluded that anomalous dominance was related to the language difficulties of DS persons.

An early decline of cognitive abilities in DS adults has long been noted (Gibson et al. 1988), although some studies indicate that mental development in DS adults continues well into the third and fourth decades of life (Berry et al. 1984, Silverstein et al. 1986). Indirect confirmation of the theory of early decline has been provided by autopsy studies of older DS persons (Zubenko and Howland 1988). In a study of 2144 adults with DS compared to 4172 age-matched DH people without DS, Zigman et al. (1989) found that Down syndrome is accompanied by age-related deficits in adaptive behavior after age 49, regardless of the level of retardation. Several studies (Solitaire and Lamarche 1966, Zigman et al. 1987, 1989) have described an early occurrence of deterioration of the type found in Alzheimer disease; such deterioration was not present in the brains of other DH children of similar age. O'Hara (1972) also found plaques (cores of hollow fibers surrounded by deteriorating cell processes) and neurofibrillary tangles similar to those of Alzheimer disease even in DS adults without clinical indications of Alzheimer disease, and Schapiro et al. (1987) demonstrated related changes in glucose metabolism. Oliver and Holland (1987) and Patterson (1987) argued that plaques contain amyloid beta protein, that the gene for the production of this protein resides on chromosome 21, and that a similar gene has been isolated on chromosome 21 of non-DS persons with familial Alzheimer disease. At this point, the notion of the susceptibility of DS adults to early Alzheimer disease still awaits conclusive confirmation (Nadel 1988).

Summary

The discussion of cognitive deficits in a neurodevelopmental context introduced first the concepts of intelligence and of general developmental handicap (DH). It was noted that DH can result from neurological defect as well as from psychosocial disadvantage, including both adverse sociocultural and psychological influences. Genetic variability must also be taken into account.

Many theories about the nature of the cognitive developmental handicap have been presented. Several of these theories assume neurological dysfunction and were discussed in some detail, although experimental and clinical evidence supporting one theory rather than another is still sparse and contradictory at times. A brief outline of the cognitive characteristics of the organically impaired DH child was offered, and the development of such children into later childhood was described. As a specific example, the development of the child with Down syndrome was discussed.

The notion of a general cognitive deficit or developmental handicap based on IQ measurements has a long history. The concept is mainly pragmatic and provides a ready label for educational, habilitation, and caregiver purposes. Unfortunately, the label has also been a hindrance to more specific research into the nature of the deficit in individuals and has obscured differences in abilities and in deficits of subgroups based on etiology, as well as other descriptive characteristics. Neuropsychological interest should guide further research into different aspects of handicap and their etiology with a view toward an accurate description of the individual.

29

Learning Disorders

Like all children, those with a history of neurological problems must face the challenge of school. For some, school entry may need to be delayed beyond the normal period because of hospitalization or remedial needs; for others, schooling may be limited to classes with learning assistance, special education classes, or special schools. What constitutes school readiness in children has been a long-standing topic of concern among educators and child psychologists. In his discussion of psychobiological influences on school readiness, Kohen-Raz (1977) outlined three aspects: (1) intellectual maturity sufficient to handle the first-grade curriculum; (2) emotional emancipation from parents, leading to an increased openness to interact with agents outside the family; and (3) control over affect and impulsiveness to the extent that the frustrations and demands of school can be handled. The child is considered prepared for school if these three conditions are met between the age of 5 to 7 years.

After entry into school a considerable proportion of children experience learning problems. For some, these problems arise because of sensory handicaps, such as extremely poor hearing or vision. A second group, described as developmentally handicapped (see Chapter 28), fails to acquire academic skills because of a general inability to learn. Other children develop problems due to deficient or poor teaching. A fourth group consists of those who, despite educational opportunity, are poorly motivated. Yet another group includes those who experience brain damage in the prenatal and perinatal periods and have learning problems. A final group includes children who are unable to make adequate progress despite intact senses, normal intelligence, proper instruction, and normal motivation. This last group of children has been designated as having specific learning disabilities (LD):

> **Learning disabilities** is a generic term that refers to a heterogeneous group of disorders manifested by significant difficulties in the acquisition and use of listening, speaking, reading, writing, reasoning, or mathematical abilities.

471

These disorders are intrinsic to the individual and presumed to be due to central nervous system dysfunction. Even though a LD may occur concomitantly with other handicapping conditions (e.g., sensory impairment, mental retardation, social and emotional disturbance) or environmental influences (e.g., cultural differences, insufficient/inappropriate instruction, psychogenic factors), it is not the direct result of those conditions or influences (National Joint Committee for Learning Disabilities 1981).

Learning-disabled children constitute between 7 and 15 per cent of the general school population (Gaddes and Edgell 1993). Because of this high prevalence and because of interest in the presumed mechanisms underlying their disabilities, this group of children has attracted considerable attention in the educational and neuropsychological literature. A distinction has been made between specific disability in reading (dyslexia) and in arithmetic (dyscalculia), although considerable overlap exists between the two. Another distinction, between verbal, nonverbal, and mixed LD, has been accepted more recently by some authors (Hooper and Willis 1989, Rourke 1989). This distinction implies additional symptomatology in psycholinguistic (verbal), visuospatial-constructional, and social (nonverbal) skills beyond dyslexia and dyscalculia and is described later in this chapter. This chapter retains the traditional division into dyslexia and dyscalculia and focuses mainly on patterns of deficit related to neuropsychological evidence and theory. Writing disorders also will be discussed. The final sections discuss the school problems of neurologically handicapped children in general.

29.1   Dyslexia

The term "dyslexia" has been applied to children who fail to acquire adequate reading skills, and the term "alexia" is used only for the impairment of already established reading skills after brain damage. In 1968, the World Federation of Neurology defined **developmental dyslexia** as "a disorder manifested in difficulties in learning to read despite conventional instruction, adequate intelligence, and socio-economic cultural opportunity. It is dependent upon fundamental cognitive disabilities which are frequently of constitutional origin" (Critchley and Critchley 1978). This definition emphasized the cognitive quality of the disorder and suggested that it results from essentially unknown factors, rather than from any physical or structural defect of the brain. The failure of this definition to include other forms of reading disability led to further subdivisions. **Primary** or specific **dyslexia** refers to a reading disability of constitutional origin and stresses possible subtle defects in cortical functions. In contrast, symptomatic or **acquired dyslexia** describes reading disabilities resulting from cerebral damage, such as perinatal or childhood brain damage or brain disease. Among adults with acquired dyslexia, "**deep dyslexia**" has been described as a special case of paralexia in which the patient makes semantic errors in single-word reading, e.g., reads inch as "ruler," paddock as "horses," boat as "captain."

Deep dyslexia is frequently accompanied by aphasia. Secondary dyslexia refers to reading disability resulting from environmental, emotional, and health factors (Quadfasel and Goodglass 1968).

A relatively rare form of reading disorder that does not fit into the usually observed groups should be mentioned: the child with **hyperlexia,** who tends to outperform normal readers in single word reading of which the child has little or no comprehension (Silberberg and Silberberg 1972, Siegel 1984). Hyperlexia usually occurs in the presence of general cognitive impairment. The performance of such children has been related to "visual information processing by the right hemisphere" (Cobrinik 1982), possibly as a result of left parietal lobe damage. The reading of such children seems to focus on the visual configuration, rather than on the phonetic and semantic content, and is comparable more to echolalia than meaningful reading. It occurs also in the presence of autism, but is not autism-specific (Snowling and Frith 1986).

One further distinction should be made: children who are generally backward in learning are frequently designated as "general reading backward children," in contrast to children who show specific reading retardation, i.e., specific dyslexia. This term is frequently used in the British and Australian literature.

The total prevalence of all forms of dyslexia combined has been estimated to be as high as 20 per cent in the United States. Lindgren et al. (1985) found that dyslexia in the strict sense of the word (i.e., with an IQ of 85 or better) occurred in Italy in 15.7 per cent and in the United States in 23.8 per cent of large samples of schoolchildren. In both countries dyslexia was closely associated with verbal processing deficits; the authors ascribed the difference in prevalence to the poor grapheme-phoneme correspondence in the English language as compared to Italian. The focus in this chapter is on primary dyslexia because it represents by far the largest proportion of all forms of dyslexia and is of specific interest for developmental neuropsychology.

Theoretical Background and Models

In one of the first descriptions of specific reading problems, Hinshelwood (1895) hypothesized that "visual word blindness," the inability to recognize words, resulted from damage to a so-called visual memory center for words, situated in the left angular gyrus. Morgan (1896) discussed the connection between acquired word blindness and problems of reading acquisition in children and suggested that a congenital form of word blindness could exist in otherwise intelligent children. The early concepts of reading disability were therefore based on case histories of acquired alexia in brain-damaged adults and the application of this model to children. Several forms of alexia have been identified and reclassified by Benson and Geschwind (1969, Table 29-1). The five major types of acquired reading disabilities are based on a disconnection hypothesis discussed in Chapter 9.

Orton's theory (1925) suggested that dyslexia resulted from incomplete or mixed cerebral dominance. He proposed that it was not a deficiency in the

Table 29-1 Summary of the Characteristics of Five Different Types of Reading Problems That Can Result from Brain Injuries to Adults with Previously Acquired Reading Skills

Type	Reading-related skills	Other language abilities	Nonlanguage abilities	Neurological dysfunction
Alexia without agraphia or aphasia (rare)	Impaired Reading words and text Unimpaired Reading letters Writing Letter naming Oral spelling Recognizing spelled words	Sometimes impaired Color naming Calculation (no other language disorders)	Unimpaired color matching and other abilities	Left medial occipital lobe *and* splenium of corpus callosum almost always from thrombosis involving the posterior cerebral artery
Alexia with agraphia and mild Wernicke's (fluent) aphasia	Impaired Reading letters, words, and text (paralexia) Letter naming Writing Oral spelling Recognizing spelled words	Mild impairment Naming Paraphasic substitutions Calculation	Sometimes impaired Right-left orientation Finger localization Constructional skills	Left angular gyrus from infarction, trauma, neoplasm, or arteriovenous malformation
Wernicke's (fluent) aphasia with alexia and agraphia	Impaired (secondary to aphasia) Reading letters, words, and text Writing	Severe impairment Comprehension and repetition of spoken language Naming Paraphasic substitutions Less impaired Fluent (but paraphasic speech)	Unimpaired	Left posterior superior temporal lobe from infarct or neoplasm

Syndrome	Reading/Writing	Speech	Visual/Motor	Localization
Broca's (nonfluent) aphasia with alexia and agraphia	Impaired: Letter reading, Letter naming, Writing, Oral spelling, Recognizing spelled words; Less Impaired: Reading words and text	Severe impairment: Nonfluent speech; Less impaired: Listening comprehension, Naming	Impaired: Eye movements	Broca's area of frontal lobe from neoplasms and from infarctions involving anterior branch of middle cerebral artery
Visual agnosia (controversial)	Impaired: Reading letters, words, and text; Writing	Unimpaired	Impaired: Visual perception and production of complex forms	Right parietal lobe

Source: Doehring et al. 1981.

center for visual images that caused reading problems, but rather a lag in the development of the left hemisphere, which is dominant for language abilities. Because of this developmental lag, mirror images stored in the nondominant hemisphere were not suppressed and hence interfered with visual perception (strephosymbolia). Orton's hypothesis has been questioned. Zangwill (1962) suggested that poorly developed cerebral dominance should result in a more general learning disorder, one that would include only a small subgroup of dyslexics. However, more recent theories by Geschwind and Galaburda (1987, Geschwind 1982) have revived a modern version of Orton's theory of cerebral asymmetry, to be discussed below.

A third explanation of dyslexia was developed by Werner and Strauss (1940), who studied the differences between mentally retarded children with and without brain damage. They proposed that children who demonstrated the behavioral patterns of brain damage did have brain damage, whether or not it was detectable by neurological examination. Their proposed concept of minimal brain damage had the effect of grouping together children who showed different behaviors, such as dyslexia or hyperactivity.

Current models of the relationship between the brain and developmental dyslexia focus around the notion that brain maturation may be either defective or delayed in these children. The deficit model proposes that cerebral dysfunction underlies the inability to acquire appropriate reading skills. The maturational lag or delay model adopts a developmental outlook and proposes that cerebral maturation is delayed in dyslexic children.

Cognitive and Associated Deficits of Dyslexia

The concept of dyslexia as a viable construct has been the focus of considerable debate (Benton 1975, Rutter 1983a, Yule and Rutter 1976). Opinions have varied from the view that it constitutes a unique, unitary condition or that there are a number of reading disabilities, each with its own specific set of characteristics and etiology, to the view that reading disability is only part of a general pattern of LD.

Much of the earlier research focused on dyslexia as a single, presumably unitary disorder. In that research, a point along the series of events involved in the extraction of meaning from print was selected, and the performance of disabled readers was compared with that of a matched control group to discover a presumably unitary cause of reading disability. In general, evidence from single-syndrome research suggested that at least some deficiencies in auditory discrimination, phonological coding, or morphophonemic processing can be found; these deficits may be associated with abnormal, possibly genetically transmitted, left hemisphere functioning.

Among the nonreading problems that might be associated with reading disability is the inadequate maturation of perceptual systems (Birch 1962). Disturbances in the development of visual perception as a primary cause of dyslexia were also proposed by de Hirsch (1957). Some reports continue to relate dyslexia to disturbances in eye movement (Rayner 1983) or refractory eye anomalies, such as myopia. Kirkpatrick and Wharry (1985, Wharry and Kirkpatrick 1986) attempted to demonstrate that myopic children do poorly in reading but well in arithmetic and spatial tasks, whereas the opposite would be true for hyperopic children. Deficits in motor proficiency in the absence of attention deficit disorder (Denckla et al. 1985b), neuromotor maturity (Wolff et al. 1985), auditory attention deficits under distracting conditions (Cherry and Kruger 1983), and even poor postural control (Kohen-Raz 1986) have been described as correlates of dyslexia. In a large-scale Australian study, Jorm et al. (1986) followed 453 children from kindergarten to second grade and found that those with specific dyslexia had more behavior problems, primarily attention deficit disorder, whereas a group of general reading-backward children did not. The authors interpreted this finding as an indication that an ADD factor "may play a causative role in their reading difficulty" (p. 33). Fein et al. (1988) described deficits in both verbal and nonverbal memory in a sample of dyslexic children, but they viewed these as manifestations of an underlying lesion largely unrelated to the dyslexia. Doehring (1968) found a group of reading-disabled children to be deficient on as many as 31 nonreading measures. However, the notion that reading disability in general is directly caused by deficiencies in visual attention, perception, or memory has been generally abandoned, as specifically stated in the definition of LD.

Deficiencies in auditory and phonological processing that could interfere with the recoding from written to spoken language have been described as a primary deficit underlying reading disability (Doehring et al. 1981, Tallal 1980, Vellutino 1982). Liberman and Shankweiler (1979) suggested that some children are unable to extract phonemes from spoken words, a step that they argue is essential in learning to read. These children may also have problems in abstracting the phonological segments corresponding to printed letters (Doehring et al. 1981). Deficiencies in morphophonemic processing at the level of spoken language occur in some reading-disabled children; these children lack the skill to combine phonemes to form units of meaning—morphemes (Vogel 1977). This deficit has been described as a lack of meta-linguistic awareness.

Factor-analytic research based on a model derived from Luria's (1966) theory and developed by Das et al. (1979) has explored the cognitive structure of poor and average readers. Two systems, verbal-successive and spatial-simultaneous processing, were derived. The first allows the reader to convert the consecutive presentation of elements into a new quality of simultaneous perceptibility, and the second allows the reader to go beyond the meaning of individual words and grasp the meaning of the sentence as a whole. Both are needed, although at different ages and levels of achievement in reading (Solan 1987). Leong (1980, Downing and Leong 1982) demonstrated that although poor readers were impaired on both the simultaneous and the successive processing factors, the difference was most pronounced for the successive factor. This factor represents a combination of tasks with a major component requiring sequential processing, which has also been ascribed to left hemisphere cognitive abilities.

Subtypes of Primary Dyslexia

Although the number varies, current research favors the notion of several reading disability subtypes, first introduced by Shankweiler (1964). Because different types of acquired reading disabilities have been found in adults, it seemed reasonable to assume that there should be more than one type of reading disability in children. Reading is also a complex act involving many component skills; it requires visuoperceptual skills involving discrimination of (1) closure, for example between "o" and "c"; (2) line-to-curve transformation, for example between "u" and "v"; and (3) rotational transformation, for example between "b," "d," "p," and "g." If these skills are defective, reading-disabled children may experience difficulties with the discrimination and/or the orientation of letters. Sequencing skills are also needed, especially at the letter and semantic levels, to recognize the differences between, for example, "pan and nap" and "cat chases mouse, mouse chases cat." Difficulties in serial thinking can be reflected in poor spelling and poor comprehension. The cross-modal transfer of information as an essential part of the reading process has been emphasized by Benson (1981) and others. For example, writing to dictation demands auditory input that is then translated into visual symbols. Reading is also a linguistic skill that requires the understanding of visual symbols used to convey meaning.

The many components of reading skills and the many different forms of dyslexia make it unlikely that a single focal lesion is responsible for all reading disabilities. Current theories of brain function, cognition, and language emphasize the complexity of these processes and stress their interactional, multifactorial role in reading (Downing and Leong 1982), which leads to a multiple-syndrome paradigm. Such a paradigm would include several different patterns of deficits in disabled readers.

Boder (1973) distinguished three types of reading disability based on the clinical-educational analysis of spelling and reading errors: a **dysphonetic reading disability,** one who shows little understanding of letter-sound relationships; a **dyseidetic reading disability,** one with an inability to read words as a whole; and a **dysphonetic-dyseidetic reading disability,** one with problems in both areas. This classification is still used widely. She found that, of the 107 dyslexic children in her study, 63 per cent were dysphonetic, 9 per cent were dyseidetic, 22 per cent were dysphonetic-dyseidetic, and 6 per cent were of an undetermined type.

Denckla's (1979) subtypes, also based on clinical reports, include a global mixed language disorder, an articulation-graphomotor type, an anomia-repetition disorder, a dysphonemic sequencing disorder, a verbal learning and memory disorder, and a correlational type in which reading was normal but low relative to IQ. The relationship among language, reading, and spelling is also stressed by Kirk (1983).

Again based on clinical studies, Myklebust (1978) described an intermodal reading disability that is divided into auditory-intermodal and visual-intermodal dyslexia, as well as into inner-language dyslexia, auditory dyslexia, and a visual-verbal alexia. Pirozzolo (1979), in contrast, described only two types—an auditory-linguistic and a visual-spatial disorder.

Experimental studies with visual evoked potentials led Bakker (1992, Bakker and Vinke 1985) to develop a two-subtype "balance model." According to this theory, in the early stages of learning to read, children use a right hemisphere strategy that emphasizes perceptual strategies. As children become more proficient in reading, this strategy shifts to a presumably faster, linguistic strategy, using left hemisphere processing. A dynamic balance between the two strategies is needed for normal reading development. Reading is impaired in children who rely too much on either the left hemisphere (**L-type dyslexia**) or the right hemisphere (**P-type dyslexia**) strategies. Bakker supported these two subtypes of dyslexia by demonstrating the imbalance of evoked potentials postulated by his theory and by using specific training and teaching strategies (e.g., right or left visual field stimulation) to improve reading in these children. A recent study showed significantly slower lexical decision making in P-type dyslexics depending on the length of the word (van Strien et al. 1993).

Lovett (1984, 1987) also proposed two subtypes of dyslexia, the accuracy-disabled and the rate-disabled reader. She presented extensive validation with a variety of reading-related measures and training strategies.

Differing from clinical subtyping, another approach to the study of subtypes is based on the multivariate analysis of tests given to samples of disabled readers. Mattis et al. (1975) identified three dyslexia syndromes in a multivariate grouping analysis: a language-disordered group, an articulation-graphomotor dyscoordination group, and a group with visuoperceptual disorders. A cross-validation study with 400 children between the ages of 8 and 10 confirmed this classification (Mattis 1978).

Doehring and Hoshko (1977) used the Q-technique of factor analysis and combined the measurement of multiple nonreading skills with several reading skills. The design analyzed the interaction of linguistic and neuropsychological deficits with reading skill deficits (Doehring et al. 1981). A battery of neuropsychological tests was administered to examine the extent to which neuropsychological deficit characterized each type of disability. Three types of reading disability were found: type O, slow oral word reading; type A, slow auditory-visual association of letters; and type S, slow auditory-visual association of words and syllables. Doehring's subgroups are strikingly similar to those found by Mattis, suggesting an emerging consensus of results from multivariate studies.

Other empirical studies with Q-type factor analysis and cluster analysis have produced a variety of subtype models (Fletcher and Satz 1985, Lyon et al. 1982, Rourke 1985, Spreen and Haaf 1986, Van der Vlugt 1989). Such analyses frequently yield more than two subtypes, but close inspection shows that the additional subtypes tend to be either generally impaired or close-to-normal readers, i.e., severely impaired or near-normal readers who in a dichotomous subtype classification would either be forced into one of two subtypes or omitted from the analysis (Spreen and Haaf 1986). Additional subtypes may also be generated if, in addition to measures of reading, results from intelligence and neuropsychological testing are included in the analyses, if normal readers are included, or if the population consists of both younger and older dyslexic children. Fletcher and Satz (1985), Lyon et al. (1982), and Spreen and Haaf (1986) also studied short-term (kindergarten to grade 5) response to treatment, and long-term (grade 4 to age 25) outcome in their research. A full discussion of the topic is presented by Hooper and Willis (1989) and in section 5 of this chapter.

Although the terminology and the theoretical models used by each of these subtype researchers vary considerably, some basic commonalities emerge at least as far as the two major subtypes are concerned: Boder's dysphonetic, Satz's and Lyon's, Mattis' general and specific language deficit, Bakker's P-type, Lovett's accuracy-disabled group, and Doehring and Hoschko's A and S types all show deficits in the auditory-linguistic area. Boder's dyseidetic, Satz's and Lyon's, as well as Mattis' visuoperceptual, Bakker's L-type, Lovett's, and Doehring and Hoschko's rate-disabled readers all show visuospatial problems. These two subtypes are also prominent in the Bergen follow-up (Gjessing and Karlsen 1989), in an empirical study by Nussbaum et al. (1986), and in the Spreen and Haaf study (Table 29–2). Dysfunction in different cortical areas may be hypothesized as the underlying basis of each type.

Other proposed subtypes often consist of only a few subjects and are not replicated in other studies. Newby and Lyon (1991) and Stanovich (1985) emphasized that this apparent dichotomy may be more appropriately seen as two continuous dimensions of reading ability. Whether future research will produce additional meaningful and replicable subtypes remains to be seen. Spreen and Haaf's research suggested that the auditory-linguistic subtype may have the more severe prognostic consequences; nearly all subjects in this group were found in a severely and generally impaired group when retested at age 25, although Gjessing and Karlsen (1989) reported that their sample's progress through the school years was not significantly related to subtype membership.

Electrophysiological differences between subtypes have been studied for some time. In addition to the work by Bakker and colleagues to be discussed below, various other ERP studies with populations of learning-disabled children have shown only inconsistent differences when compared to normal learning subjects. A review of ERP studies by Dool et al. (1993) indicated that such

Table 29-2   Empirically Derived Subtypes of Learning Disability

1. Minimally impaired with articulo-graphomotor or dysphonetic components (N = 14)
2. Minimally impaired with some arithmetic problems (N = 16)
3. Arithmetic disabled subtype (N = 6)
4. Severely language disabled subtype (N = 7)
5. Visuo-perceptual subtype (N = 14)
6. Severely disabled in all areas (N = 15)
7. Normal in reading and arithmetic (N = 6)

Source: Spreen and Haaf 1986.

studies are likely to be more successful if ERPs are used for the analysis of well-defined subtypes with clear cut hypotheses about the reason for electro-physiological response differences. In addition, ERPs are likely to produce better results if the experimental task for ERP measurements pertains directly to the hypothesized processing deficit, rather than being a passive task unrelated to the reading process. A semantic priming task (i.e., reading of words that are not semantically consistent with previously read words) seems promising in differentiating subtypes as it affects a specific part of the ERP, the N400 wave (Bentin et al. 1985, Kutas and van Petten 1988).

29.2 Causes of Dyslexia

The Genetic Hypothesis

The notion that some forms of reading disability may be genetic has been raised since 1905 (Thomas 1905). The evidence includes family history, the presence of reading disability in monozygotic and dyzygotic twins, and the likelihood that a genetically determined reading disability will persist through a lifetime (De-Fries et al. 1991, Pennington and Smith 1983). Byring and Michelsson (1984) reported dyslexia in relatives of 77 per cent of their group of 97 Swedish-speaking Finnish children. They also reported that dyslexia persisted in 85 per cent of their subjects in a 7- to 10-year follow-up to the age of 17 years. DeFries et al. (1991) estimated that heritable factors account for 60 per cent of the variance in dyslexics. There is no agreement, however, on the form of genetic transmission.

Co-morbidity with other disorders has stimulated further research into the genetic transmission of dyslexia. Geschwind and Behan (1982, 1984) postulated a linkage between dyslexia, left-handedness, and autoimmune and allergic disorders, based on a major theory of prenatal testosterone exposure in utero (see Chapter 5). Subsequent studies by Pennington et al. (1987) and Burke et al. (1988) confirmed this finding, but studies by Hansen et al. (1986, 1987) showed that, in addition, dyslexia was negatively associated with diabetes in the family, i.e., that learning problems occur less frequently in diabetic children or children of insulin-dependent parents. This finding suggests that the genetics of diabetes "protects" such children or that children of nondiabetic parents are more vulnerable to dyslexia. The linkage with immune system disorders was partially confirmed by Hugdahl et al. (1990), but the authors warned that it would be misleading to assume that testosterone is a major etiological substrate of either dyslexia or left-handedness.

The genetic basis of handedness has also been associated with dyslexia. Vernon (1971) claimed that left- or mixed handedness occurs more frequently in clinical cases of dyslexia. Yule and Rutter (1976) and Hardyck and Petrinovich (1977) did not find an association between handedness and dyslexia, but

Geschwind and Behan (1982, 1984) again stressed the relationship between left-handedness and dyslexia (see below).

The argument for genetic involvement in dyslexia would be strengthened if the pattern of reading disability were found to be consistent within families. Following this line of reasoning, Omenn and Weber (1978) reported cases of similar dysphonetic spelling errors in some families. Finucci et al. (1976) found that 45 per cent of 75 first-degree relatives of dyslexics and significantly more males than females were affected. Although Finucci concluded that dyslexia is "genetically heterogeneous," Pennington and Smith (1983) stated in their critical review of the literature:

> Some forms of dyslexia are transmitted genetically, and there are likely to be several forms of familial dyslexia involving different forms of transmission. Dyslexia does not appear to be a sex-linked disorder, but there is a sex difference in expression, likely due, in part, to normal, genetically based sex differences in language skills. There are different dyslexia phenotypes, developmental changes within a phenotype, and phenotypic variability across family members of similar ages (p. 377).

Perinatal Stress Factors and Neurological Abnormalities

Few prospective studies of the relationship between pre- and perinatal events and learning disabilities explore the relation between perinatal stress and specific learning disorders. Spreen (1978c) noted that, if the distinction between primary (congenital, no overt causes) and symptomatic (due to brain damage or dysfunction) forms of dyslexia is valid, one would expect to find differing neurobehavioral variables. Rourke (1978) went further and stated that, if brain dysfunction interferes with reading acquisition, then it is necessary to investigate the relationship between reading acquisition and birth events that pose risks to normal brain development.

The first autopsy report of a 12-year-old dyslexic boy (Drake 1968) showed "anomalies in the convolutional pattern of the parietal lobes bilaterally. The pattern was disrupted by penetrating deep gyri that appeared disconnected. Related areas of the corpus callosum appeared thin" (p. 496). Rosen et al. (1986) found lack of asymmetry in the planum temporale area in four consecutive autopsy studies of dyslexics, suggesting that such anomalies may be the neural base for dyslexia.

Kawi and Pasamanick (1958) provided one of the earliest studies of the relationship between birth history and reading disorders. They found that 16 per cent of infants exposed to two or more complications during birth (especially fetal anoxia) had reading problems later in life. The authors suggested that a continuum of reproductive casualty arises from stress factors at birth that may extend from fetal death to behavior and learning problems. Gesell (Goldberg and Schiffman 1972) also suggested that unrecognized minimal birth injury could express itself in speech difficulty and later in reading problems.

Investigating the effect of mothers' smoking during pregnancy, Butler and Goldstein (1973) found that children of such mothers were 4 months behind in reading at the age of 7 years. Dunn and McBurney (1977) found significant differences in favor of non-smokers' children in 14 of 48 psychological tests given at the age of 6½ years.

The relationship between premature birth and reading disability was examined in a study by DeHirsch et al. (1966), who found an association between prematurity and reading readiness, but failed to equate their premature and full-term groups for IQ levels. Taub et al. (1977) found no differences in scholastic performance between prematures and controls at the ages of 7 and 9½ years. They noted a weakness in perceptual organization among premature children that is probably overcome in later stages when verbal skills become more important (Dalby 1979). The many inconsistencies in the literature on prematurity and reading disability can be attributed to methodological differences (Caputo and Mandell 1970).

A retrospective study of several pre-, peri- and postnatal variables by Lyle (1970) of 54 6- to 12-year-old middle-class reading-retarded boys matched with 54 normal readers found two factors of reading performance: "freedom from perceptual and perceptual-motor distortions" (relating to letter and sequence reversal and memory for design errors) and "formal learning" (loading mostly on academic achievement and WISC intelligence test variables, such as arithmetic, digit span, information and coding). The first factor was significantly predicted by birth variables, including birth injury, prenatal complications, birth weight, short labor, and speech development at 6 and 24 months, whereas the second factor was best predicted by postnatal developmental criteria. Lyle noted that low birth weight and toxemia of pregnancy were not related to later reading performance.

La Benz et al. (1980) looked at a large number of early predictors of deficits in reading, writing, and spelling in the context of the Collaborative Perinatal Study. The most reliable predictors were variables measured after the first year of life, but also included birth weight, gestational age, neonatal distress, and complications of pregnancy and delivery; however, these latter variables were not predictive by themselves. The authors concluded that deficits in written communication are the result of multiple causes and that environmental and later developmental factors, particularly speech and language delay, play a more predictive role. In contrast, some studies (Galante et al. 1972, Smith et al. 1972) demonstrated a correlation between reading disability and such minor deficits as unusual birth history, abnormal EEG, and soft neurological signs.

EEG abnormalities tend to occur more frequently in LD children than in age-matched control groups of normal learners, but tend to be nonspecific both in respect to the type of LD and the locus of EEG abnormality.

Balow et al. (1976) reviewed the relationship between perinatal events and reading disability and discussed problems of methodology, such as different outcomes studied and varying research designs. They concluded that the hypothesis that very low birth weight and certain pregnancy and birth complications (particularly anoxic episodes) are related to impaired reading ability is adequately supported. However, the majority of studies of hypoxic children show more general learning deficits, rather than dyslexia alone (Gottfried 1973, Sechzer et al. 1973). Although neurological dysfunction in the newborn may play a role in some children with dyslexia, the occurrence of such complications is neither a necessary nor a sufficient explanation for reading disability (Rourke 1978). A retrospective study by Austin (1978) examined children between 6 and 16 years of age with dyslexia (n = 48) or dyscalculia (n = 67) who had an average IQ, no history of seizure disorders, cerebral palsy, hearing or visual loss and did not suffer from severe emotional disorder or environmental or cultural deprivation. Perinatal complications were found to be more frequent and more serious among children with dyscalculia (62 per cent) than among children with dyslexia (43 per cent) or children without learning difficulty (7 per cent). Delays in the attainment of many developmental milestones (sitting, walking, speaking sentences, toilet training) were evident for children with dyscalculia, whereas dyslexic children were delayed only in the onset of speaking. Neurological soft signs and abnormal EEGs were also more frequent in the dyscalculic group than in the dyslexic group or the group with no learning disorders.

Dyslexia and Cerebral Asymmetry

Orton's (1937) theory that reading disability may be linked to atypical brain asymmetry has been investigated with dichotic listening and visual half-field techniques in normal and impaired readers. It was expected that less lateralization of language in the left hemisphere would be reflected in a smaller right-ear or right visual half-field advantage. Dyslexics may also be expected to show abnormal lateral preference in the form of ambilaterality and left-handedness, extreme right- or left-handedness, and discrepancies between lateral preference and performance, although left-handedness has also been related to various other disorders in addition to dyslexia. However, no consistent differences between good and poor readers have been found (Bryden 1988, Porac and Coren 1978, Satz 1972, Witelson 1976b). Wellman and Allen (1983) did report a higher incidence of inverted hand position during writing and drawing for 7- to 9-year-old poor readers, although their lateralization on dichotic listening and visual field experiments with verbal and visuospatial material did not differ significantly from that of good readers. An experiment by Broman et al. (1986) explored reaction times and errors for the right and left hand to single-letter stimuli presented in the right and left visual fields in 8- to 13-year-old dyslexic and normal readers of similar intelligence: reaction times were slower in dyslexics for all four conditions, but not specifically impaired in the crossed (e.g., left hand-right visual field, or right hand-left visual field) conditions. Rather, they found that more errors were made in the right ipsilateral condition. The authors interpreted this finding as suggesting that interhemispheric transfer is not specifically impaired, but that processing of linguistic stimuli in the left hemisphere is the main source of dyslexic problems.

One reason for the inconsistent findings about lateral differences in poor readers may be developmental. In children who are learning academic skills, hemispheric specialization is less clear-cut than after this learning has been completed. Accumulating evidence suggests that the right hemisphere is more involved in the initial stages because of the visuoperceptual demands of beginning reading (Fletcher and Satz 1980, Hinshaw et al 1986, Licht et al. 1986) or because the right hemisphere is better at handling novel, unpracticed tasks (Goldberg and Costa 1981). As reading skills become more practiced, advancing from decoding to extracting meaning from the text, the left hemisphere becomes predominant. Hence, studies of lateral asymmetries may show different results at different ages or persisting different hemispheric deficits dependent on the type of dyslexia.

Bakker (1979) recorded visually evoked potentials (ERPs, see Chapter 3) from the right and left parietal areas of young children with reading problems. His results suggested two types of dyslexic readers as mentioned earlier: L- and P-type dyslexics. L-type dyslexics are characterized by speech mediated by the left hemisphere, but show a weak right hemisphere specialization for visual perception (predominant left ERPs). They read quickly, miss some of the perceptual features of the script, and make substitution errors. P-type dyslexics show an overdevelopment of right hemisphere functions as shown in visuospatial tasks and a depression of the left-hemisphere-mediated linguistic capabilities (predominant right ERPs). They are sensitive to the perceptual features of script, read slowly, and make presuming errors. Using a different paradigm, Segalowitz et al. (1992) found a lack of expected visual and auditory asymmetries among poor readers, although these did not account for the variation in reading skills; variations in reading skills in poor readers (but not in good readers), however, were more closely related to the frontally generated contingent negative variation of ERPs. Another ERP study from Bakker's laboratory (Licht et al. 1988) showed that the focus of lateral differences shifts to the temporal region in older children. Consistent with this finding, Wood et al. (1988, Flowers et al. 1991) found less activation of the left temporal perisylvian region during an orthographic task in adults who were childhood dyslexics using regional cerebral blood flow techniques (PET scans), and Gross-Glenn et al. (1988, 1991) reported similar findings, as well as less asymmetry in prefrontal and inferior occipital activity. Another study (Hynd and Willis 1987) based on PET techniques, however, found less activation on the right side and bilaterally in a deep dyslexic subject. Despite the inconsistencies, these results can be interpreted as inadequate hemispheric integration or inefficient simultaneous allocation of resources. Duffy and McAnulty (1990) raised the possibility that electrophysiological studies reflect compensatory mechanisms, rather than pathological change.

Anatomical evidence for a relationship between brain asymmetry and reading disability was reported by Hier et al. (1978). CT scans were obtained for 24 developmentally dyslexic patients between 14 and 47 years of age. The width of the brain at the intersection of the parietal and occipital lobes on the right was wider than on the left in 42 per cent (i.e., a reversal from the greater width of the left hemisphere commonly found in normal readers) and 33 per cent of the subjects showed virtually no asymmetry. Hier et al. (1978) estimated that individuals with reversed brain asymmetry are at risk for reading disability five times greater than persons with normal asymmetry. The authors suggested that reversed cerebral asymmetry results in language lateralization to a hemisphere that is structurally less suited to support language. This finding is supported by an EEG study of Rumsey et al. (1986); by an autopsy study of eight dyslexics who all showed symmetry of the planum temporale together with cortical anomalies in the perisylvian region of the left hemisphere (Galaburda 1989); and by a MRI study of Hynd et al. (1990b), which found that symmetry or reversed asymmetry was present in 90 per cent of dyslexics, but only in 30 per cent of children with ADHD and controls. A review of these and other studies concludes that "the available evidence is highly suggestive and justifies further, more carefully controlled studies" (Hynd et al. 1991, p. 504). However, since brain lateralization is only one aspect of the neurological substrate for reading, it is probable that reversal or absence of the normal asymmetry interacts with other factors to produce reading disability.

A case history of acquired reading disability in a 6-year-old boy who underwent left temporal lobectomy revealed that, despite the lesion, speech remained strongly lateralized to the left hemisphere (Levine et al. 1981). The authors noted that some patients with developmental dyslexia may have dysfunction of the dominant left hemisphere, rather than a reversal, delay, or incompleteness of language lateralization.

Indirect support for the poor development of lateralization and interhemispheric connections comes from studies of nootropic drugs (e.g., piracetam), which have been described as "left hemisphere specific" and as facilitating interhemispheric transfer because they seem to selectively improve abilities usually associated with the left hemisphere. Wilsher (1986) reviewed 13 double-blind studies with LD subjects, all of which seemed to demonstrate improvement of reading and reading-related skills when piracetam is administered.

The disproportionately higher incidence of reading problems among boys has been known for some time (Ansara et al. 1981, Buffery 1976, Rourke 1978, Singer et al. 1968). Lansdell (1964) and Critchley and Critchley (1978) proposed that myelination rates for boys are generally delayed and that myelination is more rapid in the left hemisphere in girls and in the right hemisphere in boys. This hypothesis has been supported in studies by Witelson (1977b), McGlone (1977), and Geschwind and Galaburda (1987). Further support comes from a study by Bakker et al. (1976), who related ear advantage on a dichotic listening task to a word-naming test. The findings suggested that girls pass through the learning-to-read stages earlier than boys. Differences in lateralization may be related to sex-linked recessive gene transmission (Aaron 1982).

Neurodevelopmental Deficit Versus Delay Models of Dyslexia

Two contrasting models for the explanation of dyslexia on the basis of neurological development have been proposed. The deficit model considers dyslexia as the result of cerebral deficit, which may take the form of faulty hemispheric organization or of abnormal development of neural cells and connections. The neurodevelopmental delay model is based on several different explanations. Some authors still accept Orton's theory that dyslexia is due to delay in the establishment of cerebral dominance. Current research has shown, however, that anatomically (Yeni-Komishian and Benson 1976), electroencephalographically (Gardiner and Walter 1977), and behaviorally (Caplan and Kinsbourne 1976), the beginnings of hemispheric specialization are present at or near birth.

Satz et al. (1974, 1978) hypothesized that the delay underlying dyslexia occurs in the early sensory perceptual and later conceptual development and is caused by disorders of central processing. This theory predicts that delays in those developmental skills that are in primary ascendance during the preschool period forecast problems in reading. However, neither reading nor the early perceptual-motor and oral language abilities are unitary abilities. Reading success depends on the interplay of a host of strengths and weaknesses related to the child's experiential and cultural background (Jansky 1978).

Language delay at age 4 has been described as an especially strong predictor of LD during school age. Tallal and Curtiss (1988) reported that, compared to IQ-matched normal controls, 85 per cent of children with language delay were found to have reading impairment at age 7 in a 5-year follow-up. Poor pattern discrimination on the Seashore Rhythm test and poor right-left discrimination have also been singled out as predictors of reading difficulties (McGivern et al. 1991). At kindergarten age, Wolf and Goodglass (1986) demonstrated that vocabulary knowledge itself is not predictive, but that word retrieval problems, as measured with the Boston Naming Test, are highly predictive of reading problems in second grade. Badian et al. (1990) and Scarborough (1991) stressed the role of phonological processing and electrophysiological measures in predicting dyslexia. Even in adulthood, dyslexics show poor non-word reading and problems with phonological awareness, and rapid naming, whereas other neuropsychological measures do not necessarily show abnormalities (Felton et al. 1990).

A neurodevelopmental delay model seems to imply that the child may eventually be able to develop these skills at a later age. Proponents of the delay model have modified this line of reasoning and asserted that further difficulties may persist during adolescence and later life because the learning history of the dyslexic child is affected (Denckla 1977). In fact, the adult outcome of reading disability, as far as it has been studied, seems to be quite poor not only for reading itself but also for general academic achievement and personal, social, and occupational adjustment (Spreen 1988a). Persistent dyslexia has also been observed in college students (Aaron 1982).

The issue of deficit or delay is akin to the nature-nurture controversy in that both factors exert considerable influence. A maturational lag could result in a neurological organization that remains deviant; a deficit or brain damage in children, which is rarely static, may result in delay. Also, children with brain damage may recover, but their catching up could be based on reorganized abilities of a different structure, not an indication of a maturational lag. Current neuropsychological models of dyslexia are probably not sophisticated enough to accommodate the many different factors involved and to relate them to specific forms of dyslexia. In the case of acquired dyslexia, the reading disability is related to specific damage, most often in the left parietal-occipital area. In developmental dyslexia, the most important primary damaging event currently reported is anoxia, which often results in diffuse damage and which could manifest itself as a delay in the early stages of development (Dalby 1979).

29.3   Writing Disorders

In addition to difficulty in learning to read, children may also have difficulty in producing written language or in performing mathematical tasks. Since writing and, to a certain extent, mathematics are dependent on the reception and comprehension of spoken and written language, many children with reading disorders also experience difficulty with these other tasks.

Writing as a means of self-expression is a highly integrative function involving language, as well as perceptual and motor processes. Writing disorders have been described as primarily related to disturbance of the language system, the visual and/or auditory perceptual system, or of the motor systems necessary for structuring and forming letters.

A useful distinction has been made between writing and handwriting (Chalfant and Scheffelin 1969). Writing refers to the commitment of one's thoughts to a written idea; it involves the ideational (or propositional) use of language, as well as the auditory and visual systems. Disturbances of any of these systems may interfere with the writing process. Handwriting, in contrast, refers to the motor aspects of writing. The term "**dysgraphia**" is often used to denote a disorder in handwriting: a child may have difficulty tracing shapes, using efficient strokes for forming letters, forming letters of appropriate size, or using a comfortable pressure in grasping a writing implement (DeQuiros and Schrager 1978). Some children may be able to produce well-formed letters, but do so extremely slowly. Others may have difficulty in beginning to write or in completing a word.

A deficit in the ability to use fine motor movements of the hands and fingers has been suggested as the basis for dysgraphic disturbances (Orton 1937); this deficit may or may not extend to the learning of other new manual activities. Goldstein (1948) suggested that difficulty in remembering motor sequences for writing or the way in which letter shapes should be constructed may be involved. Berninger and Rutberg (1992) believed that similar basic processes are forerunners of writing problems. Sandler et al. (1992) proposed four subtypes of writing disorder based on a cluster analysis of 99 9- to-15-year-old children: (1)

with fine motor and linguistic deficit, (2) with visuospatial deficit, (3) with attention and memory deficit, and (4) with sequencing problems. This subtyping is more comprehensive and deserves further validational study.

29.4 Arithmetic and Nonverbal Learning Disorders

Most dyslexia research does not report whether the children exhibited other learning problems. Some researchers have noted that only a small minority of children exhibit relatively specific learning problems other than in reading. Surveys by McAllister (1981) and Tuokko (1982) found that in both clinic and school samples as few as 7 per cent of LD children exhibit difficulty in learning to read when their learning of other subject material is adequate and that only 5 per cent experience difficulty with writing or arithmetic without difficulty in learning to read. Yet, it has been suggested that the various patterns of learning problems represent different disorders that may be distinguishable on the basis of qualitative characteristics, associated cognitive weaknesses, and, perhaps, etiology (Nelson and Warrington 1976).

Arithmetic Disorders

Arithmetic is a branch of mathematics that involves real numbers and their computations. The term "**developmental dyscalculia**" is used to denote difficulties in performing arithmetic operations, e.g., reading or writing of numbers or series of numbers, recognizing the categorical structure of numbers. Developmental dyscalculia is differentiated from dyscalculia acquired after brain lesions and **acalculia** (a complete failure of mathematical ability). Acquired calculation disturbances are most frequently related to posterior left hemisphere lesions (Grafman et al. 1982), but a spatial type of acquired dyscalculia with damage in the right parietal region has also been described (Levin and Eisenberg 1979). Kosc (1974) considered developmental dyscalculia to be a complex disorder defined as "a structural disorder of mathematical abilities which has its origins in a genetic or congenital disorder of those parts of the brain that are the direct anatomico-physiological substrates of the maturation of the mathematical abilities adequate to age, without simultaneous disorder of general mental functions" (p. 47).

Developmental dyscalculia has been further classified into subtypes. The most frequently used subtypes of dyscalculia are (1) a language-based dyscalculia with difficulty in the comprehension of verbal problems and instructions, difficulties memorizing facts and step-by-step procedures, and inexperience with subject material, frequently associated with reading problems and (2) dyscalculia associated with spatial-temporal difficulties, including number reversals, number order reversals, and carrying out operations in the wrong sequence. The second subtype is further discussed below as nonverbal LD. It is generally recognized that both the right and the left hemisphere make specific contributions to arithmetic abilities and that either or both of these two subtypes may be involved (Troup et al. 1993).

Neuropsychological Significance of Patterns of Deficit

GERSTMANN SYNDROME

Although developmental disorders of reading, writing, and arithmetic in children do not necessarily appear in the same form as acquired disorders in adults, the knowledge gained from the study of calculation disorders in brain-damaged adults has led to speculation about the possible organic bases of developmental problems. In adults, for example, dysgraphia and dyscalculia occurring in conjunction with right-left confusion and finger agnosia constitute the **Gerstmann syndrome,** which frequently has been associated with damage to the parietal lobe of the dominant hemisphere. The term "**developmental Gerstmann syndrome**" has been applied to denote the occurrence of several or all of these four behavioral deficits in children. Kinsbourne and Warrington (1963) described seven children with finger agnosia who, in every instance, exhibited two or more of the other elements of the Gerstmann syndrome. Both difficulty with spelling (five of the seven) and handwriting (four) were noted. Number concepts were not impaired, but difficulty with place value concepts was noted. The authors speculated that the underlying defect of the developmental Gerstmann syndrome is an inability to correctly order serial parts of a whole. Five of the seven children had sustained perinatal injury, but the neurological abnormalities found on examination seemed to reflect scattered disease, rather than specific structural abnormality. Benson and Geschwind (1970) presented two "pure" cases of children who showed the full tetrad of the Gerstmann syndrome and preserved reading ability. Pebenito (1987) described a boy with the full syndrome with superior intelligence and normal neurological findings; he suggested that such cases are rare.

Spellacy and Peter (1978) examined two groups of seven dyscalculic children differing in reading ability (adequate versus impaired readers). None of the children showed deficits limited to the four elements of the developmental Gerstmann syndrome. Five children did show impairment on all four elements of the syndrome, in addition to other deficits that were found among adequate and poor readers. The authors suggested that "since the presence or absence of the four Gerstmann behavioral elements does not describe a behaviorally homogeneous group, the value of the developmental Gerstmann syndrome as a behavioral description seems limited" (p. 202). No neurological examination was available for the children in this study. However, on the basis of the behavioral abnormalities exhibited by these children, bilateral involvement was proposed. Whether or not dominant parietal lobe abnormality is indicated when all four elements of the syndrome are present in children remains an open question. After reviewing several studies, Benton (1985) argued that "this aggregate is (not) anything more than an arbitrary grouping of deficits without a distinctive neuropsychological significance" (p. 206).

Nonverbal Learning Disabilities

Rourke (1978) and Rourke and Finlayson (1978) examined qualitative and quantitative differences between two groups of 15 children matched for deficient arithmetic performance but differing with respect to achievement in reading and spelling. The group of children characterized by adequate word recognition and spelling but poor arithmetic ability exhibited defective visual perception, tactile perception, and impaired psychomotor ability (Rourke and Finlayson 1978, Rourke and Strang 1978). Their arithmetic errors revealed that they attempted calculations for which they had little understanding of the task requirements (Rourke and Strang 1981). They also tended to misread mathematical signs and showed disorganized work and faulty alignment of rows and columns; occasionally, entire steps in the calculation were omitted. The authors suggested that early impairment of sensorimotor experience may have led to poor development of abstract conceptualization, which affected the basic understanding of mathematical operations. Children with poor word recognition and spelling skills but better arithmetic performance exhibited poor psycholinguistic abilities, but their visual perception, tactile perception, and sensorimotor coordination were well developed. These children avoided unfamiliar arithmetic operations. Errors usually reflected some difficulty in remembering arithmetic tables or steps in the procedure for solving a problem. Verbal memory impairment was raised as a possible underlying cognitive weakness affecting arithmetic performance. Summarizing his findings, Rourke (1982) suggested that

> the reading and spelling disability group exhibits performance that would be expected were they to be suffering from deficiencies in left hemisphere systems, whereas the arithmetic disability group exhibits performances that would be expected were they to be experiencing the untoward consequences of deficiencies in systems thought to be subserved by the right cerebral hemisphere (p. 10).

Further work by Rourke (Casey et al. 1991, Fuerst et al. 1990, Hernadek and Rourke 1994, Rourke 1989, Rourke et al. 1990, Rourke and Fuerst 1992) described this **nonverbal learning disability** (**NVLD**), a term first used by Myklebust (1975), as a white matter right hemisphere deficit. The right hemisphere deficit leads to basic problems in visuospatial organizational skills, psychomotor coordination, complex tactile-perceptual skills, reasoning, concept formation, mechanical arithmetic, and scientific reasoning. Children with NVLD can be discriminated from children with reading and spelling disabilities with high accuracy (Hernadek and Rourke 1994). These deficits are also the basis for defective social judgment, poor recognition of faces and emotional expressions, and poor adaptability to novel interpersonal situations.

Rourke described subgroups of LD children demonstrating arithmetic and social skill deficits, as well as internalizing psychopathology (Fuerst and Rourke 1993). A higher-than-average incidence of depression, motor clumsiness, and co-occurrence of attention deficit disorder was also noted. Independent reports by Voeller (1986) and Nussbaum et al. (1990) described a similar type of deficit. Solan (1987) demonstrated that arithmetic achievement was more highly correlated with measures of spatial than with verbal skills in normally achieving children. In support of the NVLD model, Loveland et al. (1990) showed that children with specific impairment in arithmetic made more errors in the comprehension and production of nonverbal puppet scenarios than in the comprehension of narrative stories, whereas children with general LD showed the opposite pattern.

A review by Semrud-Clikeman and Hynd (1991), however, warned that a specific NVLD subtype has not been verified in group research using DSM-III-R psychiatric diagnostic criteria and needs further study. Inconsistent results, for example, were obtained by Landau et al. (1987) in a study of peer and teacher ratings of LD children with higher Verbal than Performance IQ and those with no difference or higher Performance IQ; the results indicated more intact interpersonal skills for the latter group. The NVLD model would predict the opposite. White et al. (in press) found that in 157 LD and normally achieving children correlations between visuospatial and socio-emotional measures failed to reach significance. Glosser and Koppell (1987) inferred lateralized brain dysfunction from neuropsychological test results and reported that in 7- to 10-year-old LD children indicators of left hemisphere impairment were associated with dysphoria, anxiety, and social withdrawal, whereas children with indicators of right hemisphere impairment had low rates of dysphoria/anxiety but increased somatic complaints; children with non-lateralized impairment showed more pervasive emotional disturbance and attention deficit disorder. These findings would seem exploratory in nature at this time because clear lateralization based on independent neurological or radiological results has only been reported for children with acquired right hemisphere lesions (Tranel et al. 1987, Voeller 1986, Weintraub and Mesulam 1983). These studies tend to support the NVLD model. Not only the expected visuospatial deficit but also difficulties in arithmetic and problems of social isolation, withdrawal, aggressiveness, and inappropriate behavior are common in these children.

29.5   Long-Term Outcome of Learning Disabilities and Associated Problems

Several studies cited earlier indicate that LD tends to persist into adulthood (see review by Spreen 1988a). Although with milder forms of dyslexia, children may acquire a functional knowledge of reading sufficient for many jobs, they often do not read for pleasure or even read daily news reports. Ingenious ways of covering up this deficit (i.e., watching TV newscasts as a substitute, displaying reading matter in the home) have been described. A major follow-up study of 203 learning-disabled children and 52 normal learners from age 10 to 25 (Spreen 1988b) confirmed these findings. Less than 40 per cent of these subjects completed grade 12 compared to 98 per cent of the control group; only 30 per cent attended an academic school program compared to 84 per cent of the control group; and only 24 per cent reported that they had no problems in reading, spelling, speaking, or writing compared to 84 per cent of the control group. Unemployment was much higher than in the control group, and 36 per cent reported difficulties in finding a job compared to 8 per cent in the control group; the level of employment and monthly salaries were considerably below those reported by the control group. In addition, social adjustment, marital problems, and delinquency were also higher in the LD group. Most importantly, the study showed a breakdown of the LD group into those with definite neurological signs, those with "soft signs," and those without neurological findings. In virtually all areas of follow-up, LD subjects with neurological signs showed a poorer outcome than those with soft signs; in turn, subjects with soft signs showed poorer outcome than those without neurological signs, although this latter group was still significantly poorer in outcome than control subjects.

Although learning problems directly related to emotional disorder are not included in the definition of LD, long-term follow-up of the development of LD children shows that emotional problems are frequent in such populations. Developmentally, they may precede the learning problems, follow them, or occur at the same time. Byring and Michelsson (1984) reported current emotional disorders in 64 per cent of their adult dyslexic population. Adaptive behavior problems in LD subjects were found with high frequency by Leigh (1987).

Rutter's Isle of Wight study demonstrated that reading retardation is strongly associated with psychiatric disorder in both brain disorder and non-organic disorder groups. The association was even more pronounced than the well-established relationship between IQ and psychiatric disorder (Rutter et al. 1970a). In another study, Rutter et al. (1970b) found that conduct disorders are more closely related to specific reading problems than are emotional disorders. One-quarter of the children with specific reading retardation showed antisocial behavior. Conversely, one-third of the children with conduct disorders were reading-retarded compared with 4 per cent of the general school-aged population. Clark (1970) reported similar findings. Rutter et al. (1970b) concluded from an analysis of individual behavior items and the specific forms of reading difficulties that antisocial retarded readers had more in common with "pure" retarded readers and less with "pure" antisocial children. It is possible, therefore, that the conduct disorder arises as a consequence of the reading difficulties, i.e., that the reduction in self-esteem from school failure engenders behavior problems. Social factors and family support are also highly influential.

Chapman (1980) focused specifically on differences between 81 LD children and 81 matched controls and found a poorer general and academic self-concept, more external academic locus of control, lower self-expectations, and lowered mothers' and teachers' expectations in LD children. Similar results were found

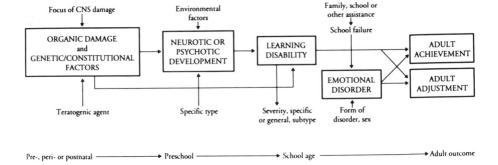

Figure 29-1. A model of interaction of causes of learning disabilities and emotional disorders (Spreen 1989a).

in a review of other studies (Spreen 1989b). Spreen discussed two major theories: (1) that emotional problems occur as a secondary reaction to the stress and frustration of the demands of years of schooling and (2) that the LD is the result of a primary disorder, i.e., an unconscious emotional block resulting from the child's failure to identify with parents, peers, or teachers. A third theory, namely that both LD and emotional problems are related to a genetic/constitutional factor or of brain dysfunction, also expressed by Livingston (1985), was proposed, and a model of interaction with environmental factors, reaction to school failure, and the ameliorating effects of family, school, or other assistance was generated (Figure 29-1). In support of this model, the social and emotional adjustment scale results, the percentage of divorced and separated parents, the behavior problems reported, the percentage of subjects with psychiatric or psychological treatment, and MMPI personality profiles all indicated that the most severe emotional problems occurred in the LD group with neurological signs, followed by those with soft signs, and then those without neurological signs, although such problems were still significantly higher than in the control group. It was also observed that after school-leaving age, some of the emotional problems (and delinquency, Waldie and Spreen 1993) subsided to some degree, whereas others continued with the same severity; this may be the result of being released from the stress of continuous school failure. The lateralization of brain dysfunction as indicated in the neurological findings did not produce significant differences in Spreen's study.

Summary

Specific learning disabilities are found in a considerable proportion of children with average intelligence, who, in spite of adequate instruction and sociocultural background, fail to acquire academic skills appropriate for their age and grade in school. The traditional subdivision into dyslexic and dyscalculic children was made in this chapter, although considerable overlap exists between the two disorders. Of greater importance is the search for reliable and valid subtypes of learning disabilities that might provide clues to the underlying specific deficits in information processing, to the neuropsychological mechanism, and ultimately to different forms of remediation appropriate for each subtype. Although this search has been promising and several models of subtyping, using both clinical and statistical approaches, have been offered, no attempts have been made to include reading, spelling, and writing, as well as arithmetic disorders at the same time. Conceivably, a more comprehensive search of this kind might point up new information useful for neurodevelopmental models. So far, most models remain in the realm of neuropsychological theory; concrete information about the actual brain dysfunction of such children is extremely rare. The relationship between specific learning disabilities and pre- and perinatal abnormalities for the most part is inconclusive.

Children with obvious neurological handicap, especially those with serious cognitive deficit, are likely to have difficulties in school achievement. These difficulties are usually best described as general learning and school problems or academic retardation, rather than as specific learning disabilities. A distinction between school problems directly related to CNS damage and those occurring secondary to health problems should be made. A few selected studies of the school performance of neurologically handicapped populations were described, suggesting that even within such populations great variability in academic performance can and does exist.

30

Psychiatric Disorders

This chapter deals both with major psychiatric disorders of childhood and adolescence that have been associated with developmental neurological deficit and the relationship between specific neurodevelopmental events and emotional and behavioral disorders. Psychiatric disorders found in children with some specific neurological syndromes were mentioned in previous chapters (e.g., low birth weight, brain injury, metabolic disorders, minor physical anomalies, vision, hearing and language disorders) and are not reviewed here.

Childhood psychopathology may be Axis II diagnoses in DSM-III-R (American Psychiatric Association 1987). These diagnoses include, in addition to topics already discussed (e.g., mental retardation, ADHD), pervasive developmental disorders (such as autistic disorders), conduct disorder, oppositional defiant disorder, and a number of disorders outside the field of this book (anxiety disorders of childhood and adolescence, gender identity disorders, and elective mutism). Other axis I and II childhood psychiatric disorders, such as depression or compulsive disorders, and specific neurodevelopmental events so far have attracted less attention from neuropsychologists and will be mentioned only briefly. The overall prevalence estimates of moderate to severe psychiatric disorders of any type range from 14 to 20 per cent (Brandenburg et al. 1990, Costello 1991).

Psychopathology in children tends to be less differentiated than in adults. In children it is unusual to find a single specific disorder, such as severe obsessions or depression, in isolation; more often they occur as part of a cluster of symptoms. Factor-analytic studies point toward two basic factors in most childhood psychiatric disturbances: emotional disturbance in which anxiety, depression, and somatic complaints predominate and conduct disorder with attendant disobedience, disruptiveness, destructiveness, aggressiveness, and delinquency (Kolvin et al. 1971a and b, Wolff 1971). However, the expression of each disorder changes considerably with the age of the child (Rutter 1986).

Children with neurological deficit have an increased prevalence of psychiatric disorder of most types. Conversely, children suffering from major psychotic dis-

496

orders have a considerably higher rate of familial incidence, neurological impairment, and early childhood trauma than those with minor behavioral or emotional problems. The presence of neurological soft signs has been reported for nearly all childhood psychiatric disorders. Mentally handicapped children have a strikingly high incidence of psychiatric disorders (64 per cent in severely, 57 per cent in mildly handicapped persons, Gillberg et al. 1986). This chapter attempts to review the evidence establishing a link between these disorders and neurological and neuropsychological deficit.

30.1   Organic Brain Disorder and Psychiatric Sequelae

The incidence of emotional disorder in children with brain damage is generally elevated and correlates with the degree of neuropsychological deficit, as in adults (Bornstein et al. 1989), although in learning-disabled children it tends to subside somewhat at school-leaving age (Figure 30-1). Rutter (1990, Rutter et al. 1970a) examined the psychiatric aspects of brain disorder in 3300 children. All children between the ages of 9 to 11 from the Isle of Wight were screened by group testing and parent and teacher interviews. Mentally retarded children educated outside the school system and children who attended private schools (5.8 per cent of the total child population) were not included. Children were divided into groups selected for more intensive study, and organically impaired children of other age groups were added as follows:

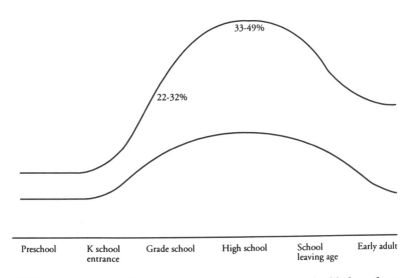

Figure 30-1. Prevalence of emotional disorders in learning-disabled students and normal learners over time. (Spreen 1989b).

- a control group of 125 neurologically normal 9- to 10-year-olds
- a neurological disorder group, subdivided into children with uncomplicated seizures, children with a definite structural lesion above the brainstem but without seizures, children with a lesion at or below the brainstem, and children with a lesion above the brainstem with seizures
- a group of blind or deaf children
- a non-neurological chronic physical disorders group (asthma, diabetes, heart disease)
- a psychiatric disorder group

The children in the target groups were given neurological and psychiatric examinations and psychological testing. Interviews with the parents and the children's teachers were conducted, and questionnaires regarding emotional, behavioral, and social adjustment were answered by parents and teachers.

The incidence of psychiatric disorder rose sharply when organic disorder was present. The general prevalence of psychiatric disorder among the school population of 10- to 11-year-olds was 6.6 per cent. The prevalence of psychopathology among children with non-neurological physical disorders was 11.5 per cent. Among children with uncomplicated epilepsy, the rate of psychopathology rose to 28.6 per cent. Children with lesions above the brainstem but without seizures had a 37.5 per cent incidence of psychiatric disorder. Among children with a confirmed lesion above the brainstem and with seizures, psychiatric disorder was found in 58.3 per cent (Graham 1971, Table 30-1).

Although children with physical handicaps alone may not seem to be more predisposed to diagnosable psychiatric disorder, it is a common clinical observation that they have low self-esteem and negative feelings, not only about the disability but about the attitudes of others toward them. Physical dependency on others, as well as considerable restriction of normal activities, requires emo-

Table 30-1 Psychiatric Disorder in Children Attending School

Diagnosis	General population (excluding neuro-epileptic children)	Neuro-epileptic children	
		With uncomplicated epilepsy	With lesions above brainstem with or without fits
Neurotic disorder	42	8	4
Antisocial or conduct disorder	41	6	3
Mixed disorder	26	3	4
Hyperkinetic syndrome	1	1	3
Psychosis	0	0	1
Other	1	0	1
Total cases	111	18	16
Total population in each group	2189	63	36

Source: Rutter et al. 1970a.

tional adjustment. Even if the family is thoughtful and careful in dealing with the child, it is not uncommon for others to treat handicapped children insensitively (Cruickshank et al. 1976b).

The finding that over half of the children with lesions above the brainstem and seizures had psychiatric disorder indicates a particular vulnerability for psychopathology. The specific effect of a brain lesion was indicated by Rutter et al.'s (1970a) finding that children with non-neurological physical disorders had an incidence of psychopathology close to average. The authors concluded that the high rate of psychiatric disorder in children with epilepsy cannot be attributed to the associated social difficulties often reported in epileptics because non-epileptic children with lesions above the brainstem showed an even higher incidence of psychopathology.

Teachers' ratings of children with brain disorders revealed more restlessness, fidgetiness, poorer concentration, greater irritability, and more fighting than in the general population (Rutter et al. 1970a). Examination of the data suggested that these behaviors were more a function of psychiatric disorder than of brain dysfunction because they were characteristic of many children with emotional and conduct disorders generally. However, children with brain pathology tended to be rated by their teachers as poorer in concentration than normal children, irrespective of the presence of psychiatric disorder. Reduced motor activity was noticed in 21 per cent of the children with brain disorder and psychopathology, but only in 3 per cent of the children with psychopathology but without brain disorder.

Psychiatric disorders in children with neurological impairment cannot be viewed in isolation. Other factors, including genetic/constitutional predisposition, environmental factors, and the effect of family and school experiences, contribute to the picture presented by the child. In contrast to the overrepresentation of boys with psychiatric disorder in the general population, the incidence of psychiatric disorder in children with neurological disorder was equal for boys and girls in the Isle of Wight study.

30.2   Pervasive Developmental Disorders

Among the pervasive developmental disorders, a distinction is made between autistic disorder and childhood schizophrenia. The prevalence of all pervasive developmental disorders has been established as 10 to 15 children in every 10,000 (DSM III-R). The male-female ratio has been reported as between 3:1 and 4:1.

Autistic Disorder

Autistic disorder, first recognized and described by Kanner (1943) as "early infantile autism," almost always begins before the age of 30 months. Following Rutter (1978), DSM-III-R identifies three universal characteristics: failure to develop social relationships ("qualitative impairment in reciprocal social interactions"; qualitative impairment in verbal and nonverbal communication and in imaginative activity, and compulsive or ritualistic behavior ("markedly restricted repertoire of activities and interests"). Asperger (1944) described a somewhat similar disorder that is still treated as a separate syndrome by some authors. Children with **Asperger syndrome,** in contrast to those with autism, have early language development and are more intelligent, but show all other signs of autism and tend to be unusually clumsy. They are also reported to be physically and neurologically normal (Nissen 1986, Rutter 1986) and show little, if any, difference from autistic children on test batteries (Szatmari et al. 1990a). Gillberg and Gillberg (1989a) estimated the prevalence of autism as 2 to 4.5 per 10,000 and that of Asperger syndrome tentatively as 10 to 26 per 10,000. In France, the prevalence of autism was reported as 5.1 per 10,000 (Cialdella and Mamelle 1989). Strikingly, March birthdays were much more common than expected on the basis of the general population birth rate in Sweden (Gillberg 1990); the author interpreted this finding as an indication of seasonal variation in gestation, attributable primarily to the males in the study.

Of all autistic children, 75 per cent have an IQ of 50 or less, although the degree of mental handicap is not necessarily related to the severity of autism, and standard intelligence test results may be misleading because of their reliance on cooperation and verbal comprehension. Special partial giftedness (e.g., rote memory, calculation ability) in autistic children has also been reported (Kanner 1943, Nissen 1986, Stevens and Moffit 1988). One-third of retarded autistic children develop epileptic seizures. Reviewing the evidence from numerous studies, Leslie and Frith (1990) concluded that autism is best described as a basic cognitive disorder rather than an affective one.

ETIOLOGY

Psychogenic, genetic, and organic factors have figured prominently in etiologic characterizations of autistic disorders.

Psychogenic Etiology.   The notion, first proposed by Kanner (1949), that autism is an acquired psychogenic disorder because of early experience with cold, anxious, solitary, intelligent, and obsessive parents has been generally abandoned. Several studies did not find evidence of more than a slightly negative attitude of parents toward their autistic children compared with parents of normal children (DeMyer et al. 1972, McAdoo and DeMyer 1978, Rutter et al. 1970a). The negativity that was present was attributed to a reaction of the parents to a difficult, withdrawn, unresponsive, and rejecting child, rather than as an unprovoked negativity that could generate autism. Cox et al. (1975) found that autism was not related to parental personality attributes, such as warmth, emotional demonstrativeness or responsiveness, or sociability, or to psychiatric disorder of the parents. To test the possibility that severe psychosocial stress precipitates infantile autism, Cox et al. (1975) compared 19 autistic boys with a group of boys with developmental receptive aphasia. All children had a normal nonverbal

IQ and no overt neurological disorder. No significant differences were found between the two groups in the amount of stress suffered during the first 2 years of life, including such events as death of relatives, divorce of parents, financial status, health, and family relationships.

Children reared in conditions of extreme physical and emotional deprivation often show some of the features of autism in infancy. General development is retarded; the infant is passive, does not respond to human contact, does not maintain eye contact, smiles little, and shows repetitive behaviors, such as rocking or head banging (Spitz and Wolf 1946). However, unlike infantile autism, this condition seems to be completely reversible (McBride 1975).

Today, many authors may agree with Cutting (1990) that autism is not an acquired, but an organic disorder, "no different, except in degree, from aphasia, agnosia, and other disturbances in higher mental function" (p. 1).

Genetic Factors.   The incidence of autism in siblings of autistic children is 50 times higher than in the general population. However, incidence rates alone do not provide conclusive evidence of heritability because patterns of child rearing cannot be ruled out. Folstein and Rutter (1977) studied 21 twin pairs, with one member in each who was autistic. Eleven pairs were monozygotic (MZ), and ten pairs were dizygotic (DZ). Half of the autistic children were severely retarded, one-quarter were mildly or moderately retarded, and one-quarter had normal intelligence. The male:female ratio was 3.4:1. When the twins of the originally selected autistic children were examined, the full syndrome of infantile autism was found in 4 of the 11 MZ pairs. Of the twins who were MZ but discordant, the non-autistic twin was in most cases cognitively impaired. None of the DZ twins showed concordance. In 6 of 17 autistic twins of the discordant pairs, evidence of brain injury at birth was found.

A study of the twins' families revealed a history of affective disorders in four families, although schizophrenia was not found in any of the families. One non-twin sibling was also autistic (Folstein and Rutter 1977). A history of speech delay in childhood was found for at least one parent in three of the families. The results suggest that a hereditary factor is not sufficient to produce autism; organic factors may play a contributory role. Konstantareas (1986) concluded that "what may be inherited is an increased vulnerability to teratogenic influences" (p. 684). He interpreted the results as indicative of a strong inherited predisposition for autism in association with cerebral injury at birth.

Similar findings were published by Ritvo et al. (1985), who hypothesized autosomal recessive inheritance in 46 families with multiple cases of autism. They had earlier proposed a lowered serotonin level as one possible cause of autism (Ritvo et al. 1983). In an epidemiological survey of Utah, Ritvo et al. (1989) found autism to be 215 times more frequent among siblings of autistic patients than in the general population. Sahley and Panksepp (1987), in contrast, suggested that "autism, at least partially, represents a disruptive overactivation or hypersensitization of neurohormone systems in the brain, such as brain opioids" (p. 201).

Controversy has existed throughout the history of the syndrome as to whether infantile autism is an early version of schizophrenia or whether it is a separate disorder. Unlike the parents of children with schizophrenia, parents of autistic children do not show a particularly high incidence of psychosis or other psychopathology. Kanner (1954) found no cases of schizophrenia among 200 parents of autistic children. Creak and Ini (1960) found schizophrenia in 2 out of 120 parents of autistic children. Lotter (1967) recorded only one psychotic parent among 60 autistic children. Kolvin et al. (1971b) detected one case of schizoaffective disorder among 92 parents of autistic children, but also found 6 parents with schizophrenia among 64 parents of children with late-onset schizophrenia. This lack of association with schizophrenia in the families suggests that the two syndromes are distinct, i.e., that autism is not an early form of schizophrenia.

Cantwell et al. (1978) concluded that the frequency of schizophrenia is not increased among parents of autistic children, but that a marked increase in schizophrenia is found in parents of children whose psychosis begins in late childhood or adolescence. However, Wolff et al. (1988) suggested that schizoid traits in parents may be a marker for one of the genetic determinants of childhood autism.

Organic Factors.   Ornitz (1973) found more frequent perinatal complications in autistic children than in controls. He argued against a genetic etiology. In his opinion, Rutter's et al. (1970) concordance rate is too low to be considered significant. He observed that autistic individuals do not usually have children; hence, a more likely explanation of autism would be early genetic damage caused by metabolic, traumatic, or infectious influences. Because both prenatal and postnatal influences might be etiologically related, organic rather than inherited factors are a more likely cause. Ornitz (1978) attempted to validate his hypothesis by examining 74 autistic children. He found that 23 per cent of the children had indications of major organic disorders, such as cerebral palsy, congenital rubella, and an abnormal EEG. An additional 17.6 per cent also showed minor neurological signs. A higher frequency of minor physical anomalies has also been found in autistic children (Konstantareas et al. 1989). Finally, a functional imbalance among monoamines in autistic children has been demonstrated in several studies (Martineau et al. 1991).

So far, no specific brain dysfunction or pathology has been associated with autism except for a general increase in neurological abnormalities. An MRI study by Garber et al. (1989) revealed no brain abnormalities. Piven et al. (1991) found micropolygyria and other general brain abnormalities in the MRIs of 13 high-functioning autistic males. Jacobson et al. (1988) found enlarged size of the third ventricle but not of the lateral ventricles on CT scans; the authors regarded this finding as an indication of selective subcortical abnormalities in autism. Their finding, however, was not replicated in a study by Kleiman et al. (1992) with a different group of 11 autistic children. Murakami et al. (1989) found a 12 per cent reduction in the size of the cerebellar hemispheres on MRI.

Aitken (1991) concluded from a review of MRI and PET studies that the later-developing aspects of the cerebellum and the limbic system are most commonly affected in autism. Ballotin et al. (1989) found that autistic children show only nonspecific rather than localized abnormalities on CT.

In contrast, one study (Hauser et al. 1975) found an association between autism and enlargement of the left temporal horn in pneumoencephalograms. Fourteen of the 17 children in this study showed enlargement. The implication of a specific left-sided brain abnormality in this study would be consistent with the language problem of autistic children. Indirect corroboration was provided by Hoffmann and Prior (1982) and by Dawson (1983), who found that a group of autistic children performed significantly more poorly than children matched for chronological age and for mental age on tests presumably tapping left hemisphere functions, although they performed at their chronological age level on right hemisphere tests. Sussman and Lenwandowski (1990), however, found bilateral neuropsychological involvement and warned that conclusions drawn from tests that presumably measure right or left hemisphere functioning are highly inferential. In contrast, Cutting (1990) argued that "many of the features of infantile autism are consistent with an underdevelopment of characteristically right-hemisphere functions relative to left-hemisphere function" (p. 410). This argument is based on the notion that the semantic, pragmatic, prosodic, and grammatic but not the phonetic components of language are disturbed in autism. Although Cutting recognized the phonetic component as a "rigid, categorical function" of the left hemisphere system, he viewed all others as associated with the right hemisphere with its "reality-based system, sensitive to variation and individuality" (p. 395). He applied a similar argument to the emotional and relationship disorder of the autistic child: "The schizophrenic retreats into a library, renouncing the uncertainties of a moving, living world; the autistic child grows up in a library, never knowing the pleasures of this world" (p. 395). Cutting's theory implicating the right frontotemporal lobe region in autism has attracted little support so far (Roberts 1992).

Still another notion is that autism is based on a defective activating system in the reticular formation (Engeland 1984, Rimland 1964). According to this theory, the brainstem and diencephalon are responsible for sensory modulation, and defects in this system would result in sensory constancy defects, sameness, hyporeactivity, and motor obsession. Limited support for this theory comes from vestibular stimulation studies (Ornitz et al. 1985) and from studies by Thievierge et al. (1989) and Wong and Wong (1991) that found prolonged interpeak latencies in brainstem evoked response potentials in autistic, but not in mentally retarded children. ERPs under focused selective attention conditions showed frontal negative difference waves that were diminished in size (Ciesielski et al. 1990, Oades et al. 1990). Fein et al. (1984) also found that the cognitive impairment in autistic children is more severe when handedness is ambiguous or mixed, rather than established on one side, suggesting bilateral brain dysfunction.

Chess (1971) examined a group of 243 children with congenital rubella to observe the incidence of infantile autism. Ten of the children showed the complete syndrome of infantile autism, and eight had partial autism, which was distinguished from the full syndrome if the child showed any recognition of another person. In a prospective study Chess (1977a and b) re-examined the children at age 8 to 9 years. At this time, all 18 were still severely disordered, although Chess considered 4 to have improved. These four children had not developed oral speech, but could use sign language.

The prevalence of infantile autism inferred from Chess' study for children with congenital rubella is 412 per 10,000 for the complete syndrome alone; the prevalence would be nearly twice as high if children with the partial syndrome were included. When compared with the prevalence in the general population, an association of the syndrome with congenital rubella seems evident. Chess did not address the incidence of other forms of psychopathology in the sample; one would expect a raised incidence of other types of psychopathology as well. Children with congenital rubella are likely to have the same predisposition for various forms of serious psychopathology as other children with organic disorders; it is unlikely that there is a specific relationship between autism and rubella, although Prior (1987) used the link between autism and rubella as evidence for a viral infection theory of autism.

Considering the evidence for a variety of etiologies and the fact that some types show significant anomalies of brain structures whereas others do not, Hooper et al. (1993) concluded that autism should no longer be viewed as a homogeneous entity, but as a heterogeneous group of disorders with specific subtypes. Gillberg (1992) made the same point, but recommended subclassification according to associated medical conditions. Neuropsychological studies may reveal how such subtypes are related to specific etiologies.

THE DEVELOPMENT OF THE CHILD WITH AUTISM

In infancy, feeding difficulties are common for autistic children. The older child is often preoccupied with one particular food. The infant or child shows a marked lack of awareness of the existence of feelings of others; does not seek comfort at times of distress or does so in an abnormal manner; does not or only rarely imitate actions of others (e.g., waving bye-bye); shows no social play or does so abnormally (e.g., does not actively participate in simple games); and is grossly impaired in making peer friendships in later childhood. Communication by babbling, facial expression, gesture, mime, or spoken language is either absent or markedly abnormal (e.g., does not anticipate being held, does not look or smile at the person approaching, has a fixed stare in social situations). Imaginative activity, such as playacting and interest in stories about imaginary events, is absent. The production, volume, rate, rhythm, and intonation of speech are markedly abnormal; and the child cannot initiate or sustain a conversation. Overactivity is common, changing to underactivity in adolescence. The attention span is short. The child shows stereotyped body movement including head banging and rocking, is preoccupied with parts of objects, insists on following daily routines in precise detail, has a markedly restricted range of interest; and is absorbed in one narrow interest, e.g., lining up objects, drawing the same object over and over again. The child reacts with temper tantrums or acute anxiety if an attempt is made to change a routine, toy, food, or location.

Affection toward the parents sometimes develops after a few years, but the child usually does not make friends with peers and shows a characteristic insensitivity and indifference when dealing with others. An interesting study examined home movies taken by the parents of 11 boys before the age of 5 and before autism was diagnosed (Adrian et al. 1992). The study confirmed early anomalies of eye contact, deficiency and variability of emotional expression, defective attention and initiation of communication, and motor abnormalities.

A characteristic pattern of language disorder distinguishes autism from developmental aphasia. Autistic children who do not develop language do not gesture to communicate and do not seem to understand gesture, in contrast to children with developmental aphasia who frequently use and understand gesture as a means of social communication. If speech is present, aphasic children tend to have more articulation problems. Echolalia, the repetition and mimicking of sounds or words, is common in autistic children, but not in children with developmental aphasia. Other differences between children with autism and with receptive language disorder have been described for abnormal brainstem evoked auditory responses (Courchesne et al. 1989) and for auditory processing deficits (short-term memory for tone sequences, Lincoln et al. 1992); both are absent in autism. A follow-up into middle childhood showed that autistic children made less progress than children with developmental receptive language disorder (Cantwell et al. 1989). Another characteristic of autistic speech is the persistent reversal of the pronouns "I" and "you." It is also monotonous and lacks expression. Impaired comprehension and poor formation of verbal concepts are common. Although autistic children may remember reasonably well, they make little use of meaning in memory and thought processes and use inflexible cognitive strategies for encoding and processing new information (Minshew and Goldstein 1993). Mechanical reading, spelling, and computation are often found unimpaired compared to controls (Minshew et al. 1994). Bartak et al. (1975) considered the severity of the language disorder as critical and "probably necessary for the development of autism" (p. 142). In addition, impaired performance on neuropsychological tests of executive functions (Prior and Hoffman 1990) and fragmentation of drawings (Fein et al. 1990) have been reported.

Long-term outcome studies show that few autistic children grow up to live independently or become capable of employment. Follow-up studies during adolescence and adulthood show continuing problems in a large number of cases, although the type of psychopathology may change (Schopler and Mesibov 1982). Wolf and Goldberg (1986) reported that in an 8- to 24-year follow-up more than 50 per cent of their 80 former clients required institutional care, that symptoms persisted, and that few developed useful speech. DeMeyer et al. (1981) reviewed the results of six autism outcome studies and reported that these studies indicated fairly consistently that 5 to 19 per cent of autistic patients have good to very good outcome, whereas the majority (55 to 74 per cent) have poor to very poor outcome. Several studies (Gillberg and Steffenburg 1987, Lotter 1978) have shown that IQ at diagnosis, communicative speech before age 6, and degree of autistic symptomatology are consistently related to good outcome, whereas the development of epilepsy contributes to further deterioration and poor outcome. Persons with fragile chromosomal sites, including fragile-X syndrome and partial trisomy of chromosome 15 (Gillberg et al. 1986, 1991, Hagerman 1990) are more severely affected. Fisher et al. (1988) examined six possible etiological variables (including prematurity and PKU) and 11 associated diagnoses in 59 autistic children from North Dakota and related them in a regression analysis to IQ, receptive language, and expressive language. The presence of hyperlexia and the child's age at diagnosis were positive predictors of improvement. Surprisingly, known etiology of any form and co-diagnosis of Tourette syndrome without seizures also contributed to a positive outcome. Whitehouse and Harris (1984) proposed that the presence of hyperlexia is an indicator of a specific subgroup of autistic children.

Schizophrenia and Related Disorders

Brief psychotic episodes may occur in childhood or adolescence in situations of extreme stress. However, the diagnosis of **schizophrenia** is reserved for a long-standing psychotic disorder with profound disturbances of thought, emotion, and behavior beginning after the age of 30 months (DSM III-R 1987) that is relatively rare in incidence during childhood. The older the child at the time of diagnosis, the more closely the pattern of schizophrenia resembles the adult syndrome. The prevalence rates for childhood and adult schizophrenia combined, given in DSM III-R, are 0.2 to 1 per cent. Yolles and Kramer (1969) reported a 3 per cent prevalence of schizophrenia using a broader definition of the disorder (schizophrenic spectrum). Milder forms of the disorder, or cases lasting only a limited period, are described as schizophreniform, schizotypal personality disorder, or schizoaffective disorders. In some studies, all are included as part of the schizophrenic spectrum.

Schizophrenia is distinguished from other psychoses principally by the type of thought disorder: speech ranges from a reflection of looseness of associations in mild cases to total disorganization, referred to as "**word salad**." Impoverished thought content with poor concept formation is evident. Delusions are common and reflect the disintegration of ego boundaries and lack of reality orientation, e.g., ideas of reference, thought intrusion, and ideas of persecution. Behavior may be bizarre with stereotyped, repetitive movements. Social inappropriateness and regression to earlier developmental stages are found. Withdrawal and other autistic tendencies are common. Affect is usually blunted, with an absence of normal emotional responses to people and events; however, there may be episodes of euphoria or anger, the latter especially if the child is frustrated or provoked. Hallucinations, especially auditory, are not uncommon. DSM III-R distinguishes between schizophrenia of the catatonic, disorganized, paranoid, residual, and undifferentiated type based on the prevailing symptoms. Crow

(1980) used a distinction between positive and negative schizophrenic symptomatology: positive schizophrenia involves symptoms, such as delusions and hallucinations, whereas negative schizophrenia shows only deficit and tends to be chronic.

Etiology

Despite numerous studies in recent decades, no clear picture of the etiology of schizophrenia has emerged, and speculative theories abound. Most likely, genetic susceptibility, brain damage, and psychosocial factors are all involved.

Genetic Factors. Among the total population of patients in New York mental hospitals with schizophrenia, Kallman (1953) found 953 patients with a twin sibling, including 268 monozygotic twins. Compared to the prevalence of schizophrenia in the general population of below 1 per cent, he found concordance rates of 14.2 per cent for ordinary siblings, 14.5 per cent for dizygotic twins, 86.2 per cent for MZ twins, and 91.5 per cent for MZ twins reared together. When both parents were schizophrenic, 68.1 per cent of the children were schizophrenic. Slater (1953) reported a 76 per cent concordance rate among 41 MZ twins. Heston (1970) pointed out that concordance rates can approach 100 per cent if the full range of the schizophrenic spectrum is included. Similar results were reported by Kety et al. (1978). In a review of three long-term studies, Mirsky and Duncan-Johnson (1984) proposed, however, that the genetic risk for schizophrenia is modified by noxious familial influences, which increase the likelihood and severity of phenotypical expression. Based on a review of these and other studies, McKusick (1992) listed the transmission of schizophrenia as irregular autosomal dominant.

The hereditary susceptibility factor for schizophrenia is thus established, although the mechanisms of genetic transmission have not been fully delineated (Kety et al. 1983).

Neurological Factors. The assumption that genetic susceptibility is a major cause of schizophrenia does not preclude the possibility that pathological cerebral processes and psychosocial factors may also contribute or interact. In fact, cerebral abnormalities may be the result of genetic transmission. Announcing "the biological Renaissance of psychiatry," Bender (1942) proposed that schizophrenia resulted from disordered neurological development: islands of primitive, poorly developed CNS organization occur together with areas of relatively normal development. According to this theory, areas subserving perception, body image, and certain aspects of cognition are affected, leading to acute anxiety in the child and poor adaptive skills, which in turn result in schizophrenia. The general neurological examination would be expected to show only soft neurological signs, such as hypotonia, choreiform movements, whirling movements, or persistence of the tonic neck reflex (Bender 1956).

Several studies have searched for neurological correlates in groups of schizophrenic children. Rutter (1965) found that one-quarter of 63 psychotic children had a major neurological disorder, most often epilepsy; another quarter had "probable neurological disease." He thought that dysfunction in the language areas of the brain led to a degree of receptive aphasia; this, together with additional perceptual deficits, resulted in insensitivity to environmental stimuli and in turn to schizophrenic signs and symptoms. He admitted that this could be only a partial explanation because children with developmental aphasia do not necessarily become schizophrenic or autistic.

Other investigators have reported similar rates of neurological abnormality in children with schizophrenia. Marcus et al. (1985, Marcus 1985, Silberman and Tassone 1985) found a strong correlation between neurological functioning and IQ in an Israeli study of schizophrenic children; 22 of the 50 index children showed neurological dysfunction as compared to only 3 of the 50 control subjects. Soft neurological signs—perceptual sensory signs, poor motor coordination, poor right-left orientation, poor balance, and motor overflow—were most common; slower galvanic skin response (GSR) to emotionally meaningful stimuli and slower GSR recovery rates were also reported (Kugelmass et al. 1985), but these findings were not replicated in a well-designed study by Erlenmeyer-Kimling et al. (1985). In the Israeli study, psychological tests revealed attentional dysfunction and basic distortion of cognitive integration (Sohlberg 1985). Because younger subjects had more pathological signs, the authors raised the question of a developmental delay in children at risk for schizophrenia. Kolakowska et al. (1985) found developmental abnormalities in 46 per cent of 42 young schizophrenics; Schroeder et al. (1991) reported similar results. A Russian study (Moskalenko 1984) of 122 pairs of twins and a Swedish study of 88 high-risk offspring (McNeil 1983) both suggested that asphyxia and other complications at birth and serious physical diseases were related to the severity of schizophrenia. Torrey and Peterson (1976) and Conrad and Scheibel (1987, Crow 1987) hypothesized a maternal infection with neuroamidase-bearing viruses during the second trimester that affects the migration of primitive neurons into the primordial hippocampus. Hyde-Thomas et al. (1992) discovered a high comorbidity with leukodystrophy with schizoid symptomatology as an early indicator of schizophrenia in the absence of neurological findings. A relationship with seizure activity in middle childhood has also been reported (Caplan et al. 1991).

Several researchers have inferred "minimal brain damage" from neuropsychological examinations of schizophrenic children and adults (Pugh and Bigler 1986, Tramontana and Sherrets 1985). For example, Craft et al. (1987) gave various tests of interhemispheric transfer (cross-localization of touch, transfer of formboard learning from one hand to the other while blindfolded, etc.) to schizophrenics and controls and concluded that a developmental dysfunction of the corpus callosum is present in patients with schizophrenia and schizoaffective disorders. However, the inference of brain damage or brain abnormalities from such studies remains questionable because of the disturbed cognitive performance of schizophrenics that by itself affects many of the test results; calculations of an "impairment index" suggesting brain damage from such tests are likely to be inconclusive or even misleading. Bornstein et al. (1990b) concluded from their study that differences in test performance between schizophrenics and age-matched controls were mostly accounted for by symptom severity and level of medication.

Neuroradiological studies have proliferated in recent years. Most frequently, ventricular enlargement (ventriculomegaly) has been found in MRI studies (Pfefferbaum et al. 1990). Raz et al. (1988) found no CT abnormalities in 14 young schizophrenics or controls, but computer-assisted volumetric analysis revealed significant enlargement of the third and the lateral ventricles in the schizophrenics. A meta-analysis of 37 studies (Raz et al 1988) confirmed ventriculomegaly in schizophrenia, regardless of whether normal or medical, neurological, and nonpsychotic psychiatric controls were used.

Silverton et al. (1988) reported a follow-up study of 311 Danish children, including 207 high-risk children of schizophrenic mothers, originally seen in 1962 and again examined in 1971 to 1981. The study included CT scans of 15 subjects diagnosed as schizophrenic, 18 diagnosed as borderline, and 25 without mental illness. The three groups did not differ with respect to socioeconomic status. The authors found an association between low birth weight and ventricular enlargement; ventricular enlargement, but not birthweight, was directly associated with schizophrenia. They also attempted to test the viral hypothesis, but found that children born in January, February, and March (from mothers at seasonal high risk for virus exposure) were not more at risk than children born in other months of the year. Severity of the mother's schizophrenia was also not related to the children's risk for schizophrenia; the authors interpreted this finding as an indication that environmental stress (caused by the mother's illness) was not a strong contributing factor.

Luchins et al. (1983) noted that the percentage of persons with neuroanatomical asymmetry in the frontal and occipital areas (measured with CT scan) was significantly higher in schizophrenics than in the general population. Lower tissue density in the hippocampus has also been reported (Suddath et al. 1990). Some PET scan studies have revealed hypofrontality, a decreased level of metabolic activity in the dorsolateral prefrontal brain region (see review by Buchsbaum 1990). However, this finding was reported in only three studies, whereas six reported hyperfrontality and five found no difference between brain regions at all.

Whether such contradictory findings reflect the effect of schizophrenia characterized by positive or negative symptomatology, respectively, remains to be explored. Most studies do, however, implicate similar brain regions: the basal ganglia, the dorsolateral prefrontal cortex, and periventricular structures including the hippocampus, the medial temporal lobes, and the medial thalamus. In a review, Seidman (1983) noted that 20 to 35 per cent of schizophrenic patients show brain impairment, but that neurodiagnostic findings indicate "a complex, variable picture, including ventricular enlargement and cerebral atrophy, and disturbances of metabolism." He suggested that there are two or more syndromes, differing in severity and type of brain anomaly, and involving to different degrees the cortico-subcortical arousal/attention system involving the frontal cortex, the limbic system, and the brainstem reticular system. Similar views were expressed by Frith and Done (1988), who postulated that negative signs of schizophrenia reflect a defect in the initiation of action, which depends on brain systems linking the prefrontal cortex and the basal ganglia; positive symptoms reflect a defect in the internal monitoring of action, which depends on the links between prefrontal cortex and the hippocampus via the parahippocampal cortex and the cingulate cortex. These and other authors have speculated that positive schizophrenia is produced by excessive activity of the neurotransmitter dopamine, and can be treated with neuroleptic medication, whereas negative schizophrenia does not respond to neuroleptics and is based on structural brain abnormalities. This distinction has been questioned on empirical grounds since both symptoms can coexist and many heterogeneous forms can be found (Pogue-Geile and Zubin 1988).

Other researchers have been concerned with the lateralization of lesions. Cutting (1990) insisted that it is "hemispheric imbalance, the diminution in the activity of the right hemisphere" (p. 409) that is responsible for schizophrenic symptomatology because, as in autism, right hemisphere dysfunction causes anomalous perceptual experiences, morbid experiences of space and time, bodily delusions, anhedonia, and a morbid sense of self, leaving the left hemisphere "starved of its provider of real-life content" (p. 410). Ulrich and Otto (1984) described a "right-posterior accentuation" in EEGs of schizophrenic patients, which they interpreted as a maturation defect that may persist into adulthood and emerge as a special category of schizophrenic behavior. In contrast, Flor-Henry (1976), Gur (1978), and Lerner et al. (1977) found dichotic listening and other test and EEG results pointing to a left hemisphere deficit. Walker et al. (1981) reinterpreted the dichotic listening results in schizophrenic patients as an indicator of faulty interhemispheric transfer.

A recent review of the evidence (Heinrichs 1993) suggests that current subtyping of schizophrenia is insufficient and that better correspondence between brain anomalies and schizophrenia can only be found by "parsing" schizophrenia to reduce heterogeneity, using a "top-down" (cluster analysis of schizophrenic behavior with an enlarged set of descriptors or tests of cognitive abilities [Goldstein 1990] related to findings of brain anomalies) or a "bottom-up" approach (subtyping of brain anomalies found by a variety of neuroradiological methods and searching for corresponding behavioral manifestations).

The origin of neurological and neuropsychological abnormalities in schizophrenics is likely to be found in prenatal development. Parkinson et al. (1981) found that slowing of head growth between 24 and 36 weeks of pregnancy (measured with serial ultrasonic encephalometry) indicated risk for schizoform development, as well as for various other disorders, such as hyperactivity and learning disability. Mednick et al. (1991) provided a balanced and detailed discussion of fetal neural development as related to schizophrenia, focusing on genetic and teratogenic disturbances.

THE DEVELOPMENT OF THE CHILD WITH SCHIZOPHRENIA

Because schizophrenic spectrum disorders seem to be heterogeneous, identifying precursors of outcome, particularly for subgroups of children, may also provide the basis for more selective treatment approaches.

In an early retrospective and prospective follow-up study, O'Neal and Robins (1958) examined 248 children between the ages of 7 and 17 referred to a child guidance clinic because of severe behavioral or emotional problems. At that time, none of the cases was diagnosed as schizophrenic. After a follow-up period of 30 years, 10 per cent were schizophrenic, and only 20 per cent were considered psychiatrically normal (called the no-disease group). The remaining patients had various personality, behavioral, and emotional disorders. Two groups were selected from the original sample for comparison: the no-disease and the schizophrenic group. In addition, a control group was chosen from public school records. When the histories at the time of the original examination in childhood for the schizophrenic and the no-disease group were compared, preschizophrenic children were found to have more infections in infancy, more physical handicaps, more hearing problems, more disfigurement, and, in boys, more feminine appearance. The early childhood histories also showed more severe infections and physical problems for the preschizophrenic group. The preschizophrenic group also manifested more acting-out behavior, pathological lying, difficulties in personal relationships, and overdependence on the mother. Developmentally, delay of walking and difficulties in feeding but not general developmental delay were different between the two groups (14 per cent of the schizophrenic group had been developmentally retarded compared to only 5 per cent of the no-disease group). Both groups had a high incidence of speech disorders and learning difficulties in school. Over 60 per cent of the children in both groups were in homes with only a single parent. Certain characteristics of thinking, such as paranoid ideation, bizarre ideas, ruminations, and obsessions, were found mainly among the preschizophrenic children. O'Neal and Robins (1958) concluded that even though all children showed severely disturbed behavior at the time of the original referral, there were differences in the type of behavioral pathology between children who later would become schizophrenic and those who would show a more normal outcome.

A prospective study by Fish and Hagin (1973, Fish 1977) followed ten infants born in 1959 to mothers institutionalized for schizophrenia in state hospitals. Nine of the ten children showed severely uneven motor development and perceptual disabilities consistent with pandevelopmental retardation. Two children who had only minimally uneven development in infancy showed no psychiatric disorder at 10 years of age. The remaining eight children showed moderate to severe emotional or behavioral impairment at the age of 10 years. Most of the children were placed with adoptive parents or foster homes. One child spent most of her early childhood with her mother; this child became psychotic at the age of 6 and entered an institution. The seven remaining children showed schizoid-type personality disorders or neurotic disorders. Of particular interest was that the neurological signs of the children with psychopathology disappeared during the second year of life; only minor visuomotor deficits remained. None of the children with psychiatric disorder had a history of perinatal complications. Fish (1977) concluded from these studies that severe to mild irregularity and retardation of physical growth, postural-motor, and visual-motor development are often followed by schizophrenia or schizoid-type personality disorder of corresponding severity. However, only for the more severely disordered cases could the outcome have been predicted by signs of pandevelopmental retardation.

Asarnow and Goldstein (1986) studied children at risk for schizophrenia and found that schizotypal symptoms, such as social isolation, inadequate social rapport, and signs of cognitive slippage, were childhood precursors of adult schizophrenia. They also investigated the premorbid adjustment of children diagnosed as schizophrenic or schizotypal personality disorder at a mean age of 10 (Asarnow and Ben-Meir 1988). Ratings based on previous hospitalizations and school records for sociability, peer relationships, scholastic performance, school adaptation, and interests were significantly low premorbidly, whereas these indicators were normal in a group of children who later developed major depression or dysthymic disorder.

Another study of childhood precursors of adult schizophrenia (Nuechterlein 1986) found relationships with attention/information processing anomalies, social functioning deficits, autonomic abnormalities, and neurological soft signs; pregnancy and birth complications were also listed as factors in individual vulnerability. Cornblatt and Erlenmeyer-Kimling (1985, Dworkin et al. 1990) found that global attentional deviance and poorer social competence ratings were childhood markers of risk for schizophrenia, in their comparison of 63 children of schizophrenic parents, 43 children of parents with affective disorder, and 100 children of normal parents. The authors pointed out that the subjects were raised in unrelated families and that two siblings whose parents were both schizophrenic were raised by different foster families. Nevertheless, the argument that such deficits may be the result of environmental factors associated with living with a schizophrenic parent cannot be completely ruled out. In fact, Walker et al. (1981) presented data demonstrating that the presence of a healthy father, especially in the second year of life, ameliorates the disruptive effects of a schizophrenic mother on vulnerable male offspring. In a review of risk factors, Walker and Emory (1983) concluded that research supports an interactional model with several subgroups, including a group of constitutionally vulnerable infants with "heightened central nervous system sensitivity to disequilibriating factors," such as pre- and perinatal complications and multiple environmental stressors in infancy and childhood.

30.3   Mood Disorders

Generally, a **mood** is a pervasive emotion that may color an individual's experience for a sustained time period, such as depression, anxiety, or anger. **Mood**

disorders are derangements of the normal emotional experience, and may reflect depression, mania, or a combined manic-depressive disorder, also called bipolar affective disorders. Depression is far more common than manic or manic-depressive disorders in children. The Ontario Child Health Study surveyed 2052 households in that province in order to obtain an estimate of the prevalence of selected psychiatric disorders in children. Table 30-2 shows the figures for emotional disorder, somatization disorder, conduct disorders, and hyperactivity (Boyle et al. 1987, Links et al. 1989, Offord et al. 1987, 1991). The figures may be somewhat inflated because they are based on a parent questionnaire, not on psychiatric diagnosis. Generally, however, parent and teacher reports tend to underestimate psychiatric disorders: children report more illness than their parents report about them (Weissman et al. 1987). Offord's figures also agree fairly well with estimates obtained from mental health care utilization statistics in the same province and with even higher estimates by Ehrenberg et al (1993); the latter authors found a combined prevalence of 31.4 per cent of mild to clinical depression in adolescents in British Columbia, with sex ratios similar to Offord's. In a longitudinal study, Verhulst and Althaus (1988) stressed that behavioral-emotional problems should not be considered static. Their follow-up study of children between the ages of 4 and 14 indicated that only 54 per cent of children originally classified as disturbed still scored in the disturbed range 2 years later; however, only 5 per cent improved to a degree that placed them in the normal category. Externalizing symptoms, especially poor peer relations, showed the least improvement over time. Co-morbidity of depression with attention deficit and anxiety disorders is high (Bernstein 1991, Biederman et al. 1991, Kovacs et al. 1990).

Beardslee et al. (1985), Uddenberg (1984b) and Cytryn (1984) found a high prevalence of depressive disorders in the mothers of depressive children. Kallman (1953) proposed dominant genetic transmission with incomplete penetrance. Whether or not the disorder occurs may depend either on the presence of modifying genes or on environmental factors. Support for this hypothesis was provided by his twin study, which showed 100 per cent concordance for MZ twins, 25.5 per cent concordance for DZ twins, and 22.7 per cent for other siblings. Winokur and Tanna (1969) suggested dominant transmission linked to

Table 30-2   Prevalence of Psychiatric Disorders in Adolescents

	Age 12–16 years		Age 16–18 years	
	Boys	Girls	Boys	Girls
Conduct disorders	6.5	1.8	10.4	4.1
Hyperactivity	10.1	3.3	7.3	3.4
Emotional disorder	10.2	10.7	4.9	13.6
Somatization disorder	—	—	4.5	10.7
One or more disorders	19.5	13.5	18.8	21.8

Source: Offord et al. 1987.

the sex chromosomes, but the evidence supporting this view is weak (McKusick 1992).

Only infrequent relationships of depression with early cerebral damage or dysfunction have been observed (Rutter 1984), although Nissen (1982) argued that pre-, peri-, or postnatal brain damage may be at least a participating factor in some forms of depression. Albert (1972) reported two cases of early childhood brain damage that led to cyclic psychoses lasting into young adulthood. Shaffer et al. (1985), Cherian and Kuruvilla (1989), Chikovani (1984), Hollander et al. (1991), and Shaffer et al. (1985) all demonstrated a relationship between depressive disorders and neurological soft signs. Shaffer et al. (1985) followed 89 seven-year olds who were found to show anxiety and affective disorder at age 17. Flor-Henry (1976) and Gur (1987) viewed depression as a right hemisphere disorder based on spectral EEG and psychological test analyses. Rourke et al. (1989) also viewed depression and suicide risk as related to a right hemisphere white matter disorder if it is associated with a learning disability. In contrast, Cantwell and Baker (Baker and Cantwell 1987, Cantwell 1982) found an association of language, but not pure speech disorders, with depression, which would argue for a left hemisphere localization. A monoamine hypothesis of depression has found considerable support (Horton and Katona 1991). Although the neurochemical studies of depression are tantalizing and are reinforced by the success of drug challenge and treatment studies, no generally accepted model of the neurochemistry of depression has emerged so far (Yaylayan et al. 1990/91). In general, however, the evidence for a biological basis of depression is nonspecific; it is certainly less well established than that for autism and schizophrenia. In fact, as mentioned above, studies of autism and schizophrenia that included comparison groups of children with affective disorders regularly found much less evidence for brain dysfunction among the latter (Conde-Lopez 1983, Szatmari et al 1990).

Manic-depressive illness rarely occurs before puberty, although reactive depression is not uncommon even in early childhood (Achenbach 1982, Nissen 1982). Child abuse has been singled out as a specific contributing factor (Kashani et al. 1987, Martin and Kempe 1976). Campbell (1952) reported that of 18 adolescents with manic-depressive psychosis only 3 developed the condition before puberty. The remaining 15 developed psychosis between the ages of 12 and 16 years. Uddenberg (1984a) described typical diagnostic features present even in childhood: psychomotor inhibition with motor function appearing sluggish and vagueness with occasional restlessness; fixed, generally immobile depressive facial expression, especially around the eyes, which does not change even when the child smiles; reduced motor tone, especially around the mouth; head hanging and wavering of arms and legs.

The etiology of manic-depressive illness seems to implicate inherited factors, although individual cases with hypothyroidism have been reported that respond to levo-thyroxine treatment (Haggerty et al. 1986). Other neuroendocrinological factors may be involved (Piccinin and Ansseau 1991, Trad 1986). Hyposecretion of growth hormone and hypersecretion of cortisol have been mentioned (Goulet 1989).

30.4   Conduct and Other Disorders

Even less clearly established is the relationship of other psychiatric disorders of childhood with neurological dysfunction. Attention deficit with or without hyperactivity, the most frequently studied disorder, has been discussed in Chapter 23.

Conduct disorders (persisting problems of stealing, runaway, lying, firesetting, truancy, property violations, cruelty to people and animals, fighting, and use of weapons) have often been associated with hyperactivity, but are now treated as a separate category of disorder that often accompanies hyperactivity (Loney and Milich 1982, Milich and Fitzgerald 1985, DSM-III-R). The maturation of neurotransmitter systems as a possible basis for psychosocial disorders has been the focus of much recent research (Rasmussen et al. 1990, Swaab 1989, Tucker 1990). Neuropsychological studies have shown test profiles consistent with neurological impairment, especially in the language area (Brickman et al. 1984, McManus et al. 1985, Yeudall et al. 1987), and academic achievement is usually low. Yeudall et al. also claimed changes in the left frontotemporal lobe on spectral EEG analysis. Neurological soft signs have been reported (Wolff et al. 1982), although McManus et al. (1985) could not relate soft signs to the severity of delinquency and violent behavior. It should be noted that all of these studies were done with convicted juvenile offenders, but did not include peers with similar predisposition who did not come to the attention of the police. The hypothesis that "biological predisposition" can be exacerbated by brain damage or cerebral birth trauma (Christiansen 1977) was also contradicted by Farrington (1983), Mednick (1973), and Schulsinger (1976), who did not find that birth complications were more frequently associated with delinquency. Spreen (1981, 1988a and b) found that the presence of learning disability or neurological abnormalities at age 10 was not related to increased delinquency at age 18 in a prospective study. One would agree with Rutter and Giller (1983) that brain dysfunction can be shown to increase the risk of psychiatric disorder and educational failure, and that because of this general link, the risk for conduct disorders is also increased, but that no specific association has been demonstrated so far.

Summary

Since the days of the German psychiatrist Griesinger, who proposed in 1845 that "all mental disease is brain disease," the search for brain abnormalities related to emotional and psychiatric disorder has continued despite periods of almost exclusively psychodynamic and behavioristic orientation in both psychiatry and psychology. If brain dysfunction and environmental influences are seen as interactive, these different approaches to psychopathology are no longer contradictory.

Early brain injury and brain disorder are often followed by psychopathology and often occur together with disorders of language and reading. Yet, the interaction with a possible genetic predisposition, with psychosocial environmental factors, and particularly with the treatment and school environment is prominent in most studies of childhood psychopathology. Only in a few instances does the type of psychopathology show a more causal relationship with any type of brain dysfunction, whereas in most studies the type of psychopathology found with a brain dysfunction follows the proportions found in the general population. A surprisingly large number of children in many studies, including those with severe brain damage, remain free of psychopathology of any kind. Invoking a lesser degree of "genetic predisposition" in such cases, as has been occasionally done, remains an unsatisfactory explanation and deserves further study.

A special case among the childhood psychiatric disorders is autism, which has found various etiological explanations. Although theories of brain dysfunction in autism are common, the relationship remains obscure. More likely, brain damage may interact with genetic factors in the causation of autism. A similar picture, though less clear, emerges for childhood schizophrenia. The biological basis of depression remains elusive, although several speculative theories have been proposed. Even less clear-cut evidence has been described for the neurological basis of conduct disorders.

References

Aaron, P.G. 1982. The neuropsychology of developmental dyslexia. In R.N. Malatesha & P.G. Aaron (Eds.), *Reading Disorders: Varieties and Treatments*. New York: Academic Press.

Aaron, P.G. & Baker, C. 1982. The neuropsychology of dyslexia in college students. In R.N. Malatesha & L.N. Hartlage (Eds.), *The Neuropsychology of Cognition*. Groningen: Sythoff & Nordhoff.

Aase, J.M. 1990. *Diagnostic Dysmorphology*. New York: Plenum Press.

Abel, E.L. (Ed.) 1981. *Fetal Alcohol Syndrome*. Boca Raton, FL: CRC Press.

Abel, E.L. 1984. Prenatal effects of alcohol. *Drug and Alcohol Dependency*, 14, 1.

Abramowicz, M. & Kass, E.H. 1966. Pathogenesis and prognosis of maturity. *New England Journal of Medicine*, 16, 878; 17, 938; 18, 1001; 19, 1053.

Achenbach, T.M. 1978. *Research in Developmental Psychology: Concepts, Strategies, Methods*. New York: The Free Press.

Achenbach, T.M. 1982. Childhood depression: A review of research. In B.B. Lahey & A.E. Kazdin (Eds.), *Advances in Clinical Child Psychology*. Vol. 5. New York: Plenum Press.

Achenbach, T.M. 1988. Integrating assessment and taxonomy. In M. Rutter, A.H. Tuma & I.S. Lann (Eds.), *Assessment and Diagnosis in Child Psychopathology*. New York: Guilford Press.

Achilles, R.F. 1956. Communicative anomalies of individuals with cerebral palsy: Part 2: Analysis of communicative processes of 90 athetoids as compared with 61 other types of cerebral palsy. *Cerebral Palsy Review*, 17, 19.

Adams, C.T.B. 1983. Hemispherectomy—A modification. *Journal of Neurology, Neurosurgery and Psychiatry*, 46, 617.

Adams, R.D. & Victor, M. 1977. Disorders contingent upon deviations in development of the nervous system. In R.D. Adams & M. Victor (Eds.), *Principles of Neurology*. New York: McGraw-Hill.

Adams, R.D. & Victor, M. (Eds.) 1993. *Principles of Neurology*, 5th ed. New York: McGraw-Hill.

Adams, R.M., Kocsis, J.J. & Estes, R.E. 1974. Soft neurological signs in learning-disabled children and controls. *American Journal for Disturbed Children*, 128, 614.

517

Adesman, A.R., Altschuler, L.A., Lipkin, P.H. & Walco, G.A. 1990. Otitis media in children with learning disabilities and in children with attention deficit disorder with hyperactivity. *Pediatrics*, 85, 442.

Adrian, J.L., Perrot, A., Sauvage, D. & Leddet, I. 1992. Early symptoms in autism from family home movies: Evaluation and comparison between 1st and 2nd year of life using I.B.S.E. scale. *Acta Paedopsychiatrica/International Journal of Child and Adolescent Psychiatry*, 55, 71.

Aicardie, J. & Chevrie, J.J. 1970. Convulsive status epilepticus in infants and children: A study of 239 cases. *Epilepsia*, 11, 187.

Aicardie, L., Lefevre, J. & Lerique-Koechlin, A. 1965. A new syndrome: spasms in flexion, callosal agenesis, ocular abnormalities. *Electroencephalography and Clinical Neurophysiology*, 19, 609.

Ainsworth, M.D.S. 1973. The development of infant-mother attachment. In B.M. Caldwell & H.N. Ricciuti (Eds.), *Review of Child Development Research*, Vol. 3. Chicago: University of Chicago Press.

Ainsworth, M.D.S., Blehar, M., Waters, E. & Wall, S. 1978. *Patterns of Attachment: A Psychological Study of the Strange Situation*. Hillsdale, NJ: Erlbaum.

Aitken, K. 1991. Examining the evidence for a common structural basis to autism. *Developmental Medicine and Child Neurology*, 33, 930.

Akshoomoff, N.A., Courchesne, E., Yeung-Courchesne, R. & Costello, J. 1991. Brainstem auditory evoked potentials in receptive developmental language disorder. *Brain and Language*, 37, 409.

Alajouanine, T. & Lhermitte, F. 1965. Acquired aphasia in childhood. *Brain*, 88, 653.

Albert, E. 1972. Üeber manisch-depressive Psychose bei Kindern mit organischen Hirnschädigungen. *Archiv für Psychiatrie und Nervenkrankheiten*, 216, 265.

Albert, M.L. 1979. Alexia. In K.M. Heilman & E. Valenstein (Eds.), *Clinical Neuropsychology*. New York: Oxford University Press.

Alberts-Corush, J., Firestone, P. & Goodman, J.T. 1986. Attention and impulsivity characteristics of the biological and adoptive parents of hyperactive and normal control children. *American Journal of Orthopsychiatry*, 56, 413.

Albrecht, P., Torrey, E.F., Boone, E., Hicks, J.T. & Daniel, N. 1980. Raised cytomegalovirus-antibody level in cerebrospinal fluid of schizophrenic patients. *Lancet*, 8198, 769.

Albright, A.L. 1993. Pediatric brain tumors. *CA—A Cancer Journal for Clinicians*, 43, 272.

Alden, E.R., Mendelkorn, T., Woodrum, D.E., Wennberg, R.P., Parks, C.R. & Hodson, W.A. 1972. Morbidity and mortality of infants weighing less than 1,000 grams in an intensive care nursery. *Pediatrics*, 50, 40.

Alexander, D., Ehrhardt, A. & Money, J. 1966. Defective figure drawing, geometric and human, in Turner's syndrome. *Journal of Nervous and Mental Disease*, 142, 161.

Alexander, G.E. & Goldman, P.S. 1978. Functional development of the dorsolateral prefrontal cortex: An analysis using reversible cryogenic depression. *Brain Research*, 143, 233.

Alexander, M.A. & Bauer, R.E. 1988. Cerebral palsy. In V.B. van Hasselt, P.S. Strain & M. Hersen (Eds.), *Handbook of Developmental and Physical Disabilities*. New York: Pergamon Press, p. 215.

Allen, N. 1975. Chemical neurotoxins in industry and environment. In D.B. Tower (Ed.), *The Nervous System, vol. 2: The Clinical Neurosciences*. New York: Raven Press.

Allison, D.S. 1993. Fatigue after closed head injury. PhD dissertation. University of Victoria.

Almli, C.R. & Finger, S. 1992. Brain injury and recovery of function: Theories and mechanisms of functional reorganization. *Journal of Head Trauma Rehabilitation,* 7, 70.

Als, H., Tronick, E., Adamson, L. & Brazelton, T. 1976. The behavior of the full-term but underweight newborn infant. *Developmental Medicine and Child Neurology,* 18, 590.

Als, H., Tronick, E., Lester, B.M. & Brazelton, T.B. 1977. The Brazelton neonatal behavioral assessment scale. *Journal of Abnormal Child Psychology,* 5, (3), 217.

Als, H., Lester, B. & Brazelton, T.B. 1979. Dynamics of the behavioural organization of the premature infant: A theoretical perspective. In T.M. Field, A.M. Sosteck, S. Goldberg, & H. H. Shumann, (Eds.), *Infants Born at Risk: Behaviour and Development.* New York: Spectrum.

Als, H., Lester, B.M., Tronick, E.C. & Brazelton, T.B. 1982. Manual for the assessment of preterm infants' behavior (APIB). In H.E. Fitzgerald, B.M. Lester & M.W. Yogman (Eds.), *Theory and Research in Behavioral Pediatrics,* Vol. 1. New York: Plenum Press, p. 65.

Als, H., Duffy, F.H. & McAnulty, G.B. 1988. Assessing functional competence in preterm and full term newborns as measured with the APIB:I. *Infant Behavior and Development,* 11, 319.

Als, H., Duffy, F.H., McAnulty, G.B. & Badian, N. 1989. Continuity of neurobehavioral functioning in preterm and full term newborns. In M.C. Bornstein & N.A. Krasnegor (Eds.), *Stability and Continuity in Mental Development. Behavioral and Biological Perspectives.* Hillsdale, NJ: Lawrence Erlbaum Associates.

Altman, J. & Bulut, F.G. 1976. Organic maturation and the development of learning capacity. In M.R. Rosenzweig & E.L. Bennett (Eds.), *Neural Mechanisms of Learning and Memory.* Cambridge, MA: MIT Press.

Altman, J., Brunner, R.L. & Bayer, S.A. 1973. The hippocampus and behavioral maturation. *Behavioral Biology,* 8, 557.

Altschuler, R.A., Bobbin, R.P., Clopton, B.M. & Hoffman, D.W. (Eds.) 1991. *Neurobiology of Hearing: The Central Auditory System.* New York: Raven Press.

Alyman, C. 1991. Sex-related differences in spatial ability: A test of ecological validity. M.A. Thesis, University of Guelph, Ontario.

Ameli, N.O. 1980. Hemispherectomy for the treatment of epilepsy and behavior disturbance. *Canadian Journal of Neurological Sciences,* 7(1), 33.

American Association on Mental Retardation (AAMR) 1992. *Mental Retardation: Definition, Classification, and Systems of Support.* Washington, D.C.

American Psychiatric Association 1987, 1994. *Diagnostic and Statistical Manual of Mental Disorders,* 3rd ed.—Revised, 4th ed. Washington: American Psychiatric Association.

Amiel-Tison, C. 1968. Neurological evaluation of the maturity of newborn infants. *Archives of Disease in Children,* 43, 89.

Amiel-Tison, C. 1976. A method for neurologic evaluation within the first year of life. In L. Gluck (Ed.), *Current Problems in Pediatrics.* New York: Year Book Publishers, p. 1.

Amiel-Tison, C. 1980. Possible acceleration of neurological maturation following high-risk pregnancy. *American Journal of Obstetrics and Gynecology,* 138, 303.

Amiel-Tison, C. 1982. Neurologic signs, aetiology, and implications. In Stratton, P. (Ed.), *Psychobiology of the Human Newborn,* New York: John Wiley & Sons, p. 75.

Anastopoulos, A.D. & Barkley, R.A. 1988. Biological factors in attention deficit-hyperactivity disorder. *Behavior Therapist,* 11, 47.

Anderson, E. 1975. Genetic mechanisms in human behavioral development. In K.W. Schaie, V.E. Anderson, G.E. McClearn, & J. Money (Eds.), *Developmental Human Behavior Genetics*. Lexington, MA: Lexington Books, p. 113.

Anderson, E. 1979. The psychological and social adjustment of adolescents with cerebral palsy or spina bifida and hydrocephalus. *International Journal of Rehabilitation Research*, 2, 245.

Andre-Thomas, A., Chesni, Y. & Saint-Anne Dargassies 1960. *The Neurological Examination of the Infant, Clinics in Developmental Medicine*, No. 1. London: Heinemann.

Andrews, E. & Cappon, D. 1957. Autism and schizophrenia in a child guidance clinic. *Canadian Psychiatric Association Journal*, 2, 1.

Andrews, R.J. & Elkins, J. 1981. The management and education of children with spina bifida and hydrocephalus. ERDC Report No. 32. Canberra: Australian Government Publishing Service.

Angle, C.R. & McIntyre, M.S. 1964. Lead poisoning during pregnancy. *American Journal of Diseases of Children*, 108, 436.

Annegers, J.F. 1983. The epidemiology of head trauma in children. In K. Shapiro (Ed.), *Pediatric Head Trauma*. Mount Kisco, NY: Futura, p. 1.

Annegers, J.F., Gradow, J.D., Kurland, L.T. & Laws, E.R. 1980. The incidence, causes, and secular trends of head trauma in Olmsted County, Minnesota, 1935–1974. *Neurology*, 30, 912.

Annegers, J.F., Hauser, W.A., Anderson, V.E. & Kurland, L.T. 1982. The risks of seizure disorders among relatives of patients with childhood onset epilepsy. *Neurology*, 32, 174.

Annett, M. 1970. Handedness, cerebral dominance and the growth of intelligence. In P. Satz & D.J. Bakker (Eds.), *Specific Reading Disability*. Rotterdam: Rotterdam University Press.

Annett, M. 1973. Laterality of childhood hemiplegia and the growth of speech and intelligence. *Cortex*, 9, 4.

Ansara, A., Geschwind, N., Galaburda, A., Albert, M. & Cartrell, N. (Eds.) 1981. *Sex Differences in Dyslexia*. Towson, MD: Orton Dyslexia Society.

Apgar, V.A. 1953. Proposal for a new method of evaluation of the newborn infant. *Anesthesia and Analgesia, Current Researches*, 22, 260.

Apgar, V. 1962. Further observations on the newborn scoring system. *American Journal of Diseases of the Child*, 104, 419.

Aram, D.M. & Horwitz, S.J. 1983. Sequential and non-speech praxic abilities in developmental verbal apraxia. *Developmental Medicine and Child Neurology*, 25, 197.

Aram, D.M., Kelman, B.L., Rose, D.F. & Whitaker, H.A. 1985. Verbal and cognitive sequelae following unilateral lesions acquired in early childhood. *Journal of Clinical and Experimental Neuropsychology*, 7, 55.

Aram, D.M., Hack, M., Hawkins, S. & Weissman, B.M. 1991. Very-low-birthweight children and speech and language development. *Journal of Speech and Hearing Research*, 34, 1169.

Arezzo, J.C., Vaughan, H.G., Kraut, M.A., Steinschneider, M. & Legatt, A.D. 1985. Intracranial generators of event-related potentials in the monkey. In J.B. Cracco, R.P. Brenner & B.F. Westmoreland (Eds.), *State of the Science in EEG-1985*. Atlanta: American Electroencephalographic Society.

Armstrong, D. & Norman, M. 1974. Periventricular leukomalacia in neonates: Complications and sequelae. *Archives of Diseases in Childhood*, 49, 367.

Arnold, A.P. 1980. Sexual differences in the brain. *American Scientist*, 68, 165.

Asanuma, H. & Arissian, K. 1984. Experiments on functional role of peripheral input to motor cortex during voluntary movements in the monkey. *Journal of Neurophysiology*, 52, 212.

Asanuma, H., Kosar, E., Tsukahara, N. & Robinson, H. 1985. Modification of the projections from the sensory cortex to the motor cortex following elimination of the thalamic projections to the motor cortex in cats. *Brain Research*, 345, 79.

Asarnow, J.R. & Ben-Meir, S. 1988. Children with schizophrenia spectrum and depressive disorders: A comparative study of premorbid adjustment, onset pattern and severity of impairment. *Journal of Child Psychology and Child Psychiatry*, 29, 477.

Asarnow, J.R. & Goldstein, M.J. 1986. Schizophrenia during adolescence and early adulthood: A developmental perspective. *Clinical Psychology Review*, 6, 211.

Asarnow, R.F., Satz, P., Light, R. & Lewis, R. 1991. Behavioral problems and adaptive functioning in children with mild and severe closed head injury. *Journal of Pediatric Psychology*, 16, 543.

Asperger, H. 1944. Die "autistischen Psychopathen" im Kindesalter. *Archiv für Psychiatrie*, 117, 1.

Astbury, J., Orgill, A.A., Bajuk, B. & Yu, V.Y.H. 1985. Neonatal and neurodevelopmental significance of behavior in very low birthweight children. *Early Human Development*, 11, 113.

Aten, J. & Davis, J. 1968. Disturbances in the perception of auditory sequence in children with minimal brain dysfunction. *Journal of Speech and Hearing Research*, 11, 236.

Atkinson, J. & Braddick, O. 1982. Sensory and perceptual capacities of the neonate. In P. Stratton (Ed.), *Psychobiology of the Newborn*. New York: Wiley.

Atkinson, J. & Braddick, O. 1989. Development of basic visual functions. In A. Slater & G. Bremner (Eds.), *Infant Development*. New York: Erlbaum, p. 7.

Austin, V.L. 1978. Discriminant and descriptive analyses of neuropsychological electroencephalographic, perinatal and developmental history correlates of children with math or reading disability. *Dissertation Abstract International*, 38 (11-B), 5554.

Aylward, G.P. 1988. Infant and early childhood assessment. In M.G. Tramontana & S.R. Hooper (Eds.), *Assessment Issues in Child Neuropsychology*. New York: Plenum Press, p. 225.

Aylward, G.P. & Kenny, T.J. 1979. Developmental follow-up: Inherent problems and a conceptual model. *Journal of Pediatric Psychology*, 4, 331.

Aylward, G.P., Verhulst, S.J. & Colliver, J.A. 1985. Development of a brief infant neurobehavioral optimality scale: Longitudinal sensitivity and specificity. *Developmental Neuropsychology*, 1, 265.

Aylward, G.P., Gustafson, N., Verhulst, S.J. & Colliver, J.A. 1987. Consistency in the diagnosis of cognitive, motor and neurologic function over the first three years. *Journal of Pediatric Psychology*, 12, 77.

Aylward, G.P., Verhulst, S.J. & Bell, S. 1989. Correlation of asphyxia and other risk factors with outcome: A contemporary view. *Developmental Medicine and Child Neurology*, 31, 329.

Ayoub, D.M., Greenough, W.T. & Juraska, J.M. 1983. Sex differences in dendritic structure in the preoptic area of the juvenile macaque monkey brain. *Science*, 219, 197.

Ayres, A.J. 1965. Patterns of perceptual-motor dysfunction in children: A factor analytic study. *Perceptual and Motor Skills*, 20, 335.

Bach-y-Rita, P. 1990. Brain plasticity as a basis for recovery of function in humans. *Neuropsychologia*, 28, 547.

Bach-y-Rita, P. & Bach-y-Rita, E.W. 1990. Biological and psychosocial factors in recovery from brain damage in humans. *Canadian Journal of Psychology*, 44, 148.

Badalyan, L.O., Zhurba, L.T. & Mastyukova, E.M. 1981. Minimal brain dysfunction in children: Neurological aspects. *Soviet Neurology and Psychiatry*, 14, 90.

Badian, N.A. 1983. Dyscalculia and nonverbal disorders of learning. In H.R. Myklebust (Ed.), *Progress in Learning Disabilities*, Vol. 5. New York: Grune & Stratton, p. 235.

Badian, N.A., McAnulty, G.B., Duffy, F.H. & Als, H. 1990. Prediction of dyslexia in kindergarten boys. *Annals of Dyslexia*, 40, 152.

Bain, J.L. 1990. Cerebral lateralization in adults with Down's syndrome. M.A. Thesis, University of Victoria.

Bain, J.L. & Spreen, O. 1991. Cerebral dominance in adults with Down's syndrome. *Journal of Clinical and Experimental Neuropsychology*, 13, 35.

Bakan, P. 1990. Nonright-handedness and the continuum of reproductive casualty. In S. Coren (Ed.), *Left-Handedness, Behavioral Implications and Anomalies*. Amsterdam: Elsevier.

Bakan, P., Dibb, G. & Reed, P. 1973. Handedness and birth stress. *Neuropsychologia*, 11, 363.

Baker, L. & Cantwell, D.P. 1987. Comparison of well, emotionally disordered, and behaviorally disordered children with linguistic problems. *Journal of the American Academy of Child and Adolescent Psychiatry*, 26, 193.

Baker, L. & Cantwell, D.P. 1992. Attention deficit disorder and speech/language disorders. *Comprehensive Mental Health Care*, 2, 3.

Bakker, D.J. 1979. Dyslexia in developmental neuropsychology—hemisphere-specific models. In D.J. Oborne, M.M. Gruneberg & J.R. Eiser (Eds.), *Research in Psychology and Medicine, Vol. I: Physical Aspects: Pain, Stress, Diagnosis and Organic Damage*. London: Academic Press, p. 347.

Bakker, D.J. 1992. Neuropsychological classification and treatment of dyslexia. *Journal of Learning Disabilities*, 25, 102.

Bakker, D.J., Teunissen, J. & Bosch, J. 1976. Development of laterality—reading patterns. In R.M. Knights & D.J. Bakker (Eds.), *The Neuropsychology of Learning Disorders: Theoretical Approaches*. Baltimore: University Park Press.

Bakker, D.J. & Vinke, J. 1985. Effects of hemisphere-specific stimulation on brain activity and reading in dyslexics. *Journal of Clinical and Experimental Neuropsychology*, 7, 505.

Bakketeig, L.S. 1977. The risk of repeated preterm or low birth weight delivery. In D. Reed & F. Stanley (Eds.), *The Epidemiology of Prematurity*. Baltimore: Urban and Schwarzenberg.

Balazs, R. 1979. Cerebellum: Certain features of its development and biochemistry. In M. Cuenod, G.W. Kreutzberg & F.E. Bloom (Eds.), *Development and Chemical Specificity of Neurons* (Progress in Brain Research, Vol. 51). Amsterdam: Elsevier/ North-Holland Biomedical Press.

Ball, R.S., Merrifield, P. & Stott, L.H. 1978. *Extended Merrill-Palmer Scales*. Chicago: Stoelting.

Ballotin, U., Bejor, M., Cecchini, A. & Martelli, A. 1989. Infantile autism and computerized tomography brain-scan findings: Specific versus nonspecific abnormalities. *Journal of Autism and Developmental Disorders*, 19, 109.

Balow, B., Rubin, R. & Rosen, M.S. 1976. Prenatal events as precursors of reading disability. *Reading Research Quarterly*, 11, 36.

Baltes, P.B. & Nesselroade, J.R. 1970. Multivariate longitudinal and cross-sectional sequences for analyzing ontogenetic and generational change: A methodological note. *Developmental Psychology*, 2, 163.

Baltes, P.B., Reese, H.W. & Nesselroade, J.R. 1977. *Life-Span Developmental Psychology: Introduction to Research Methods.* Monterey, CA: Brooks/Cole Publishing Co.

Banker, A. & Larroche, J.C. 1962. Periventricular leukomalacia in infancy. *Archives of Neurology*, 7, 386.

Barclay, A. & Walton, O. 1988. Phenylketonuria: Implications of initial serum phenylalanine levels on cognitive development. *Psychological Reports*, 63, 135.

Barkley, R.A. 1977. A review of stimulant drug research with hyperactive children. *Journal of Child Psychology and Psychiatry*, 18, 137.

Barkley, R.A. 1981. *Hyperactive Children: A Handbook for Diagnosis and Treatment.* New York: Guilford Press.

Barkley, R.A. 1986. Tic disorders and Tourette's syndrome. In E.G. Mash & L.D. Terdal (Eds.), *Behavioral Assessment of Childhood Disorders,* 2nd ed. New York: Guilford Press.

Barkley, R.A. 1990. *Attention Deficit Hyperactivity Disorder: A Handbook for Diagnosis and Treatment,* 2nd ed. New York: Guiford Press.

Barkley, R.A. & Cunningham, C.E. 1979. Stimulant drugs and activity level in hyperactive children. *American Journal of Orthopsychiatry*, 49(3), 491.

Barlow, C.F. 1974. Soft signs in children with learning disorders. *American Journal of Diseases of Children,* 128, 605.

Barnard, K.E. & Douglas, H.B. (Eds.) 1974. *Child Health Assessment. Part 1: Literature Review.* Bethesda, MD: US Department of Health, Education and Welfare, (DHEW HRA 75-30).

Barnes, M.A. & Dennis, M. 1992. Reading in children and adolescents after early-onset hydrocephalus and in normally developing age-peers: Phonological analysis, word recognition, word comprehension, and passage comprehension skills. *Journal of Pediatric Psychology,* 17, 315.

Barnet, A.P., Manson, J.I. & Wilner, E. 1970. Acute cerebral blindness in childhood. *Neurology*, 20, 1147.

Barnet, A.P., Weiss, I.P., Sotillio, M.V., Ohlrich, E.S., Shkurovich, Z. & Cravioto, J. 1978. Abnormal auditory evoked potentials in early infancy malnutrition. *Science*, 201, 450.

Barnet, A.P., Friedman, S.L., Weiss, J.I., Ohlrich, E.S., Shanks, B. & Lodge, A. 1980. Visual evoked potential development in infancy and early childhood: A longitudinal study. *Electroencephalography and Clinical Neurophysiology*, 1980, 49, 476.

Barr, D.F. 1972. *Auditory Perceptual Disorders: An Introduction.* Springfield, IL: Charles C Thomas.

Barros, F.C., Huttly, S.R.A., Victora, C.G., Kirkwood, B.R. & Vaughan, J.P. 1992. Comparison of the causes and consequences of prematurity and interuterine growth retardation: A longitudinal study in Southern Brazil. *Pediatrics*, 90, 2, 238.

Bartak, L., Rutter, M. & Cox, A. 1975. A comparative study of infantile autism and specific receptive language disorder: I. The children. *British Journal of Psychiatry*, 126, 127.

Bartel, P.R., Griesel, R.D. & Burnett, L.S. 1977a. *Long-Term Effect of Kwashiorkor on Psychomotor Ability.* Johannesburg, South Africa: Council of Scientific and Industrial Research.

Bartel, P.R., Griesel, R.D. & Burnett, L.S. 1977b. *Psychometric Assessment of the Long-Term Effects of Kwashiorkor.* Johannesburg, South Africa: Council of Scientific and Industrial Research.

Bartel, P.R., Burnett, L.S., Griesel, R.D., Freiman, I., Rosen, E.U. & Geefhuysen, J. 1978. The visual evoked potential in children after kwashiorkor. *South African Medical Journal,* 54, 857.

Bartel, P.R., Griesel, R.D., Freiman, I., Rosen, E.U. & Geefhuysen, J. 1979. Long-term effects of kwashiorkor on the electroencephalogram. *American Journal of Clinical Nutrition,* 32, 753.

Basser, L.S. 1962. Hemiplegia of early onset and the faculty of speech with special reference to the effects of hemispherectomy. *Brain,* 85, 427.

Basso, A. & Scarpa, M.T. 1990. Traumatic aphasia in children and adults: A comparison of clinical features and evolution. *Cortex,* 26, 502.

Bates, E., Bretherton, I. & Snyder, L. 1988. *From the First Words of Grammar.* New York: Cambridge Press.

Baumeister, A.A. & Bartlett, C.J. 1962. A comparison of the factor structure of normals and retardates on the WISC. *American Journal of Mental Deficiency,* 66, 641.

Bawden, H.N., Knights, R.M. & Winogron, H.W. 1985. Speeded performance following head injury in children. *Journal of Clinical and Experimental Neuropsychology,* 7, 39.

Bay, E. 1962. Sprache und Denken. *Deutsche Medizinische Wochenschrift,* 87, 1845.

Bayley, N. 1933. Mental growth during the first three years. *Genetic Psychology Monographs,* 14, 1.

Bayley, N. 1969. *Bayley Scales of Infant Development.* New York: The Psychological Corporation.

Bayley, N. 1970. Development of mental abilities. In P.H. Mussen (Ed.), *Carmichael's Manual of Child Psychology,* Vol. 1. New York: Wiley.

Beaconsfield, P., Birdwood, G. & Beaconsfield, R. 1980. The placenta. *Scientific American,* 243(2), 95.

Beardslee, W.K., Keller, M.B. & Klerman, G.D. 1985. Children of parents with affective disorder. *International Journal of Family Psychiatry,* 6, 283.

Beardsworth, E.D. & Adams, C.B. 1988. Modified hemispherectomy for epilepsy: Early results in 10 cases. *British Journal of Neurosurgery,* 2, 73.

Beasley, D.S. & Rintelmann, A.K. 1979. Central auditory processing. In W.F. Rintelmann (Ed.), *Hearing Assessment.* Baltimore: University Park Press.

Beattie, A.D., Moore, M.R., Goldberg, A., Finlayson, M.J.W., Mackie, E.M., Graham, J.F., McLaren, D.A., Murdock, R.M. & Stewart, G.T. 1975. Role of chronic low-level lead exposure in the etiology of mental retardation. *Lancet,* 1, 589.

Behrman, G. 1992. *Textbook of Pediatrics,* 14th ed. Philadelphia: W.B. Saunders.

Beitchman, J.H., Nair, R., Clegg, M. & Patel, P.G. 1986. Prevalence of speech and language disorders in 5-year-old kindergarten children in the Ottawa-Carlton region. *Journal of Speech and Hearing Disorders,* 51, 98.

Beitchman, J.H., Hood, J., Rochon, J. & Paterson, M. 1989. Empirical classification of speech-language impairment in children: II. Behavioral characteristics. *Journal of the American Academy of Child and Adolescent Psychiatry,* 28, 118.

Bell, W.L., Davis, D.L., Morgan-Fisher, A. & Ross, E.D. 1990. Acquired aprosodia in children. *Journal of Child Neurology,* 5, 19.

Bellugi, U., Sabo, H. & Vaid, J. 1988. Spatial deficits in children with Williams syndrome. In J. Styles-Davis, M. Kritchevsky & U. Bellugi (Eds.), *Spatial Cognition: Brain Bases and Development.* Hillsdale, NJ: Erlbaum. p. 273.

Belman, A.L., Lantos, G. & Horoupian, D. 1986. AIDS: Calcification of the basal ganglia in infants and children. *Neurology,* 36, 1192.

Belman, A.L., Diamond, G., Dickson, D., Horoupian, D., Liena, J., Lantos, G. & Rubinstein, A. 1988. Pediatric acquired immunodeficiency syndrome. *American Journal of Diseases in Children,* 142, 29.

Belmont, I.B., Birch, H.G. & Belmont, L. 1967. The organization of intelligence test performance in educable mentally subnormal children. *American Journal of Mental Deficiency,* 71, 969.

Belmont, J.M. 1971. Medical-behavioral research in retardation. In N.R. Ellis (Ed.), *International Review of Research in Mental Retardation,* Vol. 5. New York: Academic Press.

Belsky, J. & Isabella, R. 1988. Maternal, infant, and social-contextual determinants of attachment security. In J. Belsy & T. Nezworski (Eds.), *Clinical Implications of Attachment.* Hillsdale, NJ: Erlbaum.

Belsky, J. & Most, R.K. 1981. From exploration to play: A cross-sectional study of infant free play behavior. *Developmental Psychology,* 17, 630.

Belsky, J., Honcir, E. & Vondra, J. 1983. *Manual for the Assessment of Performance, Competence, and Executive Capacity in Infant Play.* Unpublished manuscript, Pennsylvania State University.

Benda, C.E. 1960. *The Child with Mongolism.* New York: Grune & Stratton.

Bender, B.G., Puck, M.H., Salbenblatt, J.A. & Robinson, A. 1986a. Dyslexia in 47, XXY boys identified at birth. *Behavior Genetics,* 16, 343.

Bender, B.G., Puck, M.H., Salbenblatt, J.A. & Robinson, A. 1986b. Cognitive development of children with sex chromosome abnormalities. In S.D. Smith (Ed.), *Genetic and Learning Disabilities.* London: Taylor & Francis. p. 175.

Bender, L. 1942. Schizophrenia in childhood. *The Nervous Child,* 1, 138.

Bender, L. 1947. Childhood schizophrenia: Clinical study of one hundred schizophrenic children. *American Journal of Orthopsychiatry,* 17, 40.

Bender, L. 1956. Schizophrenia in childhood: Its recognition, description and treatment. *American Journal of Orthopsychiatry,* 26, 499.

Bender, M.B. 1945. Extinction and precipitation of cutaneous sensations. *Archives of Neurology and Psychiatry,* 54, 1.

Bendersky, M. & Lewis, M. 1990. Early language ability as a function of ventricular dilation associated with intraventricular hemorrhage. *Journal of Developmental and Behavioral Pediatrics,* 11, 17.

Benes, V. 1982. Sequelae of transcallosal surgery. *Child's Brain,* 9, 69.

Benjamins, J.A. & McKhann, G.M. 1976. Development, regeneration, and aging. In G.J. Siegel, R.W. Albers, R. Katzman & B.W. Agranoff (Eds.), *Basic Neurochemistry,* 2nd ed. Boston: Little, Brown.

Bennett, E.L., Diamond, M.C., Krech, D. & Rosenzweig, M.R. 1964. Chemical and anatomical plasticity of the brain. *Science,* 146, 610.

Bennett, G. 1987. Changes in the intermediate filament composition during neurogenesis. In R.K. Hunt (Ed.), *Neural Development, Part IV: Cellular and Molecular Differentiation.* New York: Academic Press. p. 151.

Bennett, K. 1987. AIDS: A generation of children at risk. *Journal of Psychosocial Nursing,* 25, 32.

Benson, D.F. 1981. The alexias. In G. Pirozzolo (Ed.), *Neuropsychological Processes in Reading.* New York: Academic Press.

Benson, D.F. & Geschwind, N. 1969. The alexias. In P.J. Vinken & G.W. Bruyn (Eds.), *Handbook of Clinical Neurology,* Vol. 4. Amsterdam: North-Holland.

Benson, D.F. & Geschwind, N. 1970. Developmental Gerstmann syndrome. *Neurology*, 20, 293.

Bentin, S., Sahar, A. & Moscovitch, M. 1984. Intermanual transfer in patients with lesions in the trunk of the corpus callosum. *Neuropsychologia*, 22, 601.

Bentin, S., McCarthy, G. & Wood, C.C. 1985. Event-related potentials, lexical decision making and semantic priming. *Journal of Clinical and Experimental Neuropsychology*, 7, 505.

Benton, A.L. 1940. Mental development of prematurely born children. *Journal of Orthopsychiatry*, 10, 719.

Benton, A.L. 1975. Developmental dyslexia: Neurological aspects. In W.J. Friedlander (Ed.), *Advances in Neurology*, Vol. 7. New York: Raven Press, p. 1.

Benton, A.L. 1978. The cognitive functioning of children with developmental dysphasia. In M.A. Wyke (Ed.), *Developmental Dysphasia*. New York: Academic Press.

Benton, A.L. 1985. Reflections on the Gerstmann syndrome. In L. Costa & O. Spreen (Eds.), *Studies in Neuropsychology: Selected Papers of Arthur Benton*. New York: Oxford University Press.

Benton, A.L. & Pearl, D. 1978. *Dyslexia: An Appraisal of Current Knowledge*. New York: Oxford University Press.

Benton, A.L., Hamsher, K., Varney, N.R. & Spreen, O. 1983. *Contributions to Neuropsychological Assessment*. New York: Oxford University Press.

Berenberg, S.R. (Ed.). 1977. *Brain—Fetal and Infant*. The Hague: Martinus Nijhoff.

Berenberg, W. & Nankervis, G. 1970. Long-term follow-up of cytomegalic inclusion disease in infancy. *Pediatrics*, 37, 403.

Berg, K. & Berg, K. 1979. Physical and psychophysiological development. In J. Ozofski (Ed.), *Handbook of Infant Development*. New York: Plenum.

Berg, W.K., Adkinson, C.D. & Strock, B.D. 1973. Duration and frequency of periods of alertness in the newborn. *Developmental Psychology*, 9, 434.

Berger, J.R. & Levy, R.M. 1993. The neurologic complications of human immunodeficiency virus infections. *Medical Clinics of North America*, 77, 1.

Bergman, M., Costeff, H., Koren, V., Koifman, N. & Reshef, A. 1984. Auditory perception in early lateralized brain damage. *Cortex*, 20, 233.

Berker, E., Goldstein, G., Lorber, J. & Priestley, B. 1992. Reciprocal neurological developments of twins discordant for hydrocephalus. *Developmental Medicine and Child Neurology*, 34, 623.

Berman, J.L. & Ford, R. 1970. Intelligence quotients and intelligence loss in patients with phenylketonuria and some variant states. *Journal of Pediatrics*, 77, 764.

Berman, J.L., Graham, F.K., Eichman, F.D. & Waisman, R.G. 1961. Development after perinatal anoxia and other potentially damaging newborn experiences. *Pediatrics*, 28, 924.

Berman, N.E. & Payne, B.R. 1988. Development and plasticity of visual interhemispheric connections. In P.G. Shinkman (Ed.), *Advances in Neural and Behavioral Development*, Vol. 3. Norwood, NJ: Ablex.

Bernal, J. 1972. Crying during the first ten days of life, and maternal responses. *Developmental Medicine and Child Neurology*, 14, 362.

Berninger, V.W. & Rutberg, J. 1992. Relationship of finger function to beginning writing: Application to diagnosis of writing disabilities. *Developmental Medicine and Child Neurology*, 34, 198.

Bernstein, G.A. 1991. Comorbidity and severity of anxiety and depressive disorders in a clinic sample. *Journal of the American Academy of Child and Adolescent Psychiatry*, 30, 43.

Berry, M. 1974. Development of the cerebral neocortex of the rat. In G. Gottlieb (Ed.), *Studies on the Development of Behavior and the Nervous System, Vol. 2: Aspects of Neurogenesis.* New York: Academic Press.

Berry, M., McConnell, P. & Sievers, J. 1980. Dendritic growth and the control of neuronal form. In R.K. Hunt (Ed.), *Neural Development,* Part I (Current Topics in Developmental Biology, Vol. 15). New York: Academic Press.

Berry, P., Groeneweg, G., Gibson, D. & Brown, R.I. 1984. Mental development of adults with Down syndrome. *American Journal of Mental Deficiency,* 89, 252.

Best, C.A. (Ed.) 1985. *Hemispheric Function and Collaboration in the Child.* New York: Academic Press.

Beverly, D.W., Smith, I.S., Beesley, P. & Jones, J. 1990. Relationship of cranial ultrasonography, visual and auditory evoked responses with neurodevelopmental outcome. *Developmental Medicine and Child Neurology,* 32, 210.

Biederman, J., Newcorn, J. & Sprich, S. 1991. Comorbidity of attention deficit hyperactivity disorder with conduct, depressive, anxiety, and other disorders. *American Journal of Psychiatry,* 148, 564.

Biglan, A.W., van Hasselt, V.B. & Simon, J. 1988. Visual impairment. In V.B. van Hasselt, P.S. Strain & M. Herson (Eds.), *Handbook of Developmental and Physical Disabilities.* New York: Pergamon.

Bigler, E.D. 1988. The neuropsychology of hydrocephalus. *Archives of Clinical Neuropsychology,* 3, 81.

Bigler, E.D. 1989. Radiological techniques in neuropsychological assessment. In C.R. Reynolds & E. Fletcher-Janzen (Eds.), *Handbook of Clinical Child Neuropsychology.* New York: Plenum Press.

Bigler, E.D., Rosenstein, L.D., Roman, M. & Nussbaum, N.L. 1988. The clinical significance of congenital agenesis of the corpus callosum. *Archives of Clinical Neuropsychology,* 3, 189.

Bihrle, A.M., Bellugi, U., Delis, D. & Marks, S. 1989. Seeing the forest or the trees: Dissociation in visuospatial processing. *Brain and Cognition,* 11, 37.

Binet, A. 1905. A propos de la mesure de l'intelligence. *Année Psychologique,* 11, 69.

Binet, A. & Simon, T. 1908. Le development de l'intelligence chez les enfants. *Année Psychologique,* 14, 1.

Birch, H.G. 1959. Summary of conference. *American Journal of Mental Deficiency,* 64, 410.

Birch, H.G. 1962. Dyslexia and the maturation of visual function. In J. Money (Ed.), *Reading Disability.* Baltimore: Johns Hopkins Press.

Birch, H.G. 1974. Some ways of viewing studies in behavioral development. In S.R. Berenberg, M. Caniaris & N.P. Masse (Eds.), *Pre- and Postnatal Development of the Brain.* Basel: S. Karger.

Birch, H.G. & Belmont, L. 1965. Auditory-visual integration in brain-damaged and normal children. *Developmental Medicine and Child Neurology,* 7, 135.

Birch, H.G. & Diller, L. 1959. Rorschach signs of organicity: A physiological basis for perceptual disturbances. *Journal of Projective Techniques,* 23, 184.

Birch, H.G., Belmont, L. & Carp, E. 1965. The prolongation of inhibition in brain-damaged patients. *Cortex,* 1, 397.

Birch, H.G., Pineiro, C., Alcalde, E., Toca, T. & Cravioto, J. 1971. Relation of kwashiorkor in early childhood and intelligence at school age. *Pediatric Research,* 5, 579.

Bishop, D.V.M. 1987. The causes of specific developmental language disorder ("Developmental aphasia"). *Journal of Child Psychology and Psychiatry,* 28, 1.

Bishop, D.V.M. 1990a. *Handedness and Developmental Disorder.* Oxford: Blackwell Scientific Publications.

Bishop, D.V.M. 1990b. Handedness, clumsiness, and developmental language disorders. *Neuropsychologia,* 28, 681.

Bishop, D.V.M. & Robson, J. 1989. Unimpaired short-term memory and rhyme judgement in congenitally speechless individuals: Implications for the notion of articulatory coding. *Quarterly Journal of Experimental Psychology,* 41A, 123.

Bishop, D.V.M., Brown, B.B. & Robson, J. 1990. The relationship between phoneme discrimination, speech production, and language comprehension in cerebral-palsied individuals. *Journal of Speech and Hearing Research,* 33, 210.

Bjorklund, D.F. & Green, B.L. 1992. The adaptive nature of cognitive immaturity. *American Psychologist,* 47, 46.

Bjorklund, D.F. & Harnishfeger, K.K. 1990. The resources concept in cognitive development: Diverse sources of evidence and a theory of inefficient inhibition. *Developmental Review,* 10, 48.

Black, F. 1972. *Neonatal Emergencies and the Problems.* London: Butterworth.

Black, P., Blumer, D., Wellner, A.M., Shepard, R.H. & Walker, A.E. 1981. Head trauma in children: Neurological behavioral and intellectual sequelae. In P. Black (Ed.), *Brain Dysfunction in Children: Etiology, Diagnosis and Management.* New York: Raven Press.

Blakemore, C. & Cooper, G.F. 1970. Development of the brain depends on the visual environment. *Nature,* 228, 477.

Bliss, L.S. & Peterson, D.M. 1975. Performance of aphasic and nonaphasic children on a sentence repetition task. *Journal of Communication Disorders,* 8, 207.

Blom, J.L., Barth, P.G. & Visser, S.L. 1980. The visual evoked potential in the first six years of life. *Electroencephalography and Clinical Neurophysiology,* 48, 395.

Boder, E. 1973. Developmental dyslexia: A diagnostic approach based on three reading-spelling patterns. *Developmental Medicine and Child Neurology,* 15, 663.

Bodis-Wollner, I., Atkin, A., Raab, E. & Wolkstein, M. 1977. Visual association cortex and vision in man. Pattern evoked potentials in a blind boy. *Science,* 198, 629.

Boer, G.J. & Swaab, D.F. 1985. Neuropeptide effects on brain development to be expected from behavioral teratology. *Peptides,* 6, 21.

Bogen, J.E. 1979. The callosal syndrome. In K.M. Heilman & E. Valenstein (Eds.), *Clinical Neuropsychology.* New York: Oxford University Press.

Boggs, T.R. Jr., Hardy, J.B. & Frazier, T.M. 1967. Correlation of neonatal serum total bilirubin concentrations and developmental status at eight months. *Journal of Pediatrics,* 71, 553.

Bohline, D.S. 1985. Intellectual and affective characteristics of attention deficit disordered children. *Journal of Learning Disabilities,* 18, 604.

Boldyrev, A.T. 1987. Deviant behavior in epileptic children. *Zhurnal Nevropatologii i Psikhiatrii,* 87, 833.

Boles, D.B. 1980. X-linkage of spatial ability: A critical review. *Child Development,* 51, 625.

Boll, T.J. 1972. Conceptual vs. perceptual vs. motor deficits in brain-damaged children. *Journal of Clinical Psychology,* 28, 157.

Boll, T.J. 1974. Behavioral correlates of cerebral damage in children age 9–14. In R.M. Reitan & L.A. Davison (Eds.), *Clinical Neuropsychology: Current Status and Application.* Washington, DC: V.H. Winston & Sons.

Boll, T.J. 1983. Neuropsychological assessment of the child: Myths, current status, and future prospects. In C.E. Walker & M.C. Roberts (Eds.), *Handbook of Clinical Child Psychology*. New York: Wiley.

Boll, T.J. & Barth, J.T. 1981. Neuropsychology of brain damage in children. In S. Filskov & T.J. Boll (Eds.), *Handbook of Clinical Neuropsychology*. New York: Wiley.

Boll, T.J. & Reitan, R.M. 1972. Motor and tactile-perceptual deficits in brain-damaged children. *Perceptual and Motor Skills*, 34, 343.

Boller, F. & Grafman, J. (Eds.) 1992. *Handbook of Neuropsychology*, Vol. 6. Amsterdam: Elsevier.

Bond, N.W. 1981. Prenatal alcohol exposure in rodents: A review of its effects on offspring activity and learning ability. *Australian Journal of Psychology*, 33, 331.

Bond, L.A., Creasey, G.L. & Abrams, C.L. 1990. Play assessment. Reflecting and promoting cognitive competence. In E.D. Gibbs & D.M. Teti (Eds.), *Interdisciplinary Assessment of Infants. A Guide for Early Intervention Professionals*. Baltimore: Paul H. Brookes, p. 113.

Bonvillian, J.D., Orlansky, M.D. & Garland, J.B. 1982. Handedness patterns in the deaf. *Brain and Cognition*, 1, 141.

Borjeson, M.C. & Lagergren, J. 1990. Life conditions of adolescents with meningomyelocele. *Developmental Medicine and Child Neurology*, 32, 698.

Borkowski, J.G. 1985. Signs of intelligence: Strategy generalization and metacognition. In S.R. Yussen (Ed.), *The Growth of Reflection in Children*. Orlando, FL: Academic Press, p. 105.

Borlund, B.L. & Heckman, H.K. 1976. Hyperactive boys and their brothers. *Archives of General Psychiatry*, 33, 669.

Bornstein, M.H. 1978. Visual behavior of the young human infant: Relationship between chromatic and spatial perception and activity of underlying brain mechanisms. *Journal of Experimental Child Psychology*, 26, 174.

Bornstein, M.H. 1990. Stability in early mental development: From attention and information processing in infancy to language and cognition in childhood. In M.H. Bornstein & N.A. Krasnegor (Eds.), *Stability and Continuity in Mental Development: Behavioral and Biological Perspectives*. Hillsdale, NJ: Erlbaum, p. 147.

Bornstein, M.H. & Krasnegor, N.A. (Eds.) 1989. *Stability and Continuity in Mental Development: Behavioral and Biological Perspectives*. New York: Plenum.

Bornstein, M.H. & Lamb, M.E. (Eds.) 1992. *Developmental Psychology: An Advanced Textbook*, 3rd ed. Hillsdale, NJ: Erlbaum.

Bornstein, M.H. & Ruddy, M. 1984. Infant attention and maternal stimulation: Prediction of cognitive and linguistic development in singletons and twins. In H. Bouma & D. Bouwhuis (Eds.), *Attention and Performance X*. London: Lawrence Erlbaum Associates, p. 433.

Bornstein, M.H. & Sigman, M.D. 1987. Continuity in mental development from infancy. *Child Development*, 57, 251.

Bornstein, R.A., King, G. & Carroll, A. 1983. Neuropsychological abnormalities in Gilles de la Tourette' syndrome. *Journal of Nervous and Mental Disease,* 171, 497.

Bornstein, R.A., Carroll, A. & King, G. 1985. Relationship of age to neuropsychological deficit in Tourette's syndrome. *Journal of Developmental and Behavioral Pediatrics,* 6, 284.

Bornstein, R.A., Pakalnis, A., Drake, M.E. & Suga, L.J. 1988. Effects of seizure type and waveform abnormality on memory and attention. *Archives of Neurology*, 45, 884.

Bornstein, R.A., Miller, H.B. & van Schoor, J.T. 1989. Neuropsychological deficit and emotional disturbance in head-injured patients. *Journal of Neurosurgery*, 70, 509.

Bornstein, R.A., Baker, G.B., Carroll, A. & King, G. 1990a. Plasma amino acids in attention deficit disorder. *Psychiatry Research*, 33, 301.

Bornstein, R.A., Nasrallah, H.A., Olson, S.C., Coffman, M.T. & Schwarzkopf, S.B. 1990b. Neuropsychological deficit in schizophrenic subtypes: Paranoid, nonparanoid, and schizoaffective subgroups. *Psychiatry Research*, 31, 15.

Bossy, J.G. 1970. Morphological study of a case of complete, isolated, and asymptomatic agenesis of the corpus callosum. *Archives d'Anatomie, d'Histologie et d'Embryologie*, 53, 289.

Bottcher, J., Jacobsen, S., Gyldensted, C., Harmsen, A. & Gloerselt-Tarp, B. 1978. Intellectual development and brain size in 13 shunted hydrocephalic children. *Neuropaediatrie*, 9, 369.

Bottos, M., della Barba, B., Stefani, D. & Pettena, G. 1989. Locomotor strategies preceding independent walking: Prospective study of neurological and language development in 424 cases. *Developmental Medicine and Child Neurology*, 31, 25.

Boucugnani, L.L. & Jones, R.W. 1989. Behaviors analogous to frontal lobe dysfunction in children with attention deficit hyperactivity disorder. *Archives of Clinical Neuropsychology*, 4, 161.

Boulder Committee. 1970. Embryonic vertebrate central nervous system: Revised terminology. *Anatomical Record*, 166, 257.

Bower, T.G.R. 1977. *A Primer of Infant Development*. San Francisco: W.H. Freeman.

Bowlby, J. 1951. *Maternal Care and Mental Health*. Monograph No. 2. Geneva: World Health Organization.

Bowlby, J. 1969/1982. *Attachment and Loss (Vol. 1). Attachment*. New York: Basic Books.

Bowmman, J.M. 1975. Rh erythroblastosis fetalis. In F.A. Oski, E.R. Jaffe & P.A. Miescher (Eds.), *Current Problems in Pediatric Hematology*. New York: Grune & Stratton, p. 29.

Boyd, T.A. 1988. Clinical assessment of memory in children: A developmental framework for practice. In M.G. Tramontana & S.R. Hooper (Eds.), *Assessment Issues in Child Neuropsychology*. New York: Plenum Press, p. 177.

Boyle, M.H., Offord, D.R., Hofmann, H.G., Catlin, G.P., Byles, J.A., Cadman, D.T., Crawford, J.W., Links, P.S., Rae-Grant, N.I. & Szatmari, P. 1987. Ontario Child Health Study: I. Methodology. *Archives of General Psychiatry*, 44, 826.

Bracco, L., Tiezzi, A., Ginanneschi, A., Campanella, C. & Amaducci, L. 1984. Lateralization of choline acetyltransferase (Ch.AT) activity in fetus and adult human brain. *Neurosciences Newsletter*, 50, 301.

Bracken, B.A. & Cato, L.A. 1986. Rate of conceptual development among deaf preschool and primary children as compared to a matched group of nonhearing impaired children. *Psychology in the Schools*, 23, 95.

Bradley, C. 1937. The behavior of children receiving benzedrine. *American Journal of Psychiatry*, 94, 577.

Bradley, R.M. & Mistretta, C.M. 1975. Fetal receptors. *Physiological Review*, 55, 352.

Bradshaw, J. & Lawton, P. 1985. 75,000 severely disabled children. *Developmental Medicine and Child Neurology*, 27, 25.

Bradshaw, J.L. & Nettleton, N.C. 1983. *Human Cerebral Asymmetry*. New York: Prentice-Hall.

Brain, R. 1985. *Diseases of the Nervous System*. 9th ed., revised by J.W. Walton. New York: Oxford.

Brandenburg, N.A., Friedman, R.M. & Silver, S.E. 1990. The epidemiology of childhood psychiatric disorders: Prevalence findings from recent studies. *Journal of the American Academy of Child and Adolescent Psychiatry*, 29, 76.

Brandt, I. 1979. Patterns of early neurological development. In F. Falkner & J.M. Tanner (Eds.), *Human Growth, Vol. 3: Neurobiology and Nutrition.* New York: Plenum Press.

Brann, A.W. & Dykes, F.D. 1977. The effects of intrauterine asphyxia on the full-term neonate. *Clinics in Perinatalogy*, 4(1), 149.

Brasel, J. 1974. Cellular changes in intrauterine malnutrition. In M. Winick (Ed.), *Nutrition and Fetal Development.* New York: John Wiley and Sons.

Brauth, S.E., Hall, W.S. & Dooling, R.J. (Eds.) 1991. *Plasticity of Development.* Cambridge, MA: MIT Press.

Brazelton, T.B. 1973. *Neonatal Behavioral Assessment Scale.* Clinics in Developmental Medicine, No. 50. London: Heinemann.

Brazelton, T.B., Koslowski, B. & Tronick, E. 1976. Study of the neonatal behavior in Zambian and American neonates. *Journal of the American Academy of Child Psychiatry*, 15, 97.

Brazier, M.A.B. & Coceani, F. (Eds.) 1978. *Brain Dysfunction in Infantile Febrile Convulsions* (International Brain Research Organization Monograph Series). New York: Raven Press.

Brennan, J.F., Pescatore, C.A. & Hallisey, P. 1990. Ontogenic factors in short- and long-term recovery of discriminative behavior in rats after selective brain damage. *Acta Neurobiologiae Experimentalis*, 50, 141.

Brenner, A. 1977. A study of the efficacy of the Feingold diet on hyperkinetic children. *Clinical Pediatrics*, 16, 652.

Brenner, M.W., Gillman, S., Zangwill, O. & Farrell, M. 1967. Visuo-motor disability in schoolchildren. *British Medical Journal*, 4, 259.

Brenner, W.E., Bruce, R.D. & Hendricks, C.A. 1974. The characteristics and perils of breech presentation. *American Journal of Obstetrics and Gynecology*, 118, 700.

Brenner, P.R. & Stehouwer, D.J. 1991. Sparing and recovery of function in spinal larval frogs (rana catesbeiana): Effect of level of transection. *Behavioral and Neural Biology*, 56, 292.

Brent, D.A. 1986. Overrepresentation of epileptics in a consecutive series of suicide attempts seen at a children's hospital. *Journal of the American Academy of Child Psychiatry*, 25, 242.

Breslau, N. 1985. Psychiatric disorders in children with physical disabilities. *Journal of the American Academy of Child Psychiatry*, 24, 87.

Brett, E.M. 1975. The prognosis of seizures in the first three years of life. *Epilepsia*, 16, 346.

Brickman, A.S., McManus, M., Grapentine, W.L. & Alessi, N. 1984. Neuropsychological assessment of seriously delinquent adolescents. *Journal of the American Academy of Child Psychiatry*, 23, 453.

Bridgeman, E. & Snowling, M. 1988. The perception of phoneme sequences: A comparison of dyspraxic and normal children. *British Journal of Disorders of Communication*, 23, 245.

Brink, J., Garrett, A., Hale, W., Woo-Sam, J. & Nickel, V. 1970. Recovery of motor and intellectual function in children sustaining severe head injuries. *Developmental Medicine and Child Neurology*, 15, 823.

Brittis, P. 1992. Molecular guardrails in the development of the optic nerve. *Science,* 256, 2201.

Brockman, L. & Ricciuti, H. 1971. Severe protein calorie malnutrition and cognitive development in infancy and early childhood. *Developmental Psychology,* 4, 312.

Broman, M., Rudel, R.G., Helfgott, E. & Krieger, J. 1986. Inter- and intra-hemispheric processing of letter stimuli by dyslexic children and normal readers. *Cortex,* 22, 447.

Broman, S. 1979. Prenatal anoxia and cognitive development in early childhood. In T. Field, A. Sostek, S. Goldberg & H. Shuman (Eds.), *Infants Born at Risk.* New York: Spectrum Press, p. 29.

Broman, S.H., Nichols, P.L. & Kennedy, W.A. 1975. *Preschool IQ: Prenatal and Early Developmental Correlates.* Hillsdale, NJ: Erlbaum.

Broman, S., Nichols, P.L., Shaughnessy, P. & Kennedy, W. 1987. *Retardation in Young Children: A Developmental Study of Cognitive Deficit.* Hillsdale, NJ: Erlbaum.

Bronner-Fraser, M.E. & Cohen, A.M. 1980. The neural crest: What can it tell us about cell migration and determination? In R.K. Hunt (Ed.), *Neural Development, Part I* (Current Topics in Developmental Biology, Vol. 15). New York: Academic Press.

Bronson, G. 1974. The postnatal growth of visual capacity. *Child Development,* 45, 873.

Bronson, G.W. 1982. Structure, status, and characteristics of the nervous system at birth. In P. Stratton (Ed.), *Psychobiology of the Human Newborn.* New York: Wiley.

Brooks, J. & Weintraub, M. 1976. A history of infant intelligence testing. In M. Lewis (Ed.), *Origins of Intelligence: Infancy and Early Childhood.* New York: Plenum Press, p. 19.

Brouwers, P., Belman, A. & Epstein, L. 1990. Organ-specific complications: Central nervous system involvement, manifestations and evaluation. In J.S. Bruner, R.R. Oliver & P.M. Greenfield (Eds.), *Studies in Cognitive Growth.* New York: Wiley.

Brown, J.K. 1973. Convulsions in the neonatal period. *Developmental Medicine and Child Neurology,* 15, 823.

Brown, E.R. & Slobogin, P. 1987. Personality changes associated with tumors of the 4th ventricle. *Journal of Clinical and Experimental Neuropsychology,* 9, 57.

Brown, J.K., Purvis, R.J., Forfar, J.O. & Cockburn, F. 1974. Neurological aspects of perinatal asphyxia. *Developmental Medicine and Child Neurology,* 16, 567.

Brown, G., Chadwick, O., Shaffer, D., Rutter, M. & Traub, M. 1981. A prospective study of children with head injuries: Psychiatric sequelae. *Psychological Medicine,* 11, 63.

Brown, G.G., Spicer, K.B. & Malik, G. 1990. Neurobehavioral correlates of arteriovenous malformations and cerebral aneurysms. In R.A. Bornstein & G.G. Brown (Eds.), *Neurobehavioral Aspects of Cerebrovascular Disease.* New York: Oxford University Press, p. 202.

Brown, J.V., Schumacher, U., Rohlmann, A. & Ettlinger, G. 1989. Aimed movements to visual targets in hemiplegic and normal children: Is the 'good' hand of children with infantile hemiplegia also normal? *Neuropsychologia,* 27, 283.

Bruner, J. 1968. The course of cognitive growth. In N.S. Endler, L.R. Boulter & H. Osser (Eds.), *Contemporary Issues in Developmental Psychology.* New York: Holt, Rinehart & Winston.

Brunner, R.L. & Altman, J. 1974. The effects of interference with the maturation of the cerebellum and hippocampus on the development of adult behavior. In D.G. Stein, J.J. Rosen & N. Butters (Eds.), *Plasticity and Recovery of Function in the Central Nervous System.* New York: Academic Press.

Brunner, R.L., Berch, D.B. & Berry, H. 1987. Phenylketonuria and complex spatial visualization: An analysis of information processing. *Developmental Medicine and Child Neurology,* 29, 460.

Brunt, D. 1984. Apraxic tendencies in children with meningomyelocele. *Adapted Physical Activity Quarterly,* 1, 61.

Bruun, R.D. 1984. Giles de la Tourette's syndrome: An overview of clinical experience. *Journal of the American Academy of Child Psychiatry,* 23, 126.

Bruyer, R. 1985. Anatomical and behavioral study of a case of asymptomatic callosal agenesis. *Cortex,* 21, 417.

Bryden, M.P. 1979. Evidence for sex-related differences in cerebral organization. In M.A. Wittig and A.C. Petersen (Eds.), *Sex-Related Differences in Cognitive Functioning: Developmental Issues.* New York: Academic Press.

Bryden, M.P. 1982. *Laterality. Functional Asymmetry in the Intact Brain.* New York: Academic Press.

Bryden, M.P. 1988. Does laterality make any difference? Thoughts on the relation between cerebral asymmetry and reading. In D.F. Molfese & S.J. Segalowitz (Eds.), *Brain Lateralization in Children: Developmental Implications.* New York: Guilford Press, p. 509.

Bryden, M.P. & Allard, F.A. 1981. Do auditory perceptual asymmetries develop? *Cortex,* 17, 313.

Bryden, M. & Zurif, E. 1970. Dichotic listening performance in a case of agenesis of the corpus callosum. *Neuropsychologia,* 8, 371.

Bryhn, G. 1991. Attention deficit: A unitary phenomenon? *Tidsscrift for Norsk Psykologforening,* 28, 665.

Buchanan, A. & Oliver, J.E. 1977. Abuse and neglect as causes of mental retardation. A study of 140 children admitted to subnormality hospitals in Wiltshire. *British Journal of Psychiatry,* 131, 458.

Buchanan, S. 1984. The most ubiquitous toxin. *American Psychologist,* 39, 1327.

Buchsbaum, M.S. 1990. The frontal lobes, basal ganglia, and temporal lobes as sites for schizophrenia. *Schizophrenia Bulletin,* 16, 379.

Buehler, C. & Hetzer, H. 1935. *Testing Children's Development from Birth to School Age.* New York: Farrar & Rinehart, Inc.

Buffery, A.W.H. 1976. Sex differences in the neuropsychological development of verbal and spatial skills. In R.M. Knights & D.J. Bakker (Eds.), *The Neuropsychology of Learning Disorders: Theoretical Approaches.* Baltimore: University Park Press.

Buffery, A.W.H. & Gray, J.A. 1972. Sex differences in the development of spatial and linguistic skills. In C. Ounsted & D.C. Taylor (Eds.), *Gender Differences: Their Ontogeny and Significance.* Edinburgh: Churchill Livingstone.

Bullock, D. & Grossberg, S. 1989. Motor skill development and neural networks for position code invariance under speed and compliance rescaling. In H. Bloch & B.I. Bertenthal (Eds.), *Sensory-Motor Organizations and Development in Infancy and Early Childhood.* Doodrecht, Netherlands: Kluwer, p. 1.

Burack, J.A. & Zigler, E. 1990. Intentional and incidental memory in organically mentally retarded, familial retarded, and nonretarded individuals. *American Journal on Mental Retardation,* 94, 532.

Burd, L., Fisher, W.W., Kerbeshian, J. & Arnold, M.E. 1987. Is development of Tourette syndrome a marker for improvement in patients with autism and other pervasive developmental disorders? *Journal of the American Academy of Child and Adolescent Psychiatry,* 26, 162.

Burg, C., Rapoport, J.L., Bartley, L.S., Quinn, D.O. & Timmins, P. 1980. Newborn minor physical anomalies and problem behaviour at age 3. *American Journal of Psychiatry,* 137, 791.

Burklund, C.W. & Smith, A. 1977. Language and the cerebral hemispheres: Observations of verbal and nonverbal responses during 18 months following left ("dominant") hemispherectomy. *Neurology,* 27, 627.

Burling, T.A., Sappington, J.T. & Mead, A.M. 1983. Lateral specialization of a perpetual calendar task by a moderately retarded adult. *American Journal of Mental Deficiency,* 88, 326.

Burstein, B., Bank, L. & Jarvik, L.F. 1980. Sex differences in cognitive functioning: Evidence, determinants, implications. *Human Development,* 23, 289.

Bushnell, I.W.R. 1980. Face perception in early infancy. Unpublished PhD dissertation. Cambridge.

Butcher, H.J. 1968. *Human Intelligence.* London: Methuen.

Butcher, R.E., Hawver, K., Bubacher, T. & Scott, W. 1975. Behavioural effects from antenatal exposure to teratogens. In N.R. Ellis (Ed.), *Aberrant Development in Infancy.* Hillsdale, NJ: Erlbaum.

Butler, N.R. & Goldstein, H. 1973. Smoking in pregnancy and subsequent child development. *British Medical Journal,* 4, 573.

Butterbaugh, G.J. 1988. Selected psychometric and clinical review of neurodevelopmental infant tests. *The Clinical Psychologist,* 2, 4, 350.

Butterfield, S.A. 1986. Gross motor profiles of deaf children. *Perceptual and Motor Skills,* 62, 68.

Butterfield, S.A. & Ersing, W.P. 1986. Influence of age, sex, etiology, and hearing loss on balance performance by deaf children. *Perceptual and Motor Skills,* 62, 659.

Byrd, S.E. 1989. Magnetic resonance imaging of supratentorial congenital malformations. *Journal of the National Medical Association,* 81, 873.

Byring, F.K. & Michelsson, D.E. 1984. Prevalence of dyslexia in relatives of dyslexic children. *Acta Psychologica Scandinavia,* 46, 105.

Byrne, J.M. & Gates, R.D. 1987. Single-case study of left cerebral hemispherectomy: Development in the first five years of life. *Journal of Clinical and Experimental Neuropsychology,* 9, 423.

Byrne, J.M., Abbeduto, L. & Brooks, P. 1990. The language of children with spina bifida and hydrocephalus: Meeting task demands and mastering syntax. *Journal of Speech and Hearing Disorders,* 55, 118.

Cadoret, R.J., Cunningham, L., Loftus, R. & Edwards, J. 1975. Studies of adoptees from psychiatrically disturbed biologic parents. II. Temperament, hyperactive, antisocial and developmental variables. *Journal of Pediatrics,* 87, 301.

Caine, E.D., McBride, M.C. & Chiverton, P. 1988. Tourette syndrome in Monroe County school children. *Neurology,* 38, 472.

Cairns, G.F. & Butterfield, E.C. 1975. Assessing infants' auditory functioning. In B.Z. Friedlander (Ed.), *Exceptional Infant, Vol. 3, Assessment and Intervention.* New York: Brunner/Mazel.

Cairns, H. & Davidson, M.A. 1951. Hemispherectomy in the treatment of infantile hemiplegia. *Lancet,* 2, 411.

Caldwell, B.M. 1962. The usefulness of the critical period hypothesis in the study of filiative behaviours. *Merrill-Palmer Quarterly of Behaviour and Development,* 8, 229.

Callaway, E. 1973. Connections between average evoked potentials and measures of intelligence. *Archives of General Psychiatry,* 29, 553.

Camman, R. & Miehlke, A. 1989. Differentiation of motor activity of normally active and hyperactive boys in schools: Some preliminary results. *Journal of Child Psychology and Psychiatry and Allied Disciplines,* 30, 899.

Campbell, B. 1960. The factor of safety in the nervous system. *Bulletin of the Los Angeles Neurological Societies,* 23, 109.

Campbell, A.L., Bogen, J.E. & Smith, A. 1981. Disorganization and reorganization of cognitive and sensorimotor functions in cerebral commissurotomy. *Brain,* 104, 493.

Campbell, J.D. 1952. Manic-depressive psychosis in children: Report of eighteen cases. *Journal of Nervous and Mental Disorders,* 116, 424.

Campbell, P.H., Leib, S.A., Vollman, J. & Gibson, M. 1989. Interaction pattern and developmental outcome of infants with severe asphyxia: A longitudinal study of the first years of life. *Topics in Early Childhood Special Education,* 9, 48.

Cantwell, D.P. 1972. Psychiatric illness in families of hyperactive children. *Archives of General Psychiatry,* 27, 414.

Cantwell, D.P. 1975. Genetics of hyperactivity. *Journal of Child Psychology and Psychiatry,* 16, 261.

Cantwell, D.P. 1982. Depression in children with speech, language, and learning disorders. *Journal of Child Health in Contemporary Society,* 15, 51.

Cantwell, D.P. & Baker, L. 1987. Clinical significance of childhood communication disorders: Perspectives from a longitudinal study. *Journal of Child Neurology,* 2, 257.

Cantwell, D.P., Baker, L. & Rutter, M. 1978. Family factors in autism. A reappraisal of concepts and treatment. In M. Rutter and E. Schopler (Eds.), *Infantile Autism.* New York: Plenum Press.

Cantwell, D.P., Baker, L., Rutter, M. & Mawhood, L. 1989. Infantile autism and developmental receptive aphasia: A comparative follow-up into middle childhood. *Journal of Autism and Developmental Disorders,* 19, 19.

Caparulo, B.K. 1982. Computerized tomographic brain scanning in children with developmental neuropsychiatric disorders. *Annual Progress in Child Psychiatry and Child Development,* 1982, 550.

Caplan, P.G. & Kinsbourne, M. 1976. Baby drops the rattle: Asymmetry of duration of grasp by infants. *Child Development,* 47, 532.

Caplan, P.J., MacPherson, G.M. & Tobin, P. 1985. Do sex-related differences in spatial abilities exist? *American Psychologist,* 40, 786.

Caplan, R., Shields, W.D., Mori, L. & Yudovin, S. 1991. Middle childhood onset of interictal psychosis. *Journal of the American Academy of Child and Adolescent Psychiatry,* 30, 893.

Caplan, R., Guthrie, D., Mundy, P. & Sigman, M.D. 1992a. Non-verbal communication skills of surgically treated children with infantile spasms. *Developmental Medicine and Child Neurology,* 34, 499.

Caplan, R., Guthrie, D., Shields, W.D. & Mori, L. 1992b. Formal thought disorder in pediatric complex partial seizure disorder. *Journal of Child Psychology and Psychiatry and Allied Disciplines,* 33, 1399.

Caplan, R., Guthrie, D., Shields, W.D. & Sigman, M. 1992c. Early onset intractable seizures: Nonverbal communication after hemispherectomy. *Journal of Developmental and Behavioral Pediatrics*, 13, 348.

Caputo, D.V. & Mandell, W. 1970. Consequences of low birth weight. *Developmental Psychology*, 3, 363.

Caputo, D.V., Goldstein, K.M. & Taub, H.B. 1979. Development of prematurely-born children through middle childhood. In T.M. Field, A. Sostek, S. Goldberg & H. Shuman (Eds.), *Infants Born at Risk*. New York: Spectrum.

Caputo, D., Goldstein, K.M. & Taub, H.B. 1981. Neonatal compromise and later psychological development: A 10-year longitudinal study. In S.L. Friedman & M. Sigman (Eds.), *Preterm Birth and Psychological Development*. New York: Academic Press.

Cardozo-Martins, C., Mervis, C.B. & Mervis, C.A. 1985. Early vocabulary acquisition by children with Down syndrome. *American Journal of Mental Deficiency*, 90, 177.

Carey, W.B. & McDevitt, S.C. 1980. Minimal brain dysfunction and hyperkinesis: A clinical viewpoint. *American Journal of Diseases of Children*, 134, 926.

Carey, W.B., McDevitt, S.C. & Baker, D. 1979. Minimal brain dysfunction and temperament. *Developmental Medicine and Child Neurology*, 21, 765.

Carhart, R. 1967. Lesions due to kernicterus. *Acta Otolaryngologica* (Stockholm), Suppl. 221, 5.

Carlsson, G., Hugdahl, K., Uvebrant, P. & Wiklund, L.M. 1992. Pathological left-handedness revisited: Dichotic listening in children with left vs. right congenital hemiplegia. *Neuropsychologia*, 30, 471.

Carmichael, A.E. 1966. The current status of hemispherectomy for infantile hemiplegia. *Clinical Proceedings of the Children's Hospital*, 22, 285.

Caron, A.J. & Caron, R.F. 1981. Processing of relational information as an index of infant risk. In S.L. Friedman and M. Sigman (Eds.), *Preterm Birth and Psychological Development*. New York: Academic Press.

Carter, C.O. 1974. Clues to the etiology of neural tube malformations. *Developmental Medicine and Child Neurology*, 16, Suppl. 32, 3.

Carter-Saltzman, L. 1979. Patterns of cognitive functioning in relation to handedness and sex-related differences. In M.A. Wittig & A.C. Petersen (Eds.), *Sex-Related Differences in Cognitive Functioning: Developmental Issues*. New York: Academic Press.

Cartwright, G., Culbertson, K., Schreiner, R. & Gary, B. 1979. Changes in clinical presentation of term infants with intracranial hemorrhage. *Developmental Medicine and Child Neurology*, 21, 730.

Casey, J.E. & Rourke, B.P. 1992. Disorders of somatosensory perception. In I. Rapin & S.J. Segalowitz (Eds.), *Handbook of Neuropsychology, Vol. 6: Child Neuropsychology*. New York: Elsevier Science Publishers.

Casey, J.E., Rourke, B.P. & Picard, E.M. 1991. Syndrome of nonverbal learning disabilities: Age differences in neuropsychological, academic, and socioemotional functioning. *Development and Psychopathology*, 3, 329.

Casiro, O.G., Moddeman, D.M., Stanwick, R.S. & Panikkar-Thiessen, V.K. 1990. Language development of very low birth weight infants and full-term controls at 12 months of age. *Early Human Development*, 24, 65.

Casiro, O.G., Moddeman, D.M., Stanwick, R.S. & Cheang, M.S. 1991. The natural history and predictive value of early language delays in very low birth weight infants. *Early Human Development*, 26, 45.

Catalano, R.A., Calhoun, J.H., Reinecke, R.D. & Cogan, D.G. 1988. Asymmetry in congenital ocular motor apraxia. *Canadian Journal of Ophthalmology*, 23, 318.

Cattell, P. 1940, 1960, 1966. *The Measurement of Intelligence of Infants and Young Children*. New York: The Psychological Corporation.

Cattell, R.B. 1963. Theory of fluid and crystalized intelligence: A critical experiment. *Journal of Educational Psychology*, 54, 1.

Cattell, R.B. 1971. *Abilities: Their Structure, Growth and Action*. Boston: Houghton Mifflin.

Cavazzuti, G.B., Ferrari, P. & Lalla, M. 1984. Follow-up study of 482 cases with convulsive disorders during the first year of life. *Developmental Medicine and Child Neurology*, 26, 425.

Caviness, V.S. & Williams, R.S. 1979. Cellular pathology of developing human cortex. In R. Katzman (Ed.), *Congenital and Acquired Cognitive Disorders*. New York: Raven Press.

Chadwick, O., Rutter, M., Brown, G., Shaffer, D. & Traub, M. 1981. A prospective study of children with head injuries: II. Cognitive sequelae. *Psychological Medicine*, 11, 49.

Chadwick, O., Rutter, M., Shaffer, D. & Shrout, P.E. 1981. A prospective study of children with head injuries: IV. Specific cognitive deficits. *Journal of Clinical Neuropsychology*, 3(2), 101.

Chalfant, J.C. & Scheffelin, M.A. 1969. *Central Processing Dysfunction in Children: A Review of Research*. NINDS Monograph No. 9. Bethesda, MD: U.S Department of Health, Education and Welfare.

Chamberlain, R., Chamberlain, C., Howlett, B. & Claireaux, A. 1976. *British Births. Vol. 1. The First Week of Life*. London: Heinemann.

Chamove, A.S. & Molinaro, T.J. 1978. Monkey retarded learning analysis. *Journal of Mental Deficiency Research*, 22, 223.

Chamove, A.S., Kerr, G.R. & Harlow, H.F. 1973. Learning in monkeys fed elevated amino acid diets. *Journal of Medical Primatology*, 2, 223.

Chan, G.H., Jr. 1975a. Drug-induced side effects. In R.D. Harley (Ed.), *Pediatric Ophthalmology*. Philadelphia: W.B. Saunders.

Chan, G.H., Jr. 1975b. Nutritional deficiency disorders. In R.D. Harley (Ed.), *Pediatric Ophthalmology*. Philadelphia: W.B. Saunders.

Chang, P., Cook, R.D. & Fisch, R.O. 1983. Prognostic factors of the intellectual outcome of phenylketonuria: On and off diet. *Journal of Psychiatric Treatment and Evaluation*, 5, 157.

Chang, P., Weisberg, S. & Fisch, R.O. 1984. Growth development and its relationship to intellectual functioning of children with phenylketonuria. *Journal of Developmental and Behavioral Pediatrics*, 5, 127.

Chapman, J.W. 1980. *Affective Correlates of Learning Disabilities*. Lisse, Netherlands: Swets & Zeitlinger.

Chase, R.A. 1972. Neurological aspects of language disorders in children. In J.V. Irwin & M. Marge (Eds.), *Principles of Childhood Language Disabilities*. New York: Appleton-Century-Crofts.

Chelune, G.J. & Edwards, P. 1981. Early brain lesions: Ontogenetic-environmental considerations. *Journal of Consulting and Clinical Psychology*, 49, 777.

Chelune, G.J., Ferguson, W., Koon, R. & Dickey, T.O. 1986. Frontal lobe disinhibition in attention deficit disorder. *Child Psychiatry and Human Development*, 16, 221.

Cherian, A. & Kruvilla, K. 1989. Prevalence of neurological "soft signs" in affective disorders and their correlation to response to treatment. *Indian Journal of Psychiatry,* 31, 224.

Cherry, R.S. & Kruger, B. 1983. Selective auditory attention abilities of learning disabled and normal achieving children. *Journal of Learning Disabilities,* 16, 202.

Chess, S. 1971. Autism in children with congenital rubella. *Journal of Autism and Childhood Schizophrenia,* 1, 33.

Chess, S. 1977a. Follow-up report on autism in congenital rubella. *Journal of Autism and Childhood Schizophrenia.* 7(1), 69.

Chess, S. 1977b. Developmental theory revisited: Findings of a longitudinal study. *Canadian Journal of Psychiatry,* 24(2), 101.

Chess, S., Fernandez, P. & Korn, S. 1978. Behavioral consequences of congenital rubella. *Journal of Pediatrics,* 93, 699.

Chess, S., Fernandez, P. & Korn, S. 1980. The handicapped child and his family: consonance and dissonance. *Journal of the American Academy of Child Psychiatry,* 1980, 19, 56.

Chevrie, J.J. & Aicardie, J. 1977. Convulsive disorders in the first year of life: Etiological factors. *Epilepsia,* 18, 489.

Chevrie, J.J. & Aicardie, J. 1978. Convulsive disorders in the first year of life: Neurological and mental outcome and mortality. *Epilepsia,* 19, 67.

Chi, J.G., Dooling, E. & Gilles, F.H. 1977. Gyral development of the human brain. *Annals of Neurology,* 1, 86.

Chiappa, K.H. 1985. *Evoked Potentials in Clinical Medicine.* New York: Raven Press.

Chiarello, C. 1980. A house divided? Cognitive functioning with callosal agenesis. *Brain and Language,* 11(1), 128.

Chikovani, M.I. 1984. Characteristics of the neuropsychological development of premature children with perinatal brain damage. *Soviet Neurology and Psychiatry,* 17, 3.

Child, C.M. 1941. *Patterns and Problems of Development.* Chicago: University of Chicago Press.

Chisholm, I.H. 1975. Cortical blindness in cranial arteritis. *British Journal of Ophthalmology,* 59, 332.

Choux, M., Lena, G. & Genitori, L. 1992. Intracranial aneurysms in children. In A.J. Raimondi, M. Choux, & C. DiRocco (Eds.), *Cerebrovascular Diseases in Children.* New York: Springer-Verlag, p. 123.

Christiansen, K.O. 1977. A review of studies of criminality among twins. In S.A. Mednick & K.O. Christiansen (Eds.), *Biosocial Bases of Criminal Behavior.* New York: Gardner Press. p. 45.

Churchill, J.A., Inga, E. & Senf, R. 1962. The association of position at birth and handedness. *Pediatrics,* 29, 307.

Churchill, J.A., Masland, R.L., Naylor, A.A. & Ashworth, M.R. 1974. The etiology of cerebral palsy in preterm infants. *Developmental Medicine and Child Neurology,* 16, 143.

Cialdella, P. & Mamelle, N. 1989. An epidemiological study of infantile autism in a French department (Rhone): A research note. *Journal of Child Psychology and Psychiatry and Allied Disciplines,* 30, 165.

Ciesielski, K.T., Courchesne, E. & Elmasian, R. 1990. Effects of focused selective attention tasks on event-related potentials in autistic and normal individuals. *Electroencephalography and Clinical Neurophysiology,* 75, 207.

Ciganek, L. 1961. The EEG response (evoked potential) to light stimulus in man. *Electroencephalography and Clinical Neurophysiology,* 13, 165.

Cioni, G. & Pellegrinetti, G. 1982. Lateralization of sensory and motor functions in human neonates. *Perceptual and Motor Skills,* 54, 1151.

Cioni, G., Biagioni, E. & Cipolloni, C. 1990. Brain before cognition: EEG maturation in preterm infants. In I. Kostovic, S. Knezevic, H. Wiesniewski & G.J. Spilich (Eds.), *Neurodevelopment, Aging and Cognition.* Boston: Birkhauser, p. 75.

Clark, C.M. & Klonoff, H. 1990. Right and left orientation in children aged 5 to 15 years. *Journal of Clinical and Experimental Neuropsychology,* 12, 459.

Clark, M.M. 1970. *Reading Difficulties in School.* Harmondsworth: Penguin.

Clark-Stewart, K.A. 1973. Interactions between mothers and their children: Characteristics and consequences. *Monographs of the Society for Research in Child Development,* 38 (6, Serial No. 153).

Clarke, J.T.R., Gates, R.D., Hogan, S.E., Barrett, M. & MacDonald, G.W. 1987. Neuropsychological studies on adolescents with phenylketonuria returned to phenylalanine-restricted diets. *American Journal of Mental Deficiency,* 92, 255.

Clarke, S., Kraftsik, R., Van der Loos, H. & Innocenti, G.M. 1989. Forms and measures of adult and developing corpus callosum: Is there sexual dimorphism? *Journal of Comparative Neurology,* 8, 213.

Clarkson, R.L., Eimas, P.D. & Marean, G.C. 1989. Speech perception in children with histories of recurrent otitis media. *Journal of the Acoustical Society of America,* 85, 926.

Clausen, J.P., Flook, M.H., Ford, B., Green, M.M. & Popiel, E.S. 1973. *Maternity Nursing Today,* New York: McGraw-Hill.

Cleland, C.C. 1979. *The Profoundly Mentally Retarded.* Englewood Cliffs, NJ: Prentice-Hall.

Clements, S.D. 1966. *Minimal Brain Dysfunction in Children.* Monographs, No. 3. Bethesda, MD: U.S. National Institute of Neurological Disease and Blindness.

Clements, S.D. & Peters, J.E. 1981. Syndromes of minimal brain dysfunction. In P. Black (Ed.), *Brain Dysfunction in Children: Etiology, Diagnosis and Management.* New York: Raven Press, 1981.

Clemmons, D.C. & Dodrill, C.B. 1983. Vocational outcomes of high school students with epilepsy. *Journal of Applied Rehabilitation Counseling,* 14, 49.

Clopton, B.M. 1981. Neurophysiological and anatomical aspects of auditory development. In R.N. Aslin, J.R. Alberts & M.R. Petersen (Eds.), *Development of Perception: Psychobiological Perspectives. Vol. 1: Audition, Somatic Perception, and the Chemical Senses.* New York: Academic Press.

Cobrinik, L. 1982. The performance of hyperlexic children on an "incomplete words" task. *Neuropsychologia,* 20(5) 569.

Cohen, A.J. & Baird, K. 1990. Acquisition of absolute pitch: The question of critical periods. *Psychomusicology,* 9, 31.

Cohen, D.J., Bruun, R.D. & Leckman, J.F. 1988. *Tourette's Syndrome and Tic Disorders: Clinical Understanding and Treatment.* New York: Wiley.

Cohen, H., Gelinas, C., Lassonde, M. & Geoffroy, G. 1991. Auditory lateralization for speech in language-impaired children. *Brain and Language,* 41, 395.

Cohen, M. 1992. Auditory-verbal and visual-spatial memory in children with complex partial epilepsy of temporal lobe origin. *Brain and Cognition,* 20, 315.

Cohen, M.E. & Duffner, P.K. 1985. Current therapy in childhood brain tumors. *Neurology Clinics,* 3, 147.

Cohen, M.J., Holmes, G.L., Campbell, R. & Smith, J.R. 1991. Cognitive functioning following anterior two-thirds corpus callosotomy in children and adolescents: A one-year prospective report. *Journal of Epilepsy*, 4, 63.

Cohen, N.J. & Lipsett, L. 1991. Recognized and unrecognized language impairment in psychologically disturbed children: Child symptomatology, maternal depression, and family dysfunction. Preliminary report. *Canadian Journal of Behavioural Science*, 23, 376.

Cohen, N.J., Sullivan, J., Minde, K., Novak, C. & Helwig, C. 1981. Evaluation of the relative effectiveness of methylphenidate and cognitive behavior modification in the treatment of kindergarten-aged hyperactive children. *Journal of Abnormal Child Psychology*, 9, 43.

Cohen, R.A. 1993. *The Neuropsychology of Attention*. New York: Plenum.

Cohen, S.A., Parmelee, A.H., Beckwith, L. & Sigman, M. 1992. Biological and social precursors of 12-year competence in children born preterm. In C.W. Greenbaum and J.G. Auerbach (Eds.), *Longitudinal Studies of Children at Psychological Risk: Cross-National Perspectives*. Norwood, NJ: Ablex Publishing Co.

Cohn, N.B., Kircher, J., Emmerson, R.Y. & Dustman, R.E. 1985. Pattern reversal evoked potentials: Age, sex and hemispheric asymmetry. *Electroencephalography and Clinical Neurophysiology*, 62, 399.

Cole, A.J., Andermann, F., Taylor, L. & Olivier, A. 1988. The Landau-Kleffner syndrome of acquired epileptic aphasia: Unusual clinical outcome, surgical experience, and absence of encephalitis. *Neurology*, 38, 31.

Collins, A.L. 1951. Epileptic intelligence. *Journal of Consulting Psychology*, 15, 393.

Collins, A.L. & Lennox, W.G. 1947. The intelligence of 300 private-patient epileptics. *Proceedings of the Association for Research in Nervous and Mental Diseases*, 26, 586.

Colombo, J. 1982. The critical period concept: Research, methodology and theoretical issues. *Psychological Bulletin*, 91(2), 260.

Colombo, J., Mitchell, D.W., O'Brien, M. & Horowitz, F.D. 1987. The stability of visual habituation during the first year of life. *Child Development*, 58, 474.

Comings, D.E. & Comings, B.G. 1984. Tourette's syndrome and attention deficit disorder with hyperactivity: Are they genetically related? *Journal of the American Academy of Child Psychiatry*, 23, 138.

Commey, J.O.O. & Fitzhardinge, P.M. 1979. Handicap in the preterm small-for-gestational age infant. *Journal of Pediatrics*, 94, 779.

Commission of the European Community. 1980. *Childhood Deafness in the European Community*. Luxembourg: CEC.

Conde-Lopez, V., delaGandara-Martin, J.J. & deSantiago-Juarez-Lopez. 1983. Signos neurologicos suave (soft-sign) en los trastornos affectivos. *Revista del Departamento de Psyquiatrica de la Facultad de Medicina de Barcelona*, 10, 390.

Condini, A., Axia, G., Cattelan, C. & D'Urso, M.R. 1991. Development of language in 18 30-month-old HIV-1-infected but not ill children. *AIDS*, 5, 735.

Conel, J. 1939–1967. *The Postnatal Development of the Human Cerebral Cortex*, Vols. 1–8. Cambridge, MA: Harvard University Press.

Conners, C.K. 1972. Psychological effects of stimulant drugs in children with minimal brain dysfunction. *Pediatrics*, 49, 702.

Conners, C.K. 1980. *Food Additives and Hyperactive Children*. New York: Plenum Press, 1980.

Conners, C.K. & Wells, K.C. 1986. *Hyperkinetic Children: A Neuropsychological Approach*. Beverly Hills: Sage.

Conners, C.K., Taylor, E., Meo, G., Kurtz, M.A., & Fournier, M. 1972. Magnesium pemoline and dextroamphetamine: A controlled study in children with minimal brain dysfunction. *Psychopharmacologica, 62,* 321.

Connolly, J.A. 1978. Intelligence levels of Down's syndrome children. *American Journal of Mental Deficiency, 83,* 193.

Connolly, K. 1973. Learning and the concept of critical periods in infancy. In S. Chess & A. Thomas (Eds.), *Annual Progress in Psychology and Child Development.* New York: Plenum Press.

Connolly, K.J. & Prechtl, H.F.R. (Eds.) 1981. *Maturation and Development: Biological and Psychological Perspectives.* London: SIMP/Heineman.

Connolly, K. & Stratton, P. 1968. Developmental changes in associated movements. *Developmental Medicine and Child Neurology, 10,* 49.

Conrad, A.J. & Scheibel, A.B. 1987. Schizophrenia and the hippocampus: The embryological hypothesis extended. *Schizophrenia Bulletin, 13,* 577.

Conte, R. 1991. Attention disorders. In B.Y.L. Wong (Ed.), *Learning About Learning Disabilities.* New York: Academic Press.

Conte, R., Kinsbourne, M., Swanson, J., Zirk, H. & Samuels, M. 1986. Presentation rate effects on paired associate learning by attention deficit disordered children. *Child Development, 57,* 681.

Cooke, J. 1980. Early organization of the central nervous system: Form and pattern. In R.K. Hunt (Ed.), *Neural Development, Part I* (Current Topics in Developmental Biology, Vol. 15). New York: Academic Press, 1980.

Coolman, R.B., Bennett, F.C., Sells, C.J., Swanson, M.W., Andrews, M.S. & Robinson, N.M. 1985. Neuromotor development of graduates of the neonatal intensive care unit: Patterns encountered in the first two years of life. *Journal of Developmental and Behavioral Pediatrics, 6,* 327.

Cooper, J.A. & Ferry, P.C. 1978. Acquired auditory verbal agnosia and seizures in childhood. *Journal of Speech and Hearing Disorders, 43,* 176.

Cooper, J.A. & Flowers, C.R. 1987. Children with a history of acquired aphasia: Residual language and academic impairments. *Journal of Speech and Hearing Disorders, 52,* 251.

Cooper, J.A. & Griffiths, P. 1978. Treatment and prognosis. In M.A. Wyke (Ed.), *Developmental Dysphasia.* New York: Academic Press.

Cooper, R.M. & Zubek, J.P. 1958. Effects of enriched and restricted early environments on the learning ability of bright and dull rats. *Canadian Journal of Psychology, 12,* 159.

Corah, N.L., Anthony, E.J., Painter, P., Stern, J. & Thurston, D. 1965. Effects of perinatal anoxia after seven years. *Psychological Monographs, 79* (whole No. 596).

Corballis, M.C. 1983. *Human Laterality.* New York: Academic Press.

Corballis, M.C. & Morgan, M.J. 1978. On the biological basis of human laterality I. Evidence for a maturational left-right gradient. *The Behavioral and Brain Sciences, 2,* 261.

Corbett, J.A., Trimble, M.R. & Nichol, T.C. 1985. Behavioral and cognitive impairments in children with epilepsy: The long-term effects of anticonvulsant therapy. *Journal of the American Academy of Child Psychiatry, 24,* 17.

Coren, S. & Halpern, D.F. 1991. Left-handedness: A marker for decreased survival fitness. *Psychological Bulletin, 109,* 90.

Coren, S. & Porac, C. 1980. Birth factors and laterality: Effects of birth order, parental age, and birth stress on four indices of lateral preference. *Behavior Genetics, 10,* 123.

Cornblatt, B.A. & Erlenmeyer-Kimling, L. 1985. Global attentional deviance as a marker of risk for schizophrenia: Specificity and predictive validity. *Journal of Abnormal Psychology*, 94, 470.

Coryell, J. & Michel, G. 1978. How supine postural preferences of infants can contribute toward the development of handedness. *Infant Behavior and Development*, 1, 245.

Costeff, H., Reshef, A., Bergman, M. & Koren, V. 1988. Eye-sighting preference of normal and hemiplegic children and adults. *Developmental Medicine and Child Neurology*, 30, 360.

Costello, E.J. 1991. Child psychiatric epidemiology: Implications for clinical research and practice. In B.B. Lahey & A.E. Kazdin (Eds.), *Advances in Clinical Child Psychology*, Vol. 13. New York: Plenum Press.

Cotman, C.W. & Banker, G.A. 1974. The making of a synapse. In S. Ehrenpreis & I.J. Kopin (Eds.), *Reviews of Neuroscience*, Vol. 1. New York: Raven Press.

Cotman, C.W. & Nieto-Sampedro, M. 1982. Brain function, synapse renewal, and plasticity. *Annual Review of Psychology*, 33, 371.

Cotman, C.W. & Nieto-Sampedro, M. 1984. Cell biology of synaptic plasticity. *Science*, 225, 1287.

Coulter, D.L. 1987. The neurology of mental retardation. In F.J. Menolascino & J.F. Stark (Eds.), *Preventative and Curative Intervention in Mental Retardation*. Baltimore: Paul H. Brookes.

Courchesne, E. 1991. Chronology of human brain development: Event-related potential, positron emission tomography, myelinogenesis, and synaptogenesis studies. In J.W. Rohrbaugh, R. Parasuraman & R. Johnson (Eds.), *Event-Related Brain Potentials: Basis Issues and Applications*. New York: Oxford University Press, p. 210.

Courchesne, E., Lincoln, A.J., Yeung-Courchesne, R. & Elmasian, R. 1989. Pathophysiologic findings in nonretarded autism and receptive developmental language disorder. *Journal of Autism and Developmental Disorders*, 19, 1.

Coursin, D.B. 1974. Electrophysiological studies in malnutrition. In J. Cravioto, L. Hambraeus & B. Vahlquist (Eds.), *Early Malnutrition and Mental Development*. Uppsala: Swedish Nutrition Foundation.

Cowan, W.M. 1979. The development of the brain. *Scientific American*, 241(3), 112.

Cowan, W.M., Stanfield, B.B. & Kishi, K. 1980. The development of the dentate gyrus. In R.K. Hunt (Ed.), *Neural Development, Part I* (Current Topics in Developmental Biology, Vol. 15). New York: Academic Press.

Cowan, W.M., Fawcett, J.W., O'Leary, D.D.M. & Stanfield, B.B. 1984. Regressive events in neurogenesis. *Science*, 225, 1258.

Cox, A., Rutter, M., Newman, S. & Bartak, L. 1975. A comparative study of infantile autism and specific developmental receptive language disorder. II. Parental characteristics. *British Journal of Psychiatry*, 126, 146.

Craft, A., Shaw, D. & Cartlidge, N. 1972. Head injuries in children. *British Medical Journal*, 4, 200.

Craft, S., Willerman, L. & Bigler, E. 1987. Collosal dysfunction in schizoaffective disorder. *Journal of Abnormal Psychology*, 96, 205.

Craft, S., Gourovitch, M.L., Dowton, S.B. & Swanson, J.M. 1992. Lateralized deficits in visual attention in males with developmental dopamine depletion. *Neuropsychologia*, 30, 341.

Cravioto, J. & Arrieta, R. 1979. Stimulation and mental development of malnourished infants. *Lancet*, 2(8148), 899.

Cravioto, J. & DeLicardie, E. 1975. Longitudinal study of language development in severely malnourished children. In G. Serban (Ed.), *Nutrition and Mental Functions. Advances in Behavioral Biology*, Vol. XIV. New York: Plenum Press.

Cravioto, J., DeLicardie, E. & Birch, H. 1966. Nutrition, growth, and neuro-integrative development: An experimental and ecologic study. *Pediatrics*, 38, 319.

Cravioto, J., Birch, H.G. & Gaona, C.E. 1967. Early malnutrition and auditory-visual integration in school-age children. *Journal of Special Education*, 2, 75.

Creak, M. & Ini, S. 1960. Families of psychotic children. *Journal of Child Psychology and Psychiatry*, 1, 156.

Creighton, D.E. & Sauve, R.S. 1988. The Minnesota Infant Developmental Inventory in the development screening of high-risk infants at eight months. *Canadian Journal of Behavioural Science*, 20, 4, 424.

Cremieux, J., Buisseret, F. & Gary-Bobo, E. 1992. Experimental evidence that rearing kittens in stroboscopic light retards maturation of the visual cortex: A new tool for studying critical periods. *Vision Research*, 32, 41.

Critchley, M., & Critchley, E.A. 1978. *Dyslexia Defined*. London: Heinemann.

Crnic, L. 1977. Effects of infantile undernutrition on adult learning in rats: Methodological and design problems. *Psychological Bulletin*, 83(4), 715.

Crome, L., Cowie, V. & Slater, E. 1966. A statistical note on the cerebellar and brain stem weight in mongolism. *Journal of Mental Deficiency Research*, 10, 69.

Cromer, R.F. 1978. The basis of childhood dysphasia: A linguistic approach. In M.A. Wyke (Ed.), *Developmental Dysphasia*. New York: Academic Press.

Crow, T.J. 1980. Positive and negative schizophrenia symptoms and the role of dopamine. *British Journal of Psychiatry*, 149, 383.

Crow, T.J. 1987. Integrated viral genes as potential pathogens in the functional psychoses. *Journal of Psychiatric Research*, 21, 470.

Crowell, D.H., Jones, R.H., Kapuniai, L.E. & Nakagawa, J.K. 1973. Unilateral cortical activity in newborn humans: An early index of cerebral dominance? *Science*, 180, 205.

Crowner, M.L., Jaeger, J., Convit, A. & Brizer, D.A. 1987. Minor physical anomalies in violent adult inpatients. *Biological Psychiatry*, 22, 1166.

Cruickshank, W.M., Hallahan, D.P. & Bice, H.V. 1976a. The evaluation of intelligence. In W.M. Cruickshank (Ed.), *Cerebral Palsy, A Developmental Disability*, 3rd ed. Syracuse, NY: Syracuse University Press.

Cruickshank, W.M., Hallahan, D.P. & Bice, H.V. 1976b. Personality and behavioral characteristics. In W.M. Cruickshank (Ed.), *Cerebral Palsy: A Developmental Disability*, 3rd ed. Syracuse, NY: Syracuse University Press.

Culatta, B. & Young, C. 1992. Linguistic performance as a function of abstract task demands in children with spina bifida. *Developmental Medicine and Child Neurology*, 34, 434.

Culp, D.M. 1989. Developmental apraxia and augmentative and alternative communication: A case example. *Augmentative and Alternative Communication*, 5, 27.

Cumming, C.E. & Rodda, M. 1985. The effects of auditory deprivation on successive processing. *Canadian Journal of Behavioral Science*, 17, 232.

Cunningham, C.C. 1979. Aspects of early development in Down's syndrome infants. Ph.D. Dissertation. University of Manchester, England.

Cunningham, C.C. & Mittler, P.J. 1981. Maturation, development and mental handicap. In K.J. Connolly & H.F.R. Prechtl (Eds.), *Maturation and Development: Biological and Psychological Perspectives*. London: Heinemann.

Curatolo, P., Libutti, G. & Matricardi, M. 1981. Infantile spasms: A neuro-ophthalmological study. *Developmental Medicine and Child Neurology*, 23, 449.

Curtiss, S. 1977. *Genie: A Psycholinguistic Study of a Modern-Day Wild Child*. New York: Academic Press.

Curtiss, S., Fromkin, V., Rigler, D., Rigler, M. & Krashen, S. 1975. An update on the linguistic development of Genie. In D.P. Dato (Ed.), *Developmental Psycholinguistics: Theory and Applications*. Washington, DC: Georgetown University Press.

Cutting, J. 1990. *The Right Cerebral Hemisphere and Psychiatric Disorders*. Oxford: Oxford University Press.

Cynader, M.S. 1982. Modifiability of visual cortex under sensory deprivation. *Neurosciences Research Program Bulletin*, 20, 549.

Cytryn, L. 1984. A developmental view of affective disturbances in the children of affectively ill parents. *American Journal of Psychiatry*, 141, 219.

Dabiri, C. 1979. Respiratory distress syndrome. In T. Field, A. Sostek, S. Goldberg & H. Shuman (Eds.), *Infants Born at Risk*. New York: Spectrum Press.

Dalby, J.T. 1979. Deficit or delay: Neuropsychological models of developmental dyslexia. *Journal of Special Education*, 13, 239.

Dalby, M.A. 1975. Air studies in language-retarded children. Evidence of early lateralization of language function. First International Congress of Child Neurology, Toronto.

Damasio, A.R., Lima, A. & Damasio, H. 1975. Nervous function after right hemispherectomy. *Neurology*, 25, 89.

Damasio, H. 1991. Neuroanatomical correlates of aphasia. In M.T. Sarno (Ed.), *Acquired Aphasia*, 2nd ed. San Diego: Academic Press.

Damasio, H. & Damasio, A. 1980. The anatomical basis of conduction aphasia. *Brain*, 103, 337.

Dandy, W.E. 1928. Removal of right cerebral hemisphere for certain tumours with hemiplegia. *Journal of the American Medical Association*, 90, 823.

Dann, M., Levine, S.Z. & New, E.V. 1958. The development of prematurely born children with minimal postnatal weights of 1000 grams or less. *Pediatrics*, 22, 1037.

Darley, F.L. & Fay, W.H. 1980. Speech mechanism. In F.M. Lassman, R.O. Fisch, D.K. Vetter & E.S. La Benz (Eds.), *Early Correlates of Speech, Language, and Hearing*. Littleton, MA: PSG Publishing, p. 199.

Das, J.P. & Varnhagen, C.K. 1986. Neuropsychological functioning and cognitive processing. In J.E. Obrzut & G.W. Hynd (Eds.), *Child Neuropsychology*, Vol. 1. Orlando, FL: Academic Press.

Das, J.P., Kirby, J.R. & Jarman, R.F. 1979. *Simultaneous and Successive Cognitive Processes*. New York: Academic Press.

David, O., Clark, J. & Voeller, K. 1972. Lead and hyperactivity. *Lancet*, 2, 900.

Davie, R., Butler, N. & Goldstein, H. 1972. *From Birth to Seven: A Report of the National Child Developmental Study*. London: Longman.

Davies, D.P., Gray, O.P. & Ellwood, P.C. 1976. Cigarette smoking in pregnancy: Associations with maternal weight gain and fetal growth. *Lancet*, 1, 385.

Davies, P. & Stewart, A.L. 1975. Low birth-weight infants: Neurological sequelae and later intelligence. *British Medical Bulletin*, 31, 85.

Davies, P. & Tizard, J.P. 1975. Very low birth weight and subsequent neurological defect. *Developmental Medicine and Child Neurology*, 17, 3.

Davis, A.E. & Wada, J. 1977. Hemispheric asymmetries in human infants: Spectral analysis of flash and click evoked potentials. *Brain and Language*, 4, 23.

Davis, D.D., McIntyre, C.W., Murray, M.E. & Mims, S.S. 1986. Cognitive styles in children with dietary-treated phenylketonuria. *Educational and Psychological Research*, 6, 9.

Davis, E., Fennoy, I., Laraque, D. & Kanem, N. 1992. Autism and developmental abnormalities in children with perinatal cocaine exposure. *Journal of the National Medical Association*, 84, 315.

Davis, J.M., Elfenbein, J., Schum, R. & Bentler, R.A. 1986. Effects of mild and moderate hearing impairment on language, educational, and psychosocial behavior of children. *Journal of Speech and Hearing Disorders*, 51, 53.

Davison, A.N. 1977. The biochemistry of brain development and mental retardation. *British Journal of Psychiatry*, 131, 565.

Davison, A.N. & Peters, A. 1970. *Myelination*. Springfield, Ill: Charles C Thomas.

Dawson, G. 1983. Lateralized brain dysfunction in autism: Evidence from the Halstead-Reitan neuropsychological battery. *Journal of Autism and Developmental Disorders*, 13, 269.

Day, N.L., Robles, N., Richardson, G. & Geva, D. 1991. The effects of prenatal alcohol use on the growth of children at three years of age. *Alcoholism, Clinical and Experimental Research*, 15, 67.

De Ajuriaguerra, J., Jaeggi, A., Guignard, F., Kocher, F., Maquard, M., Roth, S. & Schmid, E. 1976. The development and prognosis of dysphasia in children. In D.M. Morehead & A.E. Morehead (Eds.), *Normal and Deficient Child Language*. Baltimore: University Park Press.

Dean, R. 1983. Neuropsychological correlates of total seizures with major motor epileptic children. *Journal of Clinical Neuropsychology*, 5, 1.

Decker, S.N. & DeFries, J.C. 1980. Cognitive abilities in families with reading disabled children. *Journal of Learning Disabilities*, 13, 9.

de Courten, G.M. & Rabinowicz, T. 1981a. Analysis of 100 infant deaths with intraventricular hemorrhage: Brain weights and risk factors. *Developmental Medicine and Child Neurology*, 23(3), 287.

de Courten, G.M. & Rabinowicz, T. 1981b. Intraventricular hemorrhage in premature infants: Reappraisal and new hypothesis. *Developmental Medicine and Child Neurology*, 23(3), 389.

DeFries, J.C., Stevenson, J., Gillis, J.J. & Wadsworth, S.J. 1991. Genetic etiology of spelling deficits in the Colorado and London twin studies of reading disability. *Reading and Writing*, 3, 271.

Deeg, K.H., Bundscherer, F. & Bowing, B. 1986. Zerebrale Ultraschall-Diagnostik bei Hirnmissbildungen. *Monatsschrift für Kinderheilkunde*, 134, 738.

de Haas, P.A. & Young, R.D. 1984. Attention styles of hyperactive and normal girls. *Journal of Abnormal Child Psychology*, 12, 531.

DeHirsch, K. 1957. Tests designed to discover potential reading difficulty. *American Journal of Orthopsychiatry*, 27, 566.

DeHirsch, K., Jansky, J. & Langford, W.S. 1966. Comparison between prematurely and maturely born children at three age levels. *American Journal of Orthopsychiatry*, 36, 616.

Dejerine, J. 1892. Contribution a l'etude anatomoclinique et clinique des differentes varietes de cecite verbale. *C.R. Societee Biologique*, 4, 61.

Dekaban, A. 1967. On clinical and epidemiological aspects of mental retardation. In G.A. Jervis (Ed.), *Mental Retardation*. Springfield, IL: Charles C Thomas.

Dekaban, A. 1970. *Neurology of Early Childhood*. Baltimore: Williams & Wilkins.

de Lacoste, M.C., Holloway, R.L. & Woodward, J. 1986. Sex differences in the fetal human corpus callosum. *Human Neurobiology,* 5, 93.

de Lacoste, M.C., Horvath, D.S. & Woodward, D.J. 1991. Possible sex differences in the developing human fetal brain. *Journal of Clinical and Experimental Neuropsychology,* 13, 831.

De Loache, J.S., Cassidy, D.J. & Brown, A.L. 1985. Where do I go next? Intelligent searching by very young children. *Developmental Psychology,* 20, 37.

DeLong, G.R. & Adams, R.D. 1975. Clinical aspects of tumors of the posterior fossa in childhood. In P.J. Vincken and G.W. Bruyn (Eds.), *Handbook of Clinical Neurology.* Vol. 18, part III. Amsterdam: North Holland.

DeMarco, S., Harbour, A., Hume, W.G. & Givens, G.D. 1989. Perception of time-altered monosyllables in a specific group of phonologically disordered children. *Neuropsychologia,* 27, 753.

DeMyer, M., Pontinis, W., Norton, J., Barton, S., Allen, J. & Steele, R. 1972. Parental practices and innate activity in autistic and brain damaged infants. *Journal of Autism and Childhood Schizophrenia,* 2, 49.

DeMyer, M.K., Hingtgen, J.N. & Jackson, R.K. 1981. Infantile autism reviewed: A decade of research. *Schizophrenia Bulletin,* 7, 388.

DeMyer, W. 1975. Congenital anomalies of the central nervous system. In D.B. Tower (Ed.), *The Nervous System. Vol. 2: The Clinical Neurosciences.* New York: Raven Press, 347.

Denbigh, K. 1979. Neurological impairment and educational achievement: A follow-up of learning-disabled children. M.A. thesis. University of Victoria.

Denckla, M.B. 1977. Minimal brain dysfunction and dyslexia—Beyond diagnosis by exclusion. In M.E. Blaw, I. Rapin & M. Kinsbourne (Eds.), *Topics in Child Neurology.* Jamaica: Spectrum Publications.

Denckla, M.B. 1978. Minimal brain dysfunction. In J.S. Chall & A.F. Mirsky (Eds.), *Education and the Brain.* Chicago: University of Chicago Press, p. 223.

Denckla, M.B. 1979. Childhood learning disabilities. In K.M. Heilman & E. Valenstein (Eds.), *Clinical Neuropsychology.* New York: Oxford University Press.

Denckla, M.B. 1985. Revised neurological examination for subtle signs. *Psychopharmacology Bulletin,* 24, 773.

Denckla, M.B., Rudel, R.B. & Broman, M. 1978. Spatial orientation skills. In D. Caplan (Ed.), *Biological Studies of Mental Processes.* Cambridge, MA: MIT Press.

Denckla, M.B., LeMay, M. & Chapman, C.A. 1985a. Few CT scan abnormalities found even in neurologically impaired learning disabled children. *Journal of Learning Disabilities,* 18, 132.

Denckla, M.B., Rudel, R.G., Chapman, C. & Krieger, J. 1985b. Motor proficiency in dyslexic children with and without attentional disorders. *Archives of Neurology,* 42, 228.

De Negri, M. 1967. Le disfunzioni pratto-gnosiche nell'eta evolutiva. *Gazetta Sanitario* (Milano), 38, 275.

Denhoff, E. 1976. Medical aspects. In W.M. Cruickshank (Ed.), *Cerebral Palsy: A Developmental Disability,* 3rd ed. Syracuse, NY: Syracuse University Press.

Denhoff, E. & Robinault, I.P. 1960. *Cerebral Palsy and Related Disorders: A Developmental Approach to Dysfunction.* New York: McGraw-Hill.

Dennenberg, V.H. 1968. A consideration of the usefulness of the critical period hypothesis as applied to the stimulation of rodents in infancy. In G. Newton and S. Levine (Eds.), *Early Experience and Behaviour.* Springfield, IL: Charles C Thomas.

Dennis, J. & Bower, B.D. 1972. The Aicardie syndrome. *Developmental Medicine and Child Neurology,* 14, 382.

Dennis, M. 1976. Impaired sensory and motor differentiation with corpus callosum agenesis: A lack of callosal inhibition during ontogeny? *Neuropsychologia,* 14, 455.

Dennis, M. 1977. Cerebral dominance in three forms of early brain disorder. In M.E. Blau, I. Rapin & M. Kinsbourne (Eds.), *Topics in Child Neurology.* New York: Spectrum Publications.

Dennis, M. 1980a. Capacity and strategy for syntactic comprehension after left or right hemidecortication. *Brain and Language,* 10, 287.

Dennis, M. 1980b. Language acquisition in a single hemisphere: Semantic organization. In D. Caplan (Ed.), *Biological Studies of Mental Processes.* Cambridge, MA: MIT Press, p. 159.

Dennis, M. 1980c. Strokes in childhood. I: Communicative intent, expression, and comprehension after left hemisphere arteriopathy in a right-handed nine year old. In R.W. Rieber (Ed.), *Language Development and Aphasia in Children.* New York: Academic Press.

Dennis, M. 1981. Language in a congenitally acallosal brain. *Brain and Language,* 12, 33.

Dennis, M. 1992. Word finding in children and adolescents with a history of brain injury. *Topics in Language Disorders,* 13, 66.

Dennis, M. & Barnes, M. 1990. Knowing the meaning, getting the point, bridging the gap, and carrying the message: Aspects of discourse following closed head injury in childhood and adolescence. *Brain and Language,* 39, 428.

Dennis, M. & Kohn, B. 1975. Comprehension of syntax in infantile hemiplegics after cerebral hemidecortication: Left-hemisphere superiority. *Brain and Language,* 2, 472.

Dennis, M. & Lovett, M.W. 1990. Discourse ability in children after brain damage. In Y. Joanette & H.H. Brownell (Eds.), *Discourse Ability and Brain Damage: Theoretical and Empirical Perspectives.* New York: Springer, p. 199.

Dennis, M. & Whitaker, H.A. 1976. Language acquisition following hemidecortication: Linguistic superiority of the left over the right hemisphere. *Brain and Language,* 3, 404.

Dennis, M. & Whitaker, H.A. 1977. Hemispheric equipotentiality and language acquisition. In S.J. Segalowitz & F.A. Gruber (Eds.), *Language Development and Neurological Theory.* New York: Academic Press.

Dennis, M., Fitz, C.R., Netley, C.T., Sugar, J., Harwood-Nash, D.C.F., Hendrick, E.B., Hoffman, H.J. & Humphreys, R.P. 1981. The intelligence of hydrocephalic children. *Archives of Neurology,* 38, 607.

Dennis, M., Hendrick, E.B., Hoffman, H.J. & Humphreys, R.P. 1987. Language of hydrocephalic children and adolescents. *Journal of Clinical and Experimental Neuropsychology,* 9, 593.

Dennis, M., Farrell, K., Hoffman, H.J. & Hendrick, E.B. 1988. Recognition memory of item, associative and serial-order information after temporal lobectomy for seizure disorder. *Neuropsychologia,* 26, 53.

Dennis, M., Spiegler, B.J., Hoffman, H.J., Hendrick, E.B., Humphreys, R.P. & Becker, L.E. 1991a. Brain tumors in children and adolescents: I. Effects on working, associative and serial-order memory of IQ, age at tumor onset and age of tumor. *Neuropsychologia,* 29, 813.

Dennis, M., Spiegler, B.J., Fitz, C.R., Hoffman, H.J., Hendrick, E.B., Humphreys, R.P. & Chuang, S. 1991b. Brain tumors in children and adolescents: II. The neuroanatomy of deficits in working, associative and serial-order memory. *Neuropsychologia,* 29, 829.

Dennis, M., Spiegler, B.J., Obonsawin, M.C., Maria, B.L., Cowell, C., Hoffman, H.J., Hendrick, E.B., Humphreys, R.P., Bailey, J.D. & Ehrlich, R.M. 1992. Brain tumors in children and adolescents: III. Effects of radiation and hormone status on intelligence and on working, associative and serial-order memory. *Neuropsychologia,* 30, 257.

Department of Health, Education and Welfare. (DHEW) 1966. *Patients in Mental Institutions. I. Public Institutions for the Mentally Retarded.* Bethesda, MD: National Institute of Mental Health.

Department of Health, Education and Welfare. (DHEW) 1973. *Children Served in Mental Retardation Clinics: Fiscal Year 1970–1972.* Washington, DC: U.S. Government Printing Office.

DeQuiros, J.B. & Schrager, O.L. 1978. *Neuropsychological Fundamentals in Learning Disabilities.* San Rafael, CA: Academic Therapy Publications.

De Renzi, E. 1982. *Disorders of Space Exploration and Cognition.* New York: Wiley.

DeSchonen, S. & Bry, I. 1987. Interhemispheric communication of visual learning: a developmental study in 3–6 month old infants. *Neuropsychologia,* 25, 601.

DeSchonen, S. & Mathivet, E. 1989. First come, first served: A scenario about the development of hemispheric specialization in face recognition during infancy. *Cahiers de Psychologie Cognitive,* 9, 3.

DesLauriers, A.M. & Carlson, C.F. 1969. *Your Child is Asleep. Early Infantile Autism.* Homewood, IL: Dorsey Press.

Desmond, W., Vermiand, W.M., Melnick, J.L. & Rawls, W.E. 1970. The early growth and development of infants with congenital rubella. In D.H.M. Woolam (Ed.), *Advances in Teratology,* vol. 4. London: Logos Press.

Desmond, M.M., Fisher, E.S., Vorderman, A.L., Schaffer, H.G., Andrew, L.P., Zion, T.E. & Catlin, F.I. 1978. The longitudinal course of congenital rubella encephalitis in nonretarded children. *Journal of Pediatrics,* 93, 584.

Desmond, M.M., Wilson, G.S., Vorderman, A.L., Murphy, M.A., Thurber, S., Fisher, E.S. & Kroulik, E.M. 1985. The health and educational status of adolescents with congenital rubella syndrome. *Developmental Medicine and Child Neurology,* 27, 721.

Deutsch, C.K., Matthysse, S., Swanson, J.M. & Farkas, L.G. 1990. Genetic latent structure analysis of dysmorphology in attention deficit disorder. *Journal of the American Academy of Child and Adolescent Psychiatry,* 29, 189.

Deutsch, M. (Ed.). 1990. *Management of Childhood Brain Tumors.* Boston: Kluwer.

Dewey, D., Roy, E.A., Square-Storer, P.A. & Hayden, D. 1988. Limb and oral praxic abilities of children with verbal sequencing deficits. *Developmental Medicine and Child Neurology,* 30, 743.

Diamond, A. (Ed.). 1990. *The Development and Neural Bases of Higher Cortical Functions.* New York: New York Academy of Sciences.

Diamond, A. 1991. Neuropsychological insights into the meaning of object concept development. In S. Carey & R. Gelman (Eds.), *The Epigenesis of Mind: Essays on Biology and Cognition.* Hillsdale, NJ: Erlbaum, p. 67.

Diamond, M.C. 1990. How the brain grows in response to experience. In R.E. Ornstein & C. Swencionis (Eds.), *The Healing Brain: A Scientific Reader.* New York: Guilford Press, p. 22.

Diamond, M.C., Dowling, G.A. & Johnson, R.E. 1981. Morphological cerebral cortical asymmetry in male and female rats. *Experimental Neurology,* 71, 261.

Diamond, R. & Carey, S. 1977. Developmental changes in the representation of faces. *Journal of Experimental Child Psychology,* 23, 1.

Diani, S. & Jancar, J. 1984. Aicardi's syndrome (agenesis of the corpus callosum, infantile spasms, and ocular anomalies). *Journal of Mental Deficiency Research,* 28, 143.

DiBenedetta, C., Balazs, R., Gombos, G. & Porcellati, G. (Eds.) 1980. *Multidisciplinary Approach to Brain Development* (Developments in Neuroscience, Vol. 9). Amsterdam: Elsevier/North Holland Biomedical Press.

Dignan, P.St. J. & Warkany, J. 1977. Congenital malformations: The corpus callosum. In J. Wortis (Ed.), *Mental Retardation and Developmental Disabilities,* Vol. IX. New York: Brunner/Mazel.

Dillon, D.J., Emory, E.K., Dave, R. & Rauch, M. 1989. Stimulus rate by intensity interaction of brainstem auditory evoked potentials in newborn infants. Paper presented at the meeting of the International Neuropsychological Society, Vancouver.

Dimond, S.J. 1972a. Hemispherectomy. In S.J. Dimond (Ed.), *The Double Brain.* Edinburgh: Churchill Livingstone.

Dimond, S.J. 1972b. *The Double Brain,* Edinburgh: Churchill Livingstone.

Dimond, S.J. 1975. The disconnection syndromes. In D. Williams (Ed.), *Modern Trends in Neurology,* Vol. 6. London: Butterworth.

Dimond, S. 1978. The infant brain. In S. Dimond (Ed.), *Introducing Neuropsychology.* Springfield, IL: Charles C Thomas.

Dingman, H.F. & Tarjan, G. 1960. Mental retardation and the normal distribution curve. *American Journal of Mental Deficiency,* 64, 991.

Dobbing, J. 1968a. Effects of experimental undernutrition on development of the nervous system. In N. Schrimshaw & J. Gordon (Eds.), *Malnutrition, Learning, and Behavior.* Cambridge, MA: MIT Press.

Dobbing, J. 1968b. Vulnerable periods in developing brain. In A.N. Davison & J. Dobbing (Eds.), *Applied Neurochemistry.* Oxford: Blackwell.

Dobbing, J. 1975. Prenatal nutrition and neurological development. In N.A. Buchwald & M.A.B. Brazier (Eds.), *Brain Mechanisms in Mental Retardation.* New York: Academic Press.

Dobbing, J. & Sands, J. 1973. Quantitative growth and development of human brain. *Archives of Disease in Childhood,* 48(1), 757.

Dobbing, J. & Smart, J.L. 1974. Vulnerability of developing brain and behaviour. *British Medical Bulletin,* 30, 164.

Dodd, B. 1976. A comparison of the phonological systems of mental age matched normal, severely subnormal and Down's syndrome children. *British Journal of Disorders of Communication,* 11, 27.

Dodge, P., Prensky, A. & Feigin, R. 1975. *Nutrition and the Developing Nervous System.* St. Louis: C.V. Mosby.

Dodrill, C.B. & Clemmons, D. 1984. Use of neuropsychological tests to identify high school students with epilepsy who later demonstrate inadequate performance in life. *Journal of Consulting and Clinical Psychology,* 52, 520.

Dodson, W.E. 1976. Neonatal drug intoxication: Local anesthetics. *Pediatric Clinics of North America,* 23, 399.

Dodson, W.E. 1989. Deleterious effects of drugs on the developing nervous system. *Clinics in Perinatology,* 16, 339.

Doehring, D.G. 1960. Visual-spatial memory in aphasic children. *Journal of Speech and Hearing Research,* 3, 138.

Doehring, D.G. 1968. *Patterns of Impairment in Specific Reading Disability*. Blooming-ton, IN: Indiana University Press.

Doehring, D.G. & Hoshko, I.M. 1977. Classification of reading problems by the Q-technique of factor analysis. *Cortex*, 13, 281.

Doehring, D.G., Trites, R.L., Patel, P.G. & Fiedorowizc, C.A.M. 1981. *Reading Dis-abilities. The Interaction of Reading, Language and Neuropsychological Deficits*. New York: Academic Press.

Donders, J. 1992. Premorbid behavioral and psychosocial adjustment of children with traumatic brain injury. *Journal of Abnormal Child Psychology*, 20, 233.

Donders, J., Canady, A.I. & Rourke, B.P. 1990. Psychometric intelligence after infantile hydrocephalus. *Child's Nervous System*, 6, 148.

Donders, J., Rourke, B.P. & Canady, A.I. 1992. Emotional adjustment of children with hydrocephalus and of their parents. *Journal of Child Neurology*, 7, 375.

Dool, C.B., Stelmack, R.M. & Rourke, B.P. 1993. Event-related potentials in children with learning disabilities. *Journal of Clinical Child Psychology*, 22, 387.

Doose, H. 1975. *Zerebrale Anfälle im Kindesalter*. Hamburg: Desitin.

Douglas, J.W.B. 1976. Medical ability and school achievement of premature children at 8 years of age. *British Medical Journal* 1, 1210.

Douglas, R.J. & Martin, K.A.C. 1991. Opening the grey box. *Trends in Neuroscience*, 14, 281.

Douglas, V.I. & Peters, K.G. 1979. Toward a clearer definition of the attentional deficit of hyperactive children. In G.A. Hale & M. Lewis (Eds.), *Attention and Cognitive Development*. New York: Plenum Publishing.

Downing, J. & Leong, C.K. 1982. *Psychology of Reading*, New York: Macmillan.

Drake, J.M., Hendrick, E.B., Becker, L.E., Chuang, S.H., Hoffman, H.J. & Humphreys, R.P. 1986. Intracranial meningiomas in children. *Pediatric Neuroscience*, 12, 134.

Drake, W.E. 1968. Clinical and pathological findings in a child with a developmental learning disability. *Journal of Learning Disabilities*, 1, 486.

Drillien, C.M. 1958. Growth and development in a group of children of very low birth weight. *Archives of Disease in Childhood*, 33, 10.

Drillien, C.M. 1961. The incidence of mental and physical handicaps in a group of children of very low birth weight. *Pediatrics*, 27, 452.

Drillien, C.M. 1974. Prenatal and perinatal factors in etiology and outcome of low birth weight. *Clinics in Perinatology*, 1, 197.

Drillien, C.M., Thomson, A.J.M. & Burgoyre, K. 1980. Low-birthweight children at early schoolage: A longitudinal study. *Developmental Medicine and Child Neurology*, 22, 26.

Dubey, D.R., O'Leary, S.G. & Kaufman, K.F. 1983. Training parents of hyperactive children in child management: A comparative outcome study. *Journal of Abnormal Child Psychology*, 11, 229.

Dublin, W.B. 1978. The auditory pathology of anoxia. *Otolaryngology*, 86(1), 27.

Dubowitz, L.M.S. 1979. Study of visual function in the premature infant. *Child: Care, Health and Development*, 5, 399.

Dubowitz, L.M.S., Bydder, G.M. & Muchin, J. 1985. Developmental sequence in peri-ventricular leukomalacia: Correlation of ultrasound, clinical, and nuclear magnetic resonance functions. *Archives of Disease in Childhood*, 60, 349.

Dubowitz, L.M.S., Dubowitz, V. & Goldberg, C. 1970. Clinical assessment of gestational age in the newborn infant. *Journal of Pediatrics*, 77, 1.

Duchowny, M.S. 1989. Surgery for intractable epilepsy: Issues and outcome. *Pediatrics*, 84, 886.

Duchowny, M.S., Weiss, I.P., Majlessi, H. & Barnet, A.B. 1974. Visual evoked responses in childhood cortical blindness after head trauma and meningitis. *Neurology, 24*, 933.

Duckett, S. 1981. Neuropathological aspects: Congenital malformations. In P. Black (Ed.), *Brain Dysfunction in Children*. New York: Raven Press.

Duffner, P.K. & Cohen, M.E. 1992. Changes in the approach to central nervous system tumors in childhood. *Pediatric Clinics of North America, 39*, 859.

Duffner, P.K., Cohen, M.E. & Parker, M.S. 1988. Prospective intellectual testing in children with brain tumors. *Annals of Neurology, 23*, 575.

Duffner, P.K., Cohen, M.E., Seidel, F.G. & Shucard, D.W. 1989. The significance of MRI abnormalities in children with neurofibromatosis. *Neurology, 39*, 373.

Duffner, P.K., Horowitz, M.E., Krisher, J.P., et al. 1993. Postoperative chemotherapy and delayed radiation in children less than three years of age with malignant brain tumors. *New England Journal of Medicine, 328*, 1725.

Duffy, F.H. & McAnulty, G.B. 1985. Brain electrical activity mapping (BEAM): The search for a physiological signature of dyslexia. In G.H. Duffy & N. Geschwind (Eds.), *Dyslexia: A Neuroscientific Approach to Clinical Evaluation*. Boston: Little, Brown.

Duffy, F.H. & McAnulty, G.B. 1990. Neurophysiological heterogeneity and the definition of dyslexia: Preliminary evidence for plasticity. *Neuropsychologia, 28*, 555.

Dumont, M.P. 1984. The nonspecificity of mental illness. *American Journal of Orthopsychiatry, 54*, 326.

Dunn, H.C. & McBurney, A.K. 1977. Cigarette smoking and the fetus and the child. *Pediatrics, 60*, 772.

DuPaul, G.J., Guevremont, D.C. & Barkley, R.A. 1991. Attention deficit disorder. In T.R. Kratochwill and R.J. Morris (Eds.), *The Practice of Child Therapy*. New York: Pergamon Press, p. 115.

Dusser, A., Gourtieres, F. & Aicardi, J. 1986. Ischemic strokes in children. *Journal of Child Neurology, 1*, 131.

Dworkin, R.H., Green, S.R., Small, N.E., Warner, M.L., Cornblatt, B.A. & Erlenmeyer-Kimling, L. 1990. Positive and negative symptoms and social competence in adolescents at risk for schizophrenia and affective disorders. *American Journal of Psychiatry, 147*, 1234.

Dykens, E.M., Hodapp, R.M. & Leckman, J.F. 1993. *Behavior and Development in Fragile X Syndrome*. Thousand Oaks, CA: Sage Publications.

Dykman, R.A. & Ackerman, P.T. 1976. The MBD problem: Attention, intention and information processing. In R.P. Anderson & C.G. Halcomb (Eds.), *Learning Disability/Minimal Brain Dysfunction Syndrome*. Springfield, IL: Charles C Thomas.

Eagle, R.S. 1985. Deprivation of early sensorimotor experience and cognition in the severely cerebral-palsied child. *Journal of Autism and Developmental Disorders, 15*, 269.

Eaton, W.O. & Yu, A.P. 1989. Are sex differences in child motor activity level a function of sex differences in maturational status? *Child Development, 60*, 1005.

Edelman, G.M. 1984. Cell-adhesion molecules: A molecular basis for animal form. *American Scientist, 250*, 118.

Edelman, G.M., Galin, W.J., Delouvee, A., Cunningham, B.A. & Thiery, J.P. 1983. Early epochal maps of two different cell adhesion molecules. *Proceedings of the National Academy of Sciences of the United States of America,* 80, 4384.

Edgell, D. 1979. An ethological study of preverbal communication: Some implications for thought and language. Unpublished manuscript, University of Victoria.

Edgell, D. 1986. The effects of mild and moderate hyperbilirubinemia on newborns and on development at eight months of age. PhD dissertation, University of Victoria.

Eeg-Olofsson, O. 1970. The development of the electroencephalogram in normal children and adolescents from the age of 1 through 21 years. *Acta Paediatrica Scandinavica,* 208, Suppl. 4.

Eeg-Olofsson, O. & Ringheim, Y. 1983. Stroke in children: Clinical characteristics and prognosis. *Acta Pediatrica Scandinavica,* 72, 391.

Efron, R. 1990. *The Decline and Fall of Hemispheric Specialization.* Hillsdale, NJ: Erlbaum.

Ehrenberg, M.F., Cox, D.N. & Koopman, R.F. 1990. The prevalence of depression in high-school students. *Adolescence,* 25, 905.

Ehrhardt, A.A. & Baker, S.W. 1974. Fetal androgens, human central nervous system differentiation, and behavior sex differences. In R.C. Friedman et al. (Eds.), *Sex Differences in Behavior.* New York: Wiley.

Eichorn, D.H. 1979. Physical development: Current foci of research. In J.D. Osofsky (Ed.), *Handbook of Infant Development.* New York: Wiley.

Eichhorn, S.K. 1982. Congenital cytomegalovirus infection: A significant cause of deafness and mental deficiency. *Journal of the American Medical Association,* 127, 838.

Eide, P.K. & Tysnes, O.B. 1992. Early and late outcome in head injury patients with radiological evidence of brain damage. *Acta Neurologica Scandinavica,* 86, 194.

Eilers, B.L., Desai, N.S., Wilson, M.A. & Cunningham, M.D. 1986. Classroom performance and social factors of children with birth weights of 1250 grams or less: Follow-up at 5 to 8 years. *Pediatrics,* 77, 203.

Eimas, P.D. 1986. The perception of speech in early infancy. *Scientific American,* 252, 46.

Eimas, P.D., Siqueland, E.R., Jusczyk, P. & Vigorito, J. 1971. Speech perception in infants. *Science,* 171, 303.

Eisenberg, L. 1971. Persistent problems in the study of the biopsychology of development. In E. Tobach, L.R. Aronson & E. Shaw (Eds.), *The Biopsychology of Development.* New York: Academic Press.

Eisenberg, R.B. 1976. *Auditory Competence in Early Life.* Baltimore: University Park Press.

Eisenhauer, G.L. & Woody, R.C. 1987. Self-mutilation and Tourette's syndrome. *Journal of Child Neurology,* 2, 265.

Eisenson, J. 1968a. Developmental aphasia (dyslogia). A postulation of a unitary concept of the disorder. *Cortex,* 4, 184.

Eisenson, J. 1968b. Developmental aphasia: A speculative view with therapeutic implications. *Journal of Speech and Hearing Disorders,* 33, 3.

Ekelman, B.L. & Aram, D.M. 1983. Syntactic findings in developmental verbal apraxia. *Journal of Communication Disorders,* 16, 237.

Ellenberg, J.G. & Nelson, K. 1978. Febrile seizures and later intellectual performance. *Archives of Neurology,* 35, 17.

Ellenberg, J.G., Hirtz, D.G. & Nelson, K.B. 1986. Do seizures in children cause intellectual deterioration? *New England Journal of Medicine,* 314, 1085.

Ellenberg, L. 1982. Cognitive recovery in pediatric medulloblastoma patients following neurosurgery and radiation therapy. Presented at the Tenth Annual Meeting of the International Neuropsychological Society, Pittsburgh.

Ellenberg, L., McComb, J.G., Siegel, S.E. & Stowe, S. 1987. Factors affecting intellectual outcome in pediatric brain tumor patients. *Neurosurgery, 21,* 638.

Elliott, D. 1985. Manual asymmetries in the performance of sequential movements by adolescents and adults with Down's syndrome. *American Journal of Mental Deficiency, 90,* 90.

Elliott, D., Weeks, D.J. & Jones, R. 1986. Lateral asymmetries in finger-tapping by adolescents and young adults with Down syndrome. *American Journal of Mental Deficiency, 90,* 472.

Elliott, D., Weeks, D.J. & Elliott, C.I. 1987. Cerebral specialization in individuals with Down syndrome. *American Journal of Mental Retardation, 92,* 363.

Ellis, H.D. & Young, A.W. 1988. Training in face-processing skills for a child with acquired prosopagnosia. *Developmental Neuropsychology, 4,* 283.

Ellis, N.R. 1963. The stimulus trace and behavioral inadequacy. In N.R. Ellis (Ed.), *Handbook of Mental Deficiency.* New York: McGraw-Hill.

Elonen, A.S. & Zwarensteyn, S.B. 1964. Appraisal of developmental lag in certain blind children. *Journal of Pediatrics, 65,* 599.

Eme, R.F. 1992. Selective female affliction in the developmental disorders of childhood: A literature review. *Journal of Clinical Child Psychology, 21,* 354.

Emory, E.K. & Noonan, J.R. 1984. Fetal cardiac responding: Maturational and behavioral correlates. *Developmental Psychology, 20,* 354.

Emory, E.K., Tynan, W.D. & Dave, R. 1989. Neurobehavioral anomalies in neonates with seizures. *Journal of Clinical and Experimental Neuropsychology, 11,* 231.

Emory, E.K., Walker, E.F. & Cruz, A. 1982. Fetal heart rate. Part II: Behavioral correlates. *Psychophysiology, 19,* 680.

Engeland, van H. 1984. The electrodermal orienting response to auditive stimuli in autistic children, normal children, mentally retarded children and child psychiatric patients. *Journal of Autism and Developmental Disorders, 14,* 261.

Engelsen, B. 1986. Neurotransmitter glutamate: Its clinical importance. *Acta Neurologica Scandinavica, 74,* 337.

Entus, A.K. 1977. Hemispheric asymmetry in processing of dichotically presented speech and nonspeech stimuli by infants. In S.J. Segalowitz and F.A. Gruber (Eds.), *Language Development and Neurological Theory.* New York: Academic Press.

Epstein, H.T. 1978. Growth spurts during brain development: Implications for educational policy and practice. In J.S. Chall and A.F. Mirsky (Eds.), *Education and the Brain.* Chicago: University of Chicago Press.

Epstein, H.T. 1986. Stages of human brain development. *Developmental Brain Research, 30,* 114.

Erickson, D.V. 1990. Mental functioning of infants with spina bifida on the Bayley Scale of Infant Development. *Canadian Journal of Rehabilitation, 3,* 159.

Erikson, E. 1963. *Childhood and Society,* 2nd ed. New York: McGraw-Hill.

Erlenmeyer-Kimling, L., Friedman, D., Cornblatt, B. & Jacobsen, R. 1985. Electrodermal recovery rate on children of schizophrenic parents. *Psychiatry Research, 14,* 149.

Ernhart, C.B., Wolf, A.D., Linn, P.L., Sokol, R.J., Kennard, M.J. & Filipovich, H.F. 1985. Alcohol-related birth defects: Syndrome anomalies, intrauterine growth retardation, and neonatal behavioral assessment. *Alcoholism: Clinical and Experimental Research, 9,* 447.

Escalona, S.K. 1982. Babies at double hazard: Early development of infants at biologic and social risk. *Pediatrics* 70, 670.

Escalona, S. & Corman, H. 1969. *Albert Einstein Scales of Sensorimotor Development.* Unpublished manuscript, Albert Einstein College of Medicine.

Espenschade, A.S. & Eckert, H.M. 1980. *Motor Development,* 2nd ed. Columbus, OH: Charles E. Merrill.

Espinosa, M.P., Sigman, M.D., Neumann, C.G. & Bwibo, N.O. 1992. Playground behaviors of school-age children in relation to nutrition, schooling, and family characteristics. *Developmental Psychology,* 28, 1188.

Ettlinger, G. 1977. Agenesis of the corpus callosum. In P.J. Vincken & G.W. Bruyn (Eds.) *Handbook of Clinical Neurology,* vol. 30. Amsterdam: North-Holland.

Ettlinger, G., Blakemore, C., Milner, A. & Wilson, J. 1972. Agenesis of the corpus callosum: A behavioral investigation. *Brain,* 95, 327.

Ettlinger, G., Blakemore, C., Milner, A. & Wilson, J. 1974. Agenesis of the corpus callosum: A further behavioral investigation. *Brain,* 97, 225.

Evans, D., Moodie, A. & Hansen, J. 1971. Kwashiorkor and intellectual development. *South African Medical Journal,* 45, 1413.

Ewing-Cobbs, L., Fletcher, J.M., Landry, S.H. & Levin, H.S. 1985. Language disorders after pediatric head injury. In J.K. Darby (Ed.), *Speech and Language Evaluation in Neurology: Childhood Disorders.* San Diego: Grune and Stratton, p. 97.

Ewing-Cobbs, L., Fletcher, J.M. & Levin, H.S. 1986. Neurobehavioral sequelae following head injury in children: Educational implications. *Journal of Head Trauma Rehabilitation,* 1, 57.

Ewing-Cobbs, L., Levin, H.S., Eisenberg, H.M. & Fletcher, J.M. 1987. Language functions following closed-head injury in children and adolescents. *Journal of Clinical and Experimental Neuropsychology,* 9, 575.

Eyler, F.D., Delgado-Hachey, M., Woods, N.S. & Carter, R.L. 1991. Quantification of the Dubowitz neurological assessment of preterm neonates: Developmental outcome. *Infant and Behavioral Development,* 14, 451.

Fagan, J.F. & McGrath, S.N. 1981. Infant recognition memory and later intelligence. *Intelligence,* 5, 121.

Fagan, J.F. & Singer, L.T. 1983. Infant recognition memory as a measure of intelligence. In L.P. Lipsitt (Ed.), *Advances in Infancy Research,* Vol. 2. Norwood, NJ: Ablex.

Fagan, J., Singer, L., Montie, J. & Shepherd, P. 1986. Selective screening device for the early detection of normal or delayed cognitive development in infants at risk for later mental retardation. *Pediatrics,* 78, 1021.

Fantz, R.L. & Fagan, J.F. 1975. Visual attention to size and number of pattern details by term and preterm infants during the first six months. *Child Development,* 46, 3.

Fantz, R.L. & Nevis, S. 1967. The predictive value of changes in visual preference in early infancy. In J. Hellmuth (Ed.), *The Exceptional Infant,* Vol. 1. Seattle: Special Publications, p. 349.

Fantz, R.L. & Ordy, J.M. 1959. A visual acuity test for infants under six months of age. *Psychological Record,* 9, 159.

Fantz, R.L., Ordy, J.M. & Udelf, M.S. 1962. Maturation of pattern vision in infants during the first six months. *Journal of Comparative Physiological Psychology,* 55(6), 907.

Farr, V., Mitchell, R.G., Neligan, G.A. & Parkin, J.M. 1966. The definition of a newborn infant. *Developmental Medicine and Child Neurology,* 8, 507.

Farrington, D.P. 1983. Offending from 10 to 25 years of age. In K.T. Van Dusen and S.A. Mednick (Eds.), *Prospective Studies of Crime and Delinquency.* Boston: Kluwer-Nijhoff, p. 17.

Farwell, J.R., Dohrmann, G.J. & Flannery, J.T. 1978. Intracranial neoplasms in infants. *Archives of Neurology,* 35, 533.

Farwell, J.R., Lee, Y.J., Hirtz, D.G., Sulzbacher, S.I., Ellenberg, J.H. & Nelson, K.B. 1990. Phenobarbital for febrile seizures: Effects on intelligence and on seizure recurrence. *New England Journal of Medicine,* p. 364.

Faust, D., Libon, D. & Pueschel, S. 1986–87. Neuropsychological functioning in treated phenylketonuria. *International Journal of Psychiatry in Medicine,* 16, 169.

Favata, I., Leuzzi, V. & Curatolo, P. 1987. Mental outcome of West syndrome: Prognostic value of some clinical factors. *Journal of Mental Deficiency Research,* 31, 9.

Fay, W.H. & Butler, B.V. 1968. Echolalia, IQ, and the developmental dichotomy of speech and language systems. *Journal of Speech and Hearing Research,* 11, 365.

Fazzi, E., Lanzi, G., Gerardo, A., Ometto, A. & Rondini, G. 1991. Correlation between clinical and ultrasound findings in preterm infants with cystic periventricular leukomalacia. *Italian Journal of Neurological Science,* 12, 199.

Feigin, R.D. & Dodge, P.R. 1976. Bacterial meningitis: Newer concepts of pathophysiology and neurologic sequelae. *Pediatric Clinics of North America,* 23, 541.

Fein, D., Humes, M., Kaplan, E., Lucci, D. & Waterhouse, L. 1984. The question of left hemisphere dysfunction in infantile autism. *Psychological Bulletin,* 95, 258.

Fein, D., Lucci, D. & Waterhouse, L. 1990. Brief report: Fragmented drawings in autistic children. *Journal of Autism and Developmental Disorders,* 20, 263.

Fein, G., Davenport, L., Vingling, C.D. & Galin, D. 1988. Verbal and nonverbal memory deficits in pure dyslexia. *Developmental Neuropsychology,* 4, 181.

Feinberg, I. 1982. Schizophrenia: Caused by a fault in programmed synaptic elimination during adolescence. *Journal of Psychiatric Research,* 17, 319.

Feingold, B.F. 1975. Hyperkinesis and learning disabilities linked to artificial food flavors and colors. *American Journal of Nursing,* 75, 797.

Feldman, H.M., Holland, A.L. & Keefe, K. 1989. Language abilities after left hemisphere brain injury: A case study of twins. *Topics in Early Childhood Special Education,* 9, 32.

Feldman, H.M., Holland, A.L., Kemp, S.S. & Janoski, J.E. 1992. Language development after unilateral brain injury. *Brain and Language,* 42, 89.

Felton, R.H., Naylor, C.E. & Wood, F.B. 1990. Neuropsychological profile of adult dyslexics. *Brain and Language,* 39, 485.

Fenichel, G.M. 1980. *Neonatal Neurology.* New York: Churchill Livingstone.

Fenichel, G.M. 1983. Hypoxic-ischemic encephalopathy in the newborn. *Archives of Neurology,* 40, 261.

Fenichel, G.M. 1988. *Clinical Pediatric Neurology,* Philadelphia: W.B. Saunders.

Ferguson-Smith, M.A. 1983. The reduction of anencephalic and spina bifida births by maternal serum alphafetoprotein screening. *British Medical Bulletin,* 39, 365.

Fernell, E., Gillberg, C. & von Wendt, L. 1991. Behavioural problems in children with infantile hydrocephalus. *Developmental Medicine and Child Neurology,* 33, 388.

Ferrari, F., Grosoli, M.V., Fontana, G. & Gravazutti, G.B. 1983. Neurobehavioral comparison of low risk preterm and fullterm infants at term conceptual age. *Developmental Medicine and Child Neurology,* 25, 720.

Ferrendelli, J. (Ed.) 1979. *Aspects of Developmental Neurobiology (Symposium IV).* Bethesda, MD: Society for Neuroscience.

Ferris, G. & Dorsen, M. 1975. Agenesis of the corpus callosum. 1. Neuropsychological studies. *Cortex,* 11, 95.

Ferro, J.M. & Martins, I.P. 1990. Some new aspects of neglect in children. *Behavioural Neurology,* 3, 1.

Ferro, J.M., Bravo-Marques, J.M., Castro-Caldas, A. & Antunes, L. 1983. Crossed optic ataxia: Possible role of the dorsal splenium. *Journal of Neurology, Neurosurgery and Psychiatry,* 46, 533.

Ferry, P.C., Hall, S.M. & Hicks, J.L. 1975. "Dilapidated" speech: Developmental verbal dyspraxia. *Developmental Medicine and Child Neurology,* 17, 749.

Field, M., Ashton, R. & White, K. 1978. Agenesis of the corpus callosum: Report of two preschool children and review of the literature. *Developmental Medicine and Child Neurology,* 20, 47.

Field, T. 1980. Supplemental stimulation of preterm neonates. *Early Human Development,* 413, 301.

Field, T., Dempsey, J.R. & Shuman, H.H. 1979. Developmental assessments of infants surviving the respiratory distress syndrome. In T. Field, A. Sostek, S. Goldberg & H.H. Shuman (Eds.), *Infants Born at Risk.* New York: Spectrum.

Field, T.M., Dempsey, J.R. & Shuman, H.H. 1981. Developmental follow-up of pre- and post-term infants. In S.L. Friedman & M. Sigman (Eds.), *Preterm Birth and Psychological Development.* New York: Academic Press.

Filskov, S.B. & Leli, D.A. 1981. Assessment of the individual in neuropsychological practice. In S.B. Filskov & T.J. Boll (Eds.), *Handbook of Clinical Neuropsychology.* New York: Wiley.

Fine, A., Meldrum, B.S. & Patel, S. 1990. Modulation of experimentally induced epilepsy by intracerebral grafts of fetal GABAergic neurons. *Neuropsychologia,* 28, 627.

Fine, S.R. 1968. *Blind and Partially Sighted Children. Education Survey No. 4. Department of Education and Science.* London: H.M. Stationery Office.

Finger, S. 1989. Reflections on the possible maladaptive consequences of injury-induced reorganization. *Neuropsychology,* 3, 41.

Finger, S. & Stein, D.G. 1982. *Brain Damage and Recovery. Research and Clinical Perspectives.* New York: Academic Press.

Finucci, J.M. & Childs, B. 1981. Are there really more dyslexic boys than girls? In A. Ansara et al. (Eds.), *Sex Differences in Dyslexia.* Towson, MD: Orton Dyslexia Society.

Finucci, J.M., Guthrie, J.T., Childs, A.L., Abbey, H. & Childs, B. 1976. The genetics of specific reading disability. *Annals of Human Genetics,* (Lond.), 40(1), 1.

Fior, R. 1972. Physiological maturation of auditory function between 3 and 13 years of age. *Audiology,* 11, 317.

Fiorentini, A. 1991. Parallel processes in human visual development. In J.R. Brannan (Ed.), *Applications of Parallel Processing in Vision. Advances in Psychology,* Vol. 86. Amsterdam: North-Holland, p. 81.

Firestone, P., Peters, S., Rivier, M. & Knights, R.M. 1978. Minor physical anomalies in hyperactive, retarded, and normal children and their families. *Journal of Child Psychology and Psychiatry,* 19, 155.

Fischer, K.W. 1987. Relations between brain and cognitive development. *Child Development,* 58, 623.

Fischer, M., Barkley, R.A., Edelbrock, C.S. & Smallish, L. 1990. The adolescent outcome of hyperactive children diagnosed by research criteria: II. Academic, attentional, and neuropsychological status. *Journal of Consulting and Clinical Psychology,* 58, 580.

Fish, B. 1977. Neurobiologic antecedents of schizophrenia in children. *Archives of General Psychiatry,* 34, 1297.

Fish, B. & Hagin, R. 1973. Visual-motor disorders in infants at risk for schizophrenia. *Archives of General Psychiatry,* 28, 900.

Fisher, M. & Zeaman, D. 1970. Growth and decline of retardate intelligence. In N.R. Ellis (Ed.), *International Review of Research in Mental Retardation,* Vol. 4. New York: Academic Press, p. 151.

Fisher, W., Burd, L. & Kerbeshian, J. 1988. Markers for improvement in children with pervasive developmental disorders. *Journal of Mental Deficiency Research,* 32, 357.

Fishler, K., Azen, C.G., Henderson, R. & Friedman, E.G. 1987. Psychoeducational findings among children treated for phenylketonuria. *American Journal of Mental Deficiency,* 92, 65.

Fishman, M.A. 1976. Recent clinical advances in the treatment of dysraphic states. *Pediatric Clinics of North America,* 23, 517.

Fishman, M.A. & Palkes, H.S. 1974. The validity of psychometric testing in children with congenital malformations of the central nervous system. *Developmental Medicine and Child Neurology,* 16, 180.

Fitzhardinge, P.M., Flodmark, O., Fitz, C.R. & Ashby, S. 1981. The prognostic value of computer tomography as an adjunct to assessment of the term infant with postasphyxial encephalopathy. *Journal of Pediatrics,* 99 (5), 777.

Fitzhardinge, P.M. & Stevens, E.M. 1972. The small-for-date infant. II. Neurological and intellectual sequelae. *Pediatrics* 50, 50.

Flavell, J. & Wellman, H. 1977. Metamemory. In R.V. Kail & J. Hagen (Eds.), *Perspectives on the Development of Memory and Cognition.* Hillsdale, NJ: Erlbaum, p. 3.

Flechsig, P. 1901. Developmental (myelogenetic) localization of the cortex in human subjects. *Lancet,* 2, 1027.

Fleischer, S.F. & Turkewitz, G. 1984. The use of animals for understanding the effects of malnutrition on human behavior: Models vs. a comparative approach. In J.R. Galler (Ed.), *Nutrition and Behavior.* New York: Plenum Press, p. 37.

Fletcher, J.M. & Copeland, D.R. 1988. Neurobehavioral effects of central nervous system prophylactic treatment of cancer in children. *Journal of Clinical and Experimental Neuropsychology,* 10, 495.

Fletcher, J.M. & Satz, P. 1980. Developmental changes in the neuropsychological correlates of reading achievement: A six-year longitudinal follow-up. *Journal of Clinical Neuropsychology,* 2, 23.

Fletcher, J.M. & Satz, P. 1983. Age, plasticity, and equipotentiality: A reply to Smith. *Journal of Consulting and Clinical Psychology,* 51, 763.

Fletcher, J.M. & Satz, P. 1985. Cluster analysis and the search for learning disability subtypes. In B.P. Rourke (Ed.), *Neuropsychology of Learning Disabilities: Essentials of Subtype Analysis.* New York: Guilford Press, p. 40.

Fletcher, J.M. & Taylor, H.G. 1984. Neuropsychological approaches to children: Towards a developmental neuropsychology. *Journal of Clinical and Experimental Neuropsychology,* 6, 39.

Fletcher, J.M., Miner, M.E. & Ewing-Cobbs, L. 1987. Age and recovery from head injury in children: Developmental issues. In H.S. Levin, J. Grafman & H.M. Eisenberg (Eds.), *Neurobehavioral Recovery from Head Injury.* New York: Oxford University Press, p. 279.

Fletcher, J.M., Francis, D.J., Pequenat, W., Raudenbusch, S.W., Bornstein, M.H., Schmitt, F., Brouwers, P. & Stover, E. 1991a. Neurobehavioral outcomes in diseases of childhood: Individual change model for pediatric immunodeficiency virus. *American Psychologist*, 46, 1267.

Fletcher, J.M., Francis, D.J., Thompson, N., Brookshire, B., Miner, M.E., Landry, S.H. & York, M. 1991b. Verbal-nonverbal skill discrepancies in hydrocephalic children. *Journal of Clinical and Experimental Neuropsychology*, 13, 97.

Fletcher, J.M., Bohan, T.P., Brandt, M.E. & Brookshire, B.L. 1992a. Cerebral white matter and cognition in hydrocephalic children. *Archives of Neurology*, 49, 818.

Fletcher, J.M., Francis, D.J., Thompson, N.M. & Brookshire, B.L. 1992b. Verbal and nonverbal skill discrepancies in hydrocephalic children. *Journal of Clinical and Experimental Neuropsychology*, 14, 593.

Flor-Henry, P. 1976. Lateralized temporal-limbic dysfunction and psychopathology, *Annals of the New York Academy of Science*, 280, 777.

Flower, R.M., Viehweg, R. & Ruzicka, W.R. 1961a. The communicative disorders of children with kernicterus athetosis: I. Auditory disorders. *Journal of Speech and Hearing Disorders*, 31, 41.

Flower, R.M., Viehweg, R. & Ruzicka, W.R. 1961b. The communicative disorders of children with kernicterus athetosis: II. Problems in language comprehension and use. *Journal of Speech and Hearing Disorders*, 31, 60.

Flowers, D.L., Wood, F.B. & Naylor, C.E. 1991. Regional cerebral blood flow correlates of language processing in reading disability. *Archives of Neurology*, 48, 637.

Fodor, J. 1983. *The Modularity of the Mind*. Cambridge, MA: MIT Press.

Fog, E. & Fog, M. 1963. Cerebral inhibition examined by associated movements. In M. Bax & R. McKeith (Eds.), *Minimal Cerebral Dysfunction*. London: Heinemann, p. 52.

Fogel, C.A., Mednick, S.A. & Michelsen, N. 1985. Hyperactive behavior and minor physical anomalies. *Acta Psychiatrica Scandinavica*, 72, 551.

Foley, G.M. 1990. Portrait of the arena of evaluation. Assessment in the transdisciplinary approach. In E.D. Gibbs & D.M. Teti (Eds.), *Interdisciplinary Assessment of Infants. A Guide for Early Intervention Professionals*. Baltimore: Paul H. Brookes, p. 271.

Folstein, S. & Rutter, M. 1977. Genetic influences and infantile autism. *Nature*, 265, 726.

Foltz, E.L. & Shurtleff, D.B. 1972. Hydrocephalus treated in the early weeks of life. In *Symposium on Myelomeningocele, American Academy of Orthopedic Surgeons*. St. Louis: C.V. Mosby.

Ford, L.M., Han, B.K., Steichen, J. & Babcock, D. 1989. Very-low-birth-weight, preterm infants with or without intracranial hemorrhage: Neurologic, cognitive, and cranial MRI correlations at 4–8 year follow-up. *Clinical Pediatrics*, 28, 302.

Fox, M.W. 1970. Overview and critique of stages and periods in canine development. *Developmental Psychobiology*, 4, 37.

Francis-Williams, J. & Davies, P.A. 1974. Very low birth weight and later intelligence. *Developmental Medicine and Child Neurology*, 16, 709.

Frank, V. & Torres, F. 1979. Visual evoked potentials in the evaluation of 'cortical blindness' in children. *Annals of Neurology*, 6, 126.

Frankenburg, W.K. 1983. Infant & preschool developmental screening. In M.D. Levine, W.B. Carey, A.C. Crocker & R.T. Gross (Eds.), *Developmental-Behavioral Pediatrics*. Philadelphia: W.B. Saunders, p. 927.

Frankenburg, W.K. & Dodds, J.B. 1967. *Denver Developmental Screening Test.* Denver: University of Colorado Press.

Frankenburg, W.K., Dodds, J.B., Fandal, A., Kazuk, E. & Cohrs, M. 1975. *Denver Developmental Screening Test: Reference Manual, Revised 1975 edition.* Denver: LADOCA Project & Publishing Foundation.

Fraser, F.C. & Sadovnick, A.D. 1976. Correlation of IQ in subjects with Down syndrome and their parents and sibs. *Journal of Mental Deficiency Research,* 20, 179.

Frazer, G.R. 1962. Our genetical load. A review of some aspects of genetical variation. *Annals of Human Genetics* (Lond.), 25, 387.

Freeman, D.G. 1964. Smiling in blind infants and the issue of innate vs. acquired. *Journal of Child Psychology,* 5, 171.

Freeman, J.M. & Nelson, K.B. 1988. Intrapartum asphyxia and cerebral palsy. *Pediatrics,* 82, 240.

Freeman, R.D. & Bonds, A.B. 1979. Cortical plasticity in monocularly deprived immobilized kittens depends on eye movements. *Science,* 206, 1093.

Freud, S. 1940. *An Outline of Psychoanalysis.* New York: Norton.

Freudenberg, D. 1968. *Leistungs- und Verhaltensstörungen bei kindlichen Epilepsien.* Basel, Switzerland: Karger.

Freudenberg, D. 1971. Die Pyknolepsie des Kindesalters: Eine psychodiagnostische Untersuchung. Ph.D. Dissertation: University of Freiburg, Germany.

Fride, E. & Weinstock, M. 1989. Alterations in behavioral and striatal dopamine asymmetries induced by prenatal stress. *Pharmacology, Biochemistry, and Behavior,* 32, 425.

Fried, P.A. 1989. Postnatal consequences of maternal marijuana use in humans. *Annals of the New York Academy of Sciences,* 562, 123.

Friedlander, S., Pothier, P., Morrison, D. & Herman, L. 1982. The role of neurological-developmental delay in childhood psychopathology. *American Journal of Orthopsychiatry,* 52, 102.

Friedman, J.H., Levy, H.L. & Boustany, R.M. 1989. Late onset of distinct neurological syndromes in galactosemic siblings. *Neurology,* 39, 741.

Friedrich, U., Dalby, M., Staehelin-Jensen, T. & Brunn-Petersen, G. 1982. Chromosomal studies of children with developmental language retardation. *Developmental Medicine and Child Neurology,* 24, 645.

Friedrich, W.N., Lovejoy, M.C., Shaffer, J. & Shurtleff, D.B. 1991. Cognitive abilities and achievement status of children with meningomyelocele: A contemporary sample. *Journal of Pediatric Psychology,* 16, 423.

Friel-Patti, S. & Finitzo, T. 1990. Language learning in a prospective study of otitis media with effusion in the first two years of life. *Journal of Speech and Hearing Research,* 33, 188.

Frith, C.D. & Done, D.J. 1988. Towards a neuropsychology of schizophrenia. *British Journal of Psychiatry,* 153, 437.

Frith, U. & Frith, C.D. 1974. Specific motor disabilities in Down's syndrome. *Journal of Child Psychology and Psychiatry,* 1974, 15, 293.

Frostig, M. 1975. The role of perception in the integration of psychological functions. In W.M. Cruickshank and D.P. Hallahan (Eds.), *Perceptual and Learning Disabilities in Children,* vol. 1. Syracuse: Syracuse University Press.

Fruehauf, K. 1976. Ergebnisse psychologischer Längsschnittuntersuchungen bei Kindern mit aktivem Hydrozephalus nach Shunt-Operation im ersten Lebensjahr. *Zeitschrift für Psychologie,* 184, 505.

Fuerst, D.R., Fisk, J.L. & Rourke, B.P. 1990. Psychosocial functioning of learning disabled children: Relations between WISC verbal IQ-performance IQ-discrepancies and personality subtypes. *Journal of Consulting and Clinical Psychology*, 58, 657.

Fuerst, D.R. & Rourke, B.P. 1993. Psychosocial functioning of children: Relations between personality subtypes and academic achievement. *Journal of Abnormal Child Psychology.*

Fujinaga, T., Kasuga, T., Uchida, N. & Saiga, H. 1990. Long-term follow-up study of children developmentally retarded by early environmental deprivation. *Genetic, Social, and General Psychology Monographs,* 116, 37.

Fuller, P.W., Guthrie, R.D. & Alvord, E.C. 1983. A proposed neuropathological basis for learning disabilities in children born prematurely. *Developmental Medicine and Child Neurology*, 25, 214.

Furth, H.G. 1964. Sequence learning in aphasic and deaf children. *Journal of Speech and Hearing Disorders*, 29, 171.

Furth, H.G. 1966. *Thinking without Language.* New York: Free Press.

Furth, H.G. & Youniss, J. 1964. Color-object paired associates in deaf and hearing children with and without response competition. *Journal of Consulting Psychology*, 1964, 28, 224.

Fusco, L., Ferracuti, S., Fariello, G. & Manfredi, M. 1992. Hemimegalencephaly and normal intellectual development. *Journal of Neurology, Neurosurgery and Psychiatry*, 55, 720.

Gaddes, W.H. & Crockett, D.J. 1975. The Spreen-Benton Aphasia test, normative data as a measure of normal language development. *Brain and Language*, 2, 257.

Gaddes, W.H. & Edgell, D. 1993. *Learning Disabilities and Brain Function,* 3rd ed. New York: Springer.

Galaburda, A.M. 1989. Ordinary and extraordinary brain development: Anatomical variation in developmental dyslexia. *Annals of Dyslexia*, 39, 67.

Galaburda, A. & Kemper, T. 1979. Cytoarchitectonic abnormalities in developmental dyslexia: A case study. *Annals of Neurology*, 6, 94.

Galaburda, A., Sanides, F. & Geschwind, N. 1978. Human brain: Cytoarchitectonic left-right asymmetries in the temporal speech region. *Archives of Neurology*, 35, 812.

Galaburda, A.M., Rosen, G.D. & Sherman, G.F. 1990. Individual variability in cortical organization: Its relationship to brain laterality and implications to function. *Neuropsychologia*, 28, 529.

Galante, M.B., Flye, M.E. & Stephens, L.S. 1972. Cumulative minor deficits: A longitudinal study of the relation of physical factors to school achievement. *Journal of Learning Disabilities*, 5, 75.

Galin, D. 1977. Lateral specialization and psychiatric issues: Speculations on development and the evolution of consciousness. *Annals of the New York Academy of Sciences*, 299, 397.

Galin, D. & Nachman, M. 1990. Story recall under monaural and binaural conditions: Patients with anterior temporal lesions. *Journal of Nervous and Mental Disease*, 178, 15.

Galin, D., Johnstone, J., Nakell, L. & Herron, J. 1979. Development of the capacity for tactile information transfer between hemispheres in normal children. *Science*, 24, 1330.

Gall, C. & Lynch, G. 1980. The regulation of fiber growth and synaptogenesis in the developing hippocampus. In R.K. Hunt (Ed.), *Neural Development*, Part I (Current Topics in Developmental Biology, Vol. 15). New York: Academic Press.

Galler, J.R. 1984. Behavioral consequences of malnutrition in early life. In J.R. Galler (Ed.), *Nutrition and Behavior.* New York: Plenum Press, p. 63.

Galler, J.R. & Ramsey, F. 1989. A follow-up study of the influence of early malnutrition on development: Behavior at home and at school. *Journal of the American Academy of Child and Adolescent Psychiatry,* 28, 254.

Galler, J.R., Ramsey, F.C., Forde, V., Salt, P. & Archer, E. 1987a. Long-term effects of early kwashiorkor compared with marasmus. II. Intellectual performance. *Journal of Pediatric Gastroenterology and Nutrition,* 6, 847.

Galler, J.R., Ramsey, F.C., Morley, D.S., Archer, E. & Salt, P. 1990. Long-term effects of early kwashiorkor compared with marasmus. IV. Performance on the National High School Entrance Examination. *Pediatric Research,* 28, 235.

Galler, J.R., Ramsey, F.C., Salt, P. & Archer, E. 1987b. Long-term effects of early kwashiorkor compared with marasmus. III. Fine motor skills. *Journal of Pediatric Gastroenterology and Nutrition,* 6, 855.

Galler, J.R., Ramsey, F. & Solimano, G. 1984. The influence of early malnutrition on subsequent behavioral development. III. Learning disabilities as a sequel to malnutrition. *Pediatric Research,* 18, 309.

Galler, J.R., Ramsey, F., Solimano, G. & Lowell, W.E. 1983b. The influence of early malnutrition on subsequent behavioral development. II. Classroom behavior. *Journal of the American Academy of Child Psychiatry,* 22, 16.

Galler, J.R., Ramsey, F., Solimano, G., Lowell, W.E. & Mason, E. 1983a. The influence of early malnutrition on subsequent behavioral development. I. Degree of impairment in intellectual performance. *Journal of the American Academy of Child Psychiatry,* 22, 8.

Garber, H.J., Ritvo, E.R., Chiu, L.C. & Griswold, V.J. 1989. A magnetic resonance imaging study of autism: Normal fourth ventricle size and absence of pathology. *American Journal of Psychiatry,* 146, 532.

Garber, H.L. 1988. *The Milwaukee Project. Preventing Mental Retardation in Children at Risk.* Washington: American Association on Mental Retardation.

Gardiner, M.F. & Walter, D.O. 1977. Evidence of hemispheric specialization from infant EEG. In S. Harnad, R.W. Doty, L. Goldstein, J. Jaynes & G. Krauthamer (Eds.), *Lateralization in the Nervous System.* New York: Academic Press.

Gardner, J., Lewkowicz, D. & Turkewitz, G. 1977. Development of postural asymmetry in premature human infants. *Developmental Psychobiology,* 10, 471.

Gardner, J.M., Karmel, B.Z., Magnano, C.L. & Norton, K.I. 1990. Neurobehavioral indicators of early brain insult in high-risk neonates. *Developmental Psychology,* 26, 563.

Gardner, L., Morse, A.R., Tulloch, D. & Trief, E. 1986. Visual impairment among children from birth to age five. *Journal of Visual Impairment and Blindness,* 1986, 535.

Gardner, R.A. 1979. *The Objective Diagnosis of Minimal Brain Dysfunction.* Creskill, NJ: Creative Therapeutics.

Gardner, W.J., Karnoch, I.J., McClure, C.C. & Gardner, A.K. 1955. Residual function following hemispherectomy for tumour and for infantile hemiplegia. *Brain,* 78, 487.

Gareware, A.F. 1990. Sensory integration and attention skills in Down's syndrome children. Ph.D. dissertation. University of British Columbia.

Garey, L.J. & Pettigrew, J.D. 1974. Ultrastructural changes in kitten visual cortex after environmental modification. *Brain Research,* 66, 165.

Garfield, J.C. 1964. Motor impersistence in normal and brain-damaged children. *Neurology,* 14, 623.

Garfinkel, B. 1986. Recent developments in attention deficit disorder. *Psychiatric Annals*, 16, 11.

Garn, S.M., Shaw, H.A. & McCabe, K.D. 1977. Effects of socioeconomic status and race on weight-defined and gestational prematurity in the United States. In D. Reed and F. Stanley (Eds.), *The Epidemiology of Prematurity*. Baltimore: Urban and Schwarzenberg.

Garrett, H.E. 1946. A developmental theory of intelligence. *American Psychologist*, 1, 372.

Garrett, W.J. & Robinson, E.E. 1971. Assessment of fetal size and growth rate in ultrasonic echoscopy. *Obstetrics and Gynecology*, 38, 534.

Garron, D.C. 1977. Intelligence among persons with Turner's syndrome. *Behavioral Genetics*, 7(2), 105.

Gartler, S.M., Liskay, R.M. & Gant, N. 1973. Two functional X chromosomes in human fetal oocytes. *Experimental Cell Research*, 82, 464.

Garvey, M. & Mutton, D.E. 1973. Sex chromosome aberrations and speech development. *Archives of Disease in Childhood*, 48, 937.

Gastaut, H., Gastaut, J.L., Regis, H., Bernard, R., Pinsard, N., Saint-Jaen, M., Roger, J. & Dravet, C. 1978. Computer tomography in the study of West's syndrome. *Developmental Medicine and Child Neurology*, 20, 21.

Gazzaniga, M.S. 1970. *The Bisected Brain*. New York: Appleton-Century-Crofts.

Gazzaniga, M.S., Steen, D. & Volpe, B.T. 1979. Principles of brain development. In M.S. Gazzaniga, D. Steen & B.T. Volpe (Eds.), *Functional Neuroscience*. New York: Harper & Row.

Gebelt, H. 1971. *Psychische und soziale Prognose der Epilepsie im Kindes-und Jugendalter,* Leipzig: Barth.

Gellner, L. 1959. *A Neurophysiological Concept of Mental Retardation and its Educational Implications*. Chicago: Julian Levinson Foundation.

Geoffroy, G., Lassonde, M., Delisle, F. & Decarie, M. 1983. Corpus callosotomy for control of intractable epilepsy in children. *Neurology*, 30, 891.

Gerrard, J. 1952. Kernicterus. *Brain*, 75, 526.

Geschwind, N. 1965. Disconnection syndromes in animals and man. *Brain*, 88, 237 and 585.

Geschwind, N. 1970. The clinical syndromes of the cortical connections. In D. Williams (Ed.), *Modern Trends in Neurology*, Vol. 5. London: Butterworth.

Geschwind, N. 1975. Le concept de disconnexion: l'histoire d'une idee banale mais importante. In F. Michel and B. Schott (Eds.), *Les Syndromes de Disconnexion Calleuse Chez L'Homme (Colloque Internationale de Lyon, 1974)*. Lyon: Hopital Neurologique.

Geschwind, N. 1982. Why Orton was right. *Annals of Dyslexia*, 32, 13.

Geschwind, N. & Behan, P. 1982. Left-handedness: association with immune disease, migraine, and developmental learning disorder. *Proceedings of the National Academy of Science*, 79, 5097.

Geschwind, N. & Galaburda, A.M. 1987. *Cerebral Lateralization: Biological Mechanisms, Associations, and Pathology*. Cambridge, MA: MIT Press.

Geschwind, N. & Kaplan, E. 1962. A human cerebral disconnection syndrome. *Neurology*, 12, 675.

Geschwind, N. & Levitsky, W. 1968. Left-right asymmetries in the temporal speech region. *Science*, 161, 166.

Gesell, A. & Amatruda, C.S. 1945. *The Embryology of Behaviour.* New York: Harper.

Gesell, A. & Amatruda, C.S. 1954. *Developmental Diagnosis: Normal and Abnormal Development: Clinical Methods and Practical Applications*. New York: Harper.

Gesell, H. & Ames, L. 1947. The development of handedness. *Journal of Genetic Psychology,* 70, 155.

Gesell, A. & Thompson, H. 1934. *Infant Behavior: Its Genesis and Growth.* New York: McGraw-Hill.

Gibbs, E.D. 1990. Assessment of infant mental ability: Conventional tests and issues of prediction. In E.D. Gibbs & D.M. Teti (Eds.), *Interdisciplinary Assessment of Infants. A Guide for Early Intervention Professionals.* Baltimore: Paul H. Brookes, p. 77.

Gibson, D. 1978. *Down's Syndrome: The Psychology of Mongolism.* Cambridge, England: Cambridge University Press.

Gibson, D., Groeneweg, G., Jerry, P. & Harris, A. 1988. Age and pattern of intellectual decline among Down syndrome and other mentally retarded adults. *International Journal of Rehabilitation Research,* 11, 47.

Gibson, K.R. & Petersen, A.C. (Eds.). 1991. *Brain Maturation and Cognitive Development: Comparative and Cross-Cultural Perspectives.* New York: De Gruyter.

Gienke, S. & Lewandowski, L.J. 1989. Anomalous dominance in Down syndrome young adults. *Cortex,* 25, 93.

Gilbert, J.N., Jones, K.L., Rorke, L.B., Chernoff, G.F. & James, H.E. 1986. Central nervous system anomalies associated with meningomyelocele, hydrocephalus, and the Arnold-Chiari malformation: Reappraisal of theories regarding the pathogenesis of posterior neural tube closure defects. *Neurosurgery,* 18, 559.

Gillberg, C. 1990. Do children with autism have March birthdays? *Acta Psychiatrica Scandinavica,* 82, 152.

Gillberg, C. 1992. Subgroups of autism: Are there behavioral phenotypes typical of underlying medical conditions? *Journal of Intellectual Disability Research,* 36, 201.

Gillberg, C. & Rasmussen, P. 1982. Perceptual, motor and attentional deficits in seven-year-old children: Background factors, *Developmental Medicine and Child Neurology,* 24, 752.

Gillberg, C. & Steffenburg, S. 1987. Outcome and prognostic factors in infantile autism and similar conditions: A population-based study of 46 cases followed through puberty. *Journal of Autism and Developmental Disorders,* 17, 273.

Gillberg, C., Matousek, M., Petersen, I. & Rasmussen, P. 1984. Perceptual, motor and attentional deficits in seven-year-old children. *Acta Paedopsychiatrica,* 50, 243.

Gillberg, C., Persson, E. & Wahlstrom, J. 1985. The autism-fragile-X-syndrome (AF-RAX): A population-based study of ten boys. *Journal of Mental Deficiency Research,* 30, 27.

Gillberg, C., Persson, E., Grufman, M. & Themner, U. 1986. Psychiatric disorders in mildly and severely mentally retarded urban children and adolescents. *British Journal of Psychiatry,* 149, 68.

Gillberg, C., Steffenburg, S., Wahlstrom, J. & Gillberg, I.C. 1991. Autism associated with marker syndrome. *Journal of the American Academy of Child and Adolescent Psychiatry,* 30, 489.

Gillberg, I.C. 1985. Children with minor neurodevelopmental disorders. III: Neurological and neurodevelopmental problems at age 10. *Developmental Medicine and Child Neurology,* 27, 3.

Gillberg, I.C. & Gillberg, C. 1989a. Asperger syndrome—Some epidemiological considerations: A research note. *Journal of Child Psychology and Psychiatry,* 30, 631.

Gillberg, I.C. & Gillberg, C. 1989b. Children with preschool minor neurodevelopmental disorders. IV: Behavior and school achievement at age 13. *Developmental Medicine and Child Neurology,* 31, 3.

Gjerris, F. 1976. Clinical aspects and long-term prognosis of intra-cranial tumours in infancy and childhood. *Developmental Medicine and Child Neurology,* 1976, 18, 145.

Gjessing, H.J. & Karlsen, B. 1989. *A Longitudinal Study of Dyslexia: Bergen's Multivariate Study of Children's Learning Disabilities.* New York: Springer.

Glanville, B., Best, C. & Levenson, R. 1977. A cardiac measure of cerebral asymmetry in infant auditory perception. *Developmental Psychology,* 13, 54.

Glick, S.D. (Ed.). 1985. *Cerebral Lateralization in Nonhuman Species.* New York: Academic Press.

Glos, J. & Pavlovkin, M. 1985. Profile of intellectual achievements in the WISC of children with hemiplegic form of cerebral palsy (their dependence on the hemispheric localization of the brain damage). *Studia Psychologica,* 27, 37.

Glosser, G. & Koppell, S. 1987. Emotional-behavioral patterns in children with learning disabilities: Lateralized hemispheric differences. *Journal of Learning Disabilities,* 20, 365.

Goethe, K.E. & Levin, H.S. 1986. Neuropsychological consequences of head injury in children. In G. Goldstein and R.E. Tarter (Eds.), *Advances in Clinical Neuropsychology,* Vol. 3. New York: Plenum Press, p. 213.

Gold, P. 1979. Suspected neurological impairment and cognitive abilities: A longitudinal study. *Psychological Reports,* 45, 215.

Goldberg, E.K. & Costa, L.D. 1981. Hemispheric differences in the acquisition and use of descriptive systems. *Brain and Language,* 14, 144.

Goldberg, H.K. & Schiffman, G.B. 1972. *Dyslexia: Problems of Reading Disabilities.* New York: Grune & Stratton.

Goldberger, M.E. 1974. Recovery of movement after CNS lesions in monkeys. In D.G. Stein, J.J. Rosen & N. Butters (Eds.), *Plasticity and Recovery of Function in the Central Nervous System.* New York: Academic Press.

Golden, C.J. 1981. The Luria-Nebraska Children's Battery: Theory and formulation. In G.W. Hynd & J.E. Obrzut (Eds.), *Neuropsychological Assessment and the School-Age Child: Issues and Procedures.* New York: Grune and Stratton.

Goldensohn, E.S. & Ward, A.A. 1975. Pathogenesis of epileptic seizures. In D.B. Tower (Ed.), *The Nervous System.* Vol. 2. New York: Raven Press, p. 249.

Goldfarb, W. 1943. Infant rearing and problem behaviour. *American Journal of Orthopsychiatry,* 13, 249.

Goldie, W. 1985. BAEP's: Applications in pediatric neurology. In J.B. Cracco, R.P. Brenner & B.F. Westmoreland (Eds.), *State of the Science in EEG-1985.* Atlanta: American Electroencephalographic Society.

Goldman, P.S. 1972. Developmental determinants of cortical plasticity. *Acta Neurobiologiae Experimentalis,* 32, 495.

Goldman, P.S. 1974. An alternative to developmental plasticity: Heterology of CNS structures in infants and adults. In D.G. Stein, J.F. Rosen & N. Butters (Eds.), *Plasticity and the Recovery of Function in the Central Nervous System.* New York: Academic Press.

Goldman, P.S. 1975. Age, sex, and experience as related to the neural basis of cognitive development. In N.A. Buchwald & M.A.B. Brazier (Eds.), *Brain Mechanisms in Mental Retardation.* New York: Academic Press.

Goldman, P.S. 1976. Maturation of the mammalian nervous system and the ontogeny of behavior. In J.S. Rosenblatt, R.A. Hinde, E. Shaw & C. Beer (Eds.), *Advances in the Study of Behavior,* Vol. 7. New York: Academic Press.

Goldman, P.S. & Lewis, M.E. 1978. Developmental biology of brain damage and experience. In C.W. Cotman (Ed.), *Neuronal Plasticity*. New York: Raven Press.

Goldman, P.S. & Nauta, W.J.H. 1977. Columnar distribution of corticocortical fibers in the frontal association, limbic, and motor cortex of the developing rhesus monkey. *Brain Research*, 122, 393.

Goldman, P.S. & Rakic, P.T. 1979. Impact of the outside world upon the developing primate brain. *Bulletin of the Menninger Clinic*, 43(1), 2.

Goldman, P.S., Rosvold, H.E. & Mishkin, M. 1970. Evidence for behavioral impairments following prefrontal lobectomy in the infant monkey. *Journal of Comparative and Physiological Psychology*, 70, 454.

Goldman, P.S., Crawford, H.T., Stokes, L.P., Galkin, T.W. & Rosvold, H.E. 1974. Sex-dependent behavioral effects of cerebral cortical lesions in the developing rhesus monkey. *Science*, 186, 540.

Goldman, R., Fristoe, M. & Woodcock, R.W. 1974. *Goldman-Fristoe-Woodcock Auditory Memory Tests*. Circle Pines, MN: American Guidance Service.

Goldman-Rakic, P.S. 1980. Morphological consequences of prenatal injury to the primate brain. In P.S. McConnell, G.J. Boer, H.J. Romijn, N.E. Van de Poll & M.A. Corner (Eds.), *Adaptive Capabilities of the Nervous System (Progress in Brain Research, Vol. 53)*. Amsterdam: Elsevier/North-Holland.

Goldman-Rakic, P.S. 1984. Modular organization of prefrontal cortex. *Trends in Neuroscience*, 7, 419.

Goldman-Rakic, P.S. 1987. Development of cortical circuitry and cognitive function. *Child Development*, 58, 601.

Goldman-Rakic, P.S. 1988. Topography of cognition: Parallel distributed networks in primate association cortex. *Annual Review of Neuroscience*, 11, 137.

Goldson, E. 1992. The longitudinal study of very low birthweight infants and its implications for interdisciplinary research and public policy. In C.W. Greenbaum & J.G. Auerbach (Eds.), *Longitudinal Studies of Children at Psychological Risk: Cross-National Perspectives*. Norwood, NJ: Ablex Publishing.

Goldstein, F.C. & Levin, H.S. 1985. Intellectual and academic outcome following closed head injury in children and adolescents: Research strategies and empirical findings. *Developmental Neuropsychology*, 1, 195.

Goldstein, G. 1990. Neuropsychological heterogeneity in schizophrenia: A consideration of abstraction and problem-solving abilities. *Archives of Clinical Neuropsychology*, 5, 251.

Goldstein, K. 1944. The mental changes due to frontal lobe damage. *Journal of Psychology*, 17, 187.

Goldstein, K. 1948. *Language and Language Disturbance*. New York: Grune & Stratton.

Goldstein, R., Landau, W.M. & Kleffner, F.R. 1960. Neurological observations on a population of deaf and aphasic children. *Annals of Otolaryngology, Rhinology, and Laryngology*, 69, 757.

Goleman, D. 1978. Special abilities of the sexes: Do they begin in the brain? *Psychology Today*, 258.

Gomez, F.R., Ramos-Galvan, R., Cravioto, J. & Frank, S. 1955. Kwashiorkor-protein malnutrition. *Advances in Pediatrics*, 7, 131.

Gomez, M.R. 1967. Minimal cerebral dysfunction (maximal neurological confusion). *Clinical Pediatrics*, 6, 589.

Goodman, C.S. & Bastiani, M.J. 1987. How embryonic nerve cells recognize one another. *Scientific American*, 249, 58.

Goodman, D. & Kelso, J.A.S. 1983. Exploring the functional significance of physiological tremor: A biospectroscopic approach. *Experimental Brain Research*, 49, 419.

Goodman, J.F. 1977a. IQ decline in mentally retarded adults: A matter of fact or methodological flaw. *Journal of Mental Deficiency Research*, 21, 199.

Goodman, J.F. 1977b. Medical diagnosis and intelligence levels in young mentally retarded children. *Journal of Mental Deficiency Research*, 21, 205.

Goodman, J.F. & Cameron, J. 1978. The meaning of IQ constancy in young retarded children. *Journal of Genetic Psychology*, 132, 109.

Goodman, R. 1986. Hemispherectomy and its alternatives in the treatment of intractable epilepsy in patients with infantile hemiplegia. *Developmental Medicine and Child Neurology*, 28, 251.

Goodman, R. 1989a. Limits to cerebral plasticity. In D.A. Johnson, D. Uttley & M. Wyke (Eds.), *Children's Head Injury: Who Cares?* London: Taylor & Francis, p. 12.

Goodman, R. 1989b. Neuronal misconnections and psychiatric disorder: Is there a link? *British Journal of Psychiatry*, 154, 292.

Goodman, R. & Stevenson, J.A. 1989. Twin study of hyperactivity. II. The etiological role of genes, family relationships and perinatal adversity. *Journal of Child Psychology and Psychiatry*, 5, 691.

Goodwin, D.W., Schulsinger, F., Hermauben, L., Guze, S.B. & Winokur, G. 1975. Alcoholism and the hyperactive child syndrome. *The Journal of Nervous and Mental Disease*, 160, 349.

Gordon, D.P. 1983. The influence of sex on the development of lateralization of speech. *Neuropsychologia*, 21, 139.

Gordon, R., White, D. & Diller, L. 1972. Performance of neurologically impaired preschool children with educational materials. *Exceptional Children*, 38(5), 428.

Gorman, J.J., Cogan, D.G. & Gellis, S.S. 1957. An apparatus for grading the visual acuity of infants on the basis of optokinetic nystagmus. *Pediatrics*, 19(6), 1088.

Gott, P.S. 1973a. Cognitive abilities following right or left hemispherectomy. *Cortex*, 9, 266.

Gott, P.S. 1973b. Language after dominant hemispherectomy. *Journal of Neurology, Neurosurgery, and Psychiatry*, 36, 1082.

Gott, P.S. & Saul, R.E. 1978. Agenesis of the corpus callosum: Limits of functional compensation. *Neurology*, 28, 1272.

Gottfried, A. 1973. Intellectual consequences of perinatal anoxia. *Psychological Bulletin*, 80, 231.

Gottfried, A.W. & Bathurst, K. 1983. Hand preference across time is related to intelligence in young girls, not boys. *Science*, 221, 1074.

Gottlieb, D.D. & Allen, W. 1985. Incidence of visual disorders in a selected population of hearing-impaired students. *Journal of the American Optometric Association*, 56, 292.

Gottlieb, G. 1971. Ontogenesis of sensory function in birds and mammals. In E. Tobach, L.R. Aronson & Shaw, E. (Eds.), *The Biopsychology of Development*. New York: Academic Press.

Gottlieb, G. & Krasnegor, N.A. (Eds.). 1985. *Measurement of Audition and Vision in the First Year of Postnatal Life: A Methodological Overview*. Norwood, NJ: Ablex.

Gould, J.B., Gluck, L. & Kulovich, M.V. 1977. The relationship between accelerated pulmonary maturity and accelerated neurological maturity in certain chronically stressed pregnancies. *American Journal of Obstetrics and Gynecology,* 127, 181.

Goulet, J. 1989. Depression majeure chez l'enfant: Validation du syndrome et traitement pharmacologique. *Canadian Journal of Psychiatry,* 34, 10.

Goy, R.W. & McEwen, B.S. 1981. *Sexual Diffentiation of the Brain.* Cambridge, MA: MIT Press, 1981.

Grad, L.R., Pelcovityz, D., Olson, M. & Matthews, M. 1987. Obsessive-compulsive symptomatology in children with Tourette's syndrome. *Journal of the American Academy of Child and Adolescent Psychiatry,* 26, 69.

Grafman, J., Passafiume, D., Faglioni, P. & Boller, F. 1982. Calculation disturbances in adults with focal hemispheric damage. *Cortex,* 18, 37.

Graham, F.K., Matarazzo, R.G. & Caldwell, B.M. 1956. Behavioral differences between normal and traumatized newborns: II. Standardization, reliability, and validity. *Psychological Monographs,* 70, 21. No. 428.

Graham, F.K., Ernhart, C.B., Thurston, D. & Craft, M. 1962. Development three years after perinatal anoxia and other potentially damaging newborn experiences. *Psychological Monographs,* 76 (Whole no., 522).

Graham, J.M., Bashir, A.S., Walzer, S., Stark, R.E. & Gerald, P.S. 1981. Communication skills among unselected XXY boys. *Pediatric Research,* 15, 562.

Graham, P.J. 1971. Pathology in the brain and anti-social disorder. In J. Hellmuth (Ed.), *Exceptional Infant,* Vol. 2, New York: Brunner/Mazel.

Grant, D.W. 1985. Right hemisphere function in hydrocephalic children. *Neuropsychologia,* 23, 285.

Grant, D.W., Goldberg, C., Guiney, E.J. & Fitzgerald, R.J. 1986. Should the tradition of right hemisphere shunting still prevail? *Zeitschrift für Kinderchirurgie,* 41, 48.

Grant, I. & Alves, W. 1987. Psychiatric and psychosocial disturbances in head injury. In H.S. Levin, J. Grafman & H.M. Eisenberg (Eds.), *Neurobehavioral Recovery from Head Injury.* New York: Oxford University Press, p. 232.

Grant, M.L., Ilai, D., Nussbaum, N.L. & Bigler, E.D. 1990. The relationship between continuous performance tasks and neuropsychological tests in children with attention-deficit-hyperactivity disorder. *Perceptual and Motor Skills,* 70, 435.

Green, A.H. 1985. Children traumatized by physical abuse. In S. Eth & R.S. Pynoos (Eds.), *Post-traumatic Stress Disorder in Children.* Washington, DC: American Psychiatric Association, p. 133.

Green, M.F., Satz, P., Soper, H.V. & Kharabi, F. 1987. Relationship between physical anomalies and age of onset of schizophrenia. *American Journal of Psychiatry,* 144, 666.

Green, R.C. 1988. Epilepsy surgery in children. *Journal of Child Neurology,* 3, 155.

Greenbaum, C.W. & Auerbach, J.G. 1992. The conceptualization of risk, vulnerability, and resilience in psychological development. In C.W. Greenbaum & J.G. Auerbach (Eds.), *Longitudinal Studies of Children at Psychological Risk: Cross-National Perspectives.* Norwood, NJ: Ablex.

Greenough, W.T. 1976. Enduring brain effects of different experience and training. In M.R. Rosenzweig & E.L. Bennett (Eds.), *Neural Mechanisms of Learning and Memory.* Cambridge, MA: MIT Press.

Greenough, W.T. 1986. What's special about development? Thoughts on the bases of experience-sensitive synaptic plasticity. In W.T. Greenough & J.M. Juraska (Eds.), *Developmental Neuropsychobiology.* New York: Academic Press, p. 387.

Greenough, W.T. & Juraska, J.M. 1979. Experience-induced changes in brain fine structure: Their behavioral implications. In M.E. Hahn, C. Jensen & B.C. Dudek (Eds.), *Development and Evolution of Brain Size: Behavioral Implications.* New York: Academic Press.

Greenough, W.T., Larson, J.R. & Withers, G.S. 1985. Effects of unilateral and bilateral training in a reaching task on dendritic branching of neurons in the rat motor-sensory forelimb cortex. *Behavioral and Neural Biology,* 44, 301.

Greenough, W.T., Black, J.E. & Wallace, C.S. 1987. Experience and brain development. *Child Development,* 58, 539.

Gregg, G.S. & Hutchinson, D.L. 1969. Developmental characteristics of infants surviving fetal transfusion. *Journal of the American Medical Association,* 209, 1059.

Griffith, H. & Davidson, M. 1966. Long-term changes in intellect and behavior after hemispherectomy. *Journal of Neurology, Neurosurgery, and Psychiatry,* 29, 571.

Griffiths, C.P. 1969. A follow-up study of children with disorders of speech. *British Journal of Disorders of Communication,* 4, 46.

Griffiths, P. 1972. *Developmental Aphasia: An Introduction.* London: Invalid Children's Aid Association.

Griffiths, R. 1954. *The Abilities of Babies.* London: University of London Press.

Griffiths, R. 1970. *The Abilities of Young Children. A Comprehensive System of Mental Measurement for the First Eight Years of Life.* London: Child Development Research Center.

Grigoroiu-Sernabescu, M. 1984. Intellectual and emotional development and school adjustment in preterm children at 6 and 7 years of age. Continuation of a follow-up study. *International Journal of Behavioral Development* 7, 307.

Groden, G. 1969. Relationships between intelligence, simple and complex motor proficiency. *American Journal of Mental Deficiency,* 74, 373.

Groenendaal, F., Van Hof Van Duin, J., Baerts, W. & Fetter, W.P. 1989. Effects of perinatal hypoxia on visual development during the first year of (corrected) age. *Early Human Development,* 20, 267.

Groenveld, M. & Jan, J.E. 1992. Intelligence profiles of low vision and blind children. *Journal of Visual Impairment and Blindness,* 86, 68.

Grogono, J. 1968. Children with agenesis of the corpus callosum. *Developmental Medicine and Child Neurology,* 10, 613.

Grossberg, S. 1980. How does a brain build a cognitive code? *Psychological Review,* 87, 1.

Gross-Glenn, K., Duara, R., Barker, W.W. & Loewenstein, D. 1991. Positron emission tomographic studies during serial word-reading by normal and dyslexic subjects. *Journal of Clinical and Experimental Neuropsychology,* 13, 531.

Grossman, H.J. (Ed.). 1983. *Manual on Terminology and Classification in Mental Retardation,* 3rd ed. Washington: American Association on Mental Deficiency.

Grossman, M. 1976. The present status of viral vaccines. In W.L. Drew (Ed.), *Viral Infections, A Clinical Approach.* Philadelphia: F.A. Davis.

Gruenewald-Zuberbier, E., Gruenwald, G. & Rasche, A. 1975. Hyperactive behavior and EEG arousal reactions in children. *Electroencephalography and Clinical Neurophysiology,* 38, 149.

Gruenewald-Zuberbier, E., Gruenwald, G., Rasche, A. & Netz, J. 1978. Contingent negative variation and alpha attenuation responses in children with different abilities to concentrate. *Electroencephalography and Clinical Neurophysiology,* 44, 37.

Grunnet, M.L. & Shields, W.D. 1976. Cerebellar hemorrhage in the premature infant. *Journal of Pediatrics*, 88(4), 605.

Gubbay, S.S. 1979. The clumsy child. In F.C. Rose (Ed.), *Pediatric Neurology*. London: Blackwell, p. 145.

Gubbay, S.S., Ellis, S., Walton, J.N. & Court, S.D.M. 1965. Clumsy children, a study of apraxic and agnosic defects in 21 children. *Brain*, 88, 295.

Gudmundsson, G. 1966. Epilepsy in Iceland. *Acta Neurologica Scandinavica*, suppl. 25.

Guerrini, R., Dravet, C., Raybaud, C. & Roger, J. 1992. Epilepsy and focal gyral anomalies detected by MRI: Electroclinico-morphological correlations and follow-up. *Developmental Medicine and Child Neurology*, 34, 706.

Guilford, J.P. 1956. The structure of intellect. *Psychological Bulletin*, 53, 267.

Gulick, W.L. 1971. *Hearing: Physiology and Psychophysics*. New York: Oxford University Press.

Gupta, D. (Ed.). 1984. *Paediatric Neuroendocrinology*. New York: A.R. Liss.

Gur, R.C. 1982. Sex and handedness differences in cerebral blood flow during rest and cognitive activity. *Science*, 217, 659.

Gur, R.E. 1978. Left hemisphere dysfunction and left hemisphere overactivity in schizophrenia. *Journal of Abnormal Psychology*, 87, 226.

Gur, R.E. 1987. Psychiatric disorders as brain dysfunction. *National Forum*, 67(2), 29.

Guttman, E. 1942. Aphasia in children. *Brain*, 65, 205.

Guy, J.D., Majorski, L.V., Wallace, C.J. & Guy, M.P. 1983. The incidence of minor physical anomalies in adult male schizophrenics. *Schizophrenia Bulletin*, 9, 571.

Habicht, J.P., Yarbrough, C. & Klein, R.E. 1974. Assessing nutritional status in a field study of malnutrition and mental development: Specificity, sensitivity, and congruity of indices of nutritional status. In J. Cravioto, L. Hambraeus & B. Vahlquist (Eds.), *Early Malnutrition and Mental Development*. Uppsala: Almquist & Wiksell.

Hack, M., Breslau, N., Aram, D. & Weissman, B. 1992. The effect of very low birth weight and social risk on neurocognitive abilities at school age. *Journal of Developmental and Behavioral Pediatrics*, 13, 412.

Hack, M., Breslau, N., Weissman, B. & Aram, D.M. 1991a. Effect of very low birth weight and subnormal head size on cognitive abilities at school age. *New England Journal of Medicine*, 325, 231.

Hack, M., Horbar, J.D., Malloy, M.H., Tryson, J.E., Wright, E. & Wright, L. 1991b. Very low birth weight outcomes of the National Institute of Child Health and Human Neonatal Network. *Pediatrics* 87, 5, 587.

Hadenius, A.M., Hagberg, B., Hyttnes-Bensch, K. & Sjogren, I. 1962. The natural prognosis of infantile hydrocephalus. *Acta Paediatrica* (Uppsala), 51, 117.

Hagberg, B. 1975. Pre-, peri-, and post-natal prevention of major neuropediatric handicaps. *Neuropaediatrie*, 6, 331.

Hagerman, R.J. 1990. The association between autism and fragile X syndrome. *Brain Dysfunction*, 3, 218.

Hagerman, R.J. & McBogg, P.M. 1983. *The Fragile X Syndrome*. Dillon, CO: Spectra.

Hagerman, R.J., Jackson, A.W., Levitas, A., Braden, M., McBogg, P., Kemper, M., McGarran, L., Berry, R., Matus, I. & Hagerman, P.J. 1986. Oral folic acid versus placebo in the treatment of males with the fragile X syndrome. *American Journal of Medical Genetics*, 23, 241.

Haggerty, J.J., Evans, D.I. & Prange, A.J. 1986. Organic brain syndromes associated with marginal hypothyroidism. *American Journal of Psychiatry*, 143, 785.

Hagne, I. 1968. Development of the waking EEG in normal infants during the first year of life. In P. Kellaway & I. Petersen (Eds.), *Clinical Electrophysiology of Children.* Stockholm: Almqvist and Wiksell (New York: Grune & Stratton).

Hahn, W.K. 1987. Cerebral lateralization of function: From infancy through childhood. *Psychological Bulletin,* 101, 376.

Haith, M.M., Bergman, T. & Moore, M.J. 1977. Eye contact and face scanning in early infancy. *Science,* 198, 853.

Hall, G.S. 1904. *Adolescence* Vols 1–2. New York: Appelton-Century-Crofts.

Hall, J.A. & Kimura, D. 1993. Morphological and functional asymmetry in homosexual males. *Society for Neuroscience Abstracts,* 19, 561.

Halperin, J.M., O'Brien, J.D., Newcorn, J.H. & Healy, J.M. 1990. Validation of hyperactive, aggressive, and mixed hyperactive/aggressive childhood disorders: A research note. *Journal of Child Psychology and Psychiatry and Allied Disciplines,* 31, 455.

Halstead, W.C. 1947. *Brain and Intelligence: A Quantitative Study of the Frontal Lobes.* Chicago: University of Chicago Press, 1947.

Hamburger, V. 1954. Trends in experimental neuroembryology. In P. Weiss (Ed.), *Biochemistry of the Developing Nervous System.* Chicago, IL: University of Chicago Press.

Hamilton, A.M. 1991. Sensory hand function of the child with spina bifida myelomeningocele. *British Journal of Occupational Therapy,* 54, 346.

Hankin, L., Heichel, G.H. & Botsford, R.A. 1973. Lead poisoning from colored printing inks. *Clinical Pediatrics,* 12, 654.

Hanley, W.B., Linsao, L., Davidson, W. & Moes, C.A.F. 1970. Malnutrition with early treatment of phenylketonuria. *Pediatric Research,* 4, 318.

Hannay, H.J. & Levin, H.S. 1988. Visual continuous recognition memory in normal and closed-head-injury adolescents. *Journal of Clinical and Experimental Neuropsychology,* 11, 444.

Hansen, O., Nerup, J. & Holbek, B. 1986. Common genetic origin of specific dyslexia and insulin-dependent diabetes mellitus? *Hereditas,* 105, 165.

Hansen, O., Nerup, J. & Holbek, B. 1987. Further indications of a common genetic origin of specific dyslexia and insulin-dependent diabetes mellitus. *Hereditas,* 107, 257.

Hanshaw, J.B., Scheiner, A.P., Moxley, A.W., Gaev, L., Abel, V. & Scheiner, B. 1976. School failure and deafness after silent congenital cytomegalovirus infection. *New England Journal of Medicine,* 295, 468.

Hanson, J.W., Streissguth, A.P. & Smith, D.W. 1978. The effects of moderate alcohol consumption during pregnancy on fetal growth and morphogenesis. *Journal of Pediatrics,* 92, 457.

Hanson, M.J. 1987. *Teaching the Infant with Down's Syndrome.* Austin TX: Pro-Ed Inc.

Harcherik, D.F. 1985. Computed tomography brain scanning in four neuropsychiatric disorders of childhood. *American Journal of Psychiatry,* 142, 731.

Harcherik, D.F., Carbonari, C.M., Shaywitz, S.E., Shaywitz, B.A. & Cohen, D.J. 1982. Attentional and perceptual disturbances in children with Tourette's syndrome, attention deficit disorder, and epilepsy. *Schizophrenia Bulletin,* 8, 356.

Hardy, J.B. 1968. Viruses and the fetus. *Postgraduate Medicine,* 43, 156.

Hardy, J.B. 1973. Clinical and developmental aspects of congenital rubella. *Archives of Otolaryngology,* 98, 230.

Hardy, J.M.B., Drage, J.S. & Jackson, E.C. 1979. *The First Year of Life: The Collaborative Perinatal Study of the National Institute of Neurological and Communicative Disorders and Stroke.* Baltimore: The Johns Hopkins University Press.

Harel, S., Kutai, M., Tomer, A., Tal-Posener, E., Leitner, Y., Fatal, A., Jaffa, A. & Yavin, E. 1989. Intrauterine growth retardation: Diagnosis and neurodevelopmental outcome. In N.J. Anastasiow and S. Harel (Eds.), *At-Risk Infants: Interventions, Families, and Research*. Baltimore: Paul H. Brookes, 145.

Harlan, R.E., Gordon, J.H. & Gorski, R.A. 1979. Sexual differentiation of the brain: Implications for neuroscience. In D.M. Schneider (Ed.), *Reviews of Neuroscience*, vol. 4. New York: Raven Press.

Harlow, H.F. & Harlow, M.K. 1965. The affectional systems. In A.M. Schrier, H.F. Harlow & F. Stollnitz (Eds.), *Behavior of the Nonhuman Primates*, Vol. 2. London: Academic Press.

Harlow, H.F., Thompson, C., Blomquist, A. & Schilte, K. 1970. Learning in Rhesus monkeys after varying amounts of prefrontal lobe destruction during infancy and adolescence. *Brain Research*, 18, 343.

Haron, M. & Henderson, A. 1985. Active and passive touch in developmentally dyspraxic and normal boys. *Occupational Therapy Journal of Research*, 5, 101.

Harper, J.R. 1967. Infantile spasms associated with cerebral agyria. *Developmental Medicine and Child Neurology*, 9, 460.

Harper, P.A. & Weiner, G. 1956. Sequelae of low birthweight. *Annual Review of Medicine*, 16, 405.

Harris, L.J. 1993. Do left-handers die sooner than right-handers? Commentary on Coren and Halpern's (1991) "Left-handedness: A marker for decreased survival fitness." *Psychological Bulletin*, 114, 203.

Harris, L.J. & Carlson, D.F. 1989. Pathological left-handedness: An analysis of theories and evidence. In *Handedness and Intellectual Development*. New York: Wiley.

Harrison, L.J. & Taylor, D.M. 1976. Child seizures: A 25-year follow-up. *Lancet*, 116, 948.

Harshman, R.A., Hampson, E. & Berenbaum, S.A. 1983. Individual differences in cognitive abilities and brain organization. Part I: Sex and handedness, differences in abilities. *Canadian Journal of Psychology*, 37, 144.

Hartlage, L.C. & Lucas, D.G. 1973. *Mental Development of the Pediatric Patient*. Springfield, IL: Charles C Thomas, 1973.

Hartlage, L.C., Green, J.B. & Offutt, L. 1972. Dependency in epileptic children. *Epilepsia*, 13, 27.

Hartley, X.Y. 1986. Lateralization of speech stimuli in young Down's syndrome children. *Cortex*, 17, 241.

Hartman, D.E. 1988. *Neuropsychological Toxicology: Identification and Assessment of Human Neurotoxic Syndromes*. Elmsford, NY: Pergamon.

Hartmann, A., Yatsu, F. & Kuschinsky, W. (Eds.) 1994. *Cerebral Ischemia and Basic Mechanisms*. New York: Springer.

Hartsough, C.S. & Lambert, N.M. 1985. Medical factors in hyperactive and normal children: Prenatal, developmental, and health history findings. *American Journal of Orthopsychiatry*, 55, 190.

Harvey, I., Goodyear, I.M. & Brown, S.W. 1988. The value of a neuropsychiatric examination of children with complex severe epilepsy. *Child: Care, Health and Development*, 14, 329.

Hassler, M. 1991. Maturation rate and spatial, verbal, and musical abilities: A seven-year longitudinal study. *International Journal of Neuroscience*, 58, 183.

Hastings, J.E. & Barkley, R.A. 1978. A review of psychophysiological research with hyperkinetic children. *Journal of Abnormal Child Psychology*, 6, 439.

Hatcher, R. 1976. The predictability of infant intelligence scales: A review and evaluation. *Mental Retardation,* 14, 16.

Hatta, T. 1977. Recognition of Japanese Kanji in the left and right visual fields. *Neuropsychologia,* 1977, 15, 685.

Hatta, T. & Dimond, S.J. 1981. The differential interference effects of environmental sounds on spoken speech in Japanese and British people. *Brain and Language,* 13, 241.

Hatta, T. & Moriya, K. 1988. Developmental changes of hemisphere collaboration for tactile sequential information. *International Journal for Behavioral Development,* 11, 451.

Hauser, S.L., DeLong, R. & Rosman, P. 1975. Pneumographic findings in the infantile autism syndrome (a correlation with temporal lobe disease). *Brain,* 98, 667.

Hawk, B.A., Schroeder, S.R., Robinson, G., Otto, D., Mushak, P., Kleinbaum, D. & Dawson, G. 1986. Relation of lead and social factors to IQ of low-SES children: A partial replication. *American Journal of Mental Deficiency,* 91, 178.

Hebb, D.O. 1949. *The Organization of Behavior.* New York: Oxford University Press.

Hecaen, H. & Albert, M.L. 1978. *Human Neuropsychology,* New York: Wiley.

Hecht, F. & MacFarlane, J.P. 1969. Mosaicism in Turner's syndrome reflects the lethality of XO. *Lancet,* 2, 1197.

Hechtman, L. & Weiss, G. 1983. Long-term outcome of hyperactive children. *American Journal of Orthopsychiatry,* 53, 532.

Hechtman, L., Weiss, G., Finklestein, J., Werner, A. & Benn, R. 1976. Hyperactives as young adults: Preliminary report. *Canadian Medical Association Journal,* 115, 625.

Hechtman, L., Weiss, G. & Metrakos, K. 1978. Hyperactive individuals as young adults: Current and longitudinal electroencephalographic evaluation and its relation to outcome. *Canadian Medical Association Journal,* 118, 919.

Hechtman, L., Weiss, G. & Perlman, T. 1984. Young adult outcome of hyperactive children who received long-term stimulant treatment. *Journal of the American Academy of Child Psychiatry,* 23, 261.

Hecox, K. 1975. Electrophysiological correlates of human auditory development. In L.B. Cohen & P. Salapatek (Eds.), *Infant Perception: From Sensation to Cognition,* Vol. 2. New York: Academic Press.

Heideman, R.L., Packer, R.J., Albright, L.A., Freeman, C.R. & Rorke, L.B. 1993. Tumors of the central nervous system. In P.A. Pizzo & D.G. Poplack (Eds.), *Principles and Practice of Pediatric Oncology,* 2nd ed. Philadelphia: J.B. Lippincott.

Heilman, K.M. 1979a. The neuropsychological basis of skilled movement in man. In M.S. Gazzaniga (Ed.), *Handbook of Behavioral Neurobiology, Vol. 2 Neuropsychology.* New York: Plenum Press.

Heilman, K.M. 1979b. Apraxia. In K.M. Heilman & E. Valenstein (Eds.), *Clinical Neuropsychology.* New York: Oxford University Press.

Heilman, K.M. & Valenstein, E. (Eds.). 1984. *Clinical Neuropsychology,* 2nd ed. New York: Oxford University Press.

Heinrichs, R.W. 1993. Schizophrenia and the brain: Conditions for a neuropsychology of madness. *American Psychologist,* 48, 221.

Held, R. 1989. Correlating perceptual and neuronal development. In J. Alegria, D. Holender, J.J. de Morais & M. Radeau (Eds.), *Analytic Approaches to Human Cognition.* Amsterdam: North-Holland, p. 19.

Helper, M.M. 1980. Follow-up of children with minimal brain dysfunctions: Outcomes and predictors. In H.E. Rie & E.D. Rie (Eds.), *Handbook of Minimal Brain Dysfunctions: A Critical Review.* New York: Wiley.

Heppenstrijdt, M. 1988. Neuropsychological outcome of neonatal jaundice: A 6-year follow-up study. Victoria, British Columbia: Arbutus Society for Children.

Hermelin, B. & O'Connor, N. 1970. *Psychological Experiments with Autistic Children.* Oxford: Pergamon.

Hermelin, B. & Connor, N. 1971. Functional asymmetry in the reading of Braille. *Neuropsychologia,* 9, 431.

Hernadek, M.C.S. & Rourke, B.P. 1994. Principal identifying features of the syndrome of nonverbal learning disabilities in children. *Journal of Learning Disabilities,* 27, 144.

Herron, J. (Ed.) 1980. *Neuropsychology of Left-Handedness.* New York: Academic Press.

Hershkowitz, J., Rosman, N.P. & Geschwind, N. 1984. Seizures induced by singing and recitation: A unique form of reflex epilepsy in childhood. *Archives of Neurology,* 41, 1102.

Hertzig, M.E. 1981. Neurological 'soft' signs in low-birthweight children. *Developmental Medicine and Child Neurology,* 23, 778.

Hertzig, M.E. 1982. Neurological "soft" signs in low-birthweight children. *Annual Progress in Child Psychiatry and Child Development,* 509.

Hertzig, M.E. 1983. Temperament and neurological status. In M. Rutter (Ed.), *Developmental Neuropsychiatry.* New York: Guilford Press, p. 164.

Hertzig, M.E. & Shapiro, T. 1987. The assessment of nonfocal neurological signs in school-aged children. In D.E. Tupper (Ed.), *Soft Neurological Signs.* Orlando: Grune & Stratton, p. 71.

Hertzig, M.E., Birch, H.G., Richardson, S.A. & Tizard, J. 1972. Intellectual levels of school children severely malnourished during the first two years of life. *Pediatrics,* 49, 814.

Hertzig, M.E., Bortner, M. & Birch, H.G. 1969. Neurologic findings in children educationally designated as "brain-damaged." *American Journal of Orthopsychiatry,* 39, 437.

Heston, L.L. 1970. The genetics of schizophrenia and schizoid disease. *Science,* 167, 249.

Hewitt, W. 1962. The development of the human corpus callosum. *Journal of Anatomy,* 96(3), 355.

Hickey, T.L. 1977. Postnatal development of the human lateral geniculate nucleus: Relationship to a critical period for the visual system. *Science,* 198, 836.

Hicks, R.A., Elliott, D., Garbesi, L. & Martin, S. 1979. Multiple birth risk factors and the distribution of handedness. *Cortex,* 15, 135.

Hicks, S.P. & D'Amato, C.J. 1966. Effects of ionizing radiation on mammalian development. In D.H.M. Woollam (Ed.), *Advances in Teratology.* London: Logos Press.

Hier, D.B. 1981. Sex differences in brain structure. In A. Ansara, et al. (Eds.), *Sex Differences in Dyslexia.* Towson, MD: The Orton Dyslexia Society.

Hier, D., Le May, M., Rosenberger, P. & Perlo, V. 1978. Developmental dyslexia. *Archives of Neurology,* 35, 90.

Hildreth, G. 1949. The development and training of hand dominance. II. Developmental tendencies in handedness. *Journal of Genetic Psychology,* 75, 221.

Hill, A. 1993. The predictive significance of clinical measures of brain injury in the newborn. *Clinical Investigative Medicine,* 16, 141.

Hill, A. & Volpe, J.J. 1989a. Perinatal asphyxia: Clinical aspects. *Clinics in Perinatology,* 16, 435.

Hill, A. & Volpe, J.J. 1989b. Hypoxic-ischemic encephalopathy of the newborn. In K.F. Swaiman (Ed.), *Pediatric Neurology, Principles and Practice.* St. Louis: C.V. Mosby, p. 373.

Hill, A. & Volpe, J.J. 1989c. Stroke and hemorrhage in the premature and term neonate. In M.S.B. Edwards and H.J. Hoffman (Eds.), *Cerebral Vascular Disorders in Children and Adolescents*. Baltimore: Williams & Wilkins, p. 179.

Hill, A.E., McKendrick, O., Poole, J.J., Pugh, R.E., Rosenbloom, L. & Turnock, R. 1986. The Liverpool visual assessment team: 10 years' experience. *Child: Care, Health and Development*, 12, 37.

Hill, A.L. 1975. An investigation of calendar calculating by an idiot savant. *American Journal of Psychiatry*, 132, 557.

Hill, A.L. 1977. Idiots savant: Rate of incidence. *Perceptual and Motor Skills*, 44, 161.

Hillier, W.F. 1954. Total left cerebral hemispherectomy for malignant glioma. *Neurology*, 4, 718.

Himwich, W.A. (Ed.). 1973. *Biochemistry of the Developing Brain*. New York: Dekker.

Hines, R.B., Minde, K., Marton, P. & Trehub, S. 1980. Behavioural development of premature infants: An ethological approach. *Developmental Medicine and Child Neurology*, 22, 623.

Hinshaw, S.P., Carte, E.T. & Morrison, D.C. 1986. Concurrent prediction of academic achievement in reading disabled children: The role of neuropsychological and intellectual measures at different ages. *International Journal of Clinical Neuropsychology*, 8, 308.

Hinshelwood, J. 1895. Word blindness and visual memory. *Lancet*, 2, 1564.

Hirata, T., Epcar, J.T., Walsh, A., Mednick, J., Harris, M., McGinnis, M.S., Sehring, S. & Papedo, G. 1983. Survival and outcome of infants 501–750 grams: A six year experience. *Journal of Pediatrics*, 102, 741.

Hirsch, H.V.B. & Jacobson, M. 1975. The perfectible brain: Principles of neuronal development. In M.S. Gazzaniga and C. Blakemore (Eds.), *Handbook of Psychobiology*. New York: Academic Press.

Hirsch, J.F., Sainte-Rose, C., Pierre-Kahn, A., Pfister, A. & Hoppe-Hirsch, E. 1989. Benign astrocytic and oligodendrocytic tumors of the cerebral hemispheres in children. *Journal of Neurosurgery*, 70, 568.

Hiscock, M. & Kinsbourne, M. 1987. Specialization of the cerebral hemispheres: Implications for learning. *Journal of Learning Disabilities*, 20, 130.

Hodapp, R.M., Dykens, E.M., Hagerman, R.J. & Schreiner, R. 1990. Developmental implications of changing trajectories of IQ in males with fragile X syndrome. *Journal of the American Academy of Child and Adolescent Psychiatry*, 29, 214.

Hoffman, H.J. 1985. Craniopharyngiomas. *Canadian Journal of Neurological Science*, 12, 348.

Hoffman, H.J., Hendrick, E.B., Dennis, M. & Armstrong, D. 1979. Hemispherectomy for Sturge-Weber Syndrome. *Child's Brain*, 5, 223.

Hoffmann, W.L. & Prior, M.R. 1982. Neuropsychological dimensions of autism in children: A test of the hemispheric dysfunction hypothesis. *Journal of Clinical Neuropsychology*, 4(1), 27.

Holborow, P.L. & Berry, P.S. 1986. Relationship between hyperactivity and learning difficulties. *Journal of Learning Disabilities*, 19, 426.

Holden, E.W., Tarnowski, K.J. & Prinz, R.J. 1982. Reliability of neurological soft signs in children: Reevaluation of the PANESS. *Journal of Abnormal Child Psychology*, 10, 163.

Holden, K.R., Freeman, J.M. & Mellits, E.D. 1980. Outcomes of infants with neonatal seizures. In J.A. Wada & J.K. Penry (Eds.), *Advances in Epileptology: 10th Epilepsy International Symposium*. New York: Raven Press.

Holdsworth, L.K. & Whitmore, K. 1974. A study of children attending ordinary schools. I: Their seizure patterns, progress and behavior at school. *Developmental Medicine and Child Neurology*, 16(6), 746.

Holland, B.A., Haas, D.K., Norman, D., Brant-Zawadzki, M. & Newton, T.H. 1986. MRI of normal brain maturation. *American Journal of Neuroscience Research*, 7, 201.

Hollander, E., DeCaria, C.M., Aronowitz, B. & Klein, D.F. 1991. A pilot follow-up study of childhood soft signs and the development of adult psychopathology. *Journal of Neuropsychiatry and Clinical Neurosciences*, 3, 186.

Holliman, R.E. 1988. Toxoplasmosis and the acquired immunodeficiency syndrome. *Journal of Infection*, 16, 121.

Hollyday, M. 1980. Motoneuron histogenesis and the development of limb innervation. In R.K. Hunt (Ed.), *Neural Development, Part I (Current Topics in Developmental Biology, Vol. 15)*. New York: Academic Press.

Holtzman, N.E., Kronmal, M.P.H.R., van Doornink, W., Azen, C. & Koch, R. 1986. Effect of age at loss of dietary control on intellectual performance and behavior of children with phenylketonuria. *New England Journal of Medicine*, 314, 593.

Honzik, M. 1976. Value and limitations of infant tests: An overview. In M. Lewis (Ed.), *Origins of Intelligence*. New York: Plenum Press, p. 59.

Hook, E.B. 1981. Prevalence of chromosome abnormalities during human gestation and implications for studies of environmental mutagens. *Lancet*, 2, 169.

Hooker, D. 1952. *The Prenatal Origin of Behavior*. Porter Lectures (Series 18). Lawrence, KS: University of Kansas Press.

Hooper, S.R., Boyd, T.A., Hynd, G.W. & Rubin, J. 1993. Definitional issues and neurobiological foundations of severe selective neurodevelopmental disorders. *Archives of Clinical Neuropsychology*, 8, 279.

Hooper, S.R. & Willis, W.G. 1989. *Learning Disability Subtyping: Neuropsychological Foundations, Conceptual Models, and Issues in Clinical Differentiation*. New York: Springer.

Hopkins, T., Bice, V. & Colton, K.C. 1954. *Evaluation and Education of the Cerebral Palsied Child—New Jersey Study*. Washington, DC: International Council for Exceptional Children.

Horton, A.M. 1993. *Behavioral Interventions with Brain-Injured Children*. New York: Plenum.

Horton, R. & Katona, C. (Eds.). 1991. *Biological Aspects of Affective Disorders*. San Diego: Academic Press.

Horwitz, W.A., Kestenbaum, C., Person, E. & Jarvik, L. 1965. Identical twins—idiots savant—calendar calculators. *American Journal of Psychiatry*, 121, 1075.

Househam, K.C. 1991. Computed tomography of the brain in kwashiorkor: A follow-up study. *Archives of Disease in Childhood*, 66, 623.

Househam, K.C. & deVilliers, J.F.K. 1987. Computed tomography in severe protein-calorie malnutrition. *Archives of Disease in Childhood*, 62, 589.

Howard, F.M. & Hill, J.M. 1979. Drugs in pregnancy. *Obstetrical and Gynecological Survey*, 34(9), 643.

Howie, V.M. 1980. Developmental sequalae of chronic otitis media: A review. *Journal of Developmental and Behavioral Pediatrics*, 1, 34.

Hoy, E., Weiss, G., Minde, K. & Cohen, N. 1978. The hyperactive child at adolescence. Cognitive, emotional and social functioning. *Journal of Abnormal Child Psychology*, 6, 311.

Hoy, E.A., Sykes, D.H., Bill, J.M. & Halliday, H.L. 1991. The effects of being born of very-low-birthweight. *Irish Journal of Psychology,* 12, 182.

Hoyt, C. 1986. Optic nerve hypoplasia: A changing perspective. In *Pediatric Ophthalmology and Strabism: Transactions of the New Orleans Academy of Ophthalmology.* New York: Raven Press.

Hubel, D.H. 1976. The visual cortex of normal and deprived monkeys. *American Scientist,* 67, 532.

Hubel, D.H. & Wiesel, T.N. 1965. Receptive fields of cells in striate cortex of very young visually inexperienced kittens. *Journal of Neurophysiology,* 28, 1041.

Huessy, H.R., Metoyer, M. & Townsend, M. 1974. 8–10 year follow-up of 84 children treated for behavioural disorder in rural Vermont. *Acta Paedopsychiatrica* 10, 230.

Hugdahl, K. & Carlsson, G. 1994. Dichotic listening and focused attention in children with hemiplegic cerebral palsy. *Journal of Clinical and Experimental Neuropsychology,* 16, 84.

Hugdahl, K., Synnevag, B. & Satz, P. 1990. Immune and autoimmune diseases in dyslexic children. *Neuropsychologia,* 28, 673.

Hughes, H.E., Pringle, G.F., Scribani, L.A. & Dow-Edwards, D. 1991. Cocaine treatment in neonatal rats affects adult behavioral response to amphetamine. *Neurotoxicology and Teratology,* 13, 335.

Hughlings Jackson, J. 1958 (1869). On localization in *Selected Writings,* Vol. 2. New York: Basic Books.

Humphrey, T. 1970. The development of human fetal activity and its relation to postnatal behavior. In H.W. Reese and L.P. Lipsitt (Eds.), *Advances in Child Development and Behavior,* Vol. 5. New York: Academic Press.

Hunt, J.M., Tooley, W.H. & Marvin, D. 1982. Learning disabilities in children with birth weights below 1500 grams. *Seminars in Perinatology,* 4, 280.

Hunt, J.V. 1981. Predicting intellectual disorders in childhood for pre-term infants with birthweights below 1501 gm. In S.L. Friedman & H. Sigman (Eds.), *Preterm Birth and Psychological Development.* New York: Academic Press.

Hunt, R.K. (Ed.) 1980. *Emergence of Specificity in Neural Histogenesis.* Current Topics in Developmental Biology, vol. 15. New York: Academic Press.

Hunt, R.K. (Ed.) 1982. *Neural Specificity, Plasticity and Patterns.* Current Topics in Developmental Biology. vol. 17. New York: Academic Press.

Hurley, A.D. & Hunt, R.K. (Eds.) 1980. *Neural Development,* Part I–IV. New York: Academic Press.

Hurley, A.D., Laatsch, L.K. & Dorman, C. 1983. Comparison of spina bifida, hydrocephalic patients and matched controls on neuropsychological tests. *Zeitschrift für Kinderchirurgie,* 38, Suppl. 2, 116.

Hurley, A.D., Dorman, C., Laatsch, L. & Bell, S. 1990. Cognitive functioning in patients with spina bifida, hydrocephalus, and "cocktail-party" syndrome. *Developmental Neuropsychology,* 6, 151.

Hutchings, D.E., Gibbon, J., Gaston, J. & Vacca, L. 1975. Critical periods in fetal development: Differential effects on learning and development produced by maternal vitamin A excess. In N.R. Ellis (Ed.), *Aberrant Development in Infancy.* Hillsdale, NJ: Erlbaum.

Hutchinson, D. 1978. The transdisciplinary approach. In J.B. Curry & K.K. Peppe (Eds.), *Mental Retardation: Nursing Approaches to Care.* St. Louis: C.V. Mosby.

Huttenlocher, P.R. 1990. Morphometric studies of human cerebral cortex development. *Neuropsychologia*, 28, 517.

Huttenlocher, P.R. 1984. Synapse elimination and plasticity in developing human cerebral cortex. *American Journal of Mental Deficiency*, 88, 488.

Huttenlocher, P.R. 1991. Dendritic and synaptic pathology in mental retardation. *Pediatric Neurology*, 7, 79.

Huttenlocher, P.R. & Hapke, R.J. 1990. A follow-up study of intractable seizures in childhood. *Annals of Neurology*, 28, 699.

Huttenlocher, P.R., de Courten, C., Garey, L.J. & Van der Loos, H. 1982. Synaptogenesis in human visual cortex—evidence for synapse elimination during normal development. *Neuroscience Letters*, 33, 247.

Hyde-Thomas, T.M., Ziegler, J.C. & Weinberger, D.R. 1992. Psychiatric disturbances in metachromatic leukodystrophy: Insights into the neurobiology of psychosis. *Archives of Neurology*, 49, 401.

Hynd, G.W. & Willis, W.G. 1987. *Pediatric Neuropsychology*. Orlando, FL: Grune & Stratton.

Hynd, G.W., Obrzut, J.E., Weed, W. & Hynd, C. 1979. Development of cerebral dominance: Dichotic listening asymmetry in normal and learning-disabled children. *Journal of Experimental Child Psychology*, 28, 445.

Hynd, G.W., Nieves, N., Connor, R.T. & Stone, P. 1989. Attention deficit disorder with and without hyperactivity: Reaction time and speed of cognitive processing. *Journal of Learning Disabilities*, 22, 573.

Hynd, G.W., Semrud-Clikeman M., Lorys, A.R., Novey, E.S. & Eliopulos, D. 1990a. Brain morphology in developmental dyslexia, attention deficit disorder/hyperactivity. *Archives of Neurology*, 47, 919.

Hynd, G.W., Semrud-Clikeman, M., Lorys, A.R., Novey, E.S., Eliopulos, D. & Lyytinen, H. 1990b. Corpus callosum morphology in attention deficit-hyperactivity disorder (ADHD): Morphometric analysis of MRI. *Journal of the American Academy of Child and Adolescent Psychiatry*, 29, 610.

Hynd, G.W., Semrud-Clikeman, M. & Lyytinen, H. 1991. Brain imaging in learning disabilities. In J.E. Obrzut and G.W. Hynd (Eds.), *Neuropsychological Foundations of Learning Disabilities*. San Diego: Academic Press.

Icenogle, D.A. & Kaplan, A.M. 1981. A review of congenital neurologic malformations. *Clinical Pediatrics*, 20, 565.

Ignelzi, R.J. & Bucy, P.C. 1968. Cerebral hemidecortication in the treatment of infantile cerebral hemiatrophy. *Journal of Nervous and Mental Diseases*, 147, 14.

Iloeje, S.O. 1988. Trophic limb changes among children with developmental apraxia. *Developmental Medicine and Child Neurology*, 30, 791.

Incagnoli, T. & Kane, R. 1983. Developmental perspective of the Gilles de la Tourette syndrome. *Perceptual and Motor Skills*, 57, 1271.

Ingraham, F.D. & Matson, D.D. *Neurosurgery of Infancy and Childhood*. Springfield, IL: Charles C Thomas, 1954.

Ingram, T.T.S. 1973. Soft signs. *Developmental Medicine and Child Neurology*, 15, 527.

Ingram, T.T.S. 1975. Speech disorders in childhood. In E.H. Lenneberg & E. Lenneberg (Eds.), *Foundations of Language Development*, Vol. 2. New York: Academic Press, p. 295.

Ireton, H.R. 1984. *The Preschool Developmental Inventory*. Minneapolis: Behavior Science Systems.

Ireton, H.R. 1988. *The Early Childhood Developmental Inventory.* Minneapolis: Behavior Science Systems.

Ireton, H.R. 1990. Developmental screening measures. In J.H. Johnson & J. Goldman (Eds.), *Developmental Assessment in Clinical Child Psychology. A Handbook.* New York: Pergamon Press, p. 78.

Ireton, H.R. & Thwing, E. 1974. *The Minnesota Child Development Inventory.* Minneapolis: Behavior Science Systems.

Irwin, J.V., Moore, J.M. & Rampp, D.L. 1972. Nonmedical diagnosis and evaluation. In J.V. Irwin & M. Marge (Eds.), *Principles of Childhood Language Disabilities.* New York: Appleton-Century-Croft.

Isaacson, R.L. 1975. The myth of recovery from early brain damage. In N.R. Ellis (Ed.), *Aberrant Development in Infancy.* Hillsdale, NJ: Erlbaum.

Isaacson, R.L. 1976. Recovery (?) from early brain damage. In T.D. Tjossen (Ed.), *Intervention Strategies for High-Risk Infants and Young Children.* Baltimore: University Park Press.

Isaacson, R.L. (Ed.) 1992. *The Vulnerable Brain and Environmental Risk,* Vol. 1 and 2. New York: Plenum.

Iversen, S.D. & Dunnett, S.B. 1990. Functional organization of striatum with neural grafts. *Neuropsychologia, 28,* 601.

Jabbari, B., Schwartz, D.M., MacNeil, D.M. & Coker, S.B. 1983. Early abnormalities of brainstem auditory evoked potentials in Friedreich's ataxia: Evidence of primary brainstem dysfunction. *Neurology, 33,* 1071.

Jacobs, P.A., Brunton, M. & Melville, M.M. 1965. Aggressive behavior, mental subnormality and the xxy male. *Nature, 208,* 1351.

Jacobson, J.W. & Janicki, M.P. 1983. Observed prevalence of multiple developmental disabilities. *Mental Retardation, 21,* 87.

Jacobson, M. 1978. *Developmental Neurobiology,* 2nd ed. New York: Plenum Press.

Jacobson, R., LeCouteur, A., Howlin, P. & Rutter, M. 1988. Selective subcortical abnormalities in autism. *Psychological Medicine, 18,* 39.

Jaffe, J., Pringle, G.F. & Anderson, S.W. 1985. Speed of color naming and intelligence: Association in girls, disassociation in boys. *Journal of Communication Disorders, 18,* 63.

Jan, J.E., Freeman, R.D. & Scott, E.P. 1977. *Visual Impairment in Children and Adolescents.* New York: Grune & Stratton.

Jan, J.E., Groenveld, M. & Connolly, M.B. 1990a. Head shaking by visually impaired children: A voluntary neurovisual adaptation which can be confused with spasmus mutans. *Developmental Medicine and Child Neurology, 32,* 1061.

Jan, J.E., Groenveld, M. & Sykanda, A.M. 1990b. Light-gazing by visually impaired children. *Developmental Medicine and Child Neurology, 32,* 755.

Jan, J.E., Groenveld, M., Sykanda, A.M. & Hoyt, C.S. 1987. Behavioral characteristics of children with permanent cortical visual impairment. *Developmental Medicine and Child Neurology, 29,* 571.

Janowsky, J.B. 1989. Sexual dimorphism in the human brain: Dispelling the myths. *Developmental Medicine and Child Neurology, 31,* 257.

Jansky, J.J. 1978. A critical review of some developmental and predictive precursors of reading disabilities. In A.L. Benton & D. Pearl (Eds.), *Dyslexia. An Appraisal of Current Knowledge,* New York: Oxford University Press.

Jeavons, P.M. & Harding, G.F.A. 1975. Photosensitivity epilepsy. A review of the literature and a study of 460 patients. *Clinics in Developmental Medicine,* no. 56. London: Heinemann.

Jeavons, P.M., Bower, B.D. & Dimitrakoudi, M. 1973. Long-term prognosis of 150 cases of West's syndrome. *Epilepsia,* 14, 153.

Jeeves, M.A. 1965. Agenesis of the corpus callosum—physiopathological and clinical aspects. *Proceedings of the Australian Association of Neurologists,* 3, 41.

Jeeves, M.A. 1972. Further psychological studies of the effects of agenesis of the corpus callosum in man and neonatal sectioning of the corpus callosum in animals. In J. Cernacek & F. Podivinsky (Eds.), *Cerebral Interhemispheric Relations.* Bratislava: Publishing House of the Slovac Academy of Sciences.

Jeeves, M.A. 1979. Some limits to interhemispheric integration in cases of callosal agenesis and partial commissurotomy. In I. Steele Russell, M.W. Van Hof & G. Berlucchi (Eds.), *Structure and Function of Cerebral Commissures.* Baltimore: University Park Press.

Jeeves, M.A., Silver, P.H. & Jacobson, I. 1988a. Bimanual coordination in callosal agenesis and partial commissurotomy. *Neuropsychologia,* 26, 833.

Jeeves, M.A., Silver, P.H. & Milne, A.B. 1988b. Role of the corpus callosum in the development of a bimanual motor skill. *Developmental Neuropsychology,* 4, 305.

Jeffrey, W.E. 1980. The developing brain and child development. In M.C. Wittrock (Ed.), *The Brain and Psychology.* New York: Academic Press.

Jenkins, J.J. 1979. Four points to remember: A tetrahedral model of memory experiments. In L.S. Cermak & F.I.M. Craik (Eds.), *Levels of Processing in Human Memory,* Hillsdale, NJ: Erlbaum, p. 429.

Jensen, P.B. 1987. Psychological aspects of myelomeningocele: A longitudinal study. *Scandinavian Journal of Psychology,* 28, 313.

Jernigan, T.L. & Bellugi, U. 1990. Anomalous morphology and magnetic resonance images in Williams syndrome and Down syndrome. *Archives of Neurology,* 47, 529.

Jervis, G.A. 1963. The clinical picture. In F.L. Lyman (Ed.), *Phenylketonuria.* Springfield, IL: Charles C Thomas, p. 52.

Jiang, Z.D., Liu, X.Y., Wu, Y.Y. & Zheng, M.S. 1990. Long-term impairments of brain and auditory functions of children recovered from purulent meningitis. *Developmental Medicine and Child Neurology,* 32, 473.

Johnson, D.A. 1991. Attention, children and head injury. In J.R. Crawford & D.M. Parker (Eds.), *Developments in Clinical and Experimental Neuropsychology.* New York: Plenum Press. p. 259.

Johnson, D.A. & Roetig-Johnson, K. 1989. Life in the slow lane: Attentional factors after head injury. In D.A. Johnson, D. Uttley & M.A. Wyke (Eds.), *Children's Head Injury: Who Cares?* London: Taylor & Francis, p. 80.

Johnson, E.M. & Kochhar, D.M. (Eds.). 1983. *Teratogenesis and Reproductive Toxicology.* New York: Springer.

Johnson, J.A. 1981. The etiology of hyperactivity. *Exceptional Children,* 47, 348.

Johnson, J.S. & Newport, E.L. 1991. Critical period effects on universal properties of language: The status of subjacency in the acquisition of a second language. *Cognition,* 39, 215.

Johnson, K.P. 1974. Viral infections of the developing nervous system. In R.A. Thompson & J.R. Green (Eds.), *Advances in Neurology,* Vol. 6. New York: Raven Press, p. 53.

Johnson, L. & Boggs, T.R. 1974. Bilirubin-dependent brain damage: Incidence and indications for treatment. In G.B. Odell, R. Schaffer & G. Simopoulos (Eds.), *Phototherapy of the Newborn: An Overview.* Washington, D.C.: National Academy of Sciences.

Johnson, M.H. 1990. Cortical maturation and perceptual development. In H. Bloch & B.I. Bertenthal (Eds.), *Sensory-motor Organizations and Development in Infancy and Childhood.* Dordrecht, Netherlands: Kluwer, p. 145.

Johnson, R.T. 1977. Viral infections and brain development. In S.R. Berenberg (Ed.), *Brain, Fetal and Infant.* The Hague: Martinus Nijhoff.

Johnson, R.T. 1982. *Viral Infections of the Nervous System.* New York: Academic Press.

Johnston, R.N. & Wessells, N.K. 1980. Regulation of the elongating nerve fiber. In R.K. Hunt (Ed.), *Neural Development, Part II (Current Topics in Developmental Biology, Vol. 16).* New York: Academic Press.

Johnston, W.H., Angara, V., Baumae, R., Hawke, W.A., Johnson, R.H., Keet, S. & Wood, M. 1967. Erythroblastosis fetalis and hyperbilirubinemia. *Pediatrics,* 39, 88.

Johnstone, B. & Bouman, D.E. 1992. Anoxic encephalopathy: A case study of an eight-year-old male with no residual cognitive deficit. *International Journal of Neuroscience,* 62, 207.

Jones, K.L. 1977. Fetal alcohol syndrome. In J.L. Rementeria (Ed.), *Drug Abuse in Pregnancy and Neonatal Effects.* St. Louis: C.V. Mosby.

Jones, K.L. 1988. *Smith's Recognizable Patterns of Human Malformation,* 4th ed. Philadelphia: Saunders.

Jorm, A.F., Share, D.L., Matthews, R. & Maclean, R. 1986. Behavior problems in specific reading retarded and general reading backward children: A longitudinal study. *Journal of Child Psychology and Psychiatry,* 27, 33.

Joschko, M. & Rourke, B.P. 1982. Neuropsychological dimensions of Tourette syndrome: Test-retest stability and implications for intervention. In A.J. Friedhoff & T.N. Chase (Eds.), *Gilles de la Tourette Syndrome. Advances of Neurology,* Vol. 35. New York: Raven Press.

Joseph, R. 1982. The neuropsychology of development: Hemispheric laterality, limbic language, and the origin of thought. *Journal of Clinical Psychology,* 38, 4.

Joseph, R. 1986. Reversal of cerebral dominance for language and emotion in a corpus callosotomy patient. *Journal of Neurology, Neurosurgery, and Psychiatry,* 49, 628.

Joynt, R.J. 1974. The corpus callosum: History of thought regarding its function. In M. Kinsbourne & W. Lynn Smith (Eds.). *Hemispheric Disconnection and Cerebral Function.* Springfield, IL: Charles C Thomas.

Kaffman, M., Sivan-Sher, A. & Carel, C. 1981. Obstetric history of kibbutz children with minimal brain dysfunction. *Israel Journal of Psychiatry and Related Sciences,* 18, 69.

Kaga, K. & Tanaka, Y. 1980. Auditory brainstem responses and behavioral audiometry: Developmental correlates. *Archives of Otolaryngology,* 106(9), 564.

Kagan, J., Kearsley, R.B. & Zelazo, P.R. 1978. *Infancy: Its Place in Human Development.* Cambridge, MA: Harvard University Press.

Kagan, J. & Moss, H.A. 1983. *Birth to Maturity.* New Haven, CT: Yale University Press.

Kail, R. & Bisanz, J. 1982. Information processing and cognitive development. In H.W. Reese (Ed.), *Advances in Child Development and Behavior,* Vol. 17. New York: Academic Press.

Kallman, F.J. 1953. *Heredity in Health and Mental Disorder.* New York: Norton.

Kalverboer, A.F. 1976. Neurobehavioral relationships in young children: Some remarks on concepts and methods. In R.M. Knights & D.J. Bakker (Eds.), *The Neuropsychology of Learning Disorders.* Baltimore: University Park Press.

Kalverboer, A.F., Touwen, B.C.L. & Prechtl, H.F.R. 1975. Follow-up of infants at risk of minor brain dysfunction. *Annals of the New York Academy of Sciences,* 173.

Kaminer, Y., Apter, A., Aviv, A. & Lerman, P. 1988. Psychopathology and temporal lobe epilepsy in adolescents. *Acta Psychiatrica Scandinavica,* 77, 640.

Kammerer, E.L., Gardner, J.K. & Wolff, A.B. 1988. Rey-Osterrieth complex figure drawings of deaf children with different etiologies of deafness. *Journal of Clinical and Experimental Neuropsychology,* 10, 43 (abstract).

Kandel, E. & Freed, D. 1989. Frontal lobe dysfunction and antisocial behavior: A review. *Journal of Clinical Psychology,* 45, 404.

Kandel, E., Brennan, P.A., Mednick, S.A. & Michelson, N.M. 1989. Minor physical anomalies and recidivistic adult violent criminal behavior. *Acta Psychiatrica Scandinavica,* 79, 103.

Kanner, L. 1943. Autistic disturbances of affective contact. *Nervous Child,* 2, 217.

Kanner, L. 1949. Problems of nosology and psychodynamics of early infantile autism. *American Journal of Orthopsychiatry,* 19, 416.

Kanner, L. 1954. To what extent is early infantile autism determined by constitutional inadequacies? *Proceedings of the Association for Research in Nervous and Mental Diseases,* 33, 378.

Kappers, J.A. 1971. On the structure, development, and connections of the limbic system. In G.B.A. Stoelinga & J.J. Van der Werff ten Bosch (Eds.), *Normal and Abnormal Development of Brain and Behavior.* Baltimore: Williams & Wilkins.

Karzon, R.G. 1985. Discrimination of polysyllabic sequences by one- to four-month-old infants. *Journal of Experimental Child Psychology,* 39, 326.

Kashani, J.H., Shekim, W.O., Burk, J.P. & Beck, N.C. 1987. Abuse as a predictor of psychopathology in children and adolescents. *Journal of Clinical Child Psychology,* 16, 43.

Kasper, J.C., Millichap, J.C., Backus, D.C., Child, D. & Schulman, J. 1971. A study of the relationship between neurological evidence of brain damage in children with hyperactivity and distractibility. *Journal of Consulting and Clinical Psychology,* 36, 329.

Kasteleijn-Nolst-Trenite, D.G.A., Bakker, D.J., Binnie, C.D., Buerman, A. & Van Raaij, M. 1988. Psychological effects of subclinical epileptoform EEG discharges. I. Scholastic skills. *Epilepsy Research,* 2, 111.

Kasteleijn-Nolst-Trenite, D.G.A., Smit, A.M., Velis, D.N. & Willemse, J. 1990. On-line detection of transient neuropsychological disturbances during EEG discharges in children with epilepsy. *Developmental Medicine and Child Neurology,* 32, 46.

Kater, S. & Letourneau, P. (Eds.). 1985. *Biology of the Nerve Growth Cone.* New York: Alan Liss.

Katona, F. & Berenyi, M. 1974. Differential reactions and habituation to acoustical and visual stimuli in neonates. *Activitas Nervosa Superior,* 16, 305.

Katz, V. 1971. Auditory stimulation and developmental behaviour of the premature infant. *Nursing Research,* 20, 196.

Kaufman, A.S. & Doppelt, J.E. 1976. Analysis of WISC-R standardization data in terms of stratification variables. *Child Development,* 47(1), 165.

Kaufman, A.S. & Kaufman, N.L. 1981. Neurological dysfunctions of children. *Clinical Neuropsychology,* 3, 26.

Kaufman, A.S. & Kaufman, N.L. 1983. *K-ABC: Kaufman Assessment Battery for Children.* Circle Pines, MN: American Guidance Service.

Kawi, A.A. & Pasamanick, B. 1958. Association of factors of pregnancy with reading disorders in childhood. *Journal of the American Medical Association,* 166, 1420.

Kaye, K. 1977. Towards the origin of dialogue. In H.R. Schaffer (Ed.), *Studies in Mother-Infant Interactions*. Amsterdam: Elsevier.

Kee, D.W., Gottfried, A.W., Bathurst, K. & Brown, K. 1987. Left-hemisphere language specialization: Consistency in hand preference and sex differences. *Child Development*, 58, 718.

Keeney, S.E., Adcock, E.W. & McArdle, C.B. 1991. Prospective observations of 100 high-risk neonates by high-field (1.5 Tesla) magnetic resonance imaging of the central nervous system: II. Lesions associated with hypoxic-ischemic encephalopathy. *Pediatrics*, 87, 431.

Keith, R.W. (Ed.). 1981. *Central Auditory and Language Disorders in Children*. San Diego: College-Hill Press.

Keller, C.A. 1981. Epidemiological characteristics of preterm births. In S.L. Friedman, & M. Sigman (Eds.), *Preterm Birth and Psychological Development*. New York: Academic Press.

Kennard, M.A. 1938. Reorganization of motor function in the cerebral cortex of monkeys deprived of motor and premotor areas in infancy, *Journal of Neurophysiology*, 1, 477.

Kennard, M.A. 1942. Cortical reorganization of motor function: Studies on a series of monkeys of various ages from infancy to maturity. *Archives of Neurology and Psychiatry*, 8, 227.

Kennard, M.A. 1960. Value of equivocal signs in neurologic diagnosis. *Neurology*, 10, 753.

Kenny, T.J. 1980. Hyperactivity. In H.E. Rie and E.D. Rie (Eds.), *Handbook of Minimal Brain Dysfunction*. New York: Wiley.

Kenny, T.J. & Clemmens, R.L. 1971. Medical and psychological correlates in children with learning disabilities. *Journal of Pediatrics*, 78, 273.

Kephart, N.C. 1975. The perceptual-motor match. In W.M. Cruickshank & D.P. Hallahan (Eds.), *Perceptual and Learning Disabilities in Children*, vol. 1. Syracuse: Syracuse University Press, p. 63.

Kerbeshian, J. 1985. Gilles de la Tourette disease in multiply disabled children. Special issue: Children with multiple disabilities. *Rehabilitation Literature*, 46, 255.

Kerbeshian, J. & Burd, L. 1988. Tourette disorder and schizophrenia in children. *Neuroscience and Biobehavioral Reviews*, 12, 267.

Kerschensteiner, M. & Huber, W. 1975. Grammatical impairment in developmental aphasia. *Cortex*, 11, 264.

Kessler, J.W. 1980. History of minimal brain dysfunction. In H.E. Rie & E.D. Rie (Eds.), *Handbook of Minimal Brain Dysfunction: A Critical View*. New York: Wiley.

Kessner, D.M., Singer, J., Kalk, C.E. & Schlesinger, E.R. 1973. Infant death: An analysis by maternal risk and health care. *Contrasts in Health Status*, vol. 1. Washington: National Academy of Sciences.

Kety, S.S., Rosenthal, D., Wender, P.H., Schulsinger, F. & Jacobsen, B. 1978. The biological and adoptive families of adopted individuals who became schizophrenic: Prevalence of mental illness and other characteristics. In L.C. Wynne, R.L. Cromwell, & S.W. Mathysse (Eds.), *The Nature of Schizophrenia*. New York: Wiley, p. 25.

Kety, S.S., Rowland, L.P., Sidman, R.L. & Matthysse, S.W. (Eds.). 1983. *Genetics of Neurological and Psychiatric Disorders*. Association for Research in Nervous and Mental Disease (ARNMD) Research Publications, Vol. 60. New York: Academic Press.

Kiessling, L.S., Denckla, M.B. & Carlton, M. 1983. Evidence for differential hemispheric function in children with hemiplegic cerebral palsy. *Developmental Medicine and Child Neurology,* 25, 727.

Kiff, R.D. & Lepard, C. 1966. Visual response of premature infants. *Archives of Ophthalmology,* 75, 631.

Kimura, D. 1967. Functional asymmetries of the brain in dichotic listening. *Cortex,* 3, 163.

Kimura, D. 1969. Spatial localization in left and right visual fields. *Canadian Journal of Psychology,* 23, 445.

Kimura, D. 1981. Neural mechanisms in manual signing. *Sign Language Studies,* 33, 291.

Kimura, D. 1987. Are men's and women's brains really different? *Canadian Psychology,* 28, 133.

Kimura, D. 1993. *Neuromotor Mechanisms in Human Communication.* New York: Oxford University Press.

Kimura, D. & Carson, M.W. 1993. Cognitive pattern and finger ridge asymmetry. *Society for Neuroscience Abstracts,* 19, 560.

Kimura, D. & Harshman, R.A. 1984. Sex differences in brain organization for verbal and nonverbal functions. In G.J. DeVries, et al. (Eds.), *Progress in Brain Research,* 61, 423.

King, A.C. & Ollendick, H. 1984. Gilles de la Tourette disorder: A review. *Journal of Clinical Child Psychology,* 13, 2.

Kinsbourne, M. 1973. Minimal brain dysfunction as a neurodevelopmental lag. *Annals of the New York Academy of Sciences,* 205, 268.

Kinsbourne, M. 1976a. The neuropsychological analysis of cognitive deficit. In R.G. Grenell & S. Gobay (Eds.), *Biological Foundations of Psychiatry.* vol. 1. New York: Raven Press.

Kinsbourne, M. 1976b. The ontogeny of cerebral dominance. In R.W. Rieber (Ed.), *The Neuropsychology of Language.* New York: Plenum Press.

Kinsbourne, M. & Hiscock, M. 1977. Does cerebral dominance develop? In S.J. Segalowitz & F.A. Gruber (Eds.), *Language Development and Neurological Theory.* New York: Academic Press.

Kinsbourne, M. & Warrington, E.K. 1963. The developmental Gerstmann syndrome. *Archives of Neurology,* 8, 490.

Kirby, J.R. & Das, J.P. 1990. A cognitive approach to intelligence: Attention, coding and planning. *Canadian Psychology,* 31, 320.

Kirk, U. (Ed.) 1982. *Neuropsychology of Language, Reading, and Spelling.* New York: Academic Press.

Kirk, U. 1992. Evidence for early acquisition of visual organizational ability: A developmental study. *Clinical Neuropsychologist,* 6, 171.

Kirkpatrick, S.W. & Wharry, R.E. 1985. Ocular anomalies: A comparison of learning disabled and nonlearning disabled elementary school children. *Perceptual and Motor Skills,* 61, 567.

Kitchen, W.H., Rickards, A., Ruan, M.M., McDougall, A.B., Billson, F.A., Keir, E.H. & Naylor, F.D. 1979. A longitudinal study of very low-birthweight infants. II: Results of controlled trials of intensive care and incidence of handicap. *Developmental Medicine and Child Neurology,* 21(5), 582.

Kitchen, W.H., Ryan, M.M., Rickards, A., McDougall, A.B., Billson, F.A., Keir, E.H. & Naylor, F.D. 1980. A longitudinal study of very low-birthweight infants. IV: An overview of performance at eight years of age. *Developmental Medicine and Child Neurology,* 22, 172.

Kitchen, W., Ford, G., Orgill, A., Rickards, A., Astbury, J., Lissenden, J., Bajuk, B., Yu, V., Drew, J. & Campbell, N. 1984. Outcome of infants with birthweight 500-900 gm: A regional study of 1979 and 1980 births. *Journal of Pediatrics*, 104, 921.

Klaus, M.H. & Kennel, J.H. 1976. *Maternal-Infant Bonding*, St. Louis: C.V. Mosby.

Klausmeier, H.J. & Allen, P.S. 1978. *Cognitive Development of Children and Youth: A Longitudinal Study*. New York: Academic Press.

Klawans, H.L., Glantz, R., Tanner, C.M. & Goetz, C.G. 1982. Primary writing tremor: A selective action tremor. *Neurology*, 32, 203.

Kleiman, M.D., Neff, S. & Rosman, P. 1992. The brain in infantile autism: Are posterior fossa structures abnormal? *Neurology*, 42, 753.

Klein, M.C., Sayre, J.W. & Kotok, D. 1974. Lead poisoning: Current status of the problem facing pediatricians. *American Journal of Diseases of Children*, 127, 805.

Klein, N., Hack, M., Gallagher, J. & Fanaroff, A.A. 1985. Preschool performance of children with normal intelligence who were very low-birth weight infants. *Pediatrics* 75, 531.

Klein, N.K., Hack, M. & Breslau, N. 1989. Children who were very low birth weight: Development and achievement at nine years of age. *Journal of Developmental and Behavioral Pediatrics*, 10, 32.

Knobloch, H. & Pasamanick, B. 1966. Prospective studies on the epidemiology of reproductive casualty. Methods, findings, and some implications. *Merrill-Palmer Quarterly of Behavior and Development*, 12, 27.

Knobloch, H., Rider, R.V. & Harper, P.A. 1956. Neuropsychiatric sequelae of prematurity. *Journal of the American Medical Association*, 161, 581.

Knobloch, H., Stevens, F. & Malone, A. 1987. *A Manual of Developmental Diagnosis*, 2nd ed. Houston, TX: Developmental Evaluation Materials, Inc.

Knox, C. & Kimura, D. 1970. Cerebral processing of non-verbal sounds in boys and girls. *Neuropsychologia* 8, 227.

Knox, G.E., Reynolds, D.W. & Alford, C. 1980. Perinatal infections caused by rubella, hepatitis B, cytomegalovirus, and herpes simplex. In E.J. Quilligan & N. Kretchmer (Eds.), *Fetal and Maternal Medicine*. New York: Wiley.

Knox, W.E. 1960. Phenylketonuria. In J.B. Stanbury, J.B. Wyngaarden & D.S. Frederickson (Eds.), *The Metabolic Basis of Inherited Disease*. New York: McGraw-Hill, p. 321.

Kohen-Raz, R. 1977. Psychobiological aspects of cognitive development in infancy. In R. Kohen-Raz (Ed.), *Psychobiological Aspects of Cognitive Growth*. New York: Academic Press.

Kohen-Raz, R. 1986. *Learning Disabilities and Postural Control*. London: Freund.

Kohn, B. & Dennis, M. 1974a. Patterns of hemispheric specialization after hemidecortication for infantile hemiplegia. In M. Kinsbourne and W. Lynn Smith (Eds.), *Hemispheric Disconnection and Cerebral Function*. Springfield, IL: Charles C Thomas.

Kohn, B. & Dennis, M. 1974b. Selective impairments of visuo-spatial abilities in infantile hemiplegics after right cerebral decortication. *Neuropsychologia*, 12, 505.

Kohn, H., Manowitz, P., Miller, M. & Kling, A. 1988. Neuropsychological deficits in obligatory heterozygotes for metachromatic leukodystrophy. *Human Genetics*, 79, 8.

Kolakowska, T., Williams, A.O., Jambor, K. & Ardern, M. 1985. Schizophrenia with good and poor outcome: III. Neurological "soft" signs, cognitive impairment and their clinical significance. *British Journal of Psychiatry*, 146, 348.

Kolb, B. 1989. Brain development, plasticity, and behavior. *American Psychologist*, 44, 1203.

Kolb, B. & Fantie, B. 1989. Development of the child's brain and behavior. In C.R. Reynolds & E. Fletcher-Janzen (Eds.), *Handbook of Clinical Child Neuropsychology*. New York: Plenum, p. 17.

Kolb, B. & Wishaw, I.Q. 1990. *Fundamentals of Human Neuropsychology*, 3rd ed. New York: Freeman.

Kolb, B. & Wishaw, I.Q. 1991. Mechanisms underlying behavioral sparing after neonatal retrosplenial cingulate lesions in rats: Spatial navigation, cortical architecture, and electroencephalographic activity. *Brain Dysfunction*, 4, 75.

Kolb, J.E. & Heaton, R.K. 1975. Lateralized neurologic deficits and psychopathology in a Turner syndrome patient. *Archives of General Psychiatry*, 32, 1198.

Kolvin, I., Ounsted, C., Humphrey, M. & McNay, A. 1971a. Studies in the childhood psychoses. II. The phenomenology of childhood psychoses. *British Journal of Psychiatry*, 118, 385.

Kolvin, I., Ounsted, C., Richardson, L. & Garside, R. 1971b. Studies in the childhood psychoses. III. The family and social background in childhood psychoses. *British Journal of Psychiatry*, 118, 396.

Konstantareas, M.M. 1986. Early developmental backgrounds of autistic and mentally retarded children: Future research directions. *Psychiatric Clinics of North America*, 9, 671.

Konstantareas, M.M., Homatidis, S. & Busch, J. 1989. Cognitive, communication, and social differences between autistic boys and girls. *Journal of Applied Developmental Psychology*, 10, 411.

Kooistra, C.A. & Heilman, K.M. 1988. Motor dominance and lateral asymmetry of the globus pallidus. *Neurology*, 38, 388.

Koops, K.L. & Harmon, R.J. 1980. Studies of long-term outcome in newborns with birth weights under 1500 grams. *Advances in Behavioral Pediatrics*, 1, 1.

Kopp, C.B. 1976. Action-scheme of 8-month-old infants. *Developmental Psychology*, 12, 361.

Kopp, C.B. & Parmelee, A.H. 1979. Prenatal and perinatal influences on infant behavior. In J.D. Osofsky (Ed.), *Handbook of Infant Development*. New York: Wiley-Interscience.

Korkman, M., Hilakivi, L.A., Granstroem, M.L. & Autti-Raemoe, I. 1989. The development of children exposed to alcohol in utero for varying lengths of time. *Journal of Clinical and Experimental Neuropsychology*, 11, 363.

Korner, A.F. 1973. Sex differences in newborns with special reference to differences in the organization of human behavior. *American Journal of Child Psychology*, 14, 19.

Korner, A.F. 1985. Preventative intervention with high-risk newborns. Theoretical, conceptual, and methodological perspectives. In J.D. Osofsky (Ed.), *Handbook for Infant Development*, 2nd ed. New York: Wiley-Interscience, p. 1006.

Korner, A.F. 1986. The use of waterbeds in the care of preterm infants. *Journal of Perinatology*, 6, 142.

Korner, A.F. & Thom, V.A. 1990. *Neurobehavioral Assessment of the Preterm Infant*. San Antonio, TX: The psychological Corporation.

Korner, A.F., Brown, B.W., Dimiceli, S. & Forest, T. 1989. Stable individual differences in developmentally changing preterm infants: A replicated study. *Child Development*, 60, 502.

Korner, A.F., Konstantinou, J., Dimiceli, S. & Brown, B.W. 1991. Establishing the reliability and developmental validity of a neurobehavioral assessment for preterm infants: A methodological process. *Child Development*, 62, 1200.

Korner, A.F., Stevenson, D.K., Kraemer, H.C., Spiker, D., Scott, D.T., Constantinou, J. & Dimiceli, S. 1993. Prediction of the development of low birth weight preterm infants by a new neonatal medical index. *Developmental and Behavioral Pediatrics,* 14, 2, 10.

Kosc, L. 1974. Developmental dyscalculia. *Journal of Learning Disabilities,* 7, 165.

Kosmetatos, N., Dinter, C., Williams, M.L., Lourie, H. & Berne, A.S. 1980. Intracranial hemorrhage in the premature. *American Journal of Diseases of Children,* 134, 855.

Kovacs, M., Gatsonia, C., Paulauskas, S.L. & Richards, C. 1990. Depressive disorders in childhood: IV. A longitudinal study of comorbidity with and risk for anxiety disorders. *Annual Progress in Child Psychiatry and Child Development,* 387.

Kracke, I. 1975. Perception of rhythmic sequences by receptive aphasic and deaf children. *British Journal of Communication Disorders,* 10, 43.

Kraft, R.H. 1981. The relationship between right-handed children's assessed and familial handedness and lateral specialization. *Neuropsychologia,* 19, 697.

Kramer, L.D., Locke, G.E., Ogunyemi, A. & Nelson, L. 1990. Neonatal cocaine-related seizures. *Journal of Child Neurology,* 5, 60.

Krashen, S.D. 1973. Lateralization, language learning, and the critical period: some new evidence. *Language Learning,* 23(1), 63.

Kraus, J.F., Fife, D. & Conroy, C. 1987. Pediatric head injuries: The nature, clinical course, and early outcomes in a defined United States' population. *Pediatrics,* 79, 501.

Krech, U. 1973. Complement-fixing antibodies against cytomegalovirus in different parts of the world. *Bulletin of the World Health Organization,* 49, 103.

Kresky, B., Buchbinder, S. & Greenberg, I.M. 1962. The incidence of neurologic residuals after recovery from bacterial meningitis. *Archives of Pediatrics,* 79, 63.

Krishnamoorthy, K., Shannon, D., DeLong, G., Todres, I. & Davis, K. 1979. Neurologic sequelae in the survivors of neonatal intraventricular hemorrhage. *Pediatrics,* 64, 233.

Krynauw, R.A. 1950. Infantile hemiplegia treated by removing one cerebral hemisphere. *Journal of Neurology, Neurosurgery, and Psychiatry,* 13, 243.

Kucharski, D. & Hall, W.G. 1988. Developmental changes in the access to olfactory memory. *Behavioral Neuroscience,* 102, 340.

Kudrjavcev, T., Schoenberg, B.S., Kurland, L.T. & Groover, R.V. 1983. Cerebral palsy: Trends and changes in concurrent neonatal mortality. *Neurology,* 33, 1433.

Kudrjavcev, T., Schoenberg, B.S., Kurland, L.T. & Groover, R.V. 1985. Cerebral palsy: Survival rates, associated handicaps, and distribution by clinical subtype (Rochester, MN, 1950–1976). *Neurology,* 35, 900.

Kugelmass, S., Marcus, J. & Schmueli, J. 1985. Psychophysiological reactivity in high-risk children. *Schizophrenia Bulletin,* 11, 66.

Kuhl, P.K. & Miller, J.D. 1975. Speech perception in the chinchilla: Voiced-voiceless distinctions in alveolar plosive consonants. *Science,* 190, 69.

Kumar, M.L., Nankervis, G.A. & Gold, E. 1973. Inapparent congenital cytomegalovirus infection: A follow-up study. *New England Journal of Medicine,* 288, 1370.

Kun, L.E., Mulhern, R.K. & Crisco, J.J. 1983. Quality of life in children treated for brain tumors: Intellectual, emotional, and academic function. *Journal of Neurosurgery,* 58, 1.

Kurlan, R., Licther, D. & Hewitt, D. 1989. Sensory tics in Tourette's syndrome. *Neurology,* 39, 731.

Kurtzberg, D., Vaughan, H.G., Daum, C., Grellong, B.A., Albin, S. & Rotkin, L. 1979. Neurobehavioral performance of low-birthweight infants at 40 weeks conceptual age: Comparison with normal full-born infants. *Developmental Medicine and Child Neurology,* 1979, 21, 590.

Kurtzburg, D., Hilpert, P., Kreuzer, J.A., & Vaughan, H.G. 1984. Differential maturation of cortical auditory evoked potentials to speech sounds in normal fullterm and very low-birthweight infants. *Developmental Medicine and Child Neurology,* 26, 466.

Kutas, M. & Van Petten, C. 1988. Event-related brain potential studies of language. In P.K. Ackles, J.R. Jennings & M.G.H. Coles (Eds.), *Advances in Psychophysiology,* Vol. 3. Greenwich CT: JAI, p. 139.

Laatsch, L.K., Dorman, C. & Hurley, A.D. 1984. Neuropsychological testing and survey forms to indicate possible loss of neurological functioning. *Zeitschrift für Kinderchirurgie,* 39, 125.

La Benz, P.J. 1980. Summary. In F.M. Lassman, R.O. Fisch, D.K. Vetter & E.S. La Benz (Eds.), *Early Correlates of Speech, Language and Hearing.* Littleton, MA: PSG Publishing, p. 404.

La Benz, E.S., Swaiman, K.F. & Sullivan, A.R. 1980. Written communication: Reading, writing and spelling. In F.M. Lassman, R.O. Fisch, D.K. Vetter & E.S. La Benz (Eds.), *Early Correlates of Speech, Language and Hearing.* Littleton, MA: PSG Publishing.

Lagerstrom, M., Bremme, K., Eneroth, P. & Magnusson, D. 1989. Sex-related differences in school performance and IQ-test scores at ages 10 and 13 for children with low birth weight. *Reports from the Department of Psychology,* University of Stockholm, No. 701.

Laget, P., Salbreux, R., Raimbault, J., d'Allest, A.M. & Mariani, J. 1976. Relationship between changes in somesthetic evoked responses and electroencephalographic findings in the child with hemiplegia. *Developmental Medicine and Child Neurology,* 18, 620.

Lamb, M.E., Thompson, R.A., Garner, W. & Charnov, E.L. 1985. *Infant-Mother Attachment: The Origins and Developmental Significance of Individual Differences in Strange Situation Behavior.* Hillsdale, NJ: Erlbaum.

Lamm, O. & Epstein, R. 1992. Are specific reading and writing difficulties causally connected with developmental spatial inability? Evidence from two cases of developmental agnosia and apraxia. *Neuropsychologia,* 30, 459.

Lancet. 1980. The fate of the baby under 1501 g at birth. *Lancet,* 1, 461 (Editorial).

Landau, S., Milich, R. & McFarland, M. 1987. Social status differences among subgroups of LD boys. *Learning Disability Quarterly,* 10, 277.

Landau, W., Goldstein, R. & Kleffner, F. 1960. Congenital aphasia: A clinicopathologic study. *Neurology,* 10, 915.

Landman, G.B., Levine, M.D., Fenton, T. & Solomon, B. 1986. Minor neurological indicators and developmental function in preschool children. *Developmental and Behavioral Pediatrics,* 7, 97.

Landrigan, P.J., Gehlbach, S.H., Rosenblum, B.F., Shoults, J.M., Candelaria, R.M., Barthel, W.F., Liddle, J.A., Smrek, A.L., Staehling, N.W. & Sanders, J. 1975. Epidemic lead absorption near an ore smelter. *New England Journal of Medicine,* 292, 123.

Landry, S.H., Fletcher, J.M., Zarling, C.L. Chapieski, L. & Francis, D.J. 1984. Differential outcomes associated with early medical complications in premature infants. *Journal of Pediatric Psychology,* 9, 385.

Landry, S.H., Schmidt, M. & Richardson, M.A. 1989. The effects of intraventricular hemorrhage on functional communication skills in preterm toddlers. *Journal of Developmental and Behavioral Pediatrics,* 10, 299.

Langman, I., Webster, W. & Rodier, P. 1975. Morphological and behavioral abnormalities caused by insults to the CNS in the perinatal periods. In C.L. Berry & D.E. Poswillo (Eds.), *Teratology: Trends and Applications.* New York: Springer.

Langset, M., Midtvedt, T. & Omland, T. 1989. Toxoplasmosis in blind and partially sighted children and adolescents. *Journal of Visual Impairment and Blindness,* 83, 355.

Langworthy, O.R. 1933. Development of behavior patterns and myelinization of the nervous system in the human fetus and infant. Carnegie Institute of Washington Publication No. 433: *Contributions to Embryology,* 139, 1.

Lanier, L.P., Dunn, A.J. & Hartesveldt, C.J. 1976. Development of neurotransmitters and their function in brain. In S. Ehrenpreis and I.J. Kopin (Eds.), *Reviews of Neuroscience,* Vol. 2. New York: Raven Press.

Lansdell, H. 1964. Sex differences in hemispheric asymmetry of the human brain. *Nature,* 203, 550.

Lansdown, R.G., Sheperd, J., Clayton, B.E., Delves, H.T., Graham, P.J. & Turner, W.C. 1974. Blood lead levels, behavior, and intelligence: A population study. *Lancet,* 1, 538.

Larroche, J.C. 1967. *Regional Development of the Brain in Early Life.* Symposium UNESCO and WHO. London: Blackwell Scientific Publications.

Larsen, S. 1984. Developmental changes in the pattern of ear asymmetry as revealed by a dichotic listening task. *Cortex,* 20, 5.

Larsen, S. & Hakonsen, K. 1983. Absence of ear asymmetry in blind children on a dichotic listening task compared to sighted controls. *Brain and Language,* 1983, 18, 192.

Lashley, K.S. 1938. Factors limiting recovery after central nervous system lesions. *Journal of Nervous and Mental Disorders,* 88, 733.

Lashley, K.S. 1951. The problem of serial order in behavior. In L.A. Jeffres (Ed.), *Cerebral Mechanisms in Behavior.* New York: Wiley.

Lassman, F.M., Fisch, R.O., Vetter, D.K. & La Benz, E.S. 1980. *Early Correlates of Language, Speech and Hearing.* Littleton, MA: PSG Publishing.

Lassonde, M., Bryden, M.P. & Demers, P. 1990. The corpus callosum and cerebral speech lateralization. *Brain and Language,* 38, 195.

Lassonde, M., Sauerwein, H., Chicoine, A.J. & Geoffroy, G. 1991. Absence of disconnection syndrome in callosal agenesis and early callosotomy: Brain reorganization or lack of structural specificity during ontogeny? *Neuropsychologia,* 29, 481.

Lassonde, M., Sauerwein, H., McCabe, N. & Laurencelle, L. 1988. Extent and limits of cerebral adjustment to early section or congenital absence of the corpus callosum. *Behavioural Brain Research,* 30, 165.

Latt, S.M., Kurnit, D.M., Bruns, G.P., Schreck, R.R., Morton, C.C., Kunkel, L.M., Lalande, M., Aldridge, J., Neve, R., Tantravahi, U., Kanda, N., Lindner, G. & Meryash, D. 1984. Molecular genetic approaches to human diseases involving mental retardation. *American Journal of Mental Deficiency,* 88, 561.

Lauder, J.M. 1983. Hormonal and humoral influences on brain development. *Psychoneuroendocrinology,* 8, 121.

Laufer, M. & Denhoff, E. 1957. Hyperkinetic behaviour syndrome in children. *Journal of Pediatrics,* 50, 463.

Laurence, K.M. & Tew, B.J. 1971. The natural history of spina bifida cystica and cranium bifidum cysticum: Major central nervous system malformations in South Wales. *Archives of Diseases in Childhood,* 46, 127.

Lavigne, J.V. & Burns, W.J. 1981. *Pediatric Psychology.* New York: Grune & Stratton.

Lawrence, D.G. & Hopkins, D.A. 1972. Developmental aspects of pyramidal motor control in the Rhesus monkey. *Brain Research,* 40, 117.

Lawson, D., Metcalfe, M. & Pampiglione, G. 1965. Meningitis in childhood. *British Medical Journal,* 1, 557.

Leary, P.M. 1978. The electro-encephalogram in childhood. *South African Medical Journal,* 53, 197.

Lebrun, Y. & Zangwill, O. 1981. *Lateralization of Language in the Child.* Lisse: Swets & Zeitlinger.

Lechtig, A. 1985. Early malnutrition, growth, and development. In M. Gracey & F. Falkner (Eds.), *Nutritional Needs and Assessment of Normal Growth.* New York: Raven Press, p. 185.

Leckliter, I.N., Matarazzo, J.D. & Silverstein, A.B. 1986. A literature review of factor analytic studies of the WAIS-R. *Journal of Clinical Psychology,* 42, 332.

Lecours, A.R. 1975. Myelogenetic correlates of the development of speech and language. In E.H. Lenneberg & E. Lenneberg (Eds.), *Foundations of Language Development,* Vol. 1. New York: Academic Press.

LeDouarin, N. 1980. Migration and differentiation of neural crest cells. In R.K. Hunt (Ed.), *Neural Development, Part II (Current Topics in Developmental Biology, Vol. 16).* New York: Academic Press.

Lee, M., Vaughn, B.E. & Kopp, C.B. 1983. The role of self-control in young children's performance on a delayed memory for location task. *Developmental Psychology,* 19, 40.

Legido, A., Clancy, R.R. & Berman, P.H. 1991. Neurologic outcome after electroencephalographically proven neonatal seizures. *Pediatrics,* 88, 583.

Lehman, H.J. & Lampe, H. 1970. Observations on the interhemispheric transmission of information in 9 patients with corpus callosum defect. *European Neurology,* 4, 129.

Lehmkuhl, G. 1984. Ideomotorische und ideatorische Apraxie im Kindesalter. *Acta Paedopsychiatrica,* 50, 97.

Leigh, J. 1987. Adaptive behavior of children with learning disabilities. *Journal of Learning Disabilities,* 20, 557.

Leisti, S. & Iivanainen, M. 1978. Growth, hypothalamic function and brain ventricle size in mentally retarded subjects. *Journal of Mental Deficiency Research,* 22(1), 1.

Lemay, M. & Culebras, A. 1972. Human brain—morphologic differences in the hemispheres demonstrable with carotid arteriography. *New England Journal of Medicine,* 287, 168.

Lemire, R.J., Loeser, J.D., Leech, R.W. & Alvord, E.C. 1975. *Normal and Abnormal Development of the Human Nervous System.* New York: Harper and Row.

Lenhardt, M.L. 1983. Effects of neonatal hyperbilirubinemia on Token Test performance of six-year-old children. *Journal of Auditory Research,* 23, 195.

Lenneberg, E.H. 1967. *Biological Foundations of Language.* New York: Wiley.

Lennox-Buchtal, M. 1973. Febrile convulsions: A reappraisal. *Electroencephalography and Clinical Neurophysiology,* 32, Suppl. 1.

Lenti, C., Radice, L., Cerioli, M. & Musetti, L. 1991. Tactile extinction in childhood hemiplegia. *Developmental Medicine and Child Neurology,* 33, 789.

Leong, C.K. 1980. Cognitive patterns of "retarded" and below-average readers. *Contemporary Educational Psychology,* 5, 101.

Lerer, R.J. & Lerer, M.D. 1976. The effects of methylphenidate on the soft neurological signs of hyperactive children. *Pediatrics,* 57, 521.

Lerner, J., Nachshon, J. & Carmon, A. 1977. Responses of paranoid and nonparanoid schizophrenics in a dichotic listening task. *Journal of Nervous and Mental Disease,* 164, 247.

Lescaudron, L. & Stein, D.G. 1990. Functional recovery following transplants of embryonic brain tissue in rats with lesions of visual, frontal and motor cortex: Problems and prospects for future research. *Neuropsychologia,* 28, 585.

Leslie, A.M. & Frith, U. 1990. Prospects for a cognitive neuropsychology of autism: Hobson's choice. *Psychological Review,* 97, 122.

Lester, B.M., Garcia-Coll, C., Valcarcel, M., Hoffman, J. & Brazelton, T.B. 1986. Effects of atypical patterns of fetal growth on newborn behavior. *Child Development,* 57, 11.

Lester, D. 1977. Idiots savant: A review. *Psychology,* 14, 70.

Letourneau, P.C., Kater, S.B. & Macagno, E.R. (Eds.) 1991. *The Nerve Growth Cone.* New York: Raven.

Levene, M.I. & Dubowitz, L.M.S. 1982. Low-birth-weight babies long-term follow-up. *British Journal of Hospital Medicine,* 24, 487.

Levin, H.S. 1983. Mutism after closed head injury. *Archives of Neurology,* 40, 601.

Levin, H.S. & Benton, A.L. 1986. Developmental and acquired dyscalculia in children. In I. Flehmig & L. Stern (Eds.), *Child Development and Learning Behavior.* Stuttgart: Gustav Fisher, p. 317.

Levin, H.S. & Eisenberg, H.M. 1979. Neuropsychological impairment after closed head injury in children and adolescents. *Journal of Pediatric Psychology,* 4, 389.

Levin, H.S. & Eisenberg, H. 1983. Recovery of memory and intellectual ability after head injury in children and adolescents: Sparing of function after early injury? Paper presented at the 11th meeting of the International Neuropsychological Society, Mexico City.

Levin, H.S. & Spiers, P.A. 1993. The acalculias. In K.M. Heilman and E. Valenstein (Eds.), *Clinical Neuropsychology,* 3rd ed. New York: Oxford University Press, p. 128.

Levin, H.S., Benton, A.L. & Grossman, R.G. (Eds.) 1982. *Neurobehavioral Consequences of Closed Head Injury.* New York: Oxford University Press.

Levin, H.S., Ewing-Cobbs, L. & Benton, A.L. 1984. Age and recovery from brain damage: A review of clinical studies. In S.W. Scheff (Ed.), *Aging and Recovery of Function in the Central Nervous System.* New York: Plenum.

Levin, H.S., Grafman, J. & Eisenberg, H.M. (Eds.). 1987. *Neurobehavioral Recovery from Brain Injury.* New York: Oxford University Press.

Levin, H.S., Aldrich, E.F. & Saydjari, C. 1992a. Severe head injury in children: Experience of the traumatic coma data bank. *Neurosurgery,* 32, 435.

Levin, H.S., Ewing-Cobbs, L. & Fletcher, J.M. 1992b. Neurobehavioral outcome of mild head injury in children. In H.S. Levin, H.M. Eisenberg & A.L. Benton (Eds.), *Mild Head Injury.* New York: Oxford University Press. p. 189.

Levin, H.S., Mendelsohn, D., Lilly, M.A., Fletcher, J.A., Culhane, K.A., Chapman, S.B., Harward, H., Kusnerik, L., Bruce, D. & Eisenberg, H.M. 1994. Tower of London performance in relation to magnetic resonance imaging following closed head injury in children. *Neuropsychology,* 8, 171.

Levine, D., Hier, D.B. & Calvanio, R. 1981. Acquired learning disability for reading after left temporal lobe damage in childhood. *Neurology,* 31, 257.

Levine, S. & Mullins, R.F. 1968. Hormones in infancy. In G. Newton & S. Levine (Eds.), *Early Experience and Behavior.* Springfield, IL: Charles C Thomas.

Levine, S.C. 1985. Developmental changes in right-hemisphere involvement in face recognition. In C. Best (Ed.), *Hemisphere Function and Collaboration in the Child.* New York: Academic Press, p. 157.

Levine, S.C., Huttenlocher, P., Banich, M.T. & Duda, E. 1987. Factors affecting cognitive functioning of hemiplegic children. *Developmental Medicine and Child Neurology,* 29, 27.

Levitsky, D.A. (Ed.) 1979. *Malnutrition, Environment, and Behavior: New Perspectives.* New York: Cornell University Press.

Levitsky, D.A. & Barnes, R.H. 1972. Nutritional and environmental interactions in the behavioral development of the rat: Long-term effects. *Science,* 176, 68.

Levon, F.M. 1990. Psychological development and the changing organization of the brain. In *The Annual of Psychoanalysis,* Vol. 18. Hillsdale, NJ: Analytic Press, p. 45.

Levy, J. 1969. Possible basis for the evolution of lateral specialization of the human brain. *Nature,* 224, 614.

Levy, J. & Nagylaki, T. 1972. A model for the genetics of handedness. *Genetics,* 72, 117.

Levy, J. & Reid, M. 1978. Variations in cerebral organization as a function of handedness, hand posture in writing, and sex. *Journal of Experimental Psychology,* 107, 119.

Levy, Y., Amir, N. & Shalev, R. 1992. Linguistic development of a child with a congenital L.H. lesion. *Cognitive Neuropsychology,* 9, 1.

Lewandowski, L.J. & deRienzo, P.J. 1985. WISC-R and K-ABC performance in hemiplegic children. *Journal of Psychoeducational Assessment,* 3, 215.

Lewandowski, L.J., Costenbader, V. & Richman, R. 1984. Neuropsychological aspects of Turner syndrome. *International Journal of Clinical Neuropsychology,* 7, 144.

Lewerenz, D.C. 1978. Visual acuity and the developing visual system. *Journal of the American Optometry Association,* 49(10), 1155.

Lewin, K. 1935. *A Dynamic Theory of Personality.* New York: McGraw-Hill.

Lewis, M. & Brooks-Gunn, J. 1981. Visual attention at three months as a predictor of cognitive functioning at two years of age. *Intelligence,* 5, 131.

Lewis, M. & Goldberg, S. 1969. Perceptual-cognitive development in infancy: A generalized expectancy model as a function of mother-infant interaction. *Merrill-Palmer Quarterly,* 15, 812.

Lewis, M., Sullivan, M.W. & Brooks-Gunn, J. 1985. Emotional behavior during the learning of a contingency in early infancy. *British Journal of Developmental Psychology,* 3, 307.

Lewis, M., Feiring, C. & McGuffog, C. 1986. Profiles of young gifted and normal children: Skills and abilities as related to sex and handedness. *Topics in Early Childhood Special Education,* 6, 9.

Lewis, R.S. & Christiansen, L. 1989. Intrahemispheric sex differences in the functional representation of language and praxic functions in normal individuals. *Brain and Cognition,* 9, 238.

Lewis, T.L., Maurer, D. & Kay, D. 1978. Newborn's central vision: Whole or hole? *Journal of Experimental Child Psychology,* 26, 193.

Liberman, I.Y. & Shankweiler, D. 1979. Speech, the alphabet, and teaching to read. In L.B. Resnick and P.A. Weaver (Eds.), *Theory and Practice of Early Reading,* Vol. 2. Hillsdale, NJ: Erlbaum.

Licht, R., Kok, A., Bakker, D.J. & Bouma, A. 1986. Hemispheric distribution of ERP components and word naming in preschool children. *Brain and Language,* 27, 101.

Lie, H.R., Lagergren, J., Rasmussen, F. & Lagerkvist, B. 1991. Bowel and bladder control of children with myelomeningocele: A Nordic study. *Developmental Medicine and Child Neurology,* 33, 1053.

Liederman, J. & Coryell, J. 1982. The origin of left hand preference: Pathological and non-pathological influences. *Neuropsychologia,* 20(6), 721.

Lienert, G.A. 1961. Überprüfung und genetische Interpretation der Divergenzhypothese von Wewetzer. *Vita Humana,* 4, 112.

Lienert, G.A. & Faber, C. 1963. Über die Faktorenstruktur des HAWIK auf verschiedenen Alters-und Intelligenzniveaus. *Diagnostica,* 9, 3.

Lilienfeld, A.M. 1969. *Epidemiology of Mongolism.* Baltimore: Johns Hopkins University Press.

Lilienfeld, A.M. & Parkhurst, E. 1951. A study of the association of factors of pregnancy and parturition with the development of cerebral palsy: A preliminary report. *American Journal of Hygiene,* 53, 262.

Lilienfeld, A.M. & Pasamanick, E. 1954. Association of maternal and fetal factors with the development of epilepsy. I. Abnormalities in the prenatal and paranatal periods. *Journal of the American Medical Association,* 155, 719.

Lincoln, A.J., Courchesne, E., Kilman, B.A. & Galambos, R. 1985. Neuropsychological correlates of information-processing by children with Down syndrome. *American Journal of Mental Deficiency,* 89, 403.

Lincoln, A.J., Dickstein, P., Courchesne, E. & Elmasian, R. 1992. Auditory processing abilities in non-retarded adolescents and young adults with developmental receptive language disorder and autism. *Brain and Language,* 43, 613.

Lindgren, S.D., De Renzi, E. & Richman, L.C. 1985. Cross-national comparisons of developmental dyslexia in Italy and the United States. *Child Development* 56, 1404.

Lindsay, J., Ounsted, C. & Richards, P. 1979. Long-term outcome in children with temporal lobe seizures. I. Social outcome and childhood factors, II. Marriage and parenthood, III. Psychiatric aspects in childhood and adult life. *Developmental Medicine and Child Neurology,* 21, 285, 433, 630.

Lindsay, J., Ounsted, C. & Richards, P. 1984. Long-term outcome in children with temporal lobe seizures. V: Indications and contra-indications for neurosurgery. *Developmental Medicine and Child Neurology,* 26, 25.

Lindsay, J., Ounsted, C. & Richards, P. 1987. Hemispherectomy for childhood epilepsy: A 36-year study. *Developmental Medicine and Child Neurology,* 29, 592.

Link, E.A., Weese-Mayer, D.W. & Byrd, S.E. 1991. Magnetic resonance imaging in infants exposed to cocaine prenatally: A preliminary report. *Clinical Pediatrics,* 30, 506.

Links, P.S., Boyle, M.H. & Offord, D.R. 1989. The prevalence of emotional disorders in children. *Journal of Nervous and Mental Disease,* 177, 85.

Lipper, E.G., Voorhies, T.M., Ross, G., Vannucci, R.C. & Auld, P.A.M. 1986. Early predictors of one-year outcome for infants asphyxiated at birth. *Developmental Medicine and Child Neurology,* 28, 303.

Lipton, H.L., Preziosi, T.J. & Moses, H. 1978. Adult onset of Dandy-Walker syndrome. *Archives of Neurology,* 35, 672.

Lis, C. 1969. Visuo-motor development and its disturbances in a sample of prematures born with birth weight below 1,250 grams. *Australian Journal on the Education of Backward Children,* 16, 73.

Litchen, W.H., Rickards, A.L., Ryan, M.M. & Ford, G.W. 1986. Improved outcome to two years of very low-birthweight infants: Fact or artefact? *Developmental Medicine and Child Neurology,* 28, 579.

Little, A.H. 1970. Eyelid conditioning in the human infant as a function of the interstimulus interval. Unpublished Master's thesis. Providence: Brown University.

Little, W.J. 1862. On the influence of abnormal parturition, difficult labours, premature birth, and asphyxia neonatorum, on the mental and physical conditions of the child, especially in relation to deformities. *Transactions of the Obstetric Society of London,* 3, 293.

Littman, B. & Parmalee, A.H. 1978. Medical correlates of infant development. *Pediatrics,* 61, 470.

Livingston, R. 1985. Depressive illness and learning disabilities: Research needs and practical implications. *Journal of Learning Disabilities,* 18, 518.

Livingston, S. 1972. Epilepsy in infancy, childhood and adolescence. In B. Wolman (Ed.), *Manual of Child Psychopathology.* New York: McGraw-Hill.

Locke, J.L. & Mather, P.L. 1989. Genetic factors in the ontogeny of spoken language: Evidence from monozygotic and dizygotic twins. *Journal of Child Language,* 16, 553.

Loeser, J.D. & Alvord, E.C. 1968a. Agenesis of the corpus callosum. *Brain,* 91, 553.

Loeser, J.D. & Alvord, E.C. 1968b. Clinicopathological correlations in agenesis of the corpus callosum. *Neurology,* 18, 745.

Lombroso, C.T. 1978. Convulsive disorders in newborns. In R.A. Thompson & J.R. Green (Eds.), *Pediatric Neurology and Neurosurgery.* New York: Spectrum.

Lombroso, C.T. 1983a. A prospective study of infantile spasms: Clinical and therapeutic correlations. *Epilepsia,* 24, 135.

Lombroso, C.T. 1983b. Prognosis in neonatal seizures. In A.V. Delgado-Sscueta, C.G. Wasterlain, D.M. Treiman & R.J. Porter (Eds.), *Status Epilepticus. Advances in Neurology,* Vol. 34. New York: Raven Press, p. 101.

Loney, J. 1980. Hyperkinesis comes of age: What do we know and where should we go? *American Journal of Orthopsychiatry,* 50, 28.

Loney, J. & Milich, R. 1982. Hyperactivity, inattention, and aggression in clinical practice. In M. Wolraich & D. Routh (Eds.), *Advances in Developmental and Behavioral Pediatrics,* Vol. 3. Greenwich CT: JAI Press, p. 113.

Lord, J., Varzos, N., Behrman, B. & Wicks, J. 1990. Implications of mainstream classrooms for adolescents with spina bifida. *Developmental Medicine and Child Neurology,* 32, 698.

Lorenz, K. 1935. Der Kumpan in der Umwelt des Vogels. *Journal of Ornithology,* 83, 335.

Lorenz, K. 1970. *Studies in Animal and Human Behaviour,* Vol. 1 (Translated by R. Martin) London: Methven.

Lott, I.T. 1986. The neurology of Down's syndrome. In C.J. Epstein (Ed.), *The Neurobiology of Down's Syndrome.* New York: Raven Press, p. 17.

Lotter, V. 1978. Follow-up studies. In M. Rutter & E. Schopler (Eds.), *Autism: A Reappraisal of Concept and Treatment.* New York: Plenum.

Lou, H.C. 1982. *Developmental Neurology.* New York: Raven Press.

Lou, H.C., Henriksen, L. & Bruhn, P. 1984. Focal cerebral hypoprofusion in children with dysphasia and/or attention deficit disorder. *Archives of Neurology,* 41, 825.

Lou, H.C., Henriksen, L., Bruhn, P., Borner, H. & Nielsen, J.B. 1989. Striatal dysfunction in attention deficit and hyperkinetic disorder. *Archives of Neurology,* 46, 48.

Loubar, J.F. 1991. Discourse on the development of EEG diagnostics and biofeedback for attention-deficit/hyperactivity disorders. *Biofeedback and Self-Regulation,* 16, 201.

Loveland, K.A., Fletcher, J.M. & Bailey, V. 1990. Verbal and nonverbal communication of events in learning-disability subtypes. *Journal of Clinical and Experimental Neuropsychology,* 12, 33.

Lovett, M.W. 1984. A developmental perspective on reading dysfunction: Accuracy and rate criteria in the subtyping of dyslexic children. *Brain and Language,* 22, 67.

Lovett, M.W. 1987. A developmental perspective on reading dysfunction: Accuracy and speed criteria of normal and deficient reading skill. *Child Development,* 58, 234.

Lowrey, G.H. 1978. *Growth and Development of Children,* 6th ed. Chicago: Year Book Publishers.

Lozoff, B. 1989. Nutrition and behavior. *American Psychologist,* 44, 231.

Lu, C.M., Su, C.W., Chen, S.M. & Jong, J.T. 1989. A study on the development of mental abilities of infants from birth to one year old. *Bulletin of Educational Psychology,* 22, 115.

Lubchenco, L. 1970. Assessment of gestational age and development at birth. *Pediatric Clinics of North America,* 17, 125.

Lubchenco, L.O. 1976. *The High Risk Infant.* Philadelphia: W.B. Saunders.

Lubchenco, L.O., Horner, F.A., Reed, L.H., Hix, I.E., Metcalf, D., Cohig, R., Elliott, H.C. & Bourg, M. 1963. Sequelae of premature birth. *American Journal of Diseases of Children,* 106, 101.

Lubs, H.A. 1969. A marker X syndrome. *American Journal of Human Genetics,* 21, 231.

Lucas, A., Morley, R., Lister, G. & Leeson-Payne, C. 1992. Effect of very low birth weight and subnormal head size on cognitive abilities at school age. *New England Journal of Medicine,* 325, 231.

Lucas, J.A., Rosenstein, L.D. & Bigler, E.D. 1989. Handedness and language among the mentally retarded: Implications for the model of pathological left-handedness and gender differences in hemispheric specialization. *Neuropsychologia,* 27, 713.

Lucas, S.A. 1984. Auditory discrimination and speech production in the blind child. *International Journal of Rehabilitation Research,* 7, 74.

Luchins, D.J., Weinberger, D.R. & Wyatt, R.J. 1983. Reversed cerebral asymmetry in schizophrenia. Paper presented at the 11th Annual Meeting of the International Neuropsychological Society, Mexico City.

Ludlow, C.L. 1979. Research directions and needs concerning the neurological bases of language disorders in children. In C.L. Ludlow & M.E. Doran-Quine (Eds.), *The Neurological Bases of Language Disorders in Children: Methods and Directions for Research.* NIH Publication 79-440. Bethesda, MD: U.S. Department of Health, Education and Welfare.

Ludlow, C.L., Cudahy, E., Caine, E., Brown, E.L. & Bassich, C. 1980. Auditory processing deficits in the absence of language disorder. Paper presented at the Annual Meeting of the Academy of Aphasia, San Diego.

Luessenhop, A.J., dela Cruz, T.C. & Fenichel, G.M. 1970. Surgical disconnection of the cerebral hemispheres for intractable seizures: Results in infancy and childhood. *Journal of the American Medical Association,* 213(10), 1630.

Luk, S.E., Leung, P.W. & Yuen, J. 1991. Clinic observations in the assessment of pervasiveness of childhood hyperactivity. *Journal of Child Psychology and Psychiatry and Allied Disciplines,* 32, 833.

Lund, R.D. 1978. *Development and Plasticity of the Brain: An Introduction.* New York: Oxford University Press.

Luria, A.R. 1966. *Higher Cortical Functions in Man,* 2nd ed. New York: Basic Books.

Luria, A.R. 1973. *The Working Brain.* New York: Basic Books.

Luria, A.R. & Yudovich, F.I. 1971. *Speech and Development of Mental Processes in the Child, An Experimental Investigation.* Harmondsworth, England: Penguin.

Lutman, M.E. & Haggard, M.P. (Eds.) 1983. *Hearing Science and Hearing Disorders.* New York: Academic Press.

Lyle, J.G. 1970. Certain antenatal, perinatal and developmental variables and reading retardation in middle-class boys. *Child Development,* 41, 481.

Lynch, G. 1974. The formation of new synaptic connections after brain damage and their possible role in recovery of function. *Neuroscience Research Progress Bulletin.* 12, 226.

Lynn, R.B., Buchanan, D.C., Fenichel, G.M. & Freemon, F.R. 1980. Agenesis of the corpus callosum. *Archives of Neurology,* 37, 444.

Lyon, G.R., Stewart, N. & Freedman, D. 1982. Neuropsychological characteristics of empirically derived subgroups of learning disabled readers. *Journal of Clinical Neuropsychology,* 4, 343.

Maccoby, E.E. & Jacklin, C.N. 1974. Intellectual abilities and cognitive styles. In E.E. Maccoby and C.N. Jacklin (Eds.), *The Psychology of Sex Differences.* Stanford: Stanford University Press.

MacKeith, R. & Bax, M. (Eds.) 1963. *Minimal Cerebral Dysfunction.* Little Club Clinics in Developmental Medicine, No. 10. London: Heinemann.

MacKeith, R.C. & Rutter, M. 1972. A note on the prevalence of speech and language disorders. In M. Rutter & J.A. Martin (Eds.), *The Child with Delayed Speech.* London: Heinemann.

Mackinnon, P.C.B. 1979. Sexual differentiation of the brain. In F. Falkner and J.M. Tanner (Eds.), *Human Growth, Vol. 3: Neurobiology and Nutrition.* New York: Plenum Press.

Mackworth, N.H., Grandstaff, N.W. & Pribram, K.H. 1973. Orientation to pictorial novelty by speech-disordered children. *Neuropsychologia,* 11, 443.

MacLean, P.D. 1970. The triune brain, emotion, and scientific bias. In F.O. Schmitt (Ed.), *The Neurosciences: Second Study Program.* New York: Rockefeller University Press.

MacLean, P.D. 1990. *The Triune Brain in Evolution: Role in Paleocerebral Functions.* New York: Plenum.

MacMillan, D. 1982. *Mental Retardation in School and Society,* 2nd ed. Boston: Little, Brown.

Magelby, F.L. & Farley, O.W. 1968. *Education for Blind Children.* Research Bulletin No. 16. New York: American Foundation for the Blind, p. 69.

Majnemer, A., Brownstein, A., Kadanoff, R. & Shevell, M.I. 1992. A comparison of neurobehavioral performance of healthy term and low-risk preterm infants at term. *Developmental Medicine and Child Neurology,* 34, 417.

Majowski, L.V. 1989. Higher cortical functions in children: A developmental perspective. In C.R. Reynolds & E. Fletcher-Janzen (Eds.), *Handbook of Clinical Child Neuropsychology.* New York: Plenum, p. 41.

Mandoki, M.W., Sumner, G.S., Hoffman, R.P. & Riconda, D.L. 1991. A review of Klinefelter's syndrome in children and adolescents. *Journal of the American Academy of Child and Adolescent Psychiatry,* 30, 167.

Mann, I.C. 1964. *The Development of the Human Eye*. London: British Medical Association.

Mann, I. 1969. *The Development of the Human Eye*. New York: Grune & Stratton.

Marcel, T. & Rajan, P. 1975. Lateral specialization for recognition of words and faces in good and poor readers. *Neuropsychologia*, 13, 489.

Marcell, M.M. & Weeks, S.L. 1988. Short-term memory difficulties and Down's syndrome. *Journal of Mental Deficiency Research*, 32, 153.

Marchman, V.A., Miller, R. & Bates, E.A. 1991. Babble and first words in children with focal brain injury. *Applied Psycholinguistics*, 12, 1.

Marcotte, A.C. & LaBarba, R.C. 1987. The effects of linguistic experience on cerebral lateralization for speech production in normal hearing and deaf adolescents. *Brain and Language*, 31, 276.

Marcus, J. 1985. Neurological findings in high-risk children: Childhood assessment and 5-year follow-up. *Schizophrenia Bulletin*, 11, 85.

Marcus, J., Hans, S.L., Byhouwer, B. & Norem, J. 1985. Relationship among neurological functioning, intelligence quotients, and physical anomalies. *Schizophrenia Bulletin*, 11, 101.

Marge, M. 1972. The general problem of language disabilities in children. In J.V. Irwin & M. Marge (Eds.), *Principles of Childhood Language Disabilities*. New York: Appleton-Century-Crofts.

Marin-Padilla, M. 1978. Dual origin of the mammalian neocortex and evolution of the cortical plate. *Anatomy and Embryology*, 152, 109.

Mariner, R., Jackson, A.W., Levitas, A. & Hagerman, R.J. 1986. Autism, mental retardation, and chromosomal abnormalities. *Journal of Autism and Developmental Disorders*, 16, 425.

Marino, R.V., Scholl, T.O., Karp, R.J. & Yanoff, J.M. 1987. Minor physical anomalies and learning disability: What is the prenatal component? *Journal of the National Medical Association*, 79, 37.

Marlowe, M., Errera, J. & Jacobs, J. 1983. Increased lead and cadmium burdens among mentally retarded children and children with borderline intelligence. *American Journal of Mental Deficiency*, 87, 477.

Marlowe, M., Cossairt, A., Moon, C., Errara, J., MacNeel, A., Peak, R., Ray, J. & Schroeder, C. 1984. Main and interaction effects of metallic toxins on classroom behavior. *Journal of Abnormal Child Psychology*, 13, 185.

Marr, D. 1982. *Vision*. San Francisco: Freeman.

Marschark, M. 1993. *Psychological Development of Deaf Children*. New York: Oxford University Press.

Marsh, H.W. 1989. Sex differences in the development of verbal mathematics constructs: The high school and beyond study. *American Education Research Journal*, 26, 191.

Marsh, R.W. 1985. Phrenoblysis: real or chimera? *Child Development*, 56, 1059.

Marshall, P. 1989. Attention deficit disorder and allergy: A neurochemical model of the relation between the illnesses. *Psychological Bulletin*, 434.

Martin, A. 1981. Visual processing in the acallosal brain: A clue to the differential functions of the anterior commissure and splenium. Presented at International Neuropsychological Society Meeting, Atlanta.

Martin, H.P. 1980. Nutrition, injury, illness, and minimal brain dysfunction. In H.E. Rie & E.D. Rie (Eds.), *Handbook of Minimal Brain Dysfunction, A Critical View*. New York: Wiley.

Martin, H.P. & Kempe, C.H. (Eds.). 1976. *The Abused Child: A Multidisciplinary Approach to Developmental Issues and Treatment.* Cambridge, MA: Ballinger.

Martin, J.A.M. 1981. *Voice, Speech and Language in the Child: Development and Disorder. Disorders of Human Communication,* Vol. 4. Berlin: Springer-Verlag.

Martineau, J., Barthelemy, C., Herault, J. & Jouve, J. 1991. Monoamines in autistic children: A study of age-related changes. *Brain Dysfunction,* 4, 141.

Martins, I.P., Ferro, J.M. & Trindade, A. 1987. Acquired crossed aphasia in a child. *Developmental Medicine and Child Neurology,* 29, 96.

Martyn, L.J. 1975. Pediatric neuro-ophthalmology. In R.D. Harley (Ed.), *Pediatric Ophthalmology.* Philadelphia: W.B. Saunders.

Massachusetts Medical Society. 1989. Rubella and congenital rubella syndrome—United States, 1985–1988. *Morbidity and Mortality Weekly Report,* 38, 173.

Mateer, C., Polen, S.B. & Ojemann, G.A. 1982. Sexual variations in cortical localization of naming as determined by stimulation mapping. *Behavioral and Brain Sciences,* 5, 310.

Matkin, N.D. & Carhart, R. 1966. Auditory profiles associated with Rh incompatibility. *Archives of Otolaryngology* (Chicago), 84, 502.

Matousek, M., Rasmussen, P. & Gillberg, C. 1984. EEG frequency analysis in children with so-called minimal brain dysfunction and related disorders. *Advances of Biological Psychiatry,* 15, 102.

Mattes, J.A. & Gittelman, R. 1981. Effects of artificial food colorings in children with hyperactive symptoms. *Archives of General Psychiatry,* 38, 414.

Matthews, C.G. & Klove, H. 1967. Differential psychological performance in major motor, psychomotor, and mixed seizure classifications of known and unknown etiology. *Epilepsia,* 8, 117.

Matthews, W.S. 1988. Attention deficits and learning disabilities in children with Tourette's syndrome. *Psychiatric Annals,* 18, 414.

Matthews, W.S. & Barabas, G. 1985. Recent advances in developmental pediatrics related to achievement and social behavior. *School Psychology Review,* 14, 182.

Matthews, W.S., Barabas, G., Cusack, E. & Ferrari, M. 1986. Social quotients of children with phenylketonuria before and after discontinuation of dietary therapy. *American Journal of Mental Deficiency,* 91, 92.

Mattis, S. 1978. Dyslexia syndromes: A working hypothesis that works. In A.L. Benton & D. Pearl (Eds.), *Dyslexia: An Appraisal of Current Knowledge.* New York: Oxford University Press.

Mattis, S., French, J.H. & Rapin, I. 1975. Dyslexia in children and young adults: Three independent neuropsychological syndromes. *Developmental Medicine and Child Neurology,* 17, 150.

Matzker, R. 1958. *Ein binauraler Hörsynthese-Test zum Nachweis zerebraler Hörstörungen.* Stuttgart: Thieme.

Maurer, D. & Salapatek, P. 1976. Developmental changes in the scanning of faces by young infants. *Child Development,* 47, 523.

Maurer, D. & Terrill, L. 1979. A physiological explanation of the infant's early visual development. *Canadian Journal of Psychology,* 33, 232.

Mayberry, R.I. 1992. The cognitive development of deaf children. In S.J. Segalowitz & I. Rapin (Eds.), *Handbook of Neuropsychology,* Vol. 7. Amsterdam: Elsevier, p. 51.

McAdoo, G. & DeMyer, M.K. 1978. Personality characteristics of parents. In M. Rutter & E. Schopler (Eds.), *Autism.* New York: Plenum Press.

McAllister, M. 1981. WISC characteristics of clinic-referred subgroups of disabled learners. Unpublished Masters thesis, University of Victoria.

McBride, H.C.G. 1975. The isolation syndrome in childhood. Part 1: The syndrome and its diagnosis. *Developmental Medicine and Child Neurology,* 17, 198.

McCall, R.B. 1976. The development of intellectual functioning in infancy and the prediction of later IQ. In J.D. Osofsky (Ed.), *Handbook of Infant Development.* New York: John Wiley, p. 707.

McCardle, P. & Wilson, B.E. 1990. Hormonal influence on language development in physically advanced children. *Brain and Language,* 38, 410.

McCarthy, D.A. 1972. *Manual for the McCarthy Scales of Children's Abilities.* New York: Psychological Corporation.

McCauley, E., Kay, T., Ito, J. & Treder, R. 1987. The Turner syndrome: Cognitive deficits, affective discrimination, and behavior problems. *Child Development,* 58, 464.

McConachie, H. 1990. Early language development and severe visual impairment. *Child: Care, Health and Development,* 16, 55.

McCormick, M.C., Bernbaum, J.C., Eisenberg, J.M., Kustra, S.L. & Finnegan, E. 1991. Costs incurred by parents of very low birth weight infants after the initial neonatal hospitalization. *Pediatrics* 88, 533.

McDaniels, J.W. & McDaniels, M.L. 1976. Visual and auditory cognitive processing affected by epilepsy. *Behavioral Neuropsychiatry,* 8, 78.

McDonald, A.D. 1973. Severely retarded children in Quebec: Prevalence, causes and care. *American Journal of Mental Deficiency,* 78, 205.

McDonnell, P.M. 1979. Patterns of eye-hand coordination in the first year of life. *Canadian Journal of Psychology,* 33, 253.

McFie, J. 1961. The effects of hemispherectomy on intellectual functioning in cases of infantile hemiplegia. *Journal of Neurology, Neurosurgery, and Psychiatry,* 24, 240.

McFie, J. 1975. Brain injury in childhood and language development. In N. O'Connor (Ed.), *Language, Cognitive Deficits, and Retardation.* London: Butterworth.

McGauhey, P.J., Starfield, B., Alexander, C. & Ensminger, M.E. 1992. Social environment and vulnerability of low birth weight children: A social-epidemiological perspective. *Pediatrics,* 88, 943.

McGee, M.G. 1979. *Human Spatial Abilities: Sources of Sex Differences.* New York: Praeger.

McGee, R., Williams, S. & Silva, P.A. 1984a. Background characteristics of aggressive, hyperactive, and aggressive-hyperactive boys. *Journal of the American Academy of Child Psychiatry,* 23, 280.

McGee, R., Williams, S. & Silva, P.A. 1984b. Behavioral and developmental characteristics of aggressive, hyperactive and hyperactive-aggressive boys. *Journal of the American Academy of Child Psychiatry,* 23, 270.

McGee, R., Williams, S. & Silva, P.A. 1987. A comparison of girls and boys with teacher-identified problems of attention. *Journal of the American Academy of Child and Adolescent Psychiatry,* 26, 711.

McGivern, R.F., Berka, C., Languis, M.L. & Chapman, S. 1991. Detection of deficits in temporal pattern discrimination using the Seashore Rhythm Test in young children with reading impairment. *Journal of Learning Disabilities,* 24, 58.

McGlone, J. 1977. Sex differences in the cerebral organization of verbal functions in patients with unilateral cerebral lesions. *Brain,* 100, 775.

McGlone, J. 1980. Sex differences in human brain asymmetry: A critical survey. *The Behavioral and Brain Sciences,* 3, 215.

McGlone, J. 1985. Can spatial deficits in Turner's syndrome be explained by focal CNS dysfunction or atypical speech lateralization? *Journal of Clinical and Experimental Neuropsychology*, 7, 375.

McGraw, M.B. 1946. Maturation of behaviour. In L. Carmichael (Ed.), *Manual of Child Psychology*. New York: Wiley.

McGuinness, D. & Morley, C. 1991. Sex differences in the development of visuo-spatial ability in pre-school children. *Journal of Mental Imagery*, 15, 143.

McGuinness, D. & Pribram, K.H. 1980. The neuropsychology of attention: Emotional and motivational controls. In M.C. Wittcock (Ed.), *The Brain and Psychology*. New York: Academic Press.

McIntosh, N. 1979. Medulloblastoma—A changing prognosis? *Archives of Disease in Childhood*, 54, 200.

McKay, H., Sinesterra, L., McKay, A., Gomez, H. & Lloreda, P. 1978. Improving cognitive ability in chronically deprived children. *Science*, 200, 270.

McKeever, W.F. 1981. Sex and cerebral organization: Is it really so simple? In A. Ansara, et al. (Eds.), *Sex Differences in Dyslexia*. Towson, MD: The Orton Dyslexia Society.

McKenzie, K.G. 1938. The present status of a patient who had the right cerebral hemisphere removed. *Journal of the American Medical Association*, 111, 168.

McKusick, V.A. 1992. *Mendelian Inheritance in Man; Catalogs of Autosomal Dominant, Autosomal Recessive, and X-Linked Phenotypes*, Vol. 1, 2. 10th ed. Baltimore: Johns Hopkins University Press.

McLaren, D.S., Yaktin, U.S., Kanawati, A., Sabbagh, S. & Kadi, Z. 1973. The subsequent mental and physical development of rehabilitated marasmic infants. *Journal of Mental Deficiency Research*, 17, 273.

McLaren, J. & Bryson, S.E. 1987. Review of recent epidemiological studies of mental retardation: Prevalence, associated disorders, and etiology. *American Journal of Mental Retardation*, 92, 243.

McLaughlin, J.F. & Kriegsman, E. 1980. Developmental dyspraxia in a family with X-linked mental retardation. *Developmental Medicine and Child Neurology*, 22, 84.

McLinden, D.J. 1988. Spatial task performance: A meta-analysis. *Journal of Visual Impairment and Blindness*, 82, 231.

McLone, D., Czyzewski, D., Raimondi, A.J. & Sommers, R.C. 1982. Central nervous system infections as a limiting factor in the intelligence of children with myelomeningocele. *Pediatrics*, 70(3), 338.

McMahon, R.C. 1980. Genetic etiology in the hyperactive child syndrome: A critical review. *American Journal of Orthopsychiatry*, 50, 145.

McMahon, S. & Greenberg, L.M. 1977. Serial neurological examination of hyperactive children. *Pediatrics*, 59, 584.

McManus, I.C. & Bryden, M.P. 1991. Geschwind's theory of lateralization: Developing a formal causal model. *Psychological Bulletin*, 110, 237.

McManus, I.C., Brickman, A., Alessi, N.E. & Grapentine, W.L. 1985. Neurological dysfunction in serious delinquents. *Journal of the American Academy of Child Psychiatry*, 24, 481.

McNeil, T.F. 1983. Offspring of women with nonorganic psychoses: Development of a longitudinal study of children at high risk. *Acta Psychiatrica Scandinavica*, 68, 234.

McVicker-Hunt, J. 1979. Psychological development: Early experience. *Annual Review of Psychology*, 36, 103.

Meadow, K.P. 1968. Towards a developmental understanding of deafness. *Journal of Rehabilitation of the Deaf*, 2, 1.

Mealey, J. 1975. Infantile subdural hematomas. *Pediatric Clinics of North America*, 22, 433.

Medina, J., Chokroverty, S. & Rubino, F.A. 1977. Syndrome of agitated delirium and visual impairment. A manifestation of medial temporo-occipital infarction. *Journal of Neurology, Neurosurgery and Psychiatry*, 40, 861.

Mednick, S.A. 1973. Breakdown in high-risk subjects: Familial and early environmental factors. *Journal of Abnormal Psychology*, 82, 469.

Mednick, S.A. & Kandel, E.S. 1988. Congenital determinants of violence. *Bulletin of the American Academy of Psychiatry and the Law*, 18, 101.

Mednick, S.A., Cannon, T.D., Barr, C.E. & Lyon, M. (Eds.) 1991. *Fetal Neural Development and Adult Schizophrenia*. New York: Oxford University Press.

Mehler, J., Jusczyk, P., Lambertz, G., Halsted, N., Bertoncini, J. & Amiel-Tyson, C. 1988. A precursor of language acquisition in young infants. *Cognition*, 29, 143.

Meisels, S.J., Plunkett, J.W., Roloff, D.W., Pasick, P.L. & Stiefel, G.S. 1986. Growth and development of preterm infants with respiratory distress syndrome and bronchopulmonary dysplasia. *Pediatrics*, 77, 345.

Melekian, B. 1981. Lateralization in the human newborn at birth: Asymmetry of the stepping reflex. *Neuropsychologia*, 19, 707.

Melish, M.E. & Hanshaw, J.B. 1973. Congenital cytomegalovirus infection. Developmental progress of infants detected by routine screening. *American Journal of Diseases of Children*, 126, 190.

Meltzoff, A.N. & Moore, M.K. 1977. Imitation of facial and manual gestures by human neonates. *Science*, 198, 75.

Mendelson, W., Johnson, W. & Stewart, M. 1971. Hyperactive children as teenagers: A follow-up study. *Journal of Nervous and Mental Diseases*, 153, 273.

Menkes, M.M., Rowe, J.S. & Menkes, J.H. 1967. A twenty-five year follow-up study on the hyperkinetic child with minimal brain dysfunction. *Pediatrics*, 39(3), 393.

Menser, M.A., Dodds, L. & Harley, J.D. 1967. A twenty-five year follow-up of congenital rubella. *Lancet*, 2, 1347.

Menyuk, P. 1978. Linguistic problems in children with developmental dysphasia. In M.A. Wyke (Ed.), *Developmental Dysphasia*. New York: Academic Press.

Merzenich, M.M. 1992. Development and maintenance of cortical somatosensory representations: Functional "maps" and neuroanatomical repertoires. In K.E. Barnard & T.B. Brazelton (Eds.), *Touch: The Foundation of Experience*. Madison, CT: International Universities Press, p. 47.

Meyer, A. 1981. Paul Flechsig's system of myelogenetic cortical localization in the light of recent research in neuroanatomy and neurophysiology. *The Canadian Journal of Neurological Sciences*, 8, 95.

Meyer, M.B., Jones, B.S. & Tonascia, J.A. 1976. Perinatal events associated with maternal smoking during pregnancy. *American Journal of Epidemiology*, 103, 464.

Meyer-Probst, B. 1974. Über kognitive Leistungsveränderungen hirngeschädigter Kinder. *Zeitschrift für Psychologie* (Leipzig), 182, 181.

Michel, G. 1981. Right handedness: A consequence of infant supine head orientation preference. *Science*, 212, 685.

Michel, G. & Goodwin, R. 1979. Intrauterine birth position predicts newborn supine head position preferences. *Infant Behavior and Child Development*, 2, 29.

Mikkelsen, E.J. 1982. Neurologic status in hyperactive, enuretic, encopretic, and normal boys. *Journal of the American Academy of Child Psychiatry,* 21, 75.

Milani-Comparetti, A. & Eldon, E.A. 1967. Routine developmental examination in normal and retarded children. *Developmental Medicine and Child Neurology,* 9, 631.

Milgram, N.A. 1973. Cognition and language in mental retardation: Distinctions and implications. In D.K. Routh (Ed.), *The Experimental Psychology of Mental Retardation.* Chicago: Aldine.

Milich, R. & Fitzgerald, G. 1985. Validation of inattention/overactivity and aggression ratings with classroom observations. *Journal of Consulting and Clinical Psychology,* 53, 139.

Milich, R., Lindgen, S. & Wolraich, M. 1986. The behavioral effects of sugar: A comment on Buchanan. *American Psychologist,* 41, 218.

Miller, E. & Sethi, L. 1971. The effects of hydrocephalus on perception. *Developmental Medicine and Child Neurology,* Suppl. 25, 77.

Miller, G., Dubowitz, L.M.S. & Palmer, P. 1984. Follow-up of preterm infants: Is correction of the developmental quotient for prematurity helpful? *Early Human Development,* 9, 137.

Miller, J.L. & Eimas, P.D. 1983. Studies on the categorization of speech by infants. *Cognition,* 13, 135.

Miller, J.S. 1978. Hyperactive children: A ten year study. *Pediatrics,* 61, 217.

Miller, R.G., Palkes, H.S. & Stewart, M.A. 1973. Hyperactive children in suburban elementary schools. *Child Psychiatry and Human Development,* 4, 121.

Mills, M. & Melhuish, E. 1974. Recognition of mother's voice in early infancy. *Nature* (London), 252, 123.

Milner, A.D., Jeeves, M.A., Silver, P.H., Lines, C.R. & Wilson, J. 1985. Reaction times to lateralized visual stimuli in callosal agenesis: Stimulus and response factors. *Neuropsychologia,* 23, 323.

Milner, B. 1975. Psychological aspects of focal epilepsy and its neurological management. *Advances in Neurology,* 8, 299.

Milner, R.J., Bloom, F.E. & Sutcliffe, J.G. 1987. Brain-specific genes: Strategies and issues. In R.K. Hunt (Ed.), *Neural Development, Part IV: Cellular and Molecular Differentiation.* New York: Academic Press, p. 117.

Milunski, A., Jick, H., Jick, S.S., Bruell, C.L., MacLaughlin, D.S., Rothman, K.J. & Willett, W. 1989. Multivitamin/folic acid supplementation in early pregnancy reduces the prevalence of neural tube defects. *Journal of the American Medical Association,* 262, 2847.

Mims, S.K., McIntyre, C.W. & Murray, M.E. 1983. An analysis of visual motor problems in children with dietary-treated phenylketonuria. *Educational and Psychological Research,* 3, 111.

Minde, K., Lewin, D., Weiss, G., Lavigueur, H., Douglas, V. & Sykes, E. 1971. The hyperactive child in elementary school: A 5-year, controlled follow-up. *Exceptional Children,* 38, 215.

Minde, K., Whitelaw, A., Brown, J. & Fitzhardinge, P. 1983. Effect of neonatal complications in premature infants on early parent-infant interactions. *Developmental Medicine and Child Neurology,* 25, 755.

Miner, M.E., Fletcher, J.M. & Ewing-Cobbs, L. 1986. Recovery versus outcome after head injury in children. In M.E. Miner & K.A. Wagner (Eds.), *Neural Trauma: Treatment, Monitoring and Rehabilitation Issues.* Stoneham, MA: Butterworth, p. 233.

Minkowski, M. 1928 (transl. 1963). On aphasia in polyglots. In L. Halpern (Ed.), *Problems of Dynamic Neurology*. Jerusalem: Jerusalem Post Press.

Minshew, N.J. & Goldstein, G. 1993. Is autism an amnesic disorder? Evidence from the California Verbal Learning Test. *Neuropsychology, 7,* 209.

Minshew, N.J., Goldstein, G., Taylor, H.G. & Siegel, D.J. 1994. Academic achievement in high functioning autistic individuals. *Journal of Clinical and Experimental Neuropsychology, 16,* 261.

Miranda, S. 1970. Visual abilities and pattern preferences of premature infants and full-term neonates. *Journal of Experimental Child Psychology, 10,* 189.

Miranda, S.B. & Fantz, R.L. 1974. Recognition memory in Down's syndrome and normal infants. *Child Development, 45,* 651.

Miranda, S.B., Hack, M., Fanta, R.L., Fanaroff, A.A. & Klaus, M.H. 1977. Neonatal pattern vision: A predictor of future mental performance? *Journal of Pediatrics, 91,* 642.

Mirmiran, M. & Uylings, H. 1983. The environmental enrichment effect upon cortical growth is neutralized by concomitant pharmacological suppression of active sleep in female rats. *Brain Research, 261,* 331.

Mirsky, A.F. & Duncan-Johnson, C.C. 1984. Nature versus nurture in schizophrenia: The struggle continues. *Integrative Psychiatry, 2,* 137.

Mitchell, C.L. (Ed.). 1982. *Nervous System Toxicology.* New York: Saunders.

Mitchell, R.G. 1980. Perinatal follow-up (Editorial). *Developmental Medicine and Child Neurology, 22,* 1.

Mitchell, W.G., Chavez, J.M., Lee, H. & Guzman, B.L. 1991. Academic underachievement in children with epilepsy. *Journal of Child Neurology, 6,* 65.

Mizrahi, E.M. & Kellaway, P. 1987. Characterization and classification of neonatal seizures. *Neurology, 37,* 1837.

Molfese, D.L. 1977. Infant cerebral asymmetry. In S.J. Segalowitz & F.A. Gruber (Eds.), *Language Development and Neurological Theory.* New York: Academic Press.

Molfese, D.L. & Molfese, V.J. 1979a. Hemispheric and stimulus differences as reflected in the cortical responses of newborn infants to speech stimuli. *Developmental Psychology, 15,* 505.

Molfese, D.L. & Molfese, V.J. 1979b. VOT distinctions in infants: Learned or innate? In H. Whitaker & H. Whitaker (Eds.), *Studies in Neurolinguistics,* Vol. 4. New York: Academic Press.

Molfese, D.L. & Segalowitz, S.J. (Eds.) 1988. *Brain Lateralization in Children: Developmental Implications.* New York: Guilford Press.

Molfese, D.L., Nunez, V., Seibert, S.M. & Ramanaiach, N.V. 1976. Cerebral asymmetry: Changes in factors affecting its development. In S.R. Harnad, H.D. Stekilis & J.B. Lancaster (Eds.), *Origins and Evolution of Language and Speech. Annals of the New York Academy of Sciences, 280,* 811.

Molfese, V.J. 1989. *Perinatal Risk and Infant Development. Assessment and Prediction.* New York: Guilford Press.

Molfese, V.J. & Betz, J.C. 1987. Language and motor development in infancy: Three views with neuropsychological implications. *Developmental Neuropsychology, 3,* 255.

Molteno, C.D., Magasiner, V., Sayed, R. & Karplus, M. 1990. Postural development in very low birth weight and normal birth weight infants. *Early Human Development, 24,* 93.

Moltz, H. 1968. An epigenetic interpretation of the imprinting phenomenon. In G. Newton, & S. Levine (Eds.), *Early Experience and Behavior.* Springfield, IL: Charles C Thomas.

Moltz, H. 1973. Some implications of the critical period hypothesis. *Annals of the New York Academy of Sciences, 223,* 144.

Money, J. 1973. Turner's syndrome and parietal lobe functions. *Cortex, 9,* 385.

Money, J. & Ehrhardt, A.A. 1972. *Man and Woman, Boy and Girl.* Baltimore: Johns Hopkins University Press.

Monif, G.R.G., Hardy, J.B. & Sever, J.L. 1966. Studies in congenital rubella, Baltimore 1964–65. I. Epidemiologic and virologic. *Bulletin of the Johns Hopkins Hospital, 118,* 85.

Monreal, F.J. 1985. Consideration of genetic factors in cerebral palsy. *Developmental Medicine and Child Neurology, 27,* 325.

Moore, A.D., Stambrook, M., Gill, D.D., Hawryluk, G.A., Peters, L.C. & Harrison, M.M. 1993. Factor structure of the Wechsler Adult Intelligence Scale—Revised in a traumatic brain injury sample. *Canadian Journal of Behavioural Science, 25,* 605.

Moore, V. & Law, J. 1990. Copying ability of preschool children with delayed language development. *Developmental Medicine and Child Neurology, 32,* 249.

Mordock, J.B. & Bogan, S. 1968. Wechsler patterns and symptomatic behaviors of children diagnosed as having minimal cerebral dysfunction. *Proceedings of the 76th Annual Convention.* Washington, DC: American Psychological Association, p. 663.

Morgan, W.P. 1896. A case of congenital word blindness. *British Medical Journal, 2,* 1378.

Morrison, J.R. 1979. Diagnosis of adult psychiatric patients with childhood hyperactivity. *American Journal of Psychiatry, 136,* 955.

Morrison, J.R. 1980. Childhood hyperactivity in an adult psychiatric population: Social factors. *Journal of Clinical Psychiatry, 41,* 40.

Morrison, J.R. & Stewart, M.A. 1971. A family study of the hyperactive syndrome. *Biological Psychiatry, 3,* 189.

Morrison, J.R. & Stewart, M.A. 1973. The psychiatric status of the legal families of adopted hyperactive children. *Archives of General Psychiatry, 28,* 888.

Morrow, J.D. & Wachs, T.D. 1992. Infants with myelomeningocele: Visual recognition memory and sensorimotor abilities. *Developmental Medicine and Child Neurology, 34,* 488.

Morse, A.R. & Trief, E. 1985. Diagnosis and evaluation of visual dysfunction in premature infants with low birth weight. *Journal of Visual Impairment and Blindness, 79,* 248.

Morselli, P.L., Lloyd, K.G., Loscher, W., Meldrum, B. & Reynolds, E.H. (Eds.) 1981. *Neurotransmitters, Seizures and Epilepsy.* New York: Saunders.

Moruzzi, G. & Magoun, H.W. 1949. Brain stem reticular formation and activation of the EEG. *Electroencephalography and Clinical Neurophysiology, 1,* 455.

Moshe, S.L., Albala, B.J., Ackermann, R.F. & Engel, J. 1982. Increased seizure susceptibility of the immature brain. *Neurology, 32,* 121.

Moskalenko, V.D. 1984. Differences in ontogeny, premorbid personality, and severity of schizophrenia in twins. *Neuroscience and Behavioral Physiology, 14,* 444.

Mosley, J.L. & Stan, E.A. 1982. Sex differences in intellectual and neurological disorders: Biological risk factors and male vulnerability. In I. Al-Issa (Ed.), *Gender and Psychopathology.* New York: Academic Press.

Mosley, J.L. & Stan, E.A. 1984. Human sexual dimorphism: Its cost and benefit. In H.W. Reese (Ed.), *Advances in Child Development and Behavior*, Vol. 18, p. 147.

Mosley, J.L. & Vrbancic, M.I. 1990. Dichotic stimulation and mental retardation. *Research in Developmental Disabilities*, 11, 139.

Movshon, J.A. & Van Sluyters, R.C. 1981. Visual neural development. *Annual Review of Psychology*, 32, 477.

Muir, D., Abraham, W., Forbes, B. & Harris, L. 1979. The ontogenesis of an auditory localization response from birth to four months of age. *Canadian Journal of Psychology*, 33, 320.

Mulligan, J., Painter, M., O'Donoghue, P., MacDonald, H., Allen, A. & Taylor, P. 1980. Neonatal asphyxia. II. Neonatal mortality and long-term sequelae. *Journal of Pediatrics*, 96(5), 903.

Munk, H. 1881. Über die Funktionen der Grosshirnrinde. *Gesammelte Mitteilungen aus den Jahren 1877–1880*. Berlin: August Hirschwald.

Munz, A. & Tolor, A. 1955. Psychological effects of major cerebral excision: Intellectual and emotional changes following hemispherectomy. *Journal of Nervous and Mental Diseases*, 14, 438.

Murakami, J.W., Courchesne, E., Press, G.A. & Yeung-Courchesne, R. 1989. Reduced cerebellar hemisphere size and its relationship to vermal hypoplasia in autism. *Archives of Neurology*, 46, 689.

Murdoch, B.E., Ozanne, A.E. & Smyth, V. 1991. Communicative impairment in neural tube disorders. In B.E. Murdoch (Ed.), *Acquired Neurologic Speech/Language Disorders in Childhood. Brain Damage, Behavior and Cognition*. London: Taylor & Francis, p. 216.

Murphy, L.B. 1972. Infants play and cognitive development. In M.W. Piers (Ed.), *Play and Development*, New York: Norton.

Musiek, F.E. & Geurkink, N.A. 1980. Auditory perceptual problems in children: Considerations for the otolaryngologist and audiologist. *Laryngoscope*, 90(6), 962.

Mutton, D.E. & Lea, J. 1980. Chromosome studies of children with specific speech and language delay. *Developmental Medicine and Child Neurology*, 22, 588.

Myklebust, H.R. 1975. Nonverbal learning disabilities: Assessment and intervention. In H.R. Myklebust (Ed.), *Progress in Learning Disabilities*, Vol. 3. New York: Grune & Stratton, p. 85.

Nachshon, I. & Denno, D. 1986. Lateral preferences and birth stress. Paper presented at the conference of the International Neuropsychological Society, Veldhoven, Netherlands.

Nadel, L. (Ed.) 1988. *The Psychobiology of Down Syndrome*. Cambridge, MA: MIT Press.

Naeye, R.L. 1977. Placental infarction leading to fetal or neonatal death: A prospective study. *Obstetrics & Gynecology*, 50, 583.

Naeye, R.L. & Peters, E.C. 1987. Antenatal hypoxia and low IQ values. *American Journal of Diseases of Children*, 141, 50.

Nagpal, R.D. 1992. Craniopharyngioma: Treatment by conservative surgery and radiation therapy. *Journal of Postgraduate Medicine*, 38, 175.

Nahmias, A.J., Visintine, A.M. & Starr, S.E. 1976. Viral infections of the fetus and newborn. In W.L. Drew (Ed.), *Viral Infections, A Clinical Approach*. Philadelphia: F.A. Davis.

Nakstad, P., Nornes, H. & Hauge, H.N. 1986. Traumatic aneurysm of the pericallosal arteries. *Neuroradiology*, 28, 335.

Nash, J. 1978. *Developmental Psychology: A Psychobiological Approach.* Englewood Cliffs, NJ: Prentice-Hall.

Nass, R., Baker, S., Speiser, P., Virdis, R., Balsamo, A., Cacciari, E., Loche, A., Dumic, M. & New, M. 1987. Hormones and handedness: Left-handed bias in female congenital adrenal hyperplasia patients. *Neurology, 37,* 711.

Nass, R., Peterson, H.D. & Koch, D. 1989. Differential effects of congenital left and right brain injury on intelligence. *Brain and Cognition, 9,* 258.

Natelson, S. & Sayers, M. 1973. The fate of children sustaining severe head trauma during birth. *Pediatrics,* 51(2), 169.

National Institutes of Health. 1981. *Cesearean Childbirth.* Bethesda, MD: NIH.

National Institute of Neurological and Communicative Disorders and Stroke. 1979. *Technical Document of the Panel on Developmental Neurological Disorders to the National Advisory Neurological and Communicative Disorders and Stroke Council.* Bethesda: US Department of Health and Human Services.

National Joint Committee for Learning Disabilities. 1987. Perspectives on Dyslexia. *Journal of Learning Disabilities, 20,* 107.

Needleman, H. (Ed.) 1980. *Low Level Lead Exposure: The Clinical Implications of Current Research.* New York: Raven Press.

Needleman, H.L., Davidson, I., Sewell, E.M. & Shapiro, I.M. 1974. Subclinical lead exposure in Philadelphia schoolchildren. *New England Journal of Medicine, 290,* 245.

Nelhaus, G. 1968. Head circumference from birth to eighteen years. *Pediatrics,* 41(1), 106.

Neligan, G.A., Kolvin, I., Scott, D.M. & Garside, R.F. 1976. Born too soon or born too small: A follow-up study to seven years of age. *Clinics in Developmental Medicine,* 61.

Nelson, H.E. & Warrington, E.K. 1976. Developmental spelling retardation. In R.M. Knights and D.J. Bakker (Eds.), *The Neuropsychology of Learning Disorders.* Baltimore: University Park Press.

Nelson, K. & Ellenberg, J.H. 1978. Prognosis in children with febrile seizures. *Pediatrics,* 61, 720.

Nelson, K. & Ellenberg, J.H. 1979. Neonatal signs as predictors of cerebral palsy. *Pediatrics,* 64(2), 225.

Nelson, K. & Ellenberg, J. 1981. Apgar scores as predictors of chronic neurologic disability. *Pediatrics,* 68(1), 36.

Nelson, K.B. & Ellenberg, J.H. 1986. Antecedents of cerebral palsy: Multivariate analysis of risk. *New England Journal of Medicine, 315,* 81.

Nelson, K.B. & Leviton, A. 1991. How much of neonatal encephalopathy is due to birth asphyxia? *American Journal of Diseases of Children, 145,* 1325.

Nesselroade, J.R. & Reese, H.W. 1973. *Life-Span Developmental Psychology: Methodological Issues.* New York: Academic Press.

Netley, C. 1972. Dichotic listening performance of hemispherectomized patients. *Neuropsychologia, 10,* 233.

Netley, C. 1976. Dichotic listening of callosal agenesis and Turner's syndrome patients. In S.J. Segalowicz, & F.A. Gruber (Eds.), *Language Development and Neurological Theory.* New York: Academic Press.

Netley, C. & Rovet, J. 1982. Atypical hemispheric lateralization in Turner syndrome subjects. *Cortex, 18,* 377.

Netley, C. & Rovet, J. 1987. Relations between a dermatoglyphic measure, hemispheric specialization, and intellectual abilities in 47, XXY males. *Brain and Cognition,* 6, 153.

Netley, C. & Rovet, J. 1988. The development of cognition and personality in X aneuploids and other subject groups. In D.L. Molfese and S.J. Segalowitz (Eds.), *Brain Lateralization in Children.* New York: Guilford Press. p. 401.

Neuhauser, G., Koch, G. & Schwanitz, G. 1981. Mikrozephalien. *Zeitschrift für die allgemeine Medizin,* 57, 1211.

Newberger, C., Newberger, E. & Harper, G. 1976. The social ecology of malnutrition in childhood. In J. Lloyd-Still (Ed.), *Malnutrition and Intellectual Development.* Lancaster, England: MTP Press.

Newborg, J., Stock, J.R., Wnek, L., Guidubaldi, J. & Svinicki, J. 1984. *Battelle Developmental Inventory.* Allen, TX: DLM Teaching Resources.

Newby, R.F. & Lyon, G.R. 1991. Neuropsychological subtypes of learning disabilities. In J.E. Obrzut & G.W. Hynd (Eds.), *Neuropsychological Foundations of Learning Disabilities.* San Diego: Academic Press, p. 355.

Newman, G.C., Buschi, A.I., Sugg, N.K., Kelly, T.E. & Miller, J.Q. 1982. Dandy-Walker syndrome diagnosed in utero by ultrasonography. *Neurology,* 32, 180.

Nichols, P. & Chen, T. 1981. *Minimal Brain Dysfunction. A Prospective Study.* Hillsdale, NJ: Erlbaum.

Nichols, P.L. 1987. Minimal brain dysfunction and soft signs: The collaborative perinatal project. In D.E. Tupper (Ed.), *Soft Neurological Signs.* Orlando: Grune & Stratton, p. 179.

Niebergall, G., Remschmidt, H. & Lingelbach, B. 1976. Neuropsychologische Untersuchungen zur Rückbildung traumatisch verursachter Aphasien. *Zeitschrift für klinische Psychologie,* 5, 194.

Niedt, G.W. & Schinella, R.A. 1985. Acquired immunodeficiency syndrome: Clinicopathological study of 56 autopsies. *Archives of Pathology and Laboratory Medicine,* 109, 727.

Nielsen, H.H. 1980. A longitudinal study of the psychological aspects of myelomeningocele. *Scandinavian Journal of Psychology,* 21, 45.

Nielsen, J. & Sillesen, I. 1981. Turner's syndrome in 115 Danish girls born between 1955 and 1966. *Acta Jutlandica,* 54, Medicine Series 22.

Niemann, H., Boenick, H.E., Schmidt, R.C. & Ettlinger, G. 1985. Cognitive development in epilepsy; The relative influence of epileptic activity and of brain damage. *European Archives of Psychiatry and Neurology,* 234, 399.

Nissen, G. 1982. Depressionen im Kinder und Jugendalter. *Triangel,* 21, 77.

Nissen, G. 1986. *Psychische Störungen im Kindes- und Jugendalter,* 2nd ed. Berlin: Springer.

Niswander, K.R. & Gordon, M. 1972. *The Women and Their Pregnancies: The Collaborative Perinatal Study of the National Institute of Neurologic Diseases and Stroke.* Baltimore: W.B. Saunders.

Niswander, K.R., Gordon, M. & Drage, J. 1975. The effect of intrauterine hypoxia on the child surviving to four years. *American Journal of Obstetrics and Gynecology,* 121, 892.

Njiokiktjien, C. 1988–93. *Pediatric Behavioural Neurology,* Vols. 1–4. Amsterdam: Suyi Publications.

Nobach, C.R. & Demarest, R.J. 1981. *The Human Nervous System,* 3rd ed., New York: McGraw-Hill.

Noetzel, M.J. & Blake, J.N. 1991. Prognosis for seizure control and remission in children with myelomeningocele. *Developmental Medicine and Child Neurology,* 33, 803.

Norden, K. 1981. Learning processes and personality development in deaf children. *American Annals of the Deaf,* 126, 4.

Nordgren, R.E., Reeves, A.G., Viguera, A.C. & Roberts, D.W. 1991. Corpus callosotomy for intractable seizures in the pediatric age group. *Archives of Neurology,* 48, 364.

Norman, M.G. 1976. Perinatal brain damage. *Perspectives in Pediatric Pathology,* 4, 41.

Northern, J.L. & Downs, M.P. 1988. *Hearing in Children,* 3rd ed. Baltimore: University Park Press.

Notter, R.H. & Shapiro, D.L. 1981. Lung surfactant in an era of replacement therapy. *Pediatrics,* 68(6), 781.

Novick, B.Z. & Arnold, M.M. 1988. *Fundamentals of Clinical Child Neuropsychology.* Philadelphia: Grune & Stratton.

Nowakovski, R.S. 1987. Basic concepts of CNS development. *Child Development,* 58, 568.

Nuechterlein, K.H. 1986. Childhood precursors of adult schizophrenia. *Journal of Child Psychology and Psychiatry and Allied Disciplines,* 27, 133.

Nussbaum, N.L., Bigler, E.D. & Koch, W. 1986. Neuropsychologically derived subgroups of learning disabled children: Personality/behavioral dimensions. *Journal of Research and Development in Education,* 19, 420.

Nussbaum, N.L., Grant, M.L., Roman, M.J., Poole, J.H. & Bigler, E.D. 1990. Attention deficit disorder and the mediating effect of age on academic and behavioral variables. *Developmental and Behavioral Pediatrics,* 11, 22.

Nyborg, H. & Nielsen, J. 1977. Sex chromosome abnormalities and cognitive performance: III. Field dependence, frame dependence, and failing development of perceptual stability in girls with Turner's syndrome. *Journal of Psychology,* 96, 205.

Oades, R.D., Stern, L.M., Walker, M.K. & Clark, C.R. 1990. Event-related potentials and monoamines in autistic children on a clinical trial of fenfluramine. *International Journal of Psychophysiology,* 8, 197.

Oberklaid, F., Prior, M. & Sanson, A. 1986. Temperament of preterm versus full-term infants. *Developmental and Behavioral Pediatrics* 7, 159.

Obrador, S. 1964. Nervous integration after hemispherectomy in man. In G. Schaltenbrand & C.N. Woolsey (Eds.), *Cerebral Localization and Organization.* Madison: University of Wisconsin Press.

Obrzut, J.E. & Hynd, G.W. 1986. *Child Neuropsychology,* Vols. 1 and 2. Orlando, FL: Academic Press.

Obrzut, J.E. Ouvrier, R. & Billson, F. 1986. Optic nerve hypoplasia: A review. *Journal of Child Neurology,* 1, 181.

O'Connor, N. & Hermelin, B. 1962. Visual and stereognostic shape recognition in normal children and mongol, and non-mongol imbeciles. *Journal of Mental Deficiency Research,* 6, 63.

O'Connor, N. & Hermelin, B. 1973. Short-term memory for the order of pictures and syllables by deaf and hearing children. *Neuropsychologia,* 11, 437.

Office of Population Censuses and Surveys. 1974. *Morbidity Statistics from General Practice. Studies on Medical and Population Subjects, No. 26,* London: H. M. Stationery Office.

Offord, D.R., Boyle, M.H. & Racine, Y.A. 1991. The epidemiology of antisocial behavior in childhood and adolescence. In D.J. Pepler & K.H. Rubin (Eds.), *The Development and Treatment of Childhood Aggression*. Hillsdale, NJ: Erlbaum, p. 31.

Offord, D.R., Boyle, M.H. & Szatmari, P. 1987. Ontario child health study: II. Six-month prevalence of disorder and rates of service utilization. *Archives of General Psychiatry*, 44, 832.

Offord, D.R., Sullivan, K., Allen, N. & Abrams, N. 1979. Delinquency and hyperactivity. *Journal of Nervous and Mental Disease*, 167, 734.

Ogden, J.A. 1988a. Language and memory functions after long recovery periods in left-hemispherectomized subjects. *Neuropsychologia*, 26, 645.

Ogden, J.A. 1988b. Visuospatial and other 'right-hemisphere' functions after long recovery periods in left-hemispherectomized subjects. *Neuropsychologia*, 26, 765.

Oguni, H., Olivier, A., Anderman, F. & Comair, J. 1991. Anterior callosotomy in the treatment of medically intractable epilepsies: A study of 43 patients with a mean follow-up of 39 months. *Annals of Neurology*, 30, 357.

Ogunmekan, A.D., Hwang, P.A. & Hoffman, H.J. 1989. Sturge-Weber-Dimitri disease: Role of hemispherectomy in prognosis. *Canadian Journal of Neurological Sciences*, 16, 78.

O'Hara, P.T. 1972. Electron microscopic study of the brain in Down's syndrome. *Brain*, 95, 681.

Ohlrich, E.S., Barnet, A.B., Weiss, I.P. & Shanks, B.I. 1978. Auditory evoked potential development in childhood: A longitudinal study. *Electroencephalography and Clinical Neurophysiology*, 44, 411.

Ohtahara, S., Yamatogi, Y., Ohtoska, Y., Oka, E. & Ishida, T. 1980. Prognosis of West syndrome with special reference to Lennox syndrome: A developmental study. In J.A. Wada and J.K. Penry (Eds.), *Advances in Epileptology: 10th Epilepsy International Symposium*. New York: Raven Press.

Oksche, A., Rodrigues, E.M. & Fernandez-Llebrez, P. (Eds.) 1993. *The Subcommisural Organ*. New York: Springer.

O'Leary, D.S., Lovell, M.R., Sackellares, J.C., Berent, S., Giordani, B., Seidenberg, M. & Boll, T.J. 1983. Effects of age of onset of partial and generalized seizures on neuropsychological performance in children. *Journal of Nervous and Mental Disease*, 171, 624.

O'Leary, D.D. & Stanfield, B.B. 1985. Cortical neurons with transient pyramidal axons extend and maintain collateral contact with intercortical but not intracortical targets. *Brain Research*, 336, 326.

Oliver, C. & Holland, A.J. 1987. Down's syndrome and Alzheimer's disease: A review. *Psychological Medicine*, 16, 2, 307.

Olton, D.S. & Shapiro, M.L. 1990. Electrophysiological correlates of recovery of function. *Acta Neurobiologiae Experimentalis*, 50, 125.

Omenn, G.S. & Weber, B.A. 1978. Dyslexia: Search for phenotypic and genetic heterogrenity. *American Journal of Medical Genetics*, 1, 333.

O'Neal, P. & Robins, L.N. 1958. Childhood patterns predictive of adult schizophrenia: A 30-year follow-up study. *American Journal of Psychiatry*, 115, 385.

O'Neill, J.F. 1980. The visually impaired child: Introduction. *Pediatric Annals*, 9(11), 412.

Oppenheim, R.W. 1981. Neuronal cell death and some related regressive phenomena during neurogenesis: A selective historical review and progress report. In W.M. Cowen (Ed.), *Studies in Developmental Neurobiology*, New York: Oxford University Press.

Orgill, A.A., Astbury, J., Bajuk, B. & Yu, V.Y.H. 1982. Early neurodevelopmental outcome of very low birthweight infants. *Australian Pediatric Journal* 18, 193.

Orlansky, H. 1949. Infant care and personality. *Psychological Bulletin*, 46, 1.

Ornitz, E.M. 1973. Childhood autism. A review of the clinical and experimental literature (Medical Progress). *California Medicine*, 118, 21.

Ornitz, E.M. 1978. Biological homogeneity or heterogeneity? In M. Rutter and E. Schopler (Eds.), *Autism: A Reappraisal of Concepts and Treatment*. New York: Plenum Press.

Ornitz, E.M., Atwell, C.W., Kaplan, A.R. & Westlake, J.R. 1985. Brain-stem dysfunction in autism: Results of vestibular stimulation. *Archives of General Psychiatry*, 42, 1018.

Orton, S. 1925. Word-blindness in school children. *Archives of Neurology and Psychiatry*, 14, 582.

Orton, S. 1937. *Reading, Writing and Speech Problems in Children*. New York: W.W. Norton.

Osborn, A.G. 1994. *Diagnostic Neuroradiology*. St. Louis: Mosby.

Ostfeld, B.M. & Gibbs, E. 1990. Use of family assessment in early intervention. In E.D. Gibbs & D.M. Teti (Eds.), *Interdisciplinary Assessment of Infants. A Guide for Early Intervention Professionals*. Baltimore: Paul H. Brookes, p. 249.

Ott, J. 1974. The eyes' dual function: Part II. *Eye, Ear, Nose & Throat Monthly*, 53, 377.

Ounsted, C. & Taylor, D. 1972. The Y-chromosome message: A point of view. In C. Ounsted & D. Taylor (Eds.), *Gender Differences: Their Ontogeny and Significance*. Edinburgh: Churchill Livingstone.

Ouvrier, R. & Billson, F. 1986. Optic nerve hypoplasia: A review. *Journal of Child Neurology*, 1, 181.

Overholser, J.C. 1990. Fetal alcohol syndrome: A review of the disorder. *Journal of Contemporary Psychotherapy*, 20, 163.

Overmann, S.R. 1977. Behavioral effects of asymptomatic lead exposure during neonatal development in rats. *Toxicology and Applied Pharmacology*, 41, 459.

Owen, D.R. 1972. The 47, xyy male: A review. *Psychological Bulletin*, 78, 209.

Owens, D., Dawson, J.C. & Losin, S. 1971. Alzheimer's disease in Down's syndrome. *American Journal of Mental Deficiency*, 75, 606.

Oxorn, H. 1980. *Human Labor and Birth*, 4th ed. New York: Appleton-Century-Crofts.

Ozanne, A.E., Krimmer, H. & Murdoch, B.E. 1990. Speech and language skills in children with early treated phenylketonuria. *American Journal on Mental Retardation*, 94, 625.

Page-El, E. & Grossman, H.J. 1973. Neurologic appraisal in learning disorders. *Pediatric Clinics of North America*, 20, 599.

Paine, R.S. 1968. Syndromes of minimal cerebral damage. *Pediatric Clinics of North America*, 15, 779.

Paine, R.S., Werry, J.S. & Quay, H.C. 1968. A study of minimal cerebral dysfunction. *Developmental Medicine and Child Neurology*, 10, 505.

Palkes, H. & Stewart, M. 1972. Intellectual ability and performance of hyperactive children. *American Journal of Orthopsychiatry*, 42, 35.

Palmer, P., Dubowitz, L.M.S., Levene, M.I. & Dubowitz, V. 1982. Developmental and neurological progress of preterm infants with intraventricular hemorrhage and ventricular dilation. *Archives of Disease in Childhood*, 57, 748.

Palmisano, P.A., Sneed, R.C. & Cassady, G. 1969. Untaxed whiskey and fetal lead exposure. *Journal of Pediatrics*, 75, 869.

Palo, J. & Kivalo, A. 1980. Calendar calculator with progressive mental deficiency. *Acta Paedopsychiatrica*, 42, 227.

Paneth, N. 1993. The causes of cerebral palsy: Recent evidence. *Clinical Investigative Medicine*, 16, 95.

Paneth, N., Bommarito, M. & Stricker, J. 1992. Electronic fetal monitoring and later outcome. In *Current Concepts: Intrapartum Fetal Surveillance*. Second International Symposium on Perinatal Asphyxia. Vancouver: Canadian Medical Protective Association.

Pansky, B. & Allen, D.J. 1980. *Review of Neuroscience*. New York: MacMillan Publishing Co.

Papanicolaou, A.C., DiScenna, A., Gillespie, L. & Aram, D. 1990. Probe-evoked potential findings following unilateral left-hemisphere lesions in children. *Archives of Neurology*, 47, 562.

Papile, L.A., Munsick-Bruno G. & Schaefer A. 1983. Relationship of cerebral intraventricular hemorrhage and early childhood neurologic handicaps. *Journal of Pediatrics* 103, 273.

Park, T.S., Hoffman, H.J., Hendrick, E.B., Humphreys, R.P. & Becker, L.E. 1983. Medulloblastoma: Clinical presentation and management, experience at the Hospital for Sick Children, Toronto, 1950–1980. *Journal of Neurosurgery*, 58, 543.

Parker, R.S. 1990. *Traumatic Brain Injury and Neuropsychological Impairment*. New York: Springer.

Parkinson, C.E., Wallis, S. & Harvey, D. 1981. School achievement and behaviour of children who were small-for-dates at birth. *Developmental Medicine and Child Neurology*, 23, 41.

Parmelee, A.H., 1974. *Newborn neurological examination*. Unpublished manuscript, August 1974.

Parmelee, A.H., Jr. 1981. Auditory function and neurological maturation in preterm infants. In S.L. Friedman and M. Sigman (Eds.), *Preterm Birth and Psychological Development*. New York: Academic Press.

Parmelee, A.H. & Michaelis, R. 1971. Neurological examination of the newborn. In J. Hellmuth (Ed.), *Exceptional Infant, Vol. 2: Studies in Abnormalities*. London: Butterworth, 3.

Parmelee, A.H. & Schulte, F.J. 1970. Developmental testing of preterm and small for date infants. *Pediatrics*, 45, 21.

Parmelee, A.H., Michaelis, R., Kopp, C.B. & Sigman, M.D. 1976. Selection of developmental assessment techniques for infants at risk. *Merrill-Palmer Quarterly of Development and Behavior*, 22, 177.

Pasamanick, B. & Knobloch, H. 1960. Brain damage and reproductive casualty. *American Journal of Orthopsychiatry*, 30, 298.

Pass, R.F., Stagno, S., Myers, G.J. & Alford, C.A. 1980. Outcome of symptomatic congenital cytomegalovirus infection: Results of long-term longitudinal follow-up. *Pediatrics*, 66, 758.

Passler, M.A., Isaac, W. & Hynd, G.W. 1985. Neuropsychological development of behavior attributed to frontal lobe functioning in children. *Developmental Neuropsychology*, 1, 349.

Patterson, D. 1987. The causes of Down syndrome. *Scientific American*, 257 (2), 52.

Paul, R.H. 1992. The relationship between fetal heart rate patterns and asphyxia in the human fetus. In *Proceedings of the Second International Symposium on Perinatal Asphyxia*. Vancouver: Canadian Medical Protective Association.

Paul, R. & Cohen, D.J. 1982. Communication development and its disorders: A psycholinguistic perspective. *Schizophrenia Bulletin*, 8, 279.

Paulhus, D.L. & Martin, C.L. 1986. Predicting adult temperament from minor physical anomalies. *Journal of Personality and Social Psychology*, 50, 1235.

Paulsen, K. & O'Donnell, J.P. 1979. Construct validation of children's behavior problem dimension: Relationship to activity level, impulsivity, and soft neurological signs. *Journal of Psychology*, 101, 273.

Paulsen, K.A. & O'Donnell, J.P. 1980. The relationship between minor physical anomalies and "soft signs" of brain damage. *Perceptual and Motor Skills*, 51, 402.

Pease, D.C. (Ed.) 1971. *Cellular Aspects of Neural Growth and Differentiation* (UCLA Forum in Medical Sciences No. 14). Los Angeles: University of California Press.

PeBenito, R. 1987. Developmental Gerstmann syndrome: Case report and review of the literature. *Developmental and Behavioral Pediatrics*, 8, 229.

PeBenito, R. & Cracco, J.B. 1988. Congenital ocular motor apraxia. Case reports and literature review. *Clinica Pediatrica Philadelphia*, 27, 27.

PeBenito, R., Fisch, C.B. & Fisch, M.L. 1988. Developmental Gerstmann syndrome. *Archives of Neurology*, 45, 977.

Peele, T.L. 1954. *The Neuroanatomical Basis for Clinical Neurology*. New York: McGraw-Hill.

Peiper, A. 1963. *Cerebral Function of Infancy and Childhood*. New York: Consultant Bureau.

Pelham, W.E. 1986. The effects of psychostimulant drugs on learning and academic achievement in children with attention-deficit disorders and learning disabilities. In J. Torgesen & B. Wong (Eds.), *Psychological and Educational Perspectives on Learning Disabilities*. New York: Academic Press, p. 259.

Pennington, B. 1991. *Diagnosing Learning Disorders*. New York: Guilford.

Pennington, B.F. & Smith, S.D. 1983. Genetic influences on learning disabilities and speech and language disorders. *Child Development*, 54, 369.

Pennington, B.F., Heaton, R.K., Karzmark, P., Pendleton, M.G., Lehman, R. & Shucard, D.W. 1985. The neuropsychological phenotype in Turner syndrome. *Cortex*, 21, 391.

Pennington, B.F., Van Doorninck, W.J., McCabe, L.L. & McCabe, E.R. 1987. Neuropsychological deficits in early treated phenylketonuric children. *American Journal of Mental Deficiency*, 89, 467.

Penrose, L.S. 1963. *The Biology of Mental Defect*, 2nd ed. London: Sidgwick & Jackson.

Peters, J.E., Romine, J.S. & Dykman, R.A. 1975. A special neurological examination of children with learning disabilities. *Developmental Medicine and Child Neurology*, 17, 63.

Peters, M. 1988. The size of the corpus callosum in males and females: Implications of a lack of allometry. *Canadian Journal of Psychology*, 42, 313.

Petersen, A.C. 1981. Sex differences in performance on spatial tasks: Biopsychosocial influences. In A. Ansara, N. Geschwind, A. Galaburda, M. Albert & N. Gartrell (Eds.), *Sex Differences in Dyslexia*. Towson, MD: The Orton Dyslexia Society.

Petit, T.L., Alfano, D.P. & LeBoutellier, J.C. 1983. Early lead exposure and the hippocampus: A review and recent advances. *NeuroToxicology*, 4, 79.

Pfefferbaum, A., Lim, K., Rosenbloom, M. & Zipursky, R.B. 1990. Brain magnetic resonance imaging: Approaches for investigating schizophrenia. *Schizophrenia Bulletin,* 16, 452.

Pfenninger, K.H. 1986. Of nerve growth cones, leukocytes and memory: Second messenger systems and growth-regulated proteins. *Trends in Neuroscience,* 9, 562.

Phibbs, R.H., Harvin, D., Jones, G., Talbot, C. Cohen, M., Crowther, D. & Tolley, W.H. 1971. Development of children who had received intrauterine transfusions. *Pediatrics,* 47, 689.

Phillips, C.J. 1968. The Illinois Test of Psycholinguistic Abilities: A report on its use with English children and a comment on the psychological sequelae of low-birth-weight. *British Journal of Disorders of Communication,* 3, 143.

Phillips, D., McCartney, K., Scarr, S. & Howes, C. 1987. Selective review of infant day care research: A cause for concern! *Zero to Three,* 7(2), 187.

Piacentini, J.C. & Hynd, G.W. 1988. Language after dominant hemispherectomy: Are plasticity of function and equipotentiality viable concepts? *Clinical Psychology Review,* 8, 595.

Piaget, J. 1952. *The Origins of Intelligence in Children.* New York: International Universities Press.

Piaget, J. 1960. *Psychology of Intelligence.* Patterson, NJ: Littlefield Adams.

Piccinin, B. & Ansseau, M. 1991. Interest du sommeil et des tests neuroendocriniens en tant que marqueurs biologiques de la depression chez l'enfant et l'adolescents. *Encephale,* 17, 457.

Pinneau, S.R. 1955. Reply to Dr. Spitz. *Psychological Bulletin,* 52, 459.

Piper, M.C., Kunos, I., Willis, D.M., Mazer, B. 1985. Effects of gestational age on neurological functioning of the very low-birth weight infant at 40 weeks. *Developmental Medicine and Child Neurology,* 27, 596.

Pirozzolo, F. 1979. *The Neuropsychology of Developmental Reading Disorders.* New York: Praeger.

Pirozzolo, F.J., Pirozzolo, P.H. & Ziman, R.B. 1979. Neuropsychological assessment of callosal agenesis: Report of a case with normal intelligence and absence of the disconnection syndrome. *Clinical Neuropsychology,* 1(1), 13.

Pisoni, D.B. 1977. Identification and discrimination of the relative onset of two component tones: Implication for the perception of voicing in stops. *Journal of the Acoustical Society of America,* 61, 1352.

Piven, J., Berthier, M.L., Starkstein, S.E. & Nehme, E. 1991. Magnetic resonance imaging evidence for a defect of cerebral cortical development in autism. *Annual Progress in Child Psychiatry and Child Development,* 455.

Pizzo, P.A. & Poplack, D.G. (Eds.) 1993. *Principles and Practice of Pediatric Oncology,* 2nd ed. Philadelphia: J.B. Lippincott.

Pizzo, P.A. & Wilfert, C.M. (Eds.) 1992. *Pediatric AIDS: The Challenge of HIV Infection in Infants.* Baltimore: Williams & Wilkins.

Placek, P. 1977. Maternal and infant health factors associated with low infant birth weight: Findings from the 1972 National Natality Survey. In D. Reed and F. Stanley (Eds.), *The Epidemiology of Prematurity.* Baltimore: Urban and Schwarzenberg.

Plante, E. 1991. MRI findings in the parents and siblings of specifically language-impaired boys. *Brain and Language,* 41, 67.

Plante, E., Swisher, L., Vance, R. & Rapcsak, S. 1991. MRI findings in boys with specific language impairment. *Brain and Language,* 41, 52.

Pliszka, S.R. 1989. Effect of anxiety on cognition, behavior, and stimulant response in ADHD. *Journal of the American Academy of Child and Adolescent Psychiatry*, 28, 882.

Plomin, R., DeFries, J.C. & McClearn, G.E. 1980. *Behavioral Genetics: A Primer.* San Francisco: W.H. Freeman and Co.

Poeck, K. 1974. *Neurologie, ein Lehrbuch für Studierende und Ärzte,* 3rd. ed. Heidelberg: Springer.

Pogue-Geile, M.F. & Zubin, J. 1988. Negative symptomatology and schizophrenia: A conceptual and empirical review. *International Journal of Mental Health*, 16, 3.

Pollitt, E. & Thompson, C. 1977. Protein-caloric malnutrition and behavior: A view from psychology. In R. Wurtman & J. Wurtman (Eds.), *Nutrition and the Brain,* vol. 2. New York: Raven Press.

Poppelreuter, W. 1990. *Disturbance of Lower and Higher Visual Capacities by Occipital Damage* (Original German 1917). Translated by J. Zihl. Oxford: Clarendon Press.

Porac, C. & Coren, S. 1978. Sighting dominance and binocular rivalry. *American Journal of Optometry*, 55(3), 208.

Porac, C. & Coren, S. 1981. *Lateral Preference and Human Behavior.* New York: Springer.

Posner, M.I. & Peterson, S.E. 1988. The attention system of the human brain. *Annual Review of Neuroscience*, 345.

Posner, M.I. & Rafal, R.D. 1987. Cognitive theories of attention and the rehabilitation of attentional deficits. In M.J. Meier, A.L. Benton & L. Diller (Eds.), *Neuropsychological Rehabilitation.* New York: Guilford Press.

Pratap, R.C. & Gururaj, A.K. 1989. Clinical and electroencephalographic features of complex partial seizures in infants. *Acta Neurologica Scandinavica*, 79, 123.

Prechtl, H.F.R. 1967. Neurological sequelae of prenatal and perinatal complications. *British Medical Journal*, 4, 763.

Prechtl, H.F.R. 1968. Neurological findings in newborn infants after pre- and perinatal complications. In J.H.P. Jonxis, H.D. Vissez, & J.A. Troelsttra (Eds.), *Dysmaturity and Prematurity.* Leiden: Drocse.

Prechtl, H.F.R. 1977. *The Neurological Examination of the Full-Term Infant,* 2nd ed. Clinics in Developmental Medicine, No. 63. London: Heinemann.

Prechtl, H.F.R. 1978. Minimal brain dysfunction syndrome and the plasticity of the nervous system. *Advances in Biological Psychiatry*, 1, 96.

Prechtl, H.F.R. 1979. Postures, motility, and respiration of low risk, preterm infants. *Developmental Medicine and Child Neurology*, 21, 1.

Prechtl, H.F.R. 1982. Assessment methods for the newborn infant, a critical evaluation. In P. Stratton (Ed.), *Psychobiology of the Human Newborn.* New York: Wiley, p. 21.

Prechtl, H.F.R. 1984. Continuity and change in early neural development. In H.F.R. Prechtl (Ed.), *Continuity of Neural Functions from Prenatal to Postnatal Life.* Clinics in Developmental Medicine, No. 94, Philadelphia: J.B. Lippincott, p. 1.

Prechtl, H.F.R. & Beintema, D. 1964. *The Neurological Examination of the Full-Term Newborn Infant.* Little Club Clinics in Developmental Medicine, No. 12. London: Spastics Society.

Prechtl, H.F.R. & O'Brien, M.J. 1982. Behavioral states of the full-term newborn. The emergence of a concept. In P. Stratton (Ed.), *Psychobiology of the Human Newborn,* New York: Wiley, p. 53.

Prechtl, H.F.R. & Stemmer, C.J. 1962. The choreiform syndrome in children. *Developmental Medicine and Child Neurology*, 4, 119.

Pribram, K.H. 1963. The new neurology: memory, novelty, thought and choice. In G.H. Glazer (Ed.), *E.E.G. and Behavior.* New York: Basic Books, p. 149.

Pribram, K.H. & Luria, A.R. 1973. *Psychophysiology of the Frontal Lobes.* New York: Academic Press.

Prior, M.R. 1987. Biological and neuropsychological approaches to childhood autism. *British Journal of Psychiatry*, 150, 8.

Prior, M. & Hoffman, W. 1990. Brief report: Neuropsychological testing of autistics through an exploration with frontal lobe tests. *Journal of Autism and Developmental Disorders*, 20, 581.

Ptito, A., Lassonde, M., Lepore, F. & Ptito, M. 1987. Visual discrimination in hemispherectomized patients. *Neuropsychologia*, 25, 869.

Pugh, M. & Bigler, E.D. 1986. Schizophrenia and prior history of "MDB": Neuropsychological findings. *International Journal of Clinical Neuropsychology*, 8, 22.

Purpura, D.P. 1975. Normal and aberrant neuronal development in the cerebral cortex of human fetus and young infant. In N.A. Buchwald & M.A.B. Brazier (Eds.), *Brain Mechanisms in Mental Retardation.* New York: Academic Press.

Purpura, D.P. 1977. Developmental pathobiology of cortical neurons in immature human brain. In L. Gluck (Ed.), *Intrauterine Asphyxia and the Developing Fetal Brain.* Chicago: Year Book Medical Publishers.

Purves, D. & Lichtman, J. 1980. Elimination of synapses in the developing nervous system. *Science*, 210, 153.

Quadfasel, F.A. & Goodglass, H. 1968. Specific reading disability and other specific disabilities. *Journal of Learning Disabilities*, 1, 590.

Quinn, K. & Geffen, G. 1986. The development of tactile transfer of information. *Neuropsychologia*, 24, 793.

Quinn, P. & Rapoport, J. 1974. Minor physical anomalies and neurologic status in hyperactive boys. *Pediatrics*, 53, 742.

Quitkin, F., Rifkin, A. & Klein, D.F. 1976. Neurological soft signs in schizophrenia and character disorders. *Archives of General Psychiatry*, 33, 845.

Rabinowicz, T. 1979. The differential maturation of the human cerebral cortex. In F. Falkner & J.M. Tanner (Eds.), *Human Growth, Vol. 3: Neurobiology and Nutrition.* New York: Plenum Press.

Rabinowicz, T., Leuba, G. & Heumann, D. 1977. Morphologic maturation of the brain: a quantitative study. In S.R. Berenberg (Ed.), *Brain—Fetal and Infant.* The Hague: Martinus Nijhoff.

Ragni, M.V., Urbach, A.H. & Taylor, S. 1987. Isolation of human immunodeficiency virus and detection deficiency syndrome and progressive encephalopathy. *Journal of Pediatrics*, 110, 892.

Raimondi, A.J., Choux, M. & DiRocco, C. (Eds.) 1992. *Cerebrovascular Diseases in Children.* New York: Springer-Verlag.

Raimondi, A.J. & Tomita, T. 1979. The disadvantages of prophylactic whole CNS postoperative radiation therapy for medulloblastoma. In P. Paoletti, G. Walker & R. Knerich (Eds.), *Multidisciplinary Aspects of Brain Tumor Therapy.* Amsterdam: Elsevier/North Holland Biomedical Press.

Rakic, P. 1972. Migrating cells and radial fibers in the developing cerebral cortex of the rhesus monkey. *Journal of Comparative Neurology*, 145, 61.

Rakic, P. 1975. Cell migration and neuronal ectopias in the brain. *Birth Defects: Original Article Series,* 11(7), 95.

Rakic, P. 1979a. Genesis of visual connections in the rhesus monkey. In R.D. Freeman (Ed.), *Developmental Neurobiology of Vision.* New York: Plenum.

Rakic, P. 1979b. Genetic and epigenetic determinants of local neuronal circuits in the mammalian central nervous system. In F.O. Schmitt & F.G. Worden (Eds.), *The Neurosciences: Fourth Study Program.* Cambridge, MA: MIT Press.

Rakic, P. 1981. Developmental events leading to laminar and areal organization of the neocortex. In F.O. Schmitt, F.G. Worden, G. Adelman & S.G. Dennis (Eds.), *The Organization of the Cerebral Cortex.* Cambridge, MA: MIT Press.

Rakic, P. 1984. Defective cell-to-cell interactions as causes of brain malformations. In E.S. Golin (Ed.), *Malformations of Development—Biological and Psychological Sources and Consequences.* New York: Academic Press, p. 239.

Rakic, P. & Goldman-Rakic, P.S. (Eds.) 1982. Development and modifiability of the cerebral cortex. *Neurosciences Research Program Bulletin,* 20, No. 4.

Rakic, P., Bourgeois, J.P., Zecevic, N., Eckenhoff, M.F. & Goldman-Rakic, P.S. 1986. Isochronic overproduction of synapses in diverse regions of the primate cerebral cortex. *Science,* 232, 232.

Ramsay, D.S. 1985. Fluctuations in unimanual hand preference in infants following onset of duplicated syllable babbling. *Developmental Psychology,* 21, 325.

Rankin, J.M., Aram, D.M. & Horwitz, S.J. 1984. Language ability and right and left hemiplegic children. *Brain and Language,* 14, 292.

Rao, J.M. 1990. A population-based study of mild mental handicap in children. Preliminary analysis of obstetric complications. *Journal of Mental Deficiency Research,* 34, 59.

Rao, S.L., Srinath, S., Aroor, S.R. & Kaliaperumal, V.G. 1992. Neuropsychological deficits in children with epilepsy. *NIMHANS Journal,* 10, 85.

Rapin, I. 1975. Children with hearing impairment. In K.E. Swaiman & F.S. Wright (Eds.), *The Practice of Pediatric Neurology.* St. Louis: C.V. Mosby.

Rapin, I. 1979. Effects of early blindness and deafness on cognition. In R. Katzman (Ed.), *Congenital and Acquired Cognitive Disorders.* New York: Raven Press.

Rapin, I. 1982. *Children with Brain Dysfunction; Neurology, Cognition, Language, and Behavior.* New York: Raven Press.

Rapin, I. & Wilson, B.C. 1978. Children with developmental language disability: Neurological aspects and assessment. In M.A. Wyke (Ed.), *Developmental Dysphasia.* New York: Academic Press.

Rapin, I., Mattis, S., Rowan, A.J. & Golden, G.G. 1977. Verbal auditory agnosia in children. *Developmental Medicine and Child Neurology,* 19(2), 192.

Rapoport, J.L. & Ferguson, H.B. 1981. Biological validation of the hyperkinetic syndrome. *Developmental Medicine and Child Neurology,* 23, 667.

Rapoport, J.L. & Ferguson, H.B. 1982. Biological validation of the hyperkinetic syndrome. *Annual Progress in Child Psychiatry and Child Development,* 569.

Rapoport, J.L. & Quinn, P.O. 1975. Minor physical anomalies (stigmata) and early developmental deviation: A major biologic subgroup of "hyperactive" children. *International Journal of Mental Health,* 4, 29.

Rappaport, L., Urion, D., Strand, K. & Fulton, A.B. 1987. Concurrence of congenital ocular motor apraxia and other motor problems: An expanded syndrome. *Developmental Medicine and Child Neurology,* 29, 85.

Rasmussen, A.M., Riddle, M.A., Leckman, J.F., Anderson, G.M. & Cohen, D.J. 1990. Neurotransmitter assessment in neuropsychiatric disorders of childhood. In S.I. Deutsch, A. Weizman & R. Weizman (Eds.), *Application of Basic Neuroscience to Child Psychiatry.* New York: Plenum, p. 33.

Rasmussen, T. 1983. Hemispherectomy for seizures revisited. *Canadian Journal of Neurological Sciences,* 10, 71.

Ratcliff, G. 1982. Disturbances in visual orientation associated with cerebral lesions. In M. Potegal (Ed.), *Spatial Abilities. Development and Physiological Foundations.* New York: Academic Press, p. 301.

Rawlings, G., Reynolds, E.O.R., Stewart, A.L. & Strang, L.B. 1971. Changing prognosis for infants of very low birthweight. *Lancet,* 1, 516.

Ray, W., Newcombe, N. Semon, J. & Cole, P.M. 1981. Spatial abilities, sex differences and EEG functioning. *Neuropsychologia,* 19(5), 719.

Rayner, K. (Ed.) 1983. *Eye Movements and Reading: Perceptual and Language Processes.* New York: Academic Press.

Raz, S., Raz, N. & Bigler, E. 1988. Ventriculomegaly in schizophrenia: Is the choice of controls important? *Psychiatric Research,* 24, 71.

Raz, S., Raz, N., Weinberger, D.R., Boronow, J., Pickar, D., Bigler, E.D. & Turkheimer, E. 1987. Morphological brain abnormalities in schizophrenia by computed tomography: A problem of measurement? *Psychiatric Research,* 22, 91.

Realmuto, G.M. 1986. Psychiatric diagnosis and behavioral characteristics of phenylketonuric children. *Journal of Nervous and Mental Diseases,* 174, 536.

Rees, N.S. 1973. Auditory processing factors in language disorders: The view from Procrustes' bed. *Journal of Speech and Hearing Disorders,* 38, 304.

Reid, D.T. & Sheffield, B. 1990. A cognitive-developmental analysis of drawing abilities in children with and without meningomyelocele. *Physical and Occupational Therapy in Pediatrics,* 10, 33.

Reigel, D.H. 1982. Spina bifida. In R.L. McLaurin (Ed.), *Pediatric Neurosurgery: Surgery of the Developing Nervous System.* Orlando, FL: Grune & Stratton.

Reinert, G. 1970. Comparative factor analytic studies of intelligence through the human life-span. In L.R. Goulet & P. Baltes (Eds.), *Life-Span Developmental Psychology: Research and Theory.* New York: Academic Press.

Reinert, G., Baltes, P.B. & Schmidt, L.R. 1965. Kritik der Differenzierungshypothese der Intelligenz: Die Leistungsdifferenzierungshypothese. *Psychologische Forschung,* 28, 246.

Reinert, G., Baltes, P.B. & Schmidt, L.R. 1966. Kritik einer Kritik der Differenzierungshypothese der Intelligenz. *Zeitschrift für Experimentelle und Angewandte Psychologie,* 13, 602.

Reinis, S. & Goldman, J.M. 1980. *The Development of the Brain: Biological and Functional Perspectives.* Springfield, IL: Charles C Thomas.

Reinisch, J.M. 1974. Fetal hormones, the brain, and human sex differences: A heuristic, integrative review of the recent literature. *Archives of Sexual Behavior,* 3(1), 51.

Reinisch, J.M., Rosenblum, L.A., Rubin, D.B. & Schulsinger, M.F. 1991a. Sex differences in developmental milestones during the first year of life. *Journal of Psychology and Human Sexuality,* 4, 19.

Reinisch, J.M., Ziemba, D.M. & Sanders, S.A. 1991b. Hormonal contributions to sexually dimorphic behavioral development in humans. *Psychoneuroendrocrinology,* 16, 213.

Reiss, A.L., Aylward, E., Freund, L.S. & Joshi, P.K. 1991. Neuroanatomy of fragile X syndrome: The posterior fossa. *Annals of Neurology,* 29, 26.

Reitan, R.M. 1974. Psychological effects of cerebral lesions in children of early school age. In R.M. Reitan and L.A. Davison (Eds.), *Clinical Neuropsychology: Current Status and Application*. Washington, DC: V.H. Winston & Sons.

Rekate, H.L. 1985. Muteness of cerebellar origin. *Archives of Neurology*, 42, 697.

Remschmidt, H. 1972. Experimentelle Untersuchungen zum Perseverationsverhalten von Epileptikern. *Archiv für Neurologie und Psychiatrie*, 215, 315.

Remschmidt, H. 1981. Neuropsychologische Befunde bei Epilepsien. In H. Remschmidt & M. Schmidt (Eds.), *Neuropsychologie des Kindesalters*. Stuttgart: Enke.

Remschmidt, H., Niebergall, G. & Geyer, M. 1980. Neuropsychologische Untersuchungen zur Rückbildung von Aphasien. In H. Remschmidt & H. Stutte (Eds.), *Neuropsychiatrische Folgen nach Schädel-Hirntrauma bei Kindern und Jugendlichen*. Berne: Huber.

Renwick, J.H. & Asker, R.L. 1983. Ethanol-sensitive times for the human conceptus. *Early Human Development*, 8, 99.

Rentz, R. 1980. Epilepsie und Psychose. *Klinische Paediatrie*, 46, 415.

Reske-Nielsen, E., Christensen, A. & Nielsen, J. 1982. A neuropathological and neuropsychological study of Turner's syndrome. *Cortex*, 18, 181.

Reynell, J. 1981. *Reynell Developmental Language Scales*, rev. ed. Windsor, England: NFER-Nelson.

Reynolds, D.M. & Jeeves, M.A. 1978. A developmental study of hemisphere specialization for recognition of faces in normal subjects. *Cortex*, 14, 511.

Reynolds, D.W., Stagno, S., Stubbs, K.G., Dahle, A.J., Livingston, M.M., Saxon, S.S. & Alford, C.A. 1974. Inapparent congenital cytomegalovirus infection with elevated cord IgM levels: Causal relation with auditory and mental deficiency. *New England Journal of Medicine*, 290, 291.

Ricci, S., Cusmai, R., Fariello, G. & Fusco, L. 1992. Double cortex: A neuronal migration anomaly as a possible cause of Lennox-Gestaut syndrome. *Archives of Neurology*, 49, 61.

Ricciuti, H.N. 1981. Adverse environmental and nutritional influences on mental development: A perspective. *Journal of the American Dietetic Association*, 79, 115.

Richardson, B.S. 1993. The fetal brain: Metabolic and circulatory response to asphyxia. *Clinical Investigative Medicine*, 16, 103.

Richter, D. 1975. Neurochemical aspects of the growth and development of the brain. In M.A.B. Brazier (Ed.), *Growth and Development of the Brain: Nutritional, Genetic, and Environmental Factors*. New York: Raven Press.

Riddle, M.A., Leckman, J.F., Anderson, G.M., Ort, S.I., Hardin, M.T., Stevenson, J. & Cohen, D.J. 1988. Tourette's syndrome: Clinical and neurochemical correlates. *Journal of the American Academy of Child and Adolescent Psychiatry*, 27, 409.

Rie, E.D., Rie, H.E., Stewart, S. & Rettemnier, S.C. 1978. An analysis of neurological soft signs in children with learning problems. *Brain and Language*, 6, 32.

Rie, H.E. & Rie, E.D. (Eds.) 1980. *Handbook of Minimal Brain Dysfunctions: A Critical View*. New York: Wiley.

Riese, M.L. 1984. Minor physical anomalies and behavior in neonates: Sex and gestational age differences. *Journal of Pediatric Psychology*, 9, 257.

Riese, M.L. 1989. Maternal alcohol and pentazocine abuse: Neonatal behavior and morphology in an opposite-sex twin pair. *Acta Genetica Medicae et Gemellologiae*, Twin Research, 38, 49.

Riesen, A.H. 1971. Problems in correlating behavioral and physiological development. In M.B. Sterman, D.J. McGinty & A.M. Adinolfi (Eds.), *Brain Development and Behavior*. New York: Academic Press.

Riesen, A.H. 1975. *The Developmental Neuropsychology of Sensory Deprivation.* New York: Academic Press.

Rigatto, H. & Brady, J.P. 1972. Periodic breathing and apnea in preterm infants. II. Hypoxia as a primary event. *Pediatrics,* 50, 219.

Riikonen, R. 1982. A long-term follow-up study of 214 children with the syndrome of infantile spasms. *Neuropediatrics,* 13, 14.

Rimland, B. 1964. *Infantile Autism: The Syndrome and its Implications for a Neural Theory of Behavior.* New York: Appleton-Century-Crofts.

Rimland, B. & Larson, G.E. 1983. Hair mineral analysis and behavior: An analysis of 51 studies. *Journal of Learning Disabilities,* 16, 279.

Rinck, C., Berg, J. & Hafeman, C. 1989. The adolescent with myelomeningocele: A review of parent experiences and expectations. *Adolescence,* 24, 699.

Ris, M.D. & Noll, R.B. 1994. Long-term neurobehavioral outcome in pediatric brain tumor patients: Review and methodological critique. *Journal of Clinical and Experimental Neuropsychology,* 16, 21.

Risser, A.H., Strauss, E.H. & Parry, P. 1985. Lateralization in attainment of neonatal head posture: Further external validation. *Perceptual and Motor Skills,* 60, 611.

Ritvo, E.O., Freeman, B.J., Geller, E. & Yuwiler, A. 1983. Effects of fenfluramine on 14 autistic outpatients. *Journal of the American Academy of Child Psychiatry,* 17, 565.

Ritvo, E.R., Jorde, L.B., Mason-Brothers, A. & Freeman, B.J. 1989. The UCLA-University of Utah epidemiological survey of autism: Recurrence risk estimates and genetic counseling. *American Journal of Psychiatry,* 146, 1032.

Ritvo, E.R., Spence, M.A., Freeman, B.J., Mason-Brothers, A., Mo, A. & Marazita, M.L. 1985. Evidence for autosomal recessive inheritance in 46 families with multiple incidences of autism. *American Journal of Psychiatry,* 142, 187.

Roach, E.S. & Riela, A.R. 1988. *Pediatric Cerebrovascular Disorders.* Mt. Kisco, NY: Futura.

Robaye, F. 1967. Approche correlationelle du developpement des gnosies et des praxies chez l'enfant de 2 a 6 ans. *Journal of Neurology* (Amsterdam) 200, 266.

Roberts, J.E., Burchinal, M.R., Koch, M.A., Footo, M.M. & Henderson, F.W. 1988. Otitis media in early childhood and its relationship to later phonological development. *Journal of Speech and Hearing Disorders,* 53, 424.

Roberts, R.J. 1992. A minority viewpoint on brain dysfunction in schizophrenia. *Contemporary Psychology,* 37, 326.

Robertson, C.M.T. & Finer, N. 1985. Term infants with hypoxic-ischemic encephalopathy: Outcome at 3.5 years. *Developmental Medicine and Child Neurology,* 27, 473.

Robertson, C.M.T., Finer, N.N. & Grace, M.G.A. 1989. School performance of survivors of neonatal encephalopathy associated with birth asphyxia at term. *Journal of Pediatrics,* 114, 753.

Robertson, C.M.T., Hrynchyshyn, P.C.E., Etches, C.P. & Pain, K. 1992. Population-based study of the incidence, complexity & severity of neurologic disability among survivors weighing 500 through 1250 grams at birth: A comparison of two birth cohorts. *Pediatrics* 90, 5, 750.

Robertson, M.M. 1989. The Gilles de la Tourette syndrome: The current status. *British Journal of Psychiatry,* 154, 147.

Robertson, M.M. & Gourdie, A. 1990. Familial Tourette's syndrome in a large British pedigree: Associated psychopathology, severity, and potential for linkage analysis. *British Journal of Psychiatry,* 156, 515.

Robertson, M.M., Trimble, M.R. & Lees, A.J. 1989. Self-injurious behavior and the Gilles de la Tourette syndrome: A clinical study and review of the literature. *Psychological Medicine,* 19, 611.

Robinson, A., Bender, B., Borelli, J. Puck, M. & Salbenblatt, J. 1983. Sex chromosomal anomalies: Prospective studies in children. *Behavior Genetics,* 13, 321.

Robinson, G.C. & Conry, R.F. 1986. Maternal age and congenital optic hypoplasia: A possible clue to etiology. *Developmental Medicine and Child Neurology,* 28, 294.

Robinson, H. & Robinson, N. 1965. *The Mentally Retarded Child.* New York: McGraw-Hill.

Robinson, H. & Robinson, N. 1976. *The Mentally Retarded Child,* 2nd ed. New York: McGraw-Hill.

Robinson, R. 1971. The small-for-date baby—II. *British Medical Journal,* 4, 480.

Robinson, R.J. 1966. Assessment of gestational age by neurological examination. *Archives of Diseases in Childhood,* 41, 437.

Robinson, R.O. 1981. Equal recovery of child and adult brain? *Developmental Medicine and Child Neurology,* 1981, 23, 379.

Rodin, E. & Rennick, P. 1979. Vocational and educational problems of epileptic patients. *Epilepsia,* 13, 149.

Rodin, E.A., Schmaltz, S. & Twitty, G. 1986. Intellectual functions of patients with childhood-onset epilepsy. *Developmental Medicine and Child Neurology,* 28, 25.

Roeltgen, M.G. & Roeltgen, D.P. 1989. Development of attention in normal children: A possible corpus callosum effect. *Developmental Neuropsychology,* 5, 127.

Roesler, H.D. 1971. Mental development of minimal brain-damaged children. *Acta Paedopsychiatrica,* 38, 71.

Rogeness, G.S., Maas, J.W., Javors, M.A. & Macedo, C.A. 1989. Attention deficit disorder symptoms and urine catecholamines. *Psychiatry Research,* 27, 241.

Rogers, R.C. & Simensen, R.J. 1987. Fragile X syndrome: A common etiology of mental retardation. *American Journal of Mental Deficiency,* 91, 445.

Roland, P.S., Finitzo, T., Friel-Patti, S. & Brown, K.C. 1989. Otitis media: Incidence, duration, and hearing status. *Archives of Otolaryngology and Head and Neck Surgery,* 115, 1049.

Rorke, L.B., Gilles, F.H., Davis, R.L. & Becker, L.E. 1985. Revision of the World Health Organization classification of brain tumors for childhood brain tumors. *Cancer,* 56, 1869.

Rose, A. 1977. Neonatal seizures. In M. Blaw, I. Rapin & M. Kinsbourne (Eds.), *Topics in Child Neurology.* New York: Spectrum Press.

Rose, F.D., Davey, M.J., Al-Khamees & Attree, E.A. 1992. General adaptive capacity and recovery of function following cortical damage in rats. *Medical Science Research,* 20, 359.

Rose, G.H. 1971. Relationship of electrophysiological and behavioral indices of visual development in mammals. In M.B. Sterman, D.J. McGinty & A.M. Adinolfi (Eds.), *Brain Development and Behavior.* New York: Academic Press.

Rose, S.A. 1981. Lags in the cognitive competence of prematurely born infants. In S.L. Friedman, & M. Sigman (Eds.), *Preterm Birth and Psychological Development.* New York: Academic Press.

Rose, S.A. 1984. Developmental changes in hemispheric specialization for tactual processing in very young children: Evidence from cross-modal transfer. *Developmental Psychology,* 20, 568.

Rose, S.A., Schmidt, K. & Bridges, W.H. 1976. Cardiac and behavioural responsivity to tactile stimulation in premature and full-term infants. *Developmental Psychology,* 12, 311.

Rose, S.W., Penry, J.K., Markrush, D., Radloff, P. & Putnam, J.K. 1973. Prevalence of epilepsy in children. *Epilepsia,* 14, 133.

Rosen, G.D., Sherman, G.F. & Galaburda, A.M. 1986. Biological interactions in dyslexia. In J.E. Obrzut and G.W. Hynd (Eds.), *Child Neuropsychology,* Vol. 1. New York: Academic Press, p. 155.

Rosenberger-Debiesse, J. & Coleman, M. 1986. Brief report: Evidence for multiple etiologies in autism. *Journal of Autism and Developmental Disorders,* 16, 385.

Rosenblith, J.F. 1961. The modified Graham behavior test for neonates: Test-retest reliability, normative data and hypotheses for future work. *Biologia Neonatorium,* 3, 174.

Rosenblith, J.F. 1974. Prognostic value of neonatal behavioral tests. In B.Z. Friedlander, G.M. Sterritt & G.E. Kirk (Eds.), *Exceptional Infant, Vol. 3: Assessment and Intervention.* New York: Brunner-Mazel.

Rosenfield, I. 1988. *The Invention of Memory: A New View of the Brain.* New York: Basic Books.

Rosenzweig, M.R. 1951. Representations of the two ears at the auditory cortex. *American Journal of Physiology,* 167, 147.

Rosett, H.L. & Sander, L.W. 1979. Effects of maternal drinking on neonatal morphology and state regulation. In J.D. Osofsky (Ed.), *Handbook of Infant Development.* New York: Wiley.

Rosinski, R.R. 1977. *The Development of Visual Perception.* Santa Monica: Goodyear Publishing Company.

Rosner, B.S. 1974. Recovery of function & localization of function in historical perspective. In D.G. Stein, J.J. Rosen & N. Butters (Eds.), *Plasticity and Recovery of Function in the Central Nervous System.* New York: Academic Press.

Rosner, J. 1990. Clinical review of neurofibromatosis. *Journal of the American Optometric Association,* 61, 613.

Ross, A.O. 1973. Conceptual issues in the evaluation of brain damage. In J.L. Khama (Ed.), *Brain Damage and Mental Retardation: A Psychological Evaluation,* 2nd ed. Springfield, IL: Charles C Thomas, p. 20.

Ross, A.O. & Pelham, W.E. 1981. Childhood psychopathology. *Annual Review of Psychology,* 32, 243.

Ross, D.M. & Ross, S.A. 1976. *Hyperactivity: Research, Theory and Action.* New York: Wiley.

Ross, D.M. & Ross, S.A. 1982. *Hyperactivity: Current Issues, Research and Theory.* New York: Wiley.

Ross, G., Lipper, E. & Auld, P.A. 1992. Hand preference, prematurity and developmental outcome at school age. *Neuropsychologia,* 30, 483.

Roth, N., Beyreiss, J., Schlenzka, K. & Beyer, H. 1991. Coincidence of attention deficit disorder and atropic disorders in children: Empirical findings and hypothetical background. *Journal of Abnormal Child Psychology,* 19, 1.

Rothlind, J.C., Posner, M.I. & Schaughency, E.A. 1991. Lateralized control of eye movements in attention deficit hyperactivity disorder. *Journal of Cognitive Neuroscience,* 3, 377.

Rourke, B.P. 1978. Neuropsychological research in reading retardation. In A.L. Benton and D. Pearl (Eds.), *Dyslexia: An Appraisal of Current Knowledge*. New York: Oxford University Press.

Rourke, B.P. 1982. Central processing deficiencies in children: Toward a developmental neuropsychological model. *Journal of Clinical Neuropsychology*, 4, 1.

Rourke, B.P. 1985. *Neuropsychology of Learning Disabilities: Essentials of Subtype Analysis*. New York: Guilford.

Rourke, B.P. 1989. *Nonverbal Learning Disabilities: The Syndrome and the Model*. New York: Guilford Press.

Rourke, B.P. & Finlayson, M.A.J. 1978. Neuropsychological significance of variations in patterns of academic performance: Verbal and visual-spatial abilities. *Journal of Abnormal Child Psychology*, 6, 121.

Rourke, B.P. & Fuerst, D.R. 1992. Psychosocial dimensions of learning disability subtypes: Neuropsychological studies in the Windsor laboratory. *School Psychology Review*, 21, 361.

Rourke, B.P. & Strang, J.D. 1978. Neuropsychological significance of variations in patterns of academic performance: Motor, psychomotor, and tactile-perceptual abilities. *Journal of Pediatric Psychology*, 3, 62.

Rourke, B.P. & Strang, J.D. 1981. Subtypes of reading and arithmetic disabilities: A neuropsychological analysis. In M. Rutter (Ed.), *Behavioral Syndromes of Brain Dysfunction in Children*. New York: Guilford Press.

Rourke, B.P., Bakker, D.J., Fisk, J.L. & Strang, J.D. 1983. *Child Neuropsychology*. New York: Guilford Press.

Rourke, B.P., Fisk, J.L. & Strang, J.D. 1986. *Neuropsychological Assessment in Children*. New York: Guilford Press.

Rourke, B.P., Young, G.C. & Leenaars, A.A. 1989. The childhood learning disability that predisposes those afflicted to adolescent and adult depression and suicide risk. *Journal of Learning Disabilities*, 22, 169.

Rourke, B.P., Del Dotto, J.E., Rourke, S.B. & Casey, J.E. 1990. Nonverbal learning disabilities: The syndrome and a case study. *Journal of School Psychology*, 28, 361.

Roussounis, S.H., Hubley, P.A. & Dear, P.R. 1993. Five-year follow-up of very low birthweight infants: Neurological and psychological outcome. *Child Care, Health and Development*, 19, 45.

Routtenberg, A. 1968. The two-arousal hypothesis: Reticular formation and limbic system. *Psychological Review*, 75, 51.

Rovee-Collier, C.K. & Lipsitt, L.P. 1982. Learning, adaptation, and memory in the newborn. In P. Stratton (Ed.), *Psychobiology of the Human Newborn*. New York: Wiley.

Rovet, J. & Netley, C. 1983. The triple X chromosome syndrome in childhood: Recent empirical findings. *Child Development*, 54, 831.

Rovet, J.F., Ehrlich, R.M. & Czuchta, D. 1990. Intellectual characteristics of diabetic children at diagnosis and one year later. *Journal of Pediatric Psychology*, 15, 775.

Rovet, J.F., Ehrlich, R.M. & Sorbara, D.L. 1992. Neurodevelopment in infants and preschool children with congenital hypothyroidism: Etiological and treatment factors affecting outcome. *Journal of Pediatric Psychology*, 17, 187.

Rovet, J.F., Sorbara, D.L. & Ehrlich, R.M. 1986. The intellectual and behavioral characteristics of children with congenital hypothyroidism identified by neonatal screening in Ontario. The Toronto prospective study. In J.F. Rovet (Ed.), *Genetic Disease: Screening and Management*. Toronto: A.R. Liss, p. 281.

Rowe, M. & Willis, W.D. (Eds.) 1985. *Development, Organization, and Processing in Somatosensory Pathways. Neurology and Neurobiology Vol. 14.* New York: A.R. Liss.

Rudel, R., Healey, J. & Denckla, M. 1984. Development of motor coordination by normal left handed children. *Developmental Medicine and Child Neurology,* 26, 104.

Ruder, K.F. & Smith, M.D. 1974. Issues in language training. In R.L. Schiefelbusch & L.L. Lloyd (Eds.), *Language Perspectives—Acquisition, Retardation, and Intervention.* Baltimore: University Park Press, p. 565.

Rudolf, M.C. & Hochberg, Z. 1990. Are boys more vulnerable to psychosocial growth retardation? *Developmental Medicine and Child Neurology,* 32, 1022.

Ruiz, M.P.D., LeFever, J.A., Hakanson, D.O., Clark, D.A. & Willimans, M.L. 1981. Early development of infants of birth weight less than 1000 grams with mechanical ventilation in the newborn period. *Pediatrics,* 68, 330.

Rumsey, J.M., Dorwart, R., Vermess, M., Denckla, M.B., Kruesi, M.J.P. & Rapoport, J.L. 1986. Magnetic resonance imaging of brain anatomy in severe developmental dyslexia. *Archives of Neurology,* 43, 1045.

Rush, D. 1981. Maternal smoking during pregnancy and child development: A review, and methodology for a new study of over 10,000 representative five year olds in Great Britain. In *Proceedings of the Third Symposium on the Prevention of Handicapping Conditions of Prenatal and Perinatal Origin.* Edmonton, Alberta: Alberta Social Services and Community Health, p. 31.

Rutledge, L.T., Wright, C. & Duncan, J. 1974. Morphological changes in pyramidal cells of mammalian neocortex associated with increased use. *Experimental Neurology,* 44, 209.

Rutter, M. 1965. The influence of organic and emotional factors in the origins, nature and outcome of child psychosis. *Developmental Medicine and Child Neurology,* 7, 518.

Rutter, M. 1978. Diagnosis and definition of childhood autism. *Journal of Autism and Childhood Schizophrenia,* 8, 139.

Rutter, M. 1980. Raised lead levels and impaired cognitive/behavioral functioning: A review of the evidence. *Developmental Medicine and Child Neurology,* Suppl. 42, 1.

Rutter, M. 1982a. Syndromes attributed to "minimal brain dysfunction" in childhood. *American Journal of Psychiatry,* 139(1), 21.

Rutter, M. 1982b. Developmental neuropsychiatry: Concepts, issues, and prospects. *Journal of Clinical Neuropsychology,* 4, 91.

Rutter, M. 1983. *Developmental Neuropsychiatry.* New York: Guilford Press.

Rutter, M. 1984. Psychopathology and development: I. Childhood antecedents of adult psychiatric disorder. *Australian and New Zealand Journal of Psychiatry,* 18, 225.

Rutter, M. 1986. Child psychiatry: The interface between clinical and developmental research. *Psychological Medicine,* 16, 151.

Rutter, M. 1990. The Isle of Wight revisited: Twenty-five years of child psychiatric epidemiology. In S. Chess & M.E. Hertzig (Eds.), *Annual Progress in Child Psychiatry and Child Development.* New York: Brunner/Mazel, p. 131.

Rutter, M. & Giller, H. 1983. *Juvenile Delinquency: Trends and Perspectives.* New York: Guilford Press.

Rutter, M., Graham, P. & Yule, W. 1970a. *A Neuropsychiatric Study in Childhood.* London: Lavenham Press.

Rutter, M., Tizard, J. & Whitmore, K. (Eds.) 1970b. *Education, Health and Behavior.* London: Longmans, Green.

Rutter, M., Graham, P., Chadwick, O. & Yule, W. 1976. Adolescent turmoil—fact or fiction? *Journal of Child Psychology and Psychiatry*, 17, 35.

Rutter, M., Tuma, A.H. & Lann, I.S. (Eds.) 1988. *Assessment and Diagnosis in Child Psychopathology*. New York: Guilford Press.

Rylov, A.L. & Anokhin, K.V. 1992. Synthesis of protein in the critical periods of early postnatal ontogenesis: Its role in the formation of intraspecies aggressive behavior in rats. *Neuroscience and Behavioral Physiology*, 22, 6.

Sackett, G.P. 1984. A nonhuman primate model of risk for deviant development. *American Journal of Mental Deficiency*, 88, 469.

Safer, D.J. 1973. A familial factor in minimal brain dysfunction. *Behavioral Genetics*, 3, 175.

Sahley, T.L. & Panksepp, J. 1987. Brain opioids and autism: An updated analysis of possible linkages. *Journal of Autism and Developmental Disorders*, 17, 201.

Saigal, S., Rosenbaum, P.L., Szatmari, P. & Campbell, D. 1991. Learning disabilities and school problems in a regional cohort of extremely low birth weight (<1000 g.) children: A comparison with term controls. *Journal of Developmental and Behavioral Pediatrics*, 12, 294.

Saigal, S., Rosenbaum, P.L., Szatmari, P. & Hoult, L. 1992. Non-right handedness among ELBW and term children at eight years in relation to cognitive function and school performance. *Developmental Medicine and Child Neurology*, 34, 425.

Saint-Anne Dargassies, S. 1966. Neurological maturation of the premature infants of 28 to 41 weeks gestational age. In F. Falkner (Ed.), *Human Development*. Philadelphia: W.B. Saunders.

Saint-Anne Dargassies, S. 1977. *Neurological Development in the Full-Term and Premature Neonate*. Amsterdam: Elsevier.

St. James-Roberts, I. 1979. Neurological plasticity, recovery from brain insult, and child development. In H.W. Reese & L.P. Lipsitt (Eds.), *Advances in Child Development and Behavior*, Vol. 14. New York: Academic Press.

St. James-Roberts, I. 1981. A reinterpretation of hemispherectomy data without functional plasticity of the brain, I. Intellectual functions. *Brain and Language*, 13, 31.

Salam, M.Z. & Adams, R.D. 1975. Research on the clinical expression and pathological basis of mental retardation. In D.B. Tower (Ed.), *The Nervous System, Vol. 2: The Clinical Neurosciences*. New York: Raven Press.

Sameroff, A.J. & Chandler, M.J. 1975. Reproductive risk and the continuum of caretaking causality. In F.D. Horowitz (Ed.), *Review of Child Development Research*, Vol. 4. Chicago: University of Chicago Press.

Sandberg, A.A. 1963. Xyy-genotype—report of a case in a male. *New England Journal of Medicine*, 268, 585.

Sanders, M., Allen, M., Alexander, G.R., Yankowitz, J., Graeber, J., Johnson, T.R.B. & Reka, M.X. 1991. Gestational age assessment in preterm neonates weighing less than 1500 grams. *Pediatrics*, 88, 3, 543.

Sanders, R.J. 1989. Sentence comprehension following agenesis of the corpus callosum. *Brain and Language*, 37, 59.

Sandler, A.D., Watson, T.E., Footo, M. & Levine, M.D. 1992. Neurodevelopmental study of writing disorders in middle childhood. *Journal of Developmental and Behavioral Pediatrics*, 13, 17.

Sarnat, H.B. 1989. Neural induction and developmental disorders of the nervous system. In N.J. Anastasiow & S. Harel (Eds.), *At-Risk Infants: Interventions, Families, and Research*. Baltimore: Paul H. Brookes, p. 191.

Sasanuma, S. & Monoi, H. 1975. The syndrome of Golgi (word-meaning) aphasia. Selective impairment of Kanji processing. *Neurology,* 25, 627.

Sass, K.J., Spencer, D.D., Spencer, S.S. & Novelly, R. 1988. Corpus callosotomy for epilepsy: II. Neurologic and neuropsychologic outcome. *Neurology,* 38, 24.

Satz, P. 1972. Pathological left-handedness: An exploratory model. *Cortex,* 8, 121.

Satz, P. 1977. Laterality tests: An inferential problem. *Cortex,* 13, 208.

Satz, P. 1982. Sex differences: Clues or myths on genetic aspects of speech and language disorders. In C. Ludlow (Ed.), *Genetic Aspects of Speech and Language Disorders.* New York: Academic Press.

Satz, P. & Bullard-Bates, C. 1981. Acquired aphasia in children. In M. Taylor Sarno (Ed.), *Acquired Aphasia.* New York: Academic Press.

Satz, P. & Fletcher, J.M. 1980. Minimal brain dysfunction: An appraisal of research concepts and methods. In H.D. Rie and E.D. Rie (Eds.), *Handbook of Minimal Brain Dysfunction.* New York: Wiley, p. 667.

Satz, P. & Soper, H.V. 1986. Left-handedness, dyslexia, and autoimmune disorder: A critique. *Journal of Clinical and Experimental Neuropsychology,* 8, 453.

Satz, P., Fried, J. & Rudegeair, R. 1974. *Differential Changes in the Acquisition of Developmental Skills in Children who Later Become Dyslexic. A Three Year Follow-Up. Recovery of Function.* New York: Academic Press.

Satz, P., Strauss, E. & Whitaker, H. 1990. The ontogeny of hemispheric specialization: Some old hypotheses revisited. *Brain and Language,* 38, 596.

Satz, P., Strauss, E., Wada, J. & Orsini, D.L. 1988. Some correlates of intra- and interhemispheric speech organization after left focal brain injury. *Neuropsychologia,* 26, 345.

Satz, P., Strauss, E., Hunter, M. & Wada, J. 1994. Re-examination of the crowding hypothesis: Effects of age of onset. *Neuropsychology,* 8, 255.

Satz, P., Taylor, H.G., Friel, J. & Fletcher, J. 1978. Some developmental and predictive precursors of reading disabilities: A six year follow up. In A.L. Benton and D. Pearl (Eds.), *Dyslexia. An Appraisal of Current Knowledge.* New York: Oxford University Press.

Sauerwein, H. & Lassonde, M.C. 1983. Intra- and interhemispheric processing of visual information in callosal agenesis. *Neuropsychologia,* 21, 167.

Saul, R.E. & Sperry, R.W. 1968. Absence of commissurotomy symptoms with agenesis of the corpus callosum. *Neurology,* 18, 307.

Saunders, J.C. & Bock, G.R. 1978. Influences of early auditory trauma on auditory development. In R. Gottlieb (Ed.), *Early Influences.* New York: Academic Press.

Saxen, L. 1980. Neural induction: Past, present, and future. In R.K. Hunt (Ed.), *Neural Development. Part 1: Current Topics in Developmental Biology,* vol. 15. New York: Academic Press.

Saxon, S. & Witriol, E. 1976. Down's syndrome and intellectual development. *Journal of Pediatric Psychology,* 1(3), 45.

Scaravilli, F. (Ed.) 1993. *The Neuropathology of HIV Infection.* New York: Springer.

Scarborough, H.S. 1991. Antecedents to reading disability: Preschool language development and literacy experiences of children from dyslexic families. *Reading and Writing,* 3, 219.

Scardafi, F.A., Field, T.M. & Schanberg, S.M. 1986. Effects of tactile/kinesthetic stimulation on the clinical course and sleep/wake behavior of preterm neonates. *Infant Behavior and Development* 9, 103.

Scarff, T.B. & Fronczak, S. 1981. Myelomeningocele: A review and update. *Rehabilitation Literature*, 42, 143.

Scarr, S. 1991. Theoretical issues in investigating intellectual plasticity. In S.E. Brauth, W.S. Hall & R.J. Dooling (Eds.), *Plasticity of Development*. Cambridge, MA: MIT Press.

Scarr-Salapatek, S. & Williams, M. 1973. The effects of early stimulation on low birth weight infants. *Child Development*, 44, 94.

Schain, R.J. 1968. Minimal brain dysfunction in children: A neurological viewpoint. *Bulletin of the Los Angeles Neurological Society*, 33, 145.

Schapiro, M.B., Haxby, J.V., Grady, C.L. & Duara, R. 1987. Decline in cerebral glucose utilization and cognitive function with aging in Down's syndrome. *Journal of Neurology, Neurosurgery and Psychiatry*, 50, 766.

Scharf, L.S. & Adams, K.M. 1984. Long-term neuropsychological impact of retrolental fibroplasia: Review and implications. *Journal of Pediatric Psychology*, 9, 303.

Schelkunov, E.L., Kenunen, O.G., Pushkov, V.V. & Charltonov, R.A. 1986. Heart rate, blood pressure regulation and neurotransmitter balance in Tourette's syndrome. *Journal of the American Academy of Child Psychiatry*, 25, 645.

Schellekens, J.M., Scholten, C.A. & Kalverboer, A.F. 1983. Visually guided hand movements in children with minor neurological dysfunction: Response time and movement organization. *Journal of Child Psychology and Psychiatry and Allied Disciplines*, 24, 89.

Schilling, F. 1970. Zur Aussagefähigkeit des Oseretzky-Tests bei normalen und hirngeschädigten Kindern. *Acta Paedopsychiatrica*, 37, 249.

Schlager, G. 1979. Bone age in children with minimal brain dysfunction. *Developmental Medicine and Child Neurology*, 21, 41.

Schleifer, M., Weiss, G., Cohen, N., Elman, M., Cvejic, H. & Kruger, E. 1975. Hyperactivity in preschoolers and the effect of methylphenidate. *American Journal of Orthopsychiatry*, 45, 38.

Schlesinger, H. & Meadows, K. 1972. *Sound and Sign: Childhood Deafness and Mental Health*. Berkeley: University of California Press.

Schlieper, A., Kiselevsky, H., Mattingly, S. & Yorke, L. 1985. Mild conductive hearing loss and language development: A one year follow-up study. *Developmental and Behavioral Pediatrics*, 6, 65.

Schmid-Rüter, E. 1977. Phenylketonurie: Früherfassung and geistige Entwicklung. Pilotstudie an 89 phenylketonurischen Kindern mit Diätbeginn im ersten bis einschliesslich zwölften Lebensmonat. *Monatsschrift für Kinderheilkunde*, 125, 479.

Schmidt, M.H., Esser, G., Allehoff, W., Geisel, B., Laucht, M. & Woerner, W. 1987. Evaluating the significance of minimal brain dysfunction: Results of an epidemiological study. *Journal of Child Psychology and Psychiatry and Allied Disciplines*, 28, 803.

Schmitt, B.D. 1975. The minimal brain dysfunction myth. *American Journal of Diseases of Childhood*, 129, 1313.

Schneider, B.A., Trehub, S.E. & Bull, D. 1979. The development of basic auditory processes in infants. *Canadian Journal of Psychology*, 33, 306.

Schneider, G.E. 1974. Anomalous axonal connections implicated in sparing and alteration of function after early lesions. In E. Eidelberg & D.G. Stein (Eds.), Function recovery after lesions of the nervous system. *Neurosciences Research Program Bulletin*, 12(2), 222.

Schneider, G.E. 1979. Is it really better to have your brain lesion early? A revision of the "Kennard Principle." *Neuropsychologia,* 17, 557.

Schoenberg, B.S., Mellinger, J.F. & Schoenberg, D.G. 1978. Cerebrovascular disease in infants and children: A study of incidence, clinical features, and survival. *Neurology,* 28, 763.

Schopler, E. & Mesibov, G. 1981. *Autism in Adolescents and Adults.* New York: Plenum Press.

Schor, D.P. 1983. PKU and temperament: Rating children three through seven years old in PKU families. *Clinical Pediatrics,* 22, 807.

Schor, D.P. 1986. Phenylketonuria and temperament in middle childhood. *Children's Health Care,* 14, 163.

Schrader, B.D. 1986. Developmental progress in very low birth weight infants during the first year of life. *Nursing Research* 35, 237.

Schroeder, J., Niethammer, R., Geider, F.J. & Reitz, C. 1991. Neurological soft signs in schizophrenia. *Schizophrenia Research,* 6, 25.

Schroeder, S. (Ed.) 1987. *Toxic Substances and Mental Retardation: Neurobehavioral Toxicology and Teratology.* Washington, DC: American Association on Mental Retardation.

Schroth, M.L. 1975. The use of IQ as a measure of problem solving ability with mongoloid and nonmongoloid retarded children. *Journal of Psychology,* 91, 49.

Schuknecht, H.F. 1974. *Pathology of the Ear.* Cambridge, MA: Harvard University Press.

Schulman-Galambos, C. & Galambos, R. 1979. Assessment of hearing. In T.M. Field, A.M. Sostek, S. Goldberg & H.H. Shuman (Eds.), *Infants at Risk: Behavior and Development.* New York: SP Medical and Scientific Books, p. 91.

Schulsinger, H. 1976. A ten-year follow-up of schizophrenic mothers. *Acta Psychiatrica Scandinavica,* 53, 371.

Schulte, F.J. & Stennert, E. 1978. Hearing defects in preterm infants. *Archives of Disease in Childhood,* 53, 269.

Schurr, P. 1969. Subdural haematomas and effusions in infancy. *Developmental Medicine and Child Neurology,* 11, 108.

Schwartz, M. 1988. Handedness, prenatal stress and pregnancy complications. *Neuropsychologia,* 26, 925.

Scott, H. 1976. Outcome of very severe birth asphyxia. *Archives of Disease in Childhood,* 51, 712.

Scott, J.P. 1958. Critical periods in the development of social behaviour in puppies. *Psychosomatic Medicine,* 20, 42.

Scott, J.P., Stewart, J.M. & DeGhett, V.J. 1974. Critical periods in the organization of systems. *Developmental Psychobiology,* 7(6), 489.

Seashore, R.H., Buxton, C.E. & McCollom, I.N. 1940. Multiple factorial analysis of fine motor skills. *American Journal of Psychology,* 53, 251.

Sechzer, J.A., Faro, M.D. & Windle, W.F. 1973. Studies of monkeys asphyxiated at birth: Implications for minimal cerebral dysfunction. *Seminars in Psychiatry,* 5, 19.

Segalowitz, S.J. & Gruber, F.A. (Eds.) 1977. *Language Development and Neurological Theory.* New York: Academic Press.

Segalowitz, S.J. & Rose-Krasnor, L. 1992. The construct of brain maturation in theories of child development. *Brain and Cognition,* 20, 1.

Segalowitz, S.J., Unsal, A. & Dywan, J. 1992. Cleverness and wisdom in 12-year-olds: Electrophysiological evidence for late maturation of the frontal lobe. *Developmental Neuropsychology,* 8, 279.

Seidel, U.P., Chadwick, O. & Rutter, M. 1975. Psychological disorders in crippled children: A comparative study of children with and without brain damage. *Developmental Medicine and Child Neurology,* 17, 563.

Seidman, L.J. 1983. Schizophrenia and brain dysfunction: An integration of recent neurodiagnostic findings. *Psychological Bulletin,* 94, 195.

Sell, S.H. 1983. Long-term sequelae of bacterial meningitis in children. *Pediatric Infectious Disease,* 2, 90.

Sell, S.H., Merrill, R.E. & Doyne, E.O. 1972a. Long-term sequelae of *Homophilus influenzae* meningitis. *Pediatrics,* 49, 206.

Sell, S.H., Webb, W.W. & Pate, J.E. 1972b. Psychological sequelae to bacterial meningitis: Two controlled studies. *Pediatrics,* 49, 212.

Selnes, O.A. & Whitaker, H.A. 1976. Morphological and functional development of the auditory system. In R.W. Rieber (Ed.), *The Neuropsychology of Language.* New York, Plenum Press.

Selzer, S.C., Lindgren, S.D. & Blackman, J.A. 1992. Long-term neuropsychological outcome of high-risk infants with intracranial hemorrhage. *Journal of Pediatric Psychology,* 17, 407.

Semrud-Clikeman, M. & Hynd, G.W. 1991. Specific nonverbal and social-skills deficits in children with learning disabilities. In J.E. Obrzut & G.W. Hynd (Eds.), *Neuropsychological Foundations of Learning Disabilities.* San Diego: Academic Press.

Sergent, J. 1986. Microgenesis of face perception. In H.D. Ellis, M.A. Jeeves, F. Newcomb & A. Young (Eds.), *Aspects of Face Processing.* Dordrecht: Martinus Nijhoff Publishers, p. 17.

Seyfort, B. & Spreen, O. 1979. Two-plated tapping performance by Down's syndrome and non-Down's syndrome retardates. *Journal of Child Psychology and Psychiatry,* 20, 351.

Seyfort, B.M.A. 1977. An investigation of syndrome-specific language impairment in Down's anomaly. Ph.D. Dissertation: University of Victoria.

Shafer, S.Q., Shaffer, D., O'Connor, P.A. & Stokman, C.J. 1983. Hard thoughts on neurological "soft signs." In M. Rutter (Ed.), *Developmental Neuropsychiatry.* New York: Guilford, p. 133.

Shaffer, D. 1978. Soft neurological signs and later psychiatric disorders—A review. *Journal of Child Psychology and Psychiatry,* 19, 63.

Shaffer, D. 1985. Neurological soft signs: Their relationship to psychiatric disorders and intelligence in childhood and adolescence. *Archives of General Psychiatry,* 42, 342.

Shaffer, D., Chadwick, O. & Rutter, M. 1975. Psychiatric outcome of localized head injury in children. In R. Porter & D. Fitzsimons (Eds.), *Outcome of Severe Damage to the Central Nervous System.* Amsterdam: CIBA Foundation Symposium No. 34, 1975.

Shaffer, J.W. 1962. A specific cognitive defect observed in gonadal aplasia (Turner's syndrome). *Journal of Clinical Psychology,* 1962, 18, 403.

Shaffer, J., Friedrich, W.N., Shurtleff, D.B. & Wolf, L. 1985. Cognitive and achievement status of children with meningomyelocele. *Journal of Pediatric Psychology,* 10, 325.

Shallice, T. 1982. Specific impairments of planning. In D.E. Broadbent and L. Weiskrantz (Eds.), *The Neuropsychology of Cognitive Function.* London: Royal Society, p. 199.

Shankweiler, D. 1964. Developmental dyslexia: A critique and review of recent evidence. *Cortex,* 1, 53.

Shapiro, A.K. & Shapiro, E. 1982. Tourette's syndrome: History and present status. In A.J. Friedhoff & T.N. Chase (Eds.), *Gilles de la Tourette Syndrome, Advances in Neurology,* Vol. 35. New York: Raven Press.

Shapiro, E., Shapiro, A.K., Fulop, G. & Hubbard, M. 1989. Controlled study of halo-peridol, pimozide, and placebo for the treatment of Gilles de la Tourette's syndrome. *Archives of General Psychiatry,* 46, 722.

Shapiro, K. 1985. Head injury in children. In D.P. Becker & J.T. Povlischock (Eds.), *Central Nervous System Trauma Status Report 1985.* Bethesda: NINCDS, p. 243.

Shapiro, K. & Smith, L.P. 1993. Special considerations for the pediatric age group. In P.R. Cooper (Ed.), *Head Injury,* 3rd ed. Baltimore: Williams & Wilkins, p. 427.

Shapiro, T., Burkes, L., Petti, T.A. & Ranz, J. 1978. Consistency of "nonfocal" neurological signs. *Journal of the American Academy of Child Psychiatry,* 17, 70.

Shapiro, T., Burkes, L., Petti, T.A. & Ranz, J. 1979. Consistency of "nonfocal" neurological signs. *Annual Progress in Child Psychiatry and Child Development,* 476.

Shaywitz, B.A., Cohen, D.J. & Shaywitz, S.E. 1979. New diagnostic terminology for minimal brain dysfunction. *Journal of Pediatrics,* 95, 734.

Shaywitz, B.A., Shaywitz, S.E., Byrne, T., Cohen, D.J. & Rothman, S. 1983. Attention deficit disorder: Quantitative analysis of CT. *Neurology,* 33, 1500.

Shaywitz, S.E. & Shaywitz, B.A. 1991. Introduction to the special series on attention deficit disorder. *Journal of Learning Disabilities,* 24, 68.

Shebilske, W.L. 1976. Extraretinal information in corrective saccades and inflow versus outflow theories of visual direction constancy. *Vision Research,* 16, 621.

Shekim, W.O., Sinclair, E., Glaser, R. & Horwitz, E. 1987. Norepinephrine and dopamine metabolites and educational variables with boys with attention deficit disorder and hyperactivity. *Journal of Child Neurology,* 2, 50.

Shepard, T.H., Miller, J.R. & Marois, D. 1975. *Methods for the Detection of Environmental Agents That Produce Congenital Defects.* New York: Elsevier.

Sheridan-Pereira, M., Ellison, P.H. & Helgeson, V. 1991. The construction of a scored neonatal neurological examination for the assessment of neurological integrity in full-term neonates. *Journal of Developmental and Behavioral Pediatrics,* 12, 25.

Shirley, M. 1933. *The First Two Years.* Minneapolis: University of Minnesota Press.

Shonkoff, J.P. & Hauser-Cram, P. 1987. Early intervention for disabled infants and their families: A quantitative analysis. *Pediatrics,* 80, 650.

Shprintzen, R.J. & Goldberg, R.B. 1986. Multiple anomaly syndromes and learning disabilities. In S.D. Smith (Ed.), *Genetics and Learning Disabilities.* London: Taylor & Francis, p. 153.

Shucard, D.W., Shucard, J.L., Clopper, R.R. & Schachter, M. 1992. Electrophysiological and neuropsychological indices of cognitive processing deficits in Turner syndrome. *Developmental Neuropsychology,* 8, 299.

Shucard, J.L., Shucard, D.W., Cummins, K.R. & Campos, J.J. 1981. Auditory evoked potentials and sex-related differences in brain development. *Brain and Language,* 13, 91.

Sidman, R.L. & Rakic, P. 1973. Neuronal migration, with special reference to the developing human brain: A review. *Brain Research,* 62, 1.

Sidtis, J.J. 1984. Music, pitch discrimination, and the mechanism of cortical hearing. In M.S. Gazzaniga (Ed.), *Handbook of Cognitive Neuroscience.* New York: Plenum Press.

Siebelink, B.M., Bakker, D.J., Binnie, C.D. & Kasteleijn-Nolst-Trenite, D.G.A. 1988. Psychological effects of subclinical epileptoform EEG discharges in children. II. General intelligence tests. *Epilepsy Research,* 2, 117.

Siegel, L. 1984. A longitudinal study of a hyperlexic child: Hyperlexia as a language disorder. *Neuropsychologia,* 22, 577.

Siegel, L. 1989. A reconceptualization of prediction from infant test scores. In M. Bornstein & N. Krasnegor (Eds.), *Stability and Continuity in Mental Development. Behavioral and Biological Perspectives.* Hillsdale, NJ: Erlbaum, p. 89.

Siegel, L. 1992. A multivariate model for the early detection of learning disabilities. In C.W. Greenbaum & J.G. Auerbach (Eds.), *Longitudinal Studies of Children at Psychological Risk: Cross-National Perspectives.* Norwood, NJ: Ablex Publishing Co.

Sigman, M.D. & Bornstein, M.H. 1986. Continuity of mental development from infancy. *Child Development,* 57, 251.

Sigman, M. & Parmelee, A.H. 1976. Visual preferences of four-month old premature and full-term infants. *Child Development,* 10, 687.

Sigman, M., Neumann, C., Jansen, A.A. & Bwibo, N. 1989. Cognitive abilities in Kenyan children in relation to nutrition, family characteristics, and education. *Child Development,* 60, 1463.

Sigman, M., McDonald, M.A., Neumann, C. & Bwibo, N. 1991. Prediction of cognitive competence in Kenyan children from toddler nutrition, family characteristics and abilities. *Journal of Child Psychology and Psychiatry and Allied Disciplines,* 32, 307.

Silber, J.H., Radcliffe, J., Peckham, V., Perilongo, G., Kishnani, P., et al. 1992. Whole-brain irradiation and decline in intelligence: The influence of dose and age on IQ score. *Journal of Clinical Oncology,* 10, 1390.

Silberberg, N.E. & Silberberg, M.C. 1972. Hyperlexia: The other end of the continuum. *Journal of Special Education,* 5, 233.

Silbergeld, E.K. 1977. Neuropharmacology of hyperkinesis. *Current Developments in Psychopharmacology,* 4, 179.

Silbergeld, E.K. & Goldberg, A.M. 1974. Lead-induced behavioral dysfunction: An animal model of hyperactivity. *Experimental Neurology,* 42, 146.

Silberman, E.K. & Tassone, E.P. 1985. The Israeli high-risk study: Statistical overview and discussion. *Schizophrenia Bulletin,* 11, 138.

Silbert, A.R., Wolff, P.H. & Lilienthal, J. 1977. Spatial and temporal processing in patients with Turner's syndrome. *Behavior Genetics,* 7, 11.

Sillanpaa, M. 1983. Social functioning and seizure status of young adults with onset of epilepsy in childhood. *Acta Neurologica Scandinavica,* 68, Suppl. No. 96.

Silva, P.A., McGee, R. & Williams, S. 1984. A longitudinal study of the intelligence and behavior of preterm and small for gestational age children. *Developmental and Behavioral Pediatrics* 5, 1.

Silverman, E. 1971. Situational variability of preschoolers' dysfluency: Preliminary study. *Perceptual and Motor Skills,* 33, 4021.

Silverstein, A.B. 1979. Mental growth from six to sixty in an institutionalized mentally retarded sample. *Psychological Reports,* 45, 643.

Silverstein, A.B., Herbs, D., Nasuta, R. & White, J.F. 1986. Effects of age on the adaptive behavior of institutionalized individuals with Down syndrome. *American Journal of Mental Deficiency,* 90, 659.

Silverstein, A.B., Legutki, G., Friedman, S.L. & Takayama, D.L. 1982. Performance of Down syndrome individuals on the Stanford-Binet Intelligence Scale. *American Journal of Mental Deficiency,* 86, 548.

Silverstein, A.B., Lozano, G.D. & White, J.F. 1989. A cluster analysis of institutionalized mentally retarded individuals. *American Journal of Mental Retardation,* 94, 1.

Silverton, L., Mednick, S.A. & Harrington, M.E. 1988. Birthweight, schizophrenia and ventricular enlargement in a high-risk sample. *Psychiatry*, 51, 272.

Simmons, F.B. 1975. Automated hearing screening for newborns. The Crib-o-gram. In G.T. Mencher (Ed.), *Early Identification of Hearing Loss*. Basel: Karger.

Simmons, F.B. & Russ, F.W. 1974. Automated hearing screening: The Crib-o-gram. *Archives of Otolaryngology*, 100, 1.

Simms, B. 1986. Learner drivers with spina bifida and hydrocephalus. The relationship between perceptual-cognitive deficit and driving performance. *Zeitschrift für Kinderchirurgie*, 41, 51.

Simonds, J.F. & Aston, L. 1980. Preterm birth, low birth weight and hyperkinetic behavior in children. *Southern Medical Journal*, 73, 1237.

Simpson, J.L. 1976. *Disorders of Sexual Differentiation*. New York: Academic Press.

Singer, J.E., Westphal, M. & Niswander, K.R. 1968. Sex differences in the incidence of neonatal abnormalities and abnormal performance of early childhood. *Child Development*, 39, 103.

Singh, V. & Ling, G.M. 1979. Amphetamines in the management of children's hyperkinesis. *Bulletin on Narcotics*, 31, 87.

Siqueland, E.R. 1973. Biological and experiential determinants of exploration in infancy. In L. Stone, H. Smith & C. Murphy (Eds.), *The Competent Infant*. New York: Basic Books.

Siqueland, E.R. 1981. Studies of visual recognition memory in preterm infants: Differences in development as a function of perinatal morbidity factors. In S.L. Friedman & M. Sigman (Eds.), *Preterm Birth and Psychological Development*. New York: Academic Press.

Skeffington, F.S. 1982. Agenesis of the corpus callosum: Neonatal ultrasound appearances. *Archives of Disease in Childhood*, 57, 713.

Sklar, R. 1986. Nutritional vitamin B_{12} deficiency in a breast-fed infant of a Vegan-diet mother. *Clinical Pediatrics*, 25, 219.

Slater, A. & Morrison, V. 1991. Visual attention and memory at birth. In M.J.S. Weiss & P.R. Zelazo (Eds.), *Newborn Attention: Biological Constraints and the Influence of Experience*. Norwood, NJ: Ablex, p. 257.

Slater, B.C. 1963. Epidemiology of congenital malformations. *Developmental Medicine and Child Neurology*, 5, 351.

Slee, P.T. 1984. The nature of mother-infant gaze during interaction as a function of emotional expression. *Journal of the American Academy of Child Psychiatry*, 21, 385.

Slooff, A.C. & Slooff, J.L. 1975. Supratentorial tumours in childhood. *Clinical Neurology and Neurosurgery*, 78, 187.

Small, L. 1982. *The Minimal Brain Dysfunctions: Diagnosis and Treatment*. New York: The Free Press.

Smith, A. 1966. Speech and other functions after left (dominant) hemispherectomy. *Journal of Neurology, Neurosurgery and Psychiatry*, 29, 467.

Smith, A. 1969. Nondominant hemispherectomy. *Neurology*, 19(5), 442.

Smith, A. 1974. Dominant and nondominant hemispherectomy. In M. Kinsbourne & W. Lynn Smith (Eds.), *Hemispheric Disconnection and Cerebral Function*. Springfield, IL: Charles C Thomas.

Smith, A. & Burklund, C. 1966. Dominant hemispherectomy: Preliminary report on neuropsychological sequelae. *Science*, 153, 1280.

Smith, A. & Sugar, O. 1975. Development of above-normal language and intelligence 21 years after left hemispherectomy. *Neurology*, 25, 813.

Smith, A., Walker, M.L. & Myers, G. 1988. Hemispherectomy and diaschisis: Rapid improvement in cerebral functions after right hemispherectomy in a six year old child. *Archives of Clinical Neuropsychology*, 3, 1.

Smith, A.C., Flick, G.L., Ferriss, G.S. & Sellmann, A.H. 1972. Prediction of developmental outcome at seven years from prenatal, perinatal, and postnatal events. *Child Development*, 43, 495.

Smith, C.A. 1975. The inner ear: Its embryological development and microstructure. In D.B. Tower (Ed.), *The Nervous System, Vol. 3: Human Communication and Its Disorders*. New York: Raven Press.

Smith, D.J. 1971. Minor malformations: Their relevance and significance. In E.B. Hook, D.T. Janerich & I.H. Porter (Eds.), *Monitoring, Birth Defects and Environment. The Problem of Surveillance*. New York: Academic Press, p. 169.

Smith, D.W. 1988. *Recognizable Patterns of Human Malformations: Genetic, Embryologic and Clinical Aspects*, 4th ed. Philadelphia: W.B. Saunders.

Smith, E.S. 1954. Purulent meningitis in infants and children. *Journal of Pediatrics*, 45, 425.

Smith, H.F. 1986. The elephant on the fence: Approaches to the psychotherapy of attention deficit disorder. *American Journal of Psychotherapy*, 40, 252.

Smith, I., Lobascher, M.E., Stevenson, J.E., Wolff, O.H., Schmidt, H., Grubel-Kaiser, S. & Bickel, H. 1978. Effect of stopping low-phenylalanine diet on intellectual progress of children with phenylketonuria. *British Medical Journal*, 2, 723.

Smith, M., Grant, L. & Sors, A.I. 1989. *Lead Exposure and Child Development, An International Assessment*. Hingham, MA: Kluwer Academic.

Smith, M.L. & Milner, B. 1988. Estimation of frequency of occurrence of abstract designs after frontal and temporal lobectomy. *Neuropsychologia*, 26, 297.

Smith, N. 1970. Replication studies. *American Psychologist*, 25, 970–975.

Smith, N.V. 1975. Universal tendencies in the child's acquisition of phonology. In N.O. O'Connor (Ed.), *Language, Cognitive Deficits and Retardation*. London: Butterworths.

Smoll, F.L. & Schutz, R.W. 1990. Quantifying gender differences in physical performance: A developmental perspective. *Developmental Psychology*, 26, 360.

Smyth, T.R. & Glencross, D.J. 1986. Information processing deficits in clumsy children. *Australian Journal of Psychology*, 38, 13.

Snart, F., O'Grady, M. & Das, J.P. 1982. Cognitive processing by subgroups of moderately mentally retarded children. *American Journal of Mental Deficiency*, 86, 465.

Snowling, M. & Frith, U. 1986. Comprehension in "hyperlexic" readers. *Journal of Experimental Child Psychology*, 42, 392.

Snyder, L.H., Schonfeld, M.D. & Offerman, E.M. 1945. A further note in the Rh factor and feeblemindedness. *Journal of Heredity*, 36, 334.

Sobotkova, D., Tautermannova, M., Dittrichova, J. & Tomanova, J. 1983. Factors affecting psychoneurological conditions of children at the age of 6 years. *Activitas Nervosa Superior*, 25, 191.

Sohlberg, S.C. 1985. Personality and neuropsychological performance of high-risk children. *Schizophrenia Bulletin*, 11, 48.

Sohns, G. 1980. Empirische Untersuchung zur visuellen Wahrnehmungsleistung von Behinderten, Hirngeschädigten, Anfallskranken Kindern und Jugendlichen. Ph.D. Dissertation, University of Bielefeld.

Sohns, G. 1981. Der Einfluss des actuellen Anfallsgeschehens auf Leistungs-und

Persönlichkeitsmerkmale bei kindlichen Epilepsien. *Archiv für Psychiatrie und Nervenkrankheiten,* 231, 111.

Solan, H.A. 1987a. A comparison of the influences of verbal-successive and spatial-simultaneous factors on achieving readers in fourth and fifth grade: A multivariate correlational study. *Journal of Learning Disabilities,* 20, 237.

Solan, H.A. 1987b. The effects of visuo-spatial and verbal skills on written and mental arithmetic. *Journal of the American Optometric Association,* 58, 88.

Solitaire, G.B. & Lamarche, J.B. 1966. Alzheimer's disease and senile dementia as seen in mongoloids: Neuropathological observations. *American Journal of Mental Deficiency,* 70, 840.

Solursh, L.P., Margulies, A., Ashem, B. & Stasiak, E. 1965. The relationship of agenesis of the corpus callosum to perception and learning. *Journal of Nervous and Mental Diseases,* 141, 180.

Sontheimer, D. 1989. Visual information processing in infancy. *Developmental Medicine and Child Neurology,* 31, 787.

Soper, H.V., Satz, P., Orsini, D.L., Van Gorp, W.G. & Green, M.F. 1987. Handedness distribution in a residential population with severe and profound mental retardation. *American Journal of Mental Deficiency,* 92, 94.

Sostek, A.M., Quinn, P.O. & Davitt, M.K. 1979. Behavior, development and neurologic status of premature and full-term infants with varying medical complications. In T. Field, A.M. Sostek, S. Goldberg & H.H. Shuman (Eds.), *Infants Born at Risk.* New York: Spectrum.

Sostek, A.M., Smith, Y.F., Katz, K.S. & Grant, E.G. 1987. Developmental outcome of preterm infants with intraventricular hemorrhage at one and two years. *Child Development,* 58, 779.

Spearman, C. 1927. *The Abilities of Man.* New York: Macmillan.

Spehlmann, R. 1981. The normal EEG from premature age to the age of 19 years. In R. Spehlmann (Ed.), *EEG Primer.* Amsterdam: Elsevier/North-Holland Biomedical Press.

Spehlmann, R., Gross, R.A., Ho, S.U., Leestma, J.E. & Norcross, K.A. 1977. Visual evoked potentials and postmortem findings in a case of cortical blindness. *Annals of Neurology,* 2, 531.

Spellacy, F. & Black, F.W. 1972. Intelligence assessment of language-impaired children by means of two nonverbal tests. *Journal of Clinical Psychology,* 28, 357.

Spellacy, F. & Peter, B. 1978. Dyscalculia and elements of the developmental Gerstmann syndrome in school children. *Cortex,* 14, 197.

Sperry, R.W. 1963. Chemoaffinity in the orderly growth of nerve fibre patterns and connections. *Proceedings of the National Academy of Sciences,* 50, 703.

Sperry, R.W. 1968. Plasticity of neural maturation. *Developmental Biology* Suppl., 2, 36.

Sperry, R.W. 1970. Perception in the absence of the neocortical commissures. Research Publications, *Association for Research in Nervous and Mental Diseases (Perception and Its Disorders),* 68, 123.

Sperry, R.W. 1971. How a developing brain gets itself properly wired for adaptive function. In E. Tobach, L.R. Aronson & E. Shaw (Eds.), *The Biopsychology of Development.* New York: Academic Press.

Sperry, R.W., Gazzaniga, M.S. & Bogen, J.E. 1969. Interhemispheric relationships: The neocortical commissures: Syndromes of hemispheric disconnection. In P.J. Vinken & G.W. Bruyn (Eds.), *Handbook of Clinical Neurology,* Vol. 4. Amsterdam: North-Holland.

Spitz, R. 1945. Hospitalism: An enquiry into the genesis of psychiatric conditions in early childhood. *Psychoanalytic Study of the Child*, 1, 53.

Spitz, R. & Wolf, K.M. 1946. Anaclitic depression: An enquiry into the genesis of psychiatric conditions in early childhood. *Psychoanalytic Study of the Child*, 2, 313.

Spreen, O. 1978a. *Learning Disabled Children Growing Up: Final Report to Canada Health and Welfare.* Victoria: University of Victoria.

Spreen, O. 1978b. The dyslexias: A discussion of neurobehavioural research. In A.L. Benton & D. Pearl (Eds.), *Dyslexia. An Appraisal of Current Knowledge,* New York: Oxford University Press.

Spreen, O. 1981. The relationship between learning disability, neurological impairment and delinquency: Results of a follow-up study. *Journal of Nervous and Mental Diseases*, 169, 791.

Spreen, O. 1988a. Prognosis of learning disability. *Journal of Consulting and Clinical Psychology*, 56, 836.

Spreen, O. 1988b. *Learning Disabled Children Growing Up: A Follow-Up into Adulthood.* New York: Oxford University Press.

Spreen, O. 1989a. The relationship between learning disability, emotional disorders, and neuropsychology: Some results and observations. *Journal of Clinical and Experimental Neuropsychology*, 11, 117.

Spreen, O. 1989b. Learning disability, neurology, and long-term outcome: Some implications for the individual and for society. *Journal of Clinical and Experimental Neuropsychology*, 11, 389.

Spreen, O. & Anderson, C.W.G. 1966. Sibling relationship and mental deficiency diagnosis as reflected in Wechsler test patterns. *American Journal of Mental Deficiency*, 71, 406.

Spreen, O., Benton, A.L. & Van Allen, M. 1966. Dissociation of visual and tactile naming in amnestic aphasia. *Neurology*, 16, 807.

Spreen, O. & Gaddes, W.H. 1969. Developmental norms for 15 neuropsychological tests, age 6 to 15. *Cortex*, 5, 171.

Spreen, O. & Haaf, R.G. 1986. Empirically derived learning disability subtypes: A replication attempt and longitudinal patterns over 15 years. *Journal of Learning Disabilities*, 19, 170.

Spreen, O. & Lawriw, I. 1980. Neuropsychological test results as predictors of outcome of learning handicap in late adolescence and early adulthood. Paper presented at the International Neuropsychological Society, San Francisco.

Sprick, U. & Sprick, C. 1991. Subcutaneous injection of carbachol enhances brain-graft induced recovery of memory function by circumventing the blood barrier. *Behavioral and Brain Research*, 43, 175.

Springer, S.P. & Deutsch, G. 1989. *Left Brain, Right Brain*, 3rd ed. San Francisco: W.H. Freeman.

Stackhouse, J. 1982. An investigation of reading and spelling performance in speech disordered children. *British Journal of Disorders of Communication*, 17, 53.

Stagno, S. 1980. Congenital toxoplasmosis. *American Journal of Diseases of Children*, 134, 635.

Stamm, J.S. & Kreder, S.V. 1979. Minimal brain dysfunction: Psychological and neurophysiological disorders in hyperkinetic children. In M.S. Gazzaniga (Ed.), *Neuropsychology.* New York: Plenum Press.

Stanovich, K.E. 1985. Cognitive processes and the reading problems of learning-disabled children: Evaluating the assumption of specificity. In J.K. Torgeson & B.Y.L. Wong

(Eds.), *Psychological and Educational Perspectives on Learning Disabilities*. New York: Academic Press, p. 87.

Starr, S.E. 1979. Cytomegalovirus. *Pediatric Clinics of North America*, 26, 283.

Stavraky, G.W. 1961. *Supersensitivity Following Lesions of the Nervous System*. Toronto: University of Toronto Press.

Stefanko, S.Z. & Schenk, V.W.D. 1979. Anatomical aspects of agenesis of the corpus callosum in man. In I. Steele Russell, M.W. Van Hof & G. Berlucchi (Eds.), *Structure and Function of Cerebral Commissures*. Baltimore: University Park Press.

Stefanotos, G.A., Green, G.G. & Ratcliff, G.G. 1989. Neurophysiological evidence of auditory channel anomalies in developmental dysphasia. *Archives of Neurology*, 46, 871.

Stein, B.E. & Gordon, B. 1981. Maturation of the superior colliculus. In R.N. Aslin, J.R. Alberts & M.R. Petersen (Eds.), *Development of Perception: Psychobiological Perspectives. Vol. 2: The Visual System*. New York: Academic Press.

Stein, L. 1988. Hearing impairment. In V.B. van Hasselt, P.S. Strain & M. Hersen (Eds.), *Handbook of Developmental and Physical Disabilities*. New York: Pergamon Press.

Stein, Z., Susser, M., Saenger, G. & Marolla, F. 1975. *Famine and Human Development. The Dutch Hunger Winter of 1944–1945*. New York: Oxford University Press.

Stein, Z.A. & Susser, M.W. 1976. Prenatal nutrition and mental competence. In J.D. Lloyd-Still (Ed.), *Malnutrition and Intellectual Development*. Littleton, MA: Publishing Sciences Group, p. 39.

Steinberg, G., Troshinsky, C. & Steinberg, H. 1971. Dextroamphetamine responsive behavior disorders in school children. *American Journal of Psychiatry*, 128, 174.

Steiner, J.E. 1979. Human facial expression in response to taste and smell stimulation. In H.W. Reese & I.P. Lipsitt (Eds.), *Advances in Child Development and Behavior*. New York: Academic Press, p. 13.

Steinhausen, H.C. 1982. Das hyperkinetische Syndrom: Klinische Befunde und Validität der Diagnose. In H.C. Steinhausen (Ed.), *Das konzentrationsgestörte und hyperaktive Kind*. Stuttgard: Kohlhammer.

Steinhausen, H.C., Goebel, D. & Nestler, V. 1984. Psychopathology in the offspring of alcoholic parents. *Journal of the American Academy of Child Psychiatry*, 23, 465.

Steinwachs, F. & Barmeyer, H. 1952. Die Beziehungen der Feinmotorik zu den puberalen Alters- und Reifungsgraden. *Zeitschrift der menschlichen Vererbungs- und Konstitutionslehre*, 31, 174.

Stern, L. 1973. The use and misuse of oxygen in the newborn infant. *Pediatric Clinics of North America*, 20(2), 447.

Stevens, D.E. & Moffit, T.E. 1988. Neuropsychological profile of an Asperger syndrome case with exceptional calculating ability. *The Clinical Neuropsychologist*, 2, 228.

Stevens, J.R. 1990. Psychiatric consequences of temporal lobectomy for intractable seizures: A 20–30-year follow-up. *Psychological Medicine*, 20, 529.

Stevens, J.R. & Hermann, B.P. 1981. Temporal lobe epilepsy, psychopathology, and violence: The state of the evidence. *Neurology*, 31, 1127.

Stevenson, A.C., Johnston, H.A., Stewart, M.I. & Golding, D.R. 1966. *Congenital Malformations*. Bulletin, Suppl. 34. Geneva: World Health Organization.

Stevenson, J.E., Hawcroft, J., Lobascher, M., Smith, I., Wolff, O.H. & Graham, P.J. 1979. Behavioral deviance in children with early treated phenylketonuria. *Archives of Disease in Childhood*, 54, 14.

Stewart, M.A. 1980. Genetic perinatal and constitutional factors in MBD. In H.E. Rie & E.D. Rie (Eds.), *Handbook of Minimal Brain Dysfunction*, New York: Wiley.

Stewart, A. 1983. Severe perinatal hazards. In M. Rutter (Ed.), *Developmental Neuro-psychiatry.* New York: Guiford Press, p. 15.

Stewart, A.L. 1986. Follow-up studies. In N.R.C. Rogerton (Ed.), *Textbook of Neona-tology,* London: Churchill Livingstone.

Stewart-Brown, S., Haslum, M.N. & Butler, N. 1985. Educational attainment of 10-year-old children with treated and untreated visual defects. *Developmental Medicine and Child Neurology,* 27, 504.

Stiles, J. & Nass, R. 1991. Spatial grouping activity in young children with congenital right or left hemisphere brain injury. *Brain and Cognition,* 15, 201.

Stimmel, B. (Ed.) 1982. *The Effects of Maternal Alcohol and Drug Abuse on the New-born.* vol. 1, no. 3 and 4. New York: Haworth Press.

Stine, O.C., Saratsiotis, J.B. & Mosser, R.S. 1975. Relationships between neurological findings and classroom behavior. *American Journal of Diseases of Children,* 129, 1036.

Stjernqvist, K. & Svenningsen, N.W. 1990. Neurobehavioral development at term of extremely low-birthweight infants (< 901 g.) *Developmental Medicine and Child Neurology,* 32, 679.

Stockard, C.R. 1921. Developmental rate and structural expression: An experimental study of twins, double monsters and single deformities and their interaction among embryonic organs during their origins and development. *American Journal of Anat-omy,* 28, 115.

Stokman, C.J., Shafer, S.Q., Shaffer, D. & Ng, S.K.C. 1986. Assessment of neurological "soft signs" in adolescents: Reliability studies. *Developmental Medicine and Child Neurology,* 28, 428.

Stores, G. 1978. School-children with epilepsy at risk for learning and behavior prob-lems. *Developmental Medicine and Child Neurology,* 20, 502.

Stores, G., Hart, J. & Piran, N. 1978. Inattentiveness in school children with epilepsy. *Epilepsia,* 19, 169.

Stratton, P. 1982. Rhythmic functions in the newborn. In P. Stratton (Ed.), *Psychobiology of the Human Newborn.* New York: Wiley.

Stratton, P. 1984. Biological preprogramming of infant behavior. In S. Chess and A. Thomas (Eds.), *Annual Progress in Child Psychiatry and Child Development 1984.* New York: Brunner/Mazel, p. 5.

Strauss, A.A. & Kephart, N.C. 1955. *Psychopathology and Education of the Brain In-jured Child. Vol. 2: Progress in Theory and Practice.* New York: Grune & Stratton.

Strauss, A.A. & Lehtinen, L.E. 1947. *Psychopathology and Education of the Brain In-jured Child,* Vol. 1. New York: Grune & Stratton.

Strauss, E. 1982. Manual persistence in infancy. *Cortex,* 18, 319.

Strauss, E., Wada, J. & Hunter, M. 1994. Callosal morphology and performance on intelligence tests. *Journal of Clinical and Experimental Neuropsychology,* 16, 79.

Strauss, M. & Davis, G.L. 1973. Viral diseases of the labyrinths: Review of the literature and discussion of the role of cytomegalovirus in congenital deafness. *Annals of Otology, Rhinology and Laryngology,* 82, 577.

Streissguth, A.P., Dwyer, S., Martin, J. & Smith, D. 1980. Teratogenic effects of alcohol in women and laboratory animals. *Science,* 209, 355.

Streissguth, A.P., Clarren, S.K. & Jones, K.L. 1985. Natural history of the fetal alcohol syndrome: A 10-year follow-up of eleven patients. *Lancet,* 2, 85.

Streissguth, A.P., Barr, H.M. & Sampson, P.D. 1992. Alcohol use during pregnancy: A longitudinal, prospective study of human behavioral teratology. In C.W. Greenbaum & J.G. Auerbach (Eds.), *Longitudinal Studies of Children at Psychological Risk: Cross-National Perspectives.* Norwood, NJ: Ablex.

Strome, M. 1977. Sudden and fluctuating hearing losses. In B.F. Jaffe (Ed.), *Hearing Loss in Children.* Baltimore: University Park Press.

Stuss, D.T. & Benson, D.F. 1986. *The Frontal Lobes.* New York: Raven Press.

Stutsman, R. 1948. *Guide for Administering the Merrill-Palmer Scale of Mental Tests.* New York: Harcourt-Brace-Jovanovich.

Styles-Davis, J. 1988. Spatial dysfunction in young children with right cerebral hemisphere injury. In J. Styles-Davis, M. Kritchevsky & U. Bellugi (Eds.), *Spatial Cognition: Brain Bases and Development.* Hillsdale, NJ: Erlbaum, p. 251.

Suddath, R.L., Christison, G.W., Torrey, E.F., Casanova, M.F. & Weiberger, D.R. 1990. Anatomical abnormalities in the brains of monozygotic twins discordant for schizophrenia. *New England Journal of Medicine, 322,* 789.

Sugar, M. 1977. Five early milestones in premature infants. *Child Psychiatry and Human Development, 8,* 11.

Suskind, R.M. 1977. Characteristics and causation of protein-caloric malnutrition in the infant and preschool child. In L.S. Greene (Ed.), *Malnutrition, Behavior, and Social Organization.* New York: Academic Press, p. 1.

Sussman, K. & Lewandowski, L. 1990. Left-hemisphere dysfunction in autism: What are we measuring? *Archives of Clinical Neuropsychology, 5,* 137.

Sutcliffe, J.G., Milner, R.J., Gottesfeld, J.M. & Reynolds, W. 1984. Control of the neuronal gene expression. *Science, 225,* 1308.

Sverd, J., Curley, A.D., Jandorf, L. & Volkersz, L. 1988. Behavior disorder and attention deficit in boys with Tourette syndrome. *Journal of the American Academy of Child and Adolescent Psychiatry, 27,* 413.

Swaab, D.F. 1989. Relation between maturation of neurotransmitter systems in the human brain and psychosocial disorders. In M. Rutter & P. Casaer (Eds.), *Biological Risk Factors for Psychosocial Disorders.* Cambridge: Cambridge University Press, p. 50.

Swaab, D.F., Boer, G.J., Boer, J., Van Leeuwen, F.W. & Visser, M. 1978. Fetal neuroendocrine mechanisms in development and partuition. In M.A. Corner, R.E. Baker, N.E. van de Poll, D.F. Swaab & H.B.M. Uylings (Eds.), *Maturation of the Nervous System. Progress in Brain Research Vol. 48.* Amsterdam: Elsevier.

Sykes, D.H., Douglas, V.I. & Morgenstern, G. 1973. Sustained attention in hyperactive children. *Journal of Child Psychology and Psychiatry, 14,* 213.

Sykes, D.H., Douglas, V.I., Weiss, G. & Minde, K.K. 1971. Attention in hyperactive children and the effect of methylphenidate (Ritalin). *Journal of Child Psychology and Psychiatry, 12,* 129.

Sylvester, P.E. 1984. Nutritional aspects of Down's syndrome with special reference to the nervous system. *British Journal of Psychiatry, 145,* 115.

Szatmari, P., Offord, D.R. & Boyle, M.H. 1989. Ontario Child Health Study: Prevalence of attention deficit disorder with hyperactivity. *Journal of Child Psychology and Psychiatry, 30,* 219.

Szatmari, P., Offord, D.R., Siegel, L.S. & Finlayson, M.A. 1990a. The clinical significance of neurocognitive impairment among children with psychiatric disorders: Diagnosis and situational specificity. *Journal of Child Psychology and Psychiatry and Allied Disciplines, 31,* 287.

Szatmari, P., Saigal, S., Rosenbaum, P. & Campbell, D. 1990b. Psychiatric disorders at five years among children with birthweights <1000 g.: A regional perspective. *Developmental Medicine and Child Neurology*, 32, 954.

Szatmari, P., Tuff, L., Finlayson, A.J. & Bartolucci, G. 1990c. Asperger syndrome and autism: Neurocognitive aspects. *Journal of the American Academy of Child and Adolescent Psychiatry*, 29, 130.

Szelag, E., Wasilewski, R. & Fersten, E. 1992. Hemispheric differences in the perception of words and faces in deaf and hearing children. *Scandinavian Journal of Psychology*, 33, 1.

Tait, P.E. 1989. Optic nerve hypoplasia: A review of the literature. *Journal of Visual Impairment and Blindness*, 1989, 207.

Takano, T., Shimoto, M., Fukuhara, Y. & Itoh, K. 1989. Galactosialidosis: Clinical and molecular analysis of 19 Japanese patients. *Brain Dysfunction*, 4, 271.

Tallal, P. 1978. An experimental investigation of the role of auditory temporal processing in normal and disordered language development. In A. Caramazzo & E.B. Zurif (Eds.), *Language Acquisition and Language Breakdown, Parallels and Divergencies*. Baltimore: Johns Hopkins University Press.

Tallal, P. 1980. Auditory temporal perception, phonics, and reading disabilities in children. *Brain and Language*, 9, 182.

Tallal, P. & Piercy, M. 1978. Defects of auditory perception in children with developmental dysphasia. In M.A. Wyke (Ed.), *Developmental Dysphasia*. London: Academic Press.

Tallal, P., Stark, R.E., Kallman, C. & Mellitis, D. 1980. Developmental dysphasia: Relation between acoustic processing deficits and verbal processing. *Neuropsychologia*, 18, 273.

Tallal, P., Stark, R. & Mellits, D. 1985. The relationship between auditory temporal analysis and receptive language development: Evidence from some studies of developmental language disorder. *Neuropsychologia*, 23, 527.

Tallal, P., Dukette, D. & Curtiss, S. 1989a. Behavioral/emotional profiles of preschool language-impaired children. *Development and Psychopathology*, 1, 51.

Tallal, P., Ross, R. & Curtiss, S. 1989b. Unexpected sex ratios in families of language/learning-impaired children. *Neuropsychologia*, 27, 987.

Tallal, P., Allard, L. & Curtiss, S. 1991a. Otitis media in language-impaired and normal children. *Journal of Speech-Language Pathology and Audiology*, 15, 33.

Tallal, P., Townsend, J., Curtiss, S. & Wulfeck, B. 1991b. Phenotypic profiles of language-impaired children based on genetic/family history. *Brain and Language*, 41, 81.

Tamaki, N. & Ehara, K. 1992. Arteriovenous malformations: Indications and strategies for surgery. In A.J. Raimondi, M. Choux & C. DiRocco (Eds.), *Cerebrovascular Diseases in Children*. New York: Springer-Verlag, p. 59.

Tamis-LeMonda, C.S. & Bornstein, M.H., 1989. Infant habituation and maternal encouragement of attention at 5 months in relation to the development of language, play, and representational competence at 13 months. *Child Development*, 60, 738.

Tan, L.E. 1985. Laterality and motor skills in four-year-olds. *Child Development*, 56, 119.

Tanabe, H., Ikeda, M., Murasawa, A., Yamada, K., Yamamoto, H. & Nakagawa, Y. 1989. A case of acquired conduction aphasia in a child. *Acta Neurologica Scandinavica*, 80, 314.

Tanguay, P.E. 1984. Toward a new classification of serious psychopathology in children. *Journal of the American Academy of Child Psychiatry*, 23, 373.

Taub, H.B., Goldstein, K.M. & Caputo, D.V. 1977. Indices of neonatal prematurity as discriminators of development in middle childhood. *Child Development*, 48, 797.

Tautermannova, M., Mandys, F., Sobotkova, D. & Dittrichova, J. 1990. Neurological findings in adolescents showing MBD signs in preschool age. *Activitas Nervosa Superior*, 32, 154.

Taylor, D.C. 1976. Developmental strategems organizing intellectual skills: Evidence from studies of temporal lobectomy for epilepsy. In R.M. Knights & D.J. Bakker (Eds.), *The Neuropsychology of Learning Disorders*. Baltimore: University Park Press.

Taylor, H.G. 1983. MBD: Meanings and misconceptions. *Journal of Clinical Neuropsychology*, 5, 271.

Taylor, H.G. 1987. The meaning and value of soft signs in the behavioral sciences. In D.E. Tupper (Ed.), *Soft Neurological Signs*. Orlando: Grune & Stratton, p. 297.

Taylor, H.G. & Fletcher, J.M. 1983. Biological foundations of "specific developmental disorders": Methods, findings, and future directions. *Journal of Clinical Child Psychology*, 12, 46.

Teasdale, G. & Jennett, B. 1974. Assessment of coma and impaired consciousness: A practical scale. *Lancet*, 2, 81.

Teele, D.W., Klein, J.O., Chase, C., Menyuk, P. & Rosner, B.A. 1990. Otitis media in infancy and intellectual ability, school achievement, speech, and language at 7 years. *Journal of Infectious Diseases*, 162, 685.

Teeter, A. & Hynd, G.W. 1981. Agenesis of the corpus callosum: A developmental study during infancy. *Clinical Neuropsychology*, 3, 29.

Teller, D.Y. 1981. Color vision in infants. In R.N. Aslin, J.R. Alberts & M.R. Petersen (Eds.), *Development of Perception: Psychobiological Perspectives, Vol. 2*. New York: Academic Press.

Teller, D.Y. & Movshon, J.A. 1986. Visual development. *Vision Research*, 26, 1483.

Telzrow, R., Snyder, D., Tronick, E., Als, H. & Brazelton, T.B. 1976. The effects of phototherapy on neonatal behavior. Paper presented at the Meeting of the American Pediatric Society, St. Louis.

Temple, C.M. & Villarroya, O. 1990. Perceptual and cognitive perspective taking in two siblings with callosal agenesis. *British Journal of Developmental Psychology*, 8, 3.

Temple, C.M., Jeeves, M.A. & Villarroya, O. 1989. Ten pen men: Rhyming skills in two children with callosal agenesis. *Brain and Language*, 37, 548.

Terman, L.M. & Merrill, M.A. 1937. *Stanford-Binet Intelligence Scale: A Manual for the third revision, Form L-M*. Boston: Houghton Mifflin.

Terr, L.X. 1985. Children traumatized in small groups. In S. Eth and R. Pynoos (Eds.), *Post-Traumatic Stress Disorder in Children*. Washington, DC: American Psychiatric Association, p. 45.

Teszner, D., Tzavaras, A., Gruner, J. & Hecaen, H. 1972. L'asymetrie droite-gauche du planum temporale: A propos de l'etude anatomique de 100 cerveaux. *Revue Neurologique*, 126, 444.

Teti, D.M. & Gibbs, E.D. 1990. Infant assessment: Historical antecedents and contemporary issues. In E.D. Gibbs and D.M. Teti (Eds.), *Interdisciplinary Assessment of Infants. A Guide for Early Intervention Professionals*. Baltimore: Paul H. Brookes, p. 3.

Teti, D.M. & Nakagawa, M. 1990. Assessing attachment in infancy: The strange situation and alternative systems. In E.D. Gibbs & D.M. Teti (Eds.), *Interdisciplinary As-*

sessment of Infants. A Guide for Early Intervention Professionals. Baltimore: Paul H. Brookes, p. 191.

Teuber, H.L. 1966. The frontal lobes and their function: Further observations on rodents, carnivores, subhuman primates and man. *International Journal of Neurology,* 5, 282.

Teuber, H.L. 1975. Recovery of function after brain injury in man. In *Outcome of Severe Damage to the Central Nervous System,* CIBA Foundation Symposium 34 (new series). Amsterdam: Elsevier.

Teuber, H.L. & Rudel, R.C. 1967. Behavior after cerebral lesions in children and adults. *Developmental Medicine and Child Neurology,* 4, 3.

Teuber, H.L. & Rudel, R.C. 1971. Spatial orientation in normal children and in children with early brain injury. *Neuropsychologia,* 9, 401.

Tew, B. & Laurence, K. M. 1975. The effects of hydrocephalus on intelligence, visual perception and school attainment. *Developmental Medicine and Child Neurology* 17, 129.

Thal, D.J., Marchman, V.A., Stiles, J. & Aram, D. 1991. Early lexical development in children with focal brain injury. *Brain and Language,* 40, 491.

Thase, M.E. 1982. Longevity and mortality in Down's syndrome. *Journal of Mental Deficiency Research,* 26, 177.

Thatcher, R.W. 1980. Neurolinguistics: Theoretical and evolutionary perspectives. *Brain and Language,* 11, 235.

Theilgaard, A. 1984. A psychological study of the personalities of XYY- and XXY-men. *Acta Psychiatrica Scandinavica,* 89, Suppl. 515.

Thieverge, J., Bedard, C., Cote, R. & Maziade, M. 1989. Brainstem auditory evoked response and subcortical abnormalities in autism. *American Journal of Psychiatry,* 147, 1609.

Thoman, E.V., Ingersoll, E.W. & Acebo, C. 1991. Premature infants seek rhythmic stimulation, and the experience facilitates neurobehavioral development. *Developmental and Behavioral Pediatrics* 12, 11.

Thomas, A. & Chess, S. 1980. *The Dynamics of Psychological Development.* New York: Brunner/Mazel.

Thomas, A., Chess, S. & Birch, H.G. 1968. *Temperament and Behavior Disorders in Children.* New York: New York University Press.

Thomas, C.J. 1905. Congenital word-blindness and its treatment. *Ophthalmoscope,* 5, 380.

Thomasius, R. 1986. Hirnorganische Veränderungen nach Lösungsmittelmissbrauch. *Nervenarzt,* 57, 596.

Thompson, J.S., Ross, R.J. & Horwitz, S.J. 1980. The role of computed axial tomography in the child with minimal brain dysfunction. *Journal of Learning Disabilities,* 13, 334.

Thompson, R.A., Cicchetti, D., Lamb, M.E. & Malkin, C. 1985. Emotional responses of Down's syndrome and normal infants in the strange situation: The organization of affective behavior in infants. *Developmental Psychology,* 21, 828.

Thompson, R.F. 1967. *Foundations of Physiological Psychology.* New York: Harper & Row.

Thompson, R.J. 1984. Behavior problems in developmentally disabled children. *Advances in Developmental and Behavioral Pediatrics,* 5, 265.

Thompson, R.J. & O'Quinn, A.N. 1979. *Developmental Disabilities: Etiologies, Manifestations, Diagnoses, and Treatments.* New York: Oxford University Press.

Thomson, J.B. 1992. *Prediction of Stimulant Response in Children with ADHD.* Ph.D. Dissertation, University of Victoria.

Thorbert, G., Alm, P., Owman, C., Sjoeberg, N.-O. & Sporrong, B. 1978. Regional changes in structural and functional integrity of myometrical adrenergic nerves in pregnant guinea-pig and their relationship to the localization of the conceptus. *Acta Physiologica Scandinavica,* 130, 120.

Thornburg, H.D. 1982. *Development in Adolescence,* 2nd ed. Monterey: Brooks/Cole Publishing Company.

Thorndike, R.L., Hapen, E.O. & Sattler, J.M. 1986. *The Stanford-Binet Ingelligence Scales,* 4th ed. Chicago, IL: Riverside Publishing Co.

Thurstone, L.L. 1938. *Primary Mental Abilities.* Chicago: University of Chicago Press.

Tieman, S.B. & Hirsch, H. 1982. Effects of lines of only one orientation mode on the morphology of cells in the visual cortex of the cat. *Journal of Comparative Neurology,* 211, 353.

Timiras, P.S., Vernadakis, A. & Sherwood, N.M. 1968. Development and plasticity of the nervous system. In N.S. Assali (Ed.), *Biology of Gestation,* Vol. II. New York: Academic Press.

Timmermans, S.R. & Christensen, B. 1991. The measurement of attention deficit in TBI children and adolescents. *Cognitive Rehabilitation,* 9, 26.

Tinbergen, N. 1951. *On the Study of Instincts.* Amsterdam: North-Holland.

Tinuper, P., Andermann, F., Villemure, J.G., Rasmussen, T.B. & Quesney, L.F. 1988. Functional hemispherectomy for treatment of epilepsy associated with hemiplegia: Rationale, indications, results, and comparison with callosotomy. *Annals of Neurology,* 24, 27.

Tischler, B. & Lowry, R.B. 1978. Phenylketonuria in British Columbia, Canada. *Monographs of Human Genetics,* 9, 102.

Tizard, B. 1968. Observations of overactive imbecile children in uncontrolled environments. *American Journal of Mental Deficiency,* 72, 540.

Tjossem, T. 1976. *Intervention Strategies for High Risk Infants and Young Children.* Baltimore: University Park Press.

Toepfer, C.F. 1980. Brain growth periodization data: Some suggestions for rethinking middle grades education. *High School Journal,* 63, 222.

Toriello, H.V. & Carey, J.C. 1988. Corpus callosum agenesis, facial anomalies, Robin sequence, and other anomalies: A new autosomal recessive syndrome? *American Journal of Medical Genetics,* 31, 17.

Torrey, E.F. & Peterson, M.R. 1976. The viral hypothesis of schizophrenia. *Schizophrenia Bulletin,* 2, 136.

Touwen, B.C.L. 1972. Laterality and dominance. *Developmental Medicine and Child Neurology,* 14, 747.

Touwen, B.C.L. 1978a. Minimal brain dysfunction and minor neurological dysfunction. In A.F. Kalverboer, H.M. van Praag & J. Mendlevicz (Eds.), *Minimal Brain Dysfunction: Fact or Fiction?* Basel: Karger, p. 55.

Touwen, B.C.L. 1978b. Variability and stereotyping in normal and deviant development. In J. Apley (Ed.), *Care of the Handicapped Child.* Clinics in Developmental Medicine, No. 67, London: Heinemann, p. 99.

Touwen, B.C.L. 1979. *Examination of the Child with Minor Neurological Dysfunction,* 2nd ed. London: Heinemann.

Touwen, B.C.L. 1980. The preterm infant in the extrauterine environment. Implications for neurology. *Early Human Development,* 413, 287.

Touwen, B.C.L. & Sporrell, T. 1979. Soft signs and MBD. *Developmental Medicine and Child Neurology*, 21, 528.

Towbin, A. 1969a. Latent spinal cord and brain stem injury in newborn infants. *Developmental Medicine and Child Neurology*, 11, 54.

Towbin, A. 1969b. Mental retardation due to germinal matrix infarction. *Science*, 164, 156.

Towbin, A. 1970. Central nervous system damage in the human fetus and the newborn infant. *American Journal of the Disabled Child*, 119, 529.

Towbin, A. 1971. Organic causes of minimal brain dysfunction: Perinatal origin of minimal cerebral lesions. *Journal of the American Medical Association*, 217(9), 1207.

Townsend, J.J., Baringer, J.R., Wolinsky, J.S., Malamud, N., Mednick, J.P., Panitch, H.S., Scott, R.A.T., Oshiro, L.S. & Cremer, N.E. 1975. Progressive rubella panencephalitis, late onset after congenital rubella. *New England Journal of Medicine*, 292, 990.

Toyama, K., Komatsu, Y., Yamamoto, N. & Kurotani, T. 1991. In vitro approach to visual cortical development and plasticity. *Neuroscience Research*, 12, 57.

Trad, P.V. 1986. *Infant Depression: Paradigms and Paradoxes*. New York: Springer Verlag.

Tramontana, M.G. & Hooper, S.R. (Eds.) 1988. *Assessment Issues in Child Neuropsychology*. New York: Plenum Press.

Tramontana, M.G. & Hooper, S.R. (Eds.) 1992. *Advances in Child Neuropsychology*. New York: Springer.

Tramontana, M.G. & Sherrets, S.D. 1985. Brain impairment in child psychiatric disorders: Correspondence between neuropsychological and CT scan results. *Journal of the American Academy of Child Psychiatry*, 24, 590.

Tranel, D., Hall, L.E., Olson, S. & Tranel, N.N. 1987. Evidence for a right-hemisphere developmental learning disability. *Developmental Neuropsychology*, 3, 113.

Tredgold, A.F. 1914. *Mental Deficiency*. New York: William Wood.

Trehub, S.E. 1973. Infant's sensitivity to vowel and tonal contrasts. *Developmental Psychology*, 9, 81.

Trehub, S.E. 1979. Reflections on the development of speech perception. *Canadian Journal of Psychology*, 33(4), 368.

Trehub, S.E., Corter, C.M. & Shosenberg, N. 1983. Neonatal reflexes: A search for lateral asymmetry. In G. Young, S.J. Segalowitz, C.M. Corter & S.E. Trehub (Eds.), *Manual Specialization and the Developing Brain*. New York: Academic Press.

Trehub, S.E., Thorpe, L.A. & Morrongiello, B.A. 1987. Organizational processes in infants' perception of auditory patterns. *Child Development*, 58, 741.

Trescher, J.H. & Ford, F.R. 1937. Sectioning of the corpus callosum in a patient with colloid cyst. *Archives of Neurology and Psychiatry*, 37, 959.

Trevarthen, C. 1970. Experimental evidence for a brainstem contribution to visual perception in man. *Brain Behavior and Evolution*, 3, 338.

Trevarthen, C.B. 1973. Behavioral embryology. In E.C. Carterette & M.P. Friedman (Eds.), *Handbook of Perception, Vol. III: Biology of Perceptual Systems*. New York: Academic Press.

Trevarthen, C.B. 1974. Cerebral embryology and the split brain. In M. Kinsbourne & W. Lynn Smith (Eds.), *Hemispheric Disconnection and Cerebral Function*. Springfield, IL: Charles C Thomas.

Trevarthen, C. 1975. Psychological activities after forebrain commissurotomy in man: Concepts, and methodological hurdles in testing. In F. Michel & B. Schott (Eds.),

Les Syndromes de Disconnexion Calleuse Chez L'Homme (Colloque Internationale de Lyon, 1974). Lyon: Hopital Neurologique.

Trevarthen, C.B. 1990. Growth and education of the hemispheres. In C.B. Trevarthen (Ed.), *Brain Circuits and Functions of the Mind*. New York: Cambridge University Press, p. 334.

Trites, R.L. 1986. The Conners teacher rating scale: Reliability, validity, and normative data. In L.M. Bloomdale (Ed.), *Attention Deficit Disorder: New Treatments, Psychopharmacology, Attention Research*. New York: Spectrum Publications.

Tronick, E. & Brazelton, T.B. 1975. Clinical uses of the Brazelton neonatal behavioral assessment. In B.Z. Friedlander, G.M. Sterritt & G.E. Kirk (Eds.), *Exceptional Infant: Assessment and Interventions*, Vol. 3. New York: Brunner/Mazel.

Tronick, E., Wise, S., Als, H., Adamson, L., Scanlon, J., & Brazelton, T.B. 1976. Regional obstetric anesthesia and newborn behavior: Effect over the first ten days of life. *Journal of Pediatrics, 58, 94.*

Troup, G.A., Bradshaw, J.L. & Nettleton, N.C. 1983. The lateralization of arithmetic and number processing: A review. *International Journal of Neuroscience, 19, 231.*

Trunca, C. 1980. The chromosome syndromes. In J. Wortis (Ed.), *Mental Retardation and Developmental Disabilities: An Annual Review*, Vol. 11. New York: Brunner/Mazel, p. 188.

Tsuboi, T. & Nielsen, J. 1976. Electroencephalographic examination of 50 women with Turner's syndrome. *Acta Neurologica Scandinavica, 54, 359.*

Tsukahara, N. 1981. Synaptic plasticity in the mammalian central nervous system. *Annual Review of Neuroscience, 4, 351.*

Tsushima, W.T. & Towne, W.S. 1977. Neuropsychological abilities of young children with questionable brain disorders. *Journal of Consulting and Clinical Psychology, 44, 757.*

Tucker, D.M. 1990. Neural and psychological maturation in a social context. In C.B. Trevarthen (Ed.), *Brain Circuits and Functions of the Mind: Essays in Honor of Roger W. Sperry*. New York: Cambridge University Press, p. 334.

Tulving, E. 1983. *Elements of Episodic Memory*. Oxford: Oxford University Press.

Tuokko, H. 1982. Cognitive correlates of arithmetic performance in clinic referred children. Ph.D. Dissertation, University of Victoria, 1982.

Tupper, D.E. 1982. Behavioral correlates of the development of interhemispheric interaction in young children. Ph.D. dissertation. University of Victoria.

Tupper, D.E. (Ed.) 1987. *Soft Neurological Signs*. Orlando, FL: Grune & Stratton.

Turkewitz, G. 1977. The development of lateral differences in the human infant. In S. Harnard, et al. (Eds.), *Lateralization in the Nervous System*. New York: Academic Press.

Turkewitz, G. 1991. Perinatal influences on the development of hemispheric specialization and complex information processing. In M.J.S. Weiss and P.R. Zelazo (Eds.), *Newborn Attention: Biological Constraints and the Influence of Experience*. Norwood, NJ: Ablex, p. 443.

Turkewitz, G. & Birch, H. 1971. Neurobehavioral organization of the human newborn. In J. Hellmuth (Ed.), *The Exceptional Infant: Studies in Abnormalities*, Vol. 2, New York: Brunner/Mazel, p. 24.

Turkewitz, G. & Kenny, P.A. 1982. Limitations on input as a basis for neural organization and perceptual development: A preliminary theoretical statement. *Developmental Psychobiology, 15, 357.*

Turner, A.M. & Greenough, W.T. 1985. Differential rearing effects on rat visual cortex synapses. I. Synaptic and neuronal density and synapses per neuron. *Brain Research*, 329, 195.

Tyler, H.R. 1968. Neurologic disorders in renal failure. *American Journal of Medicine*, 44, 734.

Uddenberg, G. 1984a. Psychiatric assessment of children: I. Diagnostic method. *Neuropsychobiology*, 11, 77.

Uddenberg, G. 1984b. Psychiatric assessment of children: II. Comparison with mothers. *Neuropsychobiology*, 11, 80.

Ueda, K., Nishida, Y., Oshima, K. & Shephard, T. 1979. Congenital rubella syndrome: Correlation of gestational age at time of maternal rubella with type of defect. *Journal of Pediatrics*, 94, 763.

Ullman, D.B., Barkley, R.A., & Brown, H.W. 1978. The behavioral symptoms of hyperkinetic children who successfully responded to stimulant drug treatment. *American Journal of Orthopsychiatry*, 48, 425.

Ullman, R.K. & Sleator, E.K. 1986. Responders, nonresponders, and placebo responders among children with attention deficit disorder: Importance of a blinded placebo evaluation. *Clinical Pediatrics*, 25, 594.

Ulrey, G. 1982a. Influences of infant behavior on assessment. In G. Ulrey & S.J. Rogers (Eds.), *Psychological Assessment of Handicapped Infants and Young Children*. New York: Thieme-Stratton, p. 1.

Ulrey, G. 1982b. Assessment of cognitive development during infancy. In G. Ulrey & S.J. Rogers (Eds.), *Psychological Assessment of Handicapped Infants and Young Children*. New York: Thieme-Stratton, p. 35.

Ulrey, G. & Rogers, S.J. (Eds.) 1982. *Psychological Assessment of Handicapped Infants and Young Children*. New York: Thieme.

Ulrich, G. & Otto, W. 1984. Zur Bedeutung intermittierender rechts-posterior betonter langsamer Wellen im EEG psychiatrischer Patienten. *Fortschritte der Neurologie und Psychiatrie*, 52, 48.

Ultmann, M.H., Belman, A.L., Ruff, H.A., Novick, B.E., Cone-Wesson, B., Cohen, H.J. & Rubinstein, A. 1985. Developmental abnormalities in infants and children with acquired immune deficiency syndrome (AIDS) and AIDS-related complex. *Developmental Medicine and Child Neurology*, 27, 563.

Upadhyay, Y. 1971. A longitudinal study of full-term neonates with hyperbilirubinemia to four years of age. *Johns Hopkins Medical Journal*, 128, 273.

Urban, L. 1994. *Cellular Mechanisms of Sensory Processing: The Somatosensory System*. New York: Springer.

U.S. Government Printing Office. 1988. *International Classification of Diseases. Ninth Revision. Clinical Modification*, 3rd ed. Washington, DC: USGPO.

Uzgiris, I.C. & Hunt, J. McV. 1975. *Assessment in Infancy: Ordinal Scales of Psychological Development*. Urbana: University of Illinois Press.

Vandenberg, S.G. & Kuse, A.R. 1979. Spatial ability: A critical review of the sex-linked major gene hypothesis. In M.A. Wittig & A.C. Petersen (Eds.), *Sex-Related Differences in Cognitive Functioning: Developmental Issues*. New York: Academic Press.

Van Der Vlugt, H. 1979. Aspects of normal and abnormal neuropsychological development. In M.S. Gazzaniga (Ed.), *Neuropsychology*. New York: Plenum Press.

Van der Vlugt, H. 1989. Classification of learning disabilities. In D.J. Bakker & H. van der Vlugt (Eds.), *Learning Disabilities: Neuropsychological Correlates and Treatment*, Vol. 1. Amsterdam: Swets & Zeitlinger, p. 71.

Van de Sandt-Koenderman, W.M., Smit, I.A. & Van Dongen, H.R. 1984. A case of acquired aphasia and convulsive disorder: Some linguistic aspects of recovery and breakdown. *Brain and Language*, 21, 174.

van Dijk, J. 1982. Rubella-handicapped children: The effects of bilateral cataract and/or hearing impairment on behaviour and learning. Lisse, Netherlands: Swets and Zeitlinger.

Van Dongen, H.R. & Visch-Brink, E.G. 1988. Naming in aphasic children: Analysis of paraphasic errors. *Neuropsychologia*, 26, 629.

Van Duyne, H.J. 1982. The development of ear-asymmetry related to cognitive growth and memory in children. In R.N. Malatesha & L.C. Hartlage (Eds.), *Neuropsychology and Cognition*, Vol. II. The Hague: Martinus Vyhoff Publishers.

Van Gelder, R.S., Dijkman, M.M.T.T., Hopkins, B., van Geijn, G.P. & Homeau-Long, D.C. 1989. Fetal head orientation preference at the gestational ages of 16 and 24 weeks. *Journal of Clinical and Experimental Neuropsychology*, 11, 364.

Van Gorp, W.G., Hinkin, C.H., Satz, P., Miller, E., Drebing, C., Weisman, J., Hoston, S., Marcotte, T. & Dixon, W. 1992. Subtypes of HIV-associated neuropsychological performance: A cluster-analytic approach. *Journal of Clinical and Experimental Neuropsychology*, 14, 101 (Abstract).

Van Hof Van Duin, J. & Mohn, G. 1984. Visual defects in children after cerebral hypoxia. *Behavioral Brain Research*, 14, 147.

Van Sluyters, R.C. & Freeman, R.D. 1977. The physiological effects of brief periods of monocular deprivation in very young kittens. *Neurosciences Abstracts*, 3, 433.

Van Strien, J.W., Bouma, A. & Bakker, D.J. 1987. Birth stress, autoimmune disease, and handedness. *Journal of Clinical and Experimental Neuropsychology*, 9, 775.

Van Strien, J.W., Bouma, A. & Bakker, D.J. 1993. Lexical decision performances in P-type dyslexic, L-type dyslexic, and normal reading boys. *Journal of Clinical and Experimental Neuropsychology*, 15, 516.

van Wendt, L., Rantakallio, P., Saukkonen, A.L., Tuisku, M. & Makinen, H. 1985. Cerebral palsy and additional handicaps in a 1-year birth cohort from Northern Finland—A prospective follow-up study to the age of 14 years. *Annals of Clinical Research*, 17, 156.

Vargha-Khadem, F. 1982. Hemispheric specialization for the processing of tactual stimuli in congenitally deaf and hearing children. *Cortex*, 18, 277.

Vargha-Khadem, F. & Corballis, M.C. 1979. Cerebral asymmetry in infants. *Brain and Language*, 8, 1.

Vargha-Khadem, F., O'Gorman, A.M. & Watters, G.V. 1985. Aphasia and handedness in relation to hemispheric side, age at injury and severity of cerebral lesion during childhood. *Brain*, 108, 677.

Varnhagen, C.K., Das, J.P. & Varnhagen, S. 1987. Auditory and visual memory span: Cognitive processing by TMR individuals with Down syndrome or other etiologies. *American Journal of Mental Deficiency*, 91, 398.

Vaughan, H.G. & Kurtzberg, D. 1989. Electrophysiological indices of human brain maturation and cognitive development. In M.R. Gunnar & C.A. Nelson (Eds.), *Developmental Behavioral Neuroscience. The Minnesota Symposia on Child Development*, Vol. 24. Hillsdale, NJ: Erlbaum, p. 1.

Vazquez, H.J. & Turner, M. 1951. Epilepsia en flexion generalizada. *Archives of Argentine Pediatrics,* 35, 111.

Vellutino, F.R. 1982. Childhood dyslexia: A language disorder. In H.R. Myklebust (Ed.), *Progress in Learning Disabilities, Vol. 5: Language Disorders.* New York: Grune & Stratton.

verEecke, W. 1989. Seeing and saying no within the theories of Spitz and Lacan. *Psychoanalysis and Contemporary Thought,* 12, 383.

Verhulst, F.C. & Althaus, M. 1988. Persistence and change in behavioral/emotional problems reported by parents of children aged 4–14: An epidemiological study. *Acta Psychiatrica Scandinavica,* 77, Suppl. 339.

Verity, C.M., Strauss, E.H., Moyes, P.D., Wada, J.A., Dunn, H.G. & Lapointe, J.S. 1982. Long term follow-up after cerebral hemispherectomy: Neurophysiological, radiological, and psychological findings. *Neurology,* 32, 629.

Vernon, M. 1976. Prematurity and deafness: The magnitude and nature of the problem among deaf children. *Exceptional Children,* 36, 289.

Vernon, M.D. 1971. *Reading and Its Difficulties.* Cambridge: Cambridge University Press.

Vernon, P.A. 1994. *The Neuropsychology of Individual Differences.* San Diego: Academic Press.

Vernon, P.E. 1950. *The Structure of Human Abilities.* London: Methuen.

Vetter, D.K., Fay, W.H. & Winitz, H. 1980. Language. In F.M. Lassman, R.O. Fisch, D.K. Vetter & E.S. La Benz (Eds.), *Early Correlates of Speech, Language, and Hearing.* Littleton, MA: PSG Publishing, p. 267.

Villar, J. & Belizan, J.M. 1982. The timing factor in the pathophysiology of the intrauterine growth retardation syndrome. *Obstetrical and Gynecological Surveys* 37, 499.

Virchow, R. 1867. Zur pathologischen Anatomie des Gehirns: I. Congenitale Encephalitis und Myelitis. *Virchow's Archiv f ur Pathologische Anatomie und Physiologie f u Klinische Medizin,* 38, 129.

Visch-Brink, E.G. & Van de Sandt-Koenderman, M. 1984. The occurrence of paraphasias in the spontaneous speech of children with an acquired aphasia. *Brain and Language,* 23, 258.

Vitiello, B., Riciuti, A.J., Stoff, D.M. & Behar, D. 1989. Reliability of subtle (soft) neurological signs in children. *Journal of the American Academy of Child and Adolescent Psychiatry,* 28, 749.

Voeller, K.S. 1986. Right hemisphere deficit syndrome in children. *American Journal of Psychiatry,* 143, 1004.

Vogel, S. 1977. Morphological ability in normal and dyslexic children. *Journal of Learning Disabilities,* 10, 41.

Vohr, B.R. & Garcia-Coll, C.T. 1985. Neurodevelopmental and school performance of very low birth weight infants: A seven year longitudinal study. *Pediatrics,* 76, 345.

Vohr, B.R., Garcia-Coll, C. & Oh, W. 1989. Language and neurodevelopmental outcome of low-birthweight infants at three years. *Developmental Medicine and Child Neurology,* 31, 582.

Vohr, B.R., Oh, W., Rosenfield, A.G. & Lowett, R.M. 1979. The preterm small-for-gestational age infant: A two year follow-up study. *American Journal of Gynecology,* 133, 425.

Volkmar, F.R. 1984. EEG abnormalities in Tourette's syndrome. *Journal of the American Academy of Child Psychiatry,* 23, 352.

Volpe, J. 1976. Perinatal hypoxic ischemic brain injury. *Pediatric Clinics of North America*, 23, 383.

Volpe, J.J. 1977. Neonatal intracranial hemorrhage: Pathophysiology, neuropathology, and clinical features. *Clinics in Perinatalogy*, 4(1), 77.

Volpe, J.J. 1987. *Neurology of the Newborn*, 2nd ed. Philadelphia: W.B. Saunders.

Volpe, J.J. 1989. Intraventricular hemorrhage in the premature infant—Current concepts. Part 1. *Annals of Neurology*, 25, 3.

von Bonin, G. 1962. Anatomical asymmetries of the cerebral hemispheres. In V.B. Mountcastle (Ed.), *Interhemispheric Relations and Cerebral Dominance*. Baltimore: Johns Hopkins Press.

Vonderhaar, W.F. & Chambers, J.F. 1975. An examination of deaf students' Wechsler performance subtest scores. *American Annals of the Deaf*, 120(6), 540.

von Economo, C. 1929. *The Cytoarchitechtonics of the Human Cerebral Cortex*. London: Oxford University Press.

von Monakow, C. 1911. Lokalisation der Hirnfunktionen. *Journal für Psychologie und Neurologie*, 17, 185 (translated in G. von Bonin *Some Papers on the Cerebral Cortex*). Springfield, IL: Charles C Thomas.

Waber, D.P. 1977. Sex differences in mental abilities, hemispheric lateralization and rate of physical growth at adolescence. *Developmental Psychology*, 13(1), 29.

Waber, D.P. 1979a. Cognitive abilities and sex-related variations in the maturation of cerebral cortical functions. In M.A. Wittig & A.C. Petersen (Eds.), *Sex-Related Differences in Cognitive Functioning: Developmental Issues*. New York: Academic Press.

Waber, D.P. 1979b. Neuropsychological aspects of Turner's syndrome. *Developmental Medicine and Child Neurology*, 21, 58.

Wada, J.A. 1964. Longitudinal analysis of chronic epileptogenic brain processes. In *Epileptology, Clinical and Basic Aspects*. Tokyo: Igaku Shoin.

Wada, J.A. 1976. Cerebral anatomical asymmetry in infant brains. Paper presented at the International Neuropsychological Society, Toronto.

Wada, J.A., Clark, R. & Hamm, A. 1975. Cerebral hemispheric asymmetry in humans. *Archives of Neurology*, 32, 239.

Wagner, M.T., Williams, J.M. & Long, C.T. 1990. The role of social networks in recovery from head trauma. *International Journal of Clinical Neuropsychology*, 12, 131.

Wald, N. 1979. Radiation injury. In P.B. Beeson, M.D. McDermott & J.B. Wyngaarden (Eds.), *Cecil Textbook of Medicine*, Vol. 1. Philadelphia: W.B. Saunders.

Waldie, K. & Spreen, O. 1993. The relationship between learning disabilities and persisting delinquency. *Journal of Learning Disabilities*, 26, 417.

Waldrop, M.F. & Goering, J.D. 1971. Hyperactivity and minor physical anomalies in elementary school children. *American Journal of Orthopsychiatry*, 41, 602.

Waldrop, M.F. & Halverson, C.E. 1971. Minor physical anomalies and hyperactive behaviour in young children. In J. Hellmuth (Ed.), *The Exceptional Infant*. New York: Brunner/Mazel.

Waldrop, M.F., Pedersen, F.A. & Bell, R.O. 1968. Minor physical abnormalities and behavior in preschool children. *Child Development*, 39, 391.

Waldrop, M.R., Bell, R.Q. & Goering, J.D. 1976. Minor physical anomalies and inhibited behavior in elementary school girls. *Journal of Child Psychology and Psychiatry*, 17, 113.

Walker, E. & Emory, E. 1983. Infants at risk for psychopathology: Offspring of schizophrenic parents. *Child Development*, 54, 1269.

Walker, E., Hoppes, E. & Emory, E. 1981a. A reinterpretation of findings of hemispheric dysfunction in schizophrenia. *Journal of Nervous and Mental Disease*, 169, 378.

Walker, E., Hoppes, E., Emory, E., Mednick, S. & Schulsinger, F. 1981b. Environmental factors related to schizophrenia in psychophysiologically labile high-risk males. *Journal of Abnormal Psychology*, 49, 313.

Walker, R.W. & Rosenblum, M.K. 1992. Childhood medulloblastoma. *Revue Neurologique*, 148, 467.

Wallace, R.B., Kaplan, R. & Werboff, J. 1977. Hippocampus and behavioral maturation. *International Journal of Neuroscience*, 7, 185.

Wallace, I.F., Gravel, J.S., McCarton, C.M. & Ruben, R.J. 1988. Otitis media and language development at 1 year of age. *Journal of Speech and Hearing Disorders*, 53, 245.

Wallace, S.J. 1984. Febrile convulsions: Their significance for later intellectual development and behaviour. *Journal of Child Psychology and Psychiatry*, 25, 15.

Wallander, J.L., Feldman, W.S. & Varni, J.W. 1989. Physical status and psychosocial adjustment in children with spina bifida. *Journal of Pediatric Psychology*, 14, 89.

Wallander, J.L. & Varni, J.W. 1989. Social support and adjustment in chronically ill and handicapped children. *American Journal of Community Psychology*, 17, 185.

Walther, B. 1982. Nährungsphosphat und Verhaltensstörung im Kindesalter—Ergebnisse einer kontrollierten Diaetstudie. In H.C. Steinhausen (Ed.), *Das konzentrationsgestörte und hyperaktive Kind.* Stuttgart: Kohlhammer, 1982.

Ward, S. & McCartney, E. 1978. Congenital auditory imperception: A follow-up study. *British Journal of Disorders of Communication*, 13(1), 3.

Warner, E.N. 1935. A survey of mongolism with a review of 100 cases. *Canadian Medical Association Journal*, 33, 495.

Watemberg, J., Cermak, S.A. & Henderson, A. 1986. Right-left discrimination in blind and sighted children. *Physical and Occupational Therapy in Pediatrics*, 6, 7.

Watkins, A., Szymonowicz, W., Jin, X. & Victor, V. 1988. Significance of seizures in very low-birth weight infants. *Developmental Medicine and Child Neurology*, 30, 162.

Watt, J.M., Robertson, C.M.T. & Grace, M.G.A. 1989. Early prognosis for ambulation of neonatal intensive care survivors with cerebral palsy. *Developmental Medicine and Child Neurology*, 31, 766.

Webster, D.B. & Webster, M. 1979. Effects of neonatal conductive hearing loss on brainstem auditory nuclei. *Annals of Otolaryngology, Rhinology and Laryngology*, 88, 684.

Wechsler, D. 1958. *The Measurement and Appraisal of Adult Intelligence.* New York: Psychological Corporation.

Wechsler, D. 1963. *Wechsler Preschool and Primary Scale of Intelligence.* New York: The Psychological Corporation.

Wegman, M.E. 1981. Annual summary of vital statistics—1980. *Pediatrics*, 68, 755.

Weil, M.L., Itabashi, H.H., Cremer, N.E., Oshiro, L.S., Lennette, E.H. & Carnay, L. 1975. Chronic progressive panencephalitis due to rubella virus simulating subacute sclerosing panencephalitis. *New England Journal of Medicine*, 292, 994.

Weinberg, W.A. & McLean, A. 1986. A diagnostic approach to developmental specific learning disorders. *Journal of Child Neurology*, 1, 158.

Weiner, G. 1970. Varying psychological sequelae of lead ingestion in children. *Public Health Report*, 85, 19.

Weintraub, S. & Mesulam, M.M. 1983. Developmental learning disability of the right hemisphere. *Archives of Neurology*, 40, 463.

Weisglass, K.N., Baerts, W., Fetter, W.P. & Sauer, P.J. 1992. Neonatal cerebral ultrasound, neonatal neurology and perinatal conditions as predictors of neurodevelopmental outcome. *Early Human Development*, 31, 131.

Weiss, B., Weisz, J.R. & Bromfield, R. 1986. Performance of retarded and nonretarded persons on information-processing tasks: Further tests of the similar structure hypothesis. *Psychological Bulletin*, 100, 157.

Weiss, G. 1980. MBD: Critical diagnostic issues. In H.E. Rie and E.D. Rie (Eds.), *Handbook of Minimal Brain Dysfunction*. New York: Wiley.

Weiss, G., Hechtman, L., Milroy, T. & Perlman, T. 1985. Psychiatric status of hyperactives as adults: A controlled prospective 15-year follow-up of 63 hyperactive children. *Journal of the American Academy of Child Psychiatry*, 24, 211.

Weiss, G., Hechtman, L. & Perlman, T. 1978. Hyperactives as young adults: School, employer, and self-rating scales obtained during ten year follow-up evaluation. *American Journal of Orthopsychiatry*, 48, 438.

Weiss, G., Hechtman, L., Perlman, T., Hopkins, J. & Wener, A. 1979. Hyperactives as young adults: A controlled prospective 10-year follow-up of 75 children. *Archives of General Psychiatry*, 36, 675.

Weiss, G., Minde, K., Werry, J.S., Douglas, V. & Nemeth, E. 1971. Studies on the hyperactive child: Five year follow-up. *Archives of General Psychiatry*, 24, 409.

Weiss, M.J.A. & Zelazo, P.R. (Eds.) 1991. *Newborn Attention: Biological Constraints and the Influence of Experience*. Norwood, NJ: Ablex.

Weiss, W. & Jackson, E.C. 1969. Maternal factors affecting birth weight. In *Perinatal Factors Affecting Human Development*. Washington, DC: Pan American Health Organization.

Weissman, M.M., Wickramaratne, P., Warner, V., John, K., Prusoff, B.A., Merikangass, K.R. & Gammon, D. 1987. Assessing psychiatric disorders in children: Discrepancies between mother and children's reports. *Archives of General Psychiatry*, 44, 747.

Wellman, M.M. & Allen, M. 1983. Variations in hand position, cerebral lateralization and reading ability among right-handed children. *Brain and Language*, 18, 277.

Welsh, M.C. & Pennington, B.F. 1988. Assessing frontal lobe functioning in children: Views from developmental psychology. *Developmental Neuropsychology*, 4, 199.

Welsh, M.C., Pennington, B.F., Ozonoff, S., Rouse, B. & McCabe, E.R.B. 1990. Neuropsychology of early treated phenylketonuria: Specific executive function deficits. *Child Development*, 61, 1697.

Wen, D.Y., Seljeskog, E.L. & Haines, S.J. 1992. Microsurgical management of craniopharyngiomas. *British Journal of Neurosurgery*, 6, 467.

Wender, P.H. 1971. *Minimal Brain Dysfunction in Children*. New York: Wiley Interscience Series.

Wender, P.H. 1977. Speculations concerning a possible biochemical basis of MBD. In J.G. Millichap (Ed.), *Learning Disabilities and Related Disorders*. Chicago: Year Book Medical Publishers, p. 13.

Wender, P.H., Reimherr, F.W. & Wood, D.R. 1981. Attention deficit disorder ('minimal brain dysfunction') in adults. *Archives of General Psychiatry*, 38, 449.

Werker, J.F. & Tees, R.C. 1984. Cross-language speech perception: Evidence for perceptual reorganization during the first year of life. *Infant Behavior and Development*, 7, 49.

Werner, E., Berman, J. & French, F. 1971. *The Children of Kauai. A Longitudinal Study from the Prenatal Period to Age 10.* Honolulu: University of Hawaii Press.

Werner, E. & Smith, R. 1977. An epidemiological perspective on some antecedents and consequences of childhood mental health problems and learning disabilities. *American Academy of Child Psychology and Psychiatry,* 293.

Werner, H. 1953. *Einführung in die Entwicklungspsychologie,* 3rd ed. Frankfurt: Fischer.

Werner, H. & Strauss, A. 1940. Causal factors in low performance. *American Journal of Mental Deficiency,* 45, 213.

Wernicke, C. 1874. *Der aphasische Symptomenkomplex.* Breslau, Germany: M. Cohn & Weigert.

Werry, J.S. & Aman, M.G. 1976. The reliability and diagnostic validity of the physical and neurological examination for soft signs (PANESS). *Journal of Autism and Childhood Schizophrenia,* 6, 253.

Werry, J.S., Minde, K., Guzman, A., Weiss, G., Dogan, K. & Hoy, E. 1972. Studies on the hyperactive child. VII: Neurological status compared with neurotic and normal children. *American Journal of Orthopsychiatry,* 42, 441.

Werry, J.S., Weiss, G. & Douglas, V. 1964. Studies on the hyperactive child. I. Some preliminary findings. *Canadian Psychiatric Association Journal,* 2, 120.

Wersh, J. & Briere, J. 1981. WISC-R subtest variability in normal Canadian children and its relationship to sex, age and IQ. *Canadian Journal of Behavioural Science,* 13, 76.

Werthmann, M.W. 1981. Medical constraints to optimal psychological development of the preterm infant. In S.L. Friedman & M. Sigman (Eds.), *Preterm Birth and Psychological Development.* New York: Academic Press.

Westerveld, M., Sass, K.J., Lencz, T., Sass, A. & Stoddard, K.R. 1991. Effects of shunt malfunction, seizure, and gender on IQ and handedness in hydrocephalic children. *Journal of Clinical and Experimental Neuropsychology,* 13, 98.

Wewetzer, K.H. 1958. Zur Differenzierung der Leistungsstrukturen bei verschiedenen Intelligenzgraden. Report, 21. *Congress of Deutsche Gesellschaft für Psychologie,* Goettingen: Hogrefe, p. 245.

Wewetzer, K.H. 1975: Zur Differenzierung des organischen Psychosyndroms nach kindlichen Hirnschäden; Kurzbericht einer experimentellen Studie. *Diagnostica,* 21, 182.

Wexler, B.E. & Lipman, A.J. 1988. Sex differences in change over time in perceptual asymmetry. *Neuropsychologia,* 26, 943.

Wharry, R.E. & Kirkpatrick, S.W. 1986. Vision and academic performance of learning disabled children. *Perceptual and Motor Skills,* 62, 323.

White, D.A., Craft, S., Hale, S. & Park, T.S. 1994. Working memory and articulation rate in children with spastic diplegic cerebral palsy. *Neuropsychology,* 8, 180.

White, J.L., Moffit, T.E. & Silva, P.A. in press. Neuropsychological and socio-emotional correlates of specific-arithmetic-disability.

White, K.D. & Brackbill, Y. 1981. Visual development in pre- and full-term infants: A review of chapters 12–15. In S.L. Friedman and M. Sigman (Eds.), *Preterm Birth and Psychological Development.* New York: Academic Press.

White, L., Johnston, H., Jones, R., Mameghan, H., Nayanar, V., et al. 1993. Postoperative chemotherapy without radiation in young children with malignant non-astrocytic brain tumours: A report from the Australia and New Zealand Childhood Cancer Study Group (ANZCCSG). *Cancer Chemotherapy and Pharmacology,* 32, 403.

White, S.H. 1970. Some general outlines of the matrix of developmental changes between five and seven years. *Bulletin of the Orton Society*, 20, 41.

Whitehouse, D. 1976. Behavior and learning problems in epileptic children. *Behavioral Neuropsychiatry*, 7, 23.

Whitehouse, D. & Harris, J.C. 1984. Hyperlexia in infantile autism. *Journal of Autism and Developmental Disorders*, 14, 281.

Whiting, S., Jan, J.E., Wong, P.K.H., Flodmark, O., Farrell, K. & McCormick, A.Q. 1985. Permanent cortical visual impairment in children. *Developmental Medicine and Child Neurology*, 27, 730.

Whitman, S., Hermann, B.P. & Gordon, A.C. 1984. Psychopathology and epilepsy; How great is the risk. *Biological Psychiatry*, 19, 213.

Whittington, A.C. & Richards, M. 1991. Handedness and mathematical ability. *Proceedings of the Orton Society*.

Wiener, G., Rider, R.V., Oppel, W.C. & Harper, P.A. 1968. Correlates of low birth weight. Psychological status at eight to ten years of age. *Pediatric Research*, 2, 110.

Wiesniewski, K.E., Laure-Kamionawska, M., Connell, F. & Wen, G.Y. 1986. Neuronal density and synaptogenesis in the postnatal stages of brain maturation in Down's syndrome. In C.J. Epstein (Ed.), *The Neurobiology of Down Syndrome*. New York: Raven Press, p. 29.

Wikler, A., Dixon, J. & Parker, J. Jr. 1970. Brain function in problem children and controls: Psychometric, neurological and electroencephalographic comparison. *American Journal of Psychiatry*, 127, 634.

Wilcox, A.J., Maxey, J. & Herbst, A.L. 1992. Prenatal diethylstilbesterol exposure and performance on college entrance examinations. *Hormones and Behavior*, 26, 433.

Wiley, J. & Goldstein, D. 1991. Sex, handedness, and allergies: Are they related to academic giftedness? *Journal for the Education of the Gifted*, 14, 412.

Willems, G., Noel, A. & Evrard, P. 1972. L'examen neuropediatrique des fonctions d'apprentissage chez l'enfant en age prescolaire. *Revue Francaise d'Hygiene et de Medicine Scolaire et Universitaire*, 32, 3.

Willerman, L. 1973. Activity level and hyperactivity in twins. *Child Development*, 44, 288.

Williams, C.A., Quinn, H., Wright, E.C., Sylvester, P.E., Gosling, P.J.H. & Dickerson, J.W.T. 1985. Xylose absorption in Down's syndrome. *Journal of Mental Deficiency Research*, 29, 173.

Williams, J.I. & Cram, D.M. 1978. Diet in the management of hyperkinesis. A review of the tests of Feingold's hypotheses. *Canadian Psychiatric Association Journal*, 23, 241.

Williamson, G.G. & Zeitlin, S. 1990. Assessment of coping and temperament. Contributions to adaptive functioning. In E.D. Gibbs and D.M. Teti (Eds.), *Interdisciplinary Assessment of Infants. A Guide for Early Intervention Professionals*. Baltimore: Paul H. Brookes, p. 215.

Williamson, M.L., Koch, R., Azen, C. & Chang, C. 1981. Correlates of intelligence test results in treated phenylketonuric children. *Pediatrics*, 68, 161.

Williamson, W.D., Desmond, M.M., Andrew, L.P. & Hicks, R.N. 1987. Visually impaired infants in the 1980s. *Clinical Pediatrics*, 1987, 241.

Wills, K.E., Holmbeck, G.N., Dillon, K. & McLone, D.G. 1990. Intelligence and achievement in children with myelomeningocele. *Journal of Pediatric Psychology*, 15, 161.

Wilsher, C.R. 1986. The nootropic concept and dyslexia. *Annals of Dyslexia*, 36, 118.

Wilson, C.B., Remington, J.S., Stagno, S. & Reynolds, D.W. 1980. Development of adverse sequelae in children born with subclinical congenital toxoplasma infection. *Pediatrics,* 66, 767.

Wilson, J.G. 1973. *Environment and Birth Defects.* New York: Academic Press.

Wilson, J.G. 1977. Environmental chemicals. In J.G. Wilson and F.C. Frazer (Eds.), *Handbook of Teratology,* Vol. 1. New York: Plenum.

Wilson, P.J.E. 1970. Cerebral hemispherectomy for infantile hemiplegia: A report of 50 cases. *Brain,* 93, 147.

Windle, W.F. 1971. Origin and early development of neural elements in the human brain. In E. Tobach, L.R. Aronsen & E. Shaw (Eds.), *The Biopsychology of Development.* New York: Academic Press.

Wing, J. 1966. Diagnosis, epidemiology and etiology. In J. Wing (Ed.), *Early Childhood Autism.* Oxford: Pergamon Press.

Winick, M. 1970. Cellular growth in intrauterine malnutrition. *Pediatric Clinics of North America,* 17, 69.

Winick, M. 1976. *Malnutrition and Brain Development.* New York: Oxford University Press.

Winick, M. & Rosso, P. 1969. The effect of severe early malnutrition on cellular growth of human brain. *Pediatric Research,* 3, 181.

Winokur, G. & Tanna, V.L. 1969. Possible role of X-linked dominant factor in manic-depressive disease. *Diseases of the Nervous System,* 30, 89.

Wishart, J.G. 1987. Performance of young nonretarded children and children with Down syndrome on Piagetian infant search tasks. *American Journal of Mental Deficiency,* 92, 169.

Witelson, S.F. 1976a. Abnormal right hemispheric specialization in developmental dyslexia. In R. Knights & D. Bakker (Eds.), The *Neuropsychology of Learning Disorders.* Baltimore: University Park Press.

Witelson, S.F. 1976b. Sex and the single hemisphere: Specialization of the right hemisphere for spatial processing. *Science,* 193, 425.

Witelson, S.F. 1977. Neural and cognitive correlates of developmental dyslexia: age and sex differences. In C. Shagass, S. Gershan & A.J. Friedhoff (Eds.), *Psychopathology and Brain Dysfunction.* New York: Raven Press.

Witelson, S.F. 1985. On hemisphere specialization and cerebral plasticity from birth: Mark II. In C. Best (Ed.), *Hemispheric Function and Collaboration in the Child.* New York: Academic Press, p. 33.

Witelson, S.F. 1987. Neurobiological aspects of language in children. *Child Development,* 58, 653.

Witelson, S.F. 1990. Neuroanatomical bases of hemispheric functional specialization in the human brain: Developmental factors. In I. Kostovic, S. Knezevic, H.M. Wisnioewski & G.J. Spilich (Eds.), *Neurodevelopment, Aging, and Cognition.* Boston, MA: Birkhauser, p. 112.

Witelson, S.F. & Pallie, W. 1973. Left hemisphere specialization for language in the newborn: Neuroanatomical evidence of asymmetry. *Brain,* 96, 641.

Witelson, S.F. & Swallow, J.A. 1988. Neuropsychological study of the development of spatial cognition. In J. Stiles-Davis, M. Kritchevsky & U. Bellugi (Eds.), *Spatial Cognition: Brain Bases and Development.* Hillsdale, NJ: Erlbaum.

Witkin, H.A., Mednick, S.A., Schulsinger, F., Bakkestrom, E., Christiansen, K.O. Goodenough, D.R., Hirschhorn, K., Lundsteen, C., Owen, D.R., Philip, J., Rubin, D.B. & Stocking, M. 1976. Criminality in XYY and XXY men. *Science,* 193, 547.

Wittig, M.A. & Petersen, A.C. (Ed.) 1979. *Sex-Related Differences in Cognitive Functioning, Developmental Issues*. New York: Academic Press.

Wolf, L. & Goldberg, B. 1986. Autistic children grow up: An eight to twenty-four year follow-up study. *Canadian Journal of Psychiatry*, 31, 550.

Wolf, M. & Goodglass, H. 1986. Dyslexia, dysnomia, and lexical retrieval: A longitudinal investigation. *Brain and Language*, 28, 154.

Wolf, S.M. & Forsythe, A. 1978. Behavior disturbance, phenobarbital, and febrile seizures. *Pediatrics*, 61, 728.

Wolff, A.B. & Thatcher, R.W. 1990. Cortical reorganization in deaf children. *Journal of Clinical and Experimental Neuropsychology*, 12, 209.

Wolff, J.R. 1978. Ontogenetic aspects of cortical architecture: Lamination. In M.A.B. Brazier & H. Petsche (Eds.), *Architectonics of the Cerebral Cortex*. New York: Raven Press.

Wolff, P.H. 1966. The causes, controls and organization of behavior in the neonate. *Psychological Issues*, 5, 1 (Monograph 17).

Wolff, P.H., Gunnoe, C. & Cohen, C. 1985. Neuromotor maturation and psychological performance: A developmental study. *Developmental Medicine and Child Neurology*, 27, 344.

Wolff, P.H. & Hurwitz, I. 1973. Functional implications of the minimal brain damage syndrome. *Seminars in Psychiatry*, 5, 105.

Wolff, P.H., Waber, D., Bauermeister, M., Cohen, C. & Ferber, R. 1982. The neuropsychological status of adolescent delinquent boys. *Journal of Child Psychology and Psychiatry*, 23, 267.

Wolff, S. 1970. Behavior of pathology of parents of disturbed children. In E.J. Anthony & C. Vioupernik (Eds.), *The Child in his Family*, Vol. 1. New York: Wiley.

Wolff, S. 1971. Dimensions and clusters of symptoms in disturbed children. *British Journal of Psychiatry*, 118, 421.

Wolff, S., Narayan, S. & Moyes, B. 1988. Personality characteristics of parents of autistic children. *Journal of Child Psychology and Psychiatry and Allied Disciplines*, 29, 143.

Wolfson, R.J., Aghamohamadi, A.M. & Berman, S.E. 1980. Disorders of hearing. In S. Gabel and M.T. Erickson (Eds.), *Child Development and Developmental Disabilities*. Boston: Little, Brown and Company.

Wong, D. & Shah, C.P. 1979. Identification of impaired hearing in early childhood. *Canadian Medical Association Journal*, 121, 529.

Wong, V. & Wong, S.N. 1991. Brainstem auditory evoked potential study in children with autistic disorder. *Journal of Autism and Developmental Disorders*, 21, 329.

Wood, N.E. 1975. Assessment of auditory processing dysfunction. *Acta Symbolica*, 6, 113.

Woods, B.T. & Carey, S. 1979. Language deficits after apparent clinical recovery from childhood aphasia. *Annals of Neurology*, 6, 405.

Woods, B.T. & Teuber, H.L. 1973. Early onset of complementary specialization of cerebral hemispheres in man. *Transactions of the American Neurological Association*, 98, 113.

Woods, B.T. & Teuber, H.L. 1978. Mirror movements after childhood hemiparesis. *Neurology*, 28, 1152.

Woollacott, M.H. 1990. Development of postural equilibrium during sitting and standing. In H. Bloch and B.I. Bertenthal (Eds.), *Sensory-motor Organizations and Development in Infancy and Childhood*. Dordrecht, Netherlands: Kluwer, p. 217.

Woolsey, T.A., Durham, D., Harris, R., Simons, D.J. & Valentino, K. 1981. Somatosensory development. In R.N. Aslin, J.R. Alberts & M.R. Petersen (Eds.), *Development of Perception: Psychological Perspectives. Vol. 1. Audition, Somatic Perception and Chemical Senses.* New York: Academic Press.

World Health Organization. 1961. *Public Health Aspects of Low Birth Weight.* Third Report of the Expert Committee on Maternal Care and Child Care. Geneva: WHO.

World Health Organization. 1983. *Infant and Young Child Nutrition* (Report by the Director General to the World Health Assembly. Document WHA 36/1983/70). Geneva: WHO.

World Health Organization. 1993. *Manual of the International Statistical Classification of Diseases, Injuries and Causes of Death,* ICD-10. Vols. 1 & 2. Geneva: World Health Organization.

Worster-Drought, C. & Allen, I.M. 1929a. Congenital auditory imperception (congenital word-deafness) with report of a case. *Journal of Neurology and Psychopathology,* 9, 193.

Worster-Drought, C. & Allen, I.M. 1929b. Congenital auditory imperception (congenital word-deafness); Investigation of a case by Head's method. *Journal of Neurology and Psychopathology,* 9, 289.

Wright, H.H., Young, S.R., Edwards, J.G., Abramson, R.K. & Duncan, J. 1986. Fragile X syndrome in a population of autistic children. *Journal of the American Academy of Child Psychiatry,* 25, 641.

Wright, L. & Jimmerson, S. 1971. Intellectual sequelae of *Homophilus influenzae* meningitis. *Journal of Abnormal Psychology,* 77, 181.

Wright, P.F., Sell, S.H., McConnell, K.B., Sitton, A.B., Thompson, J., Vaughn, W.K. & Bess, F.H. 1988. Impact of recurrent otitis media on middle ear function, hearing, and language. *Journal of Pediatrics,* 113, 581.

Wright, S.W. & Tarjan, G. 1957. Phenylketonuria. *American Journal of Diseases of Children,* 93, 405.

Wunderlich, C. 1970. *Das mongoloide Kind. Möglichkeiten der Erkennung und Betreuung.* Stuttgart: Enke.

Wyke, M.A. 1968. The effect of brain lesions in the performance of an arm-hand precision task. *Neuropsychologia,* 6, 125.

Wyllie, E., Rothner, A.D. & Luders, H. 1989. Partial seizures in children: Clinical features, medical treatment, and surgical considerations. *Pediatric Clinics of North America,* 36, 343.

Yakovlev, P.I. 1962. Morphological criteria of growth and maturation of the nervous system in man. *Association for Research in Nervous and Mental Diseases,* 39, 3.

Yakovlev, P.I. & Lecours, A.R. 1967. The myelogenetic cycles of regional maturation of the brain. In A. Minkowski (Ed.), *Regional Development of the Brain in Early Life.* Oxford: Blackwell Scientific Publications.

Yamamoto, M. 1990. Birth order, gender differences, and language development in modern Japanese pre-school children. *Psychologia—An International Journal of Psychology in the Orient,* 33, 185.

Yamasaki, D.S. & Wurtz, R.H. 1991. Recovery of function after lesions in the superior temporal sulcus in the monkey. *Journal of Neurophysiology,* 66, 651.

Yang, R.K. 1979. Infant assessment. In J.D. Osofsky (Ed.), *Handbook of Infant Development.* New York: Wiley, p. 165.

Yarrow, L.J. & Pederson, F.A. 1976. The interplay between motivation and cognition in infancy. In M. Lewis (Ed.), *Origins of Intelligence: Infancy and Early Childhood.* New York: Plenum Press, p. 379.

Yaylayan, S.A., Weller, E.B. & Weller, R.A. 1990. Biology of depression in children and adolescents. *Journal of Child and Adolescent Psychopharmacology,* 1, 215.

Yeates, K.O. & Mortensen, M.E. 1994. Acute and chronic neuropsychological consequences of mercury vapor poisoning in two early adolescents. *Journal of Clinical and Experimental Neuropsychology,* 16, 209.

Yeni-Komishian, G.H. & Benson, D.A. 1976. Anatomical study of cerebral asymmetry in the temporal lobe of humans, chimpanzees and rhesus monkeys. *Science,* 192, 387.

Yeudall, L.T., Fedora, O. & Fromm, D. 1987. A neuropsychosocial theory of persistent criminality: Implications for assessment and treatment. In R.W. Rieber (Ed.), *Advances in Forensic Psychology and Psychiatry,* Vol. 2. Norwood NJ: Ablex, p. 119.

Ylvisaker, M. (Ed.) 1986. *Head Injury Rehabilitation: Children and Adolescents* San Diego: College-Hill Press, p. 71.

Yolles, S.F. & Kramer, M. 1969. Vital statistics. In L. Bellak and L. Loeb (Eds.), *The Schizophrenic Syndrome.* New York: Grune & Stratton.

Yoss, K.A. & Darley, F.L. 1974. Developmental apraxia of speech in children with defective articulation. *Journal of Speech and Hearing Research,* 17, 399.

Young, A.W. & Ellis, H.D. 1989. Childhood prosopagnosia. *Brain and Cognition,* 9, 16.

Young, G. 1977. Manual specialization in infancy: Implications for lateralization of brain functions. In S.G. Segalowitz & F.A. Gruber (Eds.), *Language Development and Neurological Theory.* New York: Academic Press.

Young, G., Segalowitz, S.J., Corter, C.M. & Trehub, S.E. (Eds.), 1983. *Manual Specialization and the Developing Brain.* New York: Academic Press.

Yu, M.L., Hsu, C.C., Gladen, B.C. & Rogan, W.J. 1991. In utero PCB/PCDF exposure: Relation of developmental delay to dysmorphology and dose. *Neurotoxicology and Teratology,* 13, 195.

Yu, V.Y.H., and Hollingsworth, E. 1979. Improving prognosis for infants weighing 1000 g or less at birth. *Archives of Disease of Childhood,* 55, 422.

Yu-Cun, S., Yu-Feng, W. & Xiao-Ling, Y. 1985. An epidemiological investigation of minimal brain dysfunction in six elementary schools in Beijing. *Journal of Child Psychology and Psychiatry,* 26, 777.

Yule, M. & Rutter, M. 1976. Epidemiology and social implications of specific reading retardation. In R.M. Knights and D.J. Bakker (Eds.), *The Neuropsychology of Learning Disorders.* Baltimore: University Park Press.

Yule, W.M., Rutter, M., Berger, M. & Thompson, J. 1974. Over- and under-achievement in reading: Distribution in the general population. *British Journal of Educational Psychology,* 44, 1.

Zagon, I.S. & Slotkin, T.A. 1992. *Maternal Substance Abuse and the Developing Nervous System.* Orlando, FL: Academic Press.

Zaide, J. 1982. Gender differences in achievement levels and intellectual functioning in learning handicapped children. Unpublished manuscript.

Zaidel, E. 1978. Auditory language comprehension in the right hemisphere following cerebral commissurotomy and hemispherectomy: A comparison with child language and aphasia. In E. Zurif & A. Caramazza (Eds.), *The Acquisition and Breakdown of Language: Parallels and Divergencies.* Baltimore: Johns Hopkins University Press.

Zaidel, E. 1979. The split and half brains as models of congenital language disability. In C.L. Ludlow & M.E. Doran-Quine (Eds.), *The Neurological Bases of Language Disorders in Children: Methods and Directions for Research*. NIH Publication No. 79-440. Bethesda, MD: U.S. Department of Health, Education and Welfare.

Zaidel, E., Clarke, J.M. & Suyenobu, B. 1990. Hemispheric independence: A paradigm case for cognitive neuroscience. In A. Scheibel and A. Wechsler (Eds.), *Neurobiological Foundations of Higher Cognitive Functions*. New York: Guilford Press.

Zamenhof, S. & van Marthens, E. 1978. Nutritional influences on prenatal brain development. In G. Gottlieb (Ed.), *Early Influences*, Vol. IV. New York: Academic Press.

Zametkin, A.J., Nordahl, T.E., Gross, M., King, A.C., Semple, W.E., Rumsey, J., Hamburger, S. & Cohen, R. 1990. Cerebral glucose metabolism in adults with hyperactivity of childhood onset. *New England Journal of Medicine*, 323, 1361.

Zametkin, A.J. & Rappaport, J.L. 1987. Neurobiology of attention deficit disorder with hyperactivity: Where have we come to in 50 years? *Journal of the American Academy of Child and Adolescent Psychiatry*, 26, 676.

Zangwill, O.L. 1962. Dyslexia in relation to cerebral dominance. In J. Money (Ed.), *Reading Disability*. Baltimore: Johns Hopkins University Press.

Zangwill, O.L. 1978. The concept of developmental aphasia. In M.A. Wyke (Ed.), *Developmental Aphasia*. New York: Academic Press.

Zeaman, D. & House, B.J. 1962. Mongoloid MA is proportional to LogCA. *Child Development*, 33, 481.

Zelazo, P. 1981. An information processing approach to infant cognitive assessment. In M. Lewis & I. Taft (Eds.), *Developmental Disabilities: Theory, Assessment and Intervention*. New York: SP Medical & Scientific Books.

Zelazo, P.R. & Kearsley, R.B. 1989. Memory for visual sequences: Evidence for increased speed of processing with age. *Infant Behavior and Development*, 5, 263.

Zelazo, P.R. & Weiss, M.J. 1990. Infant information processing: An alternative approach. In E.D. Gibbs & D.M. Teti (Eds.), *Interdisciplinary Assessment of Infants. A Guide for Early Intervention Professionals*. Baltimore: Paul H. Brookes, p. 129.

Zeskind, P.S. & Ramey, C.T. 1981. Preventing intellectual and interactional sequelae of fetal malnutrition: A longitudinal, transactional, and synergistic approach to development. *Child Development*, 52, 213.

Zhang, L. & Jiang, Z.D. 1992. Development of the brainstem auditory pathway in low birthweight and perinatally asphyxiated children with neurological sequelae. *Early Human Development*, 30, 61.

Zigman, W.B., Schupf, N., Lubin, R.A. & Silverman, W.P. 1987. Premature regression of adults with Down syndrome. *American Journal of Mental Deficiency*, 92, 161.

Zigman, W.B., Schupf, N., Silverman, W.P. & Sterling, R.C. 1989. Changes in adaptive functioning of adults with developmental disabilities. *Australia and New Zealand Journal of Developmental Disabilities*, 15, 277.

Ziring, P.R. 1977. Congenital rubella: The teenage years. *Pediatric Annals*, 6, 762.

Ziviani, J., Hayes, A. & Chant, D. 1990. Handwriting: A perceptual-motor disturbance in children with myelomeningocele. *Occupational Therapy Journal of Research*, 10, 12.

Zollinger, R. 1935. Removal of left cerebral hemisphere: Report of a case. *Archives of Neurology and Psychiatry*, 34, 1055.

Zubenko, G.S. & Howland, R. 1988. Marked increased platelet membrane fluidity in Down syndrome with a (14q, 21q) translocation. *Journal of Geriatric Psychiatry and Neurology*, 1, 218.

Zuckerman, B.S. & Hingson, R. 1986. Alcohol consumption during pregnancy: A critical review. *Developmental Medicine and Child Neurology*, 28, 649.

Zulch, K.J. 1974. Motor and sensory findings after hemispherectomy: Ipsi- or contralateral functions? *Clinical Neurology and Neurosurgery*, 77(1), 3.

Zur, J. & Yule, W. 1990. Chronic solvent abuse: I. Cognitive sequelae. *Child Care, Health and Development*, 16, 1.

Index

Page numbers in italic refer to bold-faced definitional entries.
Page numbers followed by a "f" refer to a figure and those
followed by a "t" refer to a table.